Manfred Heidenreich

Birds of Prey

Medicine and Management

Manfred Heidenreich

Birds of Prey

Medicine and Management

With 334 illustrations, including 295 in colour

English translation by Dr Yvonne Oppenheim

Blackwell Science

First published 1997

Set in 9.5/11 pt Times
by Filmsatz Schröter, Munich
Lithography: Findl & Partners, Icking
Printed and bound in Spain by Grafos SA, Barcelona

DISTRIBUTORS

Marston Book Services Ltd
PO Box 269
Abingdon
Oxon OX14 4YN
(*Orders:* Tel: 01235-465500
                Fax: 01235-465555)

USA
Blackwell Science, Inc.
Commerce Place
350 Main Street
Malden, MA 02148
USA
(*Orders:* Tel: 617 388 82 50
                Fax: 617 388 82 55)

Canada
Copp Clark, Ltd
2775 Matheson Blvd East
Mississauga, Ontario
Canada, L4W 4P7
(*Orders:* Tel: 800 263-4374
                905 238-6074)

Australia
Blackwell Science Pty Ltd
54 University Street
Carlton, Victoria 3053
(*Orders:* Tel: 03 9347-0300
                Fax: 03 9347-5001)

A catalogue record for this title is available from the British
Library.

ISBN 0-632-04186-2

Preface

Birds of prey have always fascinated man. Initially they were symbols of freedom, strength and courage, kept as living status symbols by early rulers. Later, they became abstract emblems of heraldic might, still to be found as such today. The national symbol of the United States is the bald eagle, the Germans have the Prussian state eagle and the United Arab Emirates display a falcon on their coat of arms and on their currency. Birds of prey played a role in ancient Egyptian mythology in the form of the holy Horus falcon and a falcon represented on King Tutankhamon's breastplate. In India, vultures are still believed to carry the souls of those they consume to heaven. The peoples of the South American Andes and the Indians of North America adorned themselves with eagle and vulture feathers. After the development of falconry in the Asian steppes, raptors also became the hunting companions of man. In this role they were valued highly, even loved, especially later in the Middle Ages. Falcons became the cause of political crises, even wars, as falconry advanced to become a true art – the "ars venandi cum avibus".

In the times that followed, this concern for birds of prey was lost. Raptors became nuisance animals that competed with armed hunters for prey. They were mercilessly pursued, decimated, and sometimes brought nearly to extinction. Eventually, man's thirst for power and exploitation of nature achieved what had been left unfinished by straightforward persecution. The worldwide use of poisons in agriculture and forestry, DDT foremost among them, gave the final blow to many raptor species. The number of bird species on the brink of extinction rose precipitously. Again, birds of prey such as the peregrine falcon and the bald eagle, at the top of the food chain and thus most strongly affected, brought public attention to what was happening. Various interest groups took up the cause of preserving these species. Falconers in the U.S. and Europe began captive breeding programs for birds of prey. Conservation groups undertook the protection of the remaining breeding habitats in an effort to protect the animals from the selfish and insane people who still pursued birds of prey. Despite their laudable common goals, many of these groups did not work together and sometimes still oppose each other, even to this day.

From the early beginnings of raptor breeding efforts

and the reintroduction of endangered species evolved a widespread program of raptor management at all levels. This includes veterinarians and falconers and many people who are both. Our knowledge in the specialized field of raptor medicine grew steadily. The credit for recognizing almost twenty years ago the importance of preventing and treating the diseases of birds of prey goes to John E. Cooper. He was the first modern veterinarian to publish a book on the diseases of these birds. Since then, there has been an overwhelming number of papers and congressional reports on this subject, but no single publication that would pull together all the developments in the field of raptor management, including captive maintenance, breeding and the diseases of birds of prey.

In my twenty years as a passionate falconer and a veterinarian, I have enjoyed the trust of many colleagues who have given their valuable animals to my care. My work with birds of prey was not limited to individual animals, but quickly evolved to include the veterinary care of large public and private breeding facilities and rehabilitation centers. During these years of service I was fortunate to learn a great deal from my colleagues and from experienced raptor breeders. My thanks to all of them for their time and patience during our long hours of discussion.

This book attempts to make my collected experiences and the most recent information from the literature available to all who care about the fate of birds of prey. In view of the diversity of the potential readership, be they practicing veterinarians or biologists, raptor breeders or falconers, ornithologists or public officials, government veterinarians or customs officials, I have avoided the use of excessively technical language. I would be pleased if this book would contribute to uniting us in our common goal of preserving and protecting all birds of prey.

I thank all those who have made this book possible: The falconers and breeders both at home and abroad who have shared so much of their knowledge and experience, thereby subordinating their own interests to those of our common goal, the representatives of state and federal authorities, who tolerated my occasionally cantankerous discussions, and above all, government counselor Annette Schmidt-Raentsch and Dr. Rainer Blanke, who graciously agreed to review the chapter on legal issues regarding birds of prey. Thanks also to Mrs. Regine Gattung-Pettith and Mr. Albert Gattung, himself a falconer in body and soul, for the outstanding scientific illustrations, to Mr. Bernd Poeppelman for supplying some figures and, above all, for his incomparably beautiful painting which brings out the aesthetic qualities of the birds in this book, so often obscured elsewhere by pictures of illness and injury. My gratitude also goes to Mr. Heinz Bruening, Mr. Rainer Hussong, Dr. Peter N. Klueh, Mr. Michael Lierz and Dr. Volker Wagner for the photographs that help enrich this book, my mentor, Professor Erhard F. Kaleta, for constructive criticism and suggestions for improvement, which were taken into account in this edition, and to Dr. med. vet. Andreas Mueller, editor with Blackwell Wissenschafts-Verlag, for his care, expertise and committment in helping put together this book. Thanks also to Dr. Axel Bedürftig, director of Blackwell Wissenschaft-Verlag, for his foresight in adding this subject to his repertoire of publications and for the generous color format, as well as for the friendly and mutual understanding we share. I would like to extend particular thanks to Dr. Yvone Oppenheim, who translated the German text into English. The completion of this difficult task was only possible due to the profound knowledge that Dr. Oppenheim has at her disposal in the fields of rearing birds of prey and the medical practices associated with these birds. Last, but not least, many thanks to my wife Christa for her endless patience, her help in editing the text, and her deep understanding and love for a man who has dedicated his life to birds of prey.

Hannover, October 1995   The author

Contents

1 Introduction

Originally this book was intended to be purely a veterinary medical textbook covering the diseases of birds of prey. However, since the majority of illnesses in these birds can be traced to problems in husbandry and diet, the information in this text is especially important to raptor breeders and others who maintain raptors in captivity. That realization expanded the scope of this book considerably. In addition, the keeping of raptors is frequently not simply a private enterprise anymore, but instead is closely tied to national and international breeding and conservation efforts. This makes the chapters on captive management, feeding and captive breeding essential. The information presented in those chapters includes my own experiences as well as a wealth of knowledge contributed by experienced breeders and falconers both in Germany and abroad.

The subsequent veterinary medical chapters were purposely written on a basic scientific level in order to keep them understandable to the broadest possible readership while retaining technical accuracy. The popular writing style of this book should not be taken as an invitation for untrained lay people to avoid consulting a veterinarian when the need arises. Instead, it should encourage the various interest groups to become as in-formed as possible and to work together in the care of birds of prey.

Interested lay people will certainly find the extensive collection of color photos helpful. Professionals will also benefit from the tables and from the diagnostic and therapeutic recommendations, as well as from the up-to-date references at the end of each chapter.

Nevertheless, this book can provide only an incomplete presentation of the knowledge that has accumulated in this field over the past decades. The author has avoided publishing individual papers in recent years, preferring to incorporate the information he has gained in the field of raptor medicine into this book. Therefore some previously unpublished diseases, surgical techniques and medical theories are presented here. It is hoped that they will provide new ideas and encouragement to scientists in the field.

Should one or the other opinion expressed in this book not conform to the established theories and thus lead to debate and discussion, then the purpose of this book has been fulfilled. It seeks to encourage the urgently necessary, objective examination of all the issues that pertain to the preservation of the fascinating creatures that are birds of prey.

2 Taxonomic classification of birds of prey

All birds of prey have certain characteristics in common. They generally have a hooked beak and more or less well-developed talons. These external characteristics formed the basis of Linnaeus' 18th Century classification scheme, which inappropriately combined various very different groups of birds. For example, under the order Accipitres, he united the genera *Vultur* (vultures), *Falco* (falcons, eagles, goshawks, harriers, etc.), *Strix* (owls) and *Lanius* (shrikes).

In the latter half of the 19th Century, more specific criteria for the taxonomic organization of bird groups were developed. Not only further obvious phenotypic traits such as foot structure, toe arrangement, and numbers of feathers were used, but internal anatomic structures were also taken into account. On the basis of physiologic data such as molting patterns, the falcons (*Falconiformes*) were separated from the hawk-like raptors (*Accipitriformes*) only in this century.

In the following system Weick (1980) lists all birds of prey under the order *Falconiformes* and differentiates among three suborders, the New World vultures, the hawk-like birds, and the falcons:

Table 2.1: Classification of birds of prey according to Weick (1980)

Order: Falconiformes

<u>**Suborder:**</u> Cathartae
      Family: Cathartidae (New World vultures)
<u>**Suborder:**</u> Accipitres
      Family: Sagittariidae (secretary bird)
      Family: Pandionidae (osprey)
      Family: Accipitridae (hawks)
          Genus: kites, eagles, Old World vultures, harriers, hawks and buzzards
<u>**Suborder:**</u> Falcones
      Family: Falconidae
          <u>Subfamily:</u> Daptriinae
              (caracaras, chimangos)
          <u>Subfamily:</u> Herpetotherinae
              (laughing falcons)
          <u>Subfamily:</u> Micrasturinae (forest falcons)
          <u>Subfamily:</u> Falconinae (true falcons)
              Tribe: Polihieracini (falconets)
              Tribe: Falconini (true falcons)
                 Genus: Falco (falcon)
                 Species: peregrinus
                    (peregrine falcon)

Disagreements persisted regarding the classification of the osprey and the secretary bird, whose taxonomic relationships remain unclear to this day (Seibold, 1994).

This uncertainty is acknowledged by Amadon and Bull (1988), who remove the secretary bird from the suborder *Accipitres* and list it under a suborder of its own in their classification scheme. The divisions among the family Falconidae are also changed by these authors, being reduced to a mere two subfamilies.

Table 2.2: Classification of birds of prey according to Amadon and Bull (1988)

Order: Falconiformes

<u>**Suborder:**</u> Cathartae
      Familiy: Cathartidae (New World vultures)
<u>**Suborder:**</u> Accipitres
      Suborder: Accipitres
          Family: Accipitridae (hawk-like birds)
              <u>Subfamily:</u> Pandioninae (osprey)
              <u>Subfamily:</u> Accipitrinae (kites, eagles, Old World vultures, harriers, hawks, buzzards)
<u>**Suborder:**</u> Sagittarii
      Family: Sagittariidae (secretary bird)
<u>**Suborder:**</u> Falcones
      Family: Falconidae (falcon-like birds)
          <u>Subfamily:</u> Polyborinae (caracaras)
          <u>Subfamily:</u> Falconinae (falcons)

Although both classification schemes clearly differentiate between New World vultures and other diurnal raptors, they nevertheless both get placed in the order Falconiformes. As early as 1873, however, Garrod pointed out that this group of birds appears to be more closely related to the storks than to other birds of prey. Koenig enumerated the most important differences between New World vultures and other birds of prey in 1982. New World vultures do not have a grasping foot, and instead have a raised hallux (turkey foot). Their nasal septum is perforated and they do not possess a syrinx, and thus no voice. In contrast to other birds of prey, male New World vultures are as big or bigger than the females. Some of their behavioral traits, such as the rubbing of beaks among paired birds (see Fig. 2.1), the chicken-like roosting posture, and their

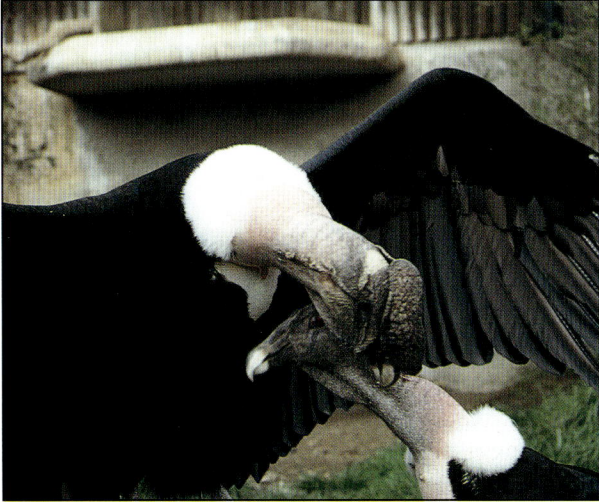

Fig. 2.1: During pair bonding and mating, Andean condors (*Vultur gryphus*) rub beaks with each other. Although this behavior is common among many types of birds, it is never seen in birds of prey. (Photo: Heidenreich)

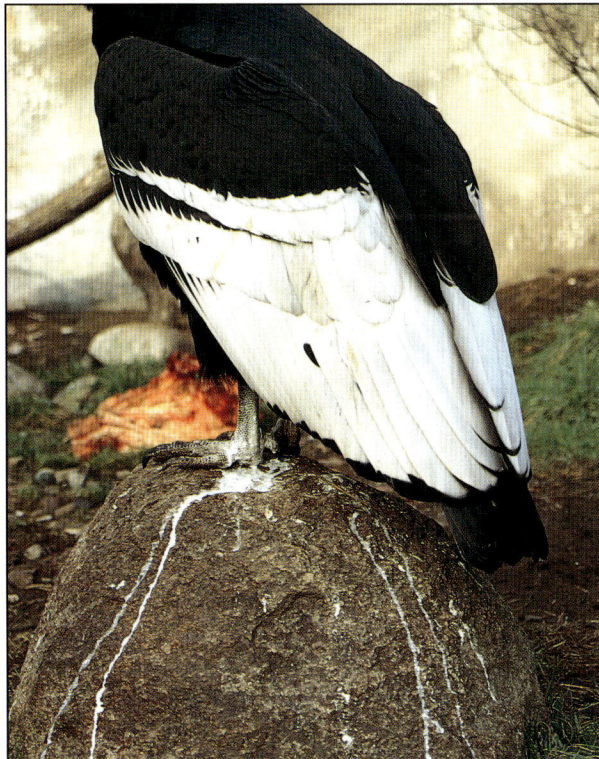

Fig. 2.2: Both condors and storks are known to defecate on their legs, a behavior that may serve in thermoregulation. (Photo: Heidenreich)

habit of defecating on their legs (see Fig. 2.2) as storks do for thermoregulation, clearly differentiate them from all other birds of prey.

Modern methods that use DNA-hybridization techniques to compare the relatedness of species within the class Aves (birds) have produced further information in recent years. Sibley and Ahlquist (1990) compared 1600 species of birds from 168 families, developing a "phylogenetic system" for classification based on their results. Birds of prey were included.

Table 2.3: Classification of birds of prey according to Sibley and Ahlquist (1990)

> **Order: Ciconiiformes**
>
> **Suborder:** Ciconii
>   **Infraorder:** Falconides
>   **Parvorder:** Accipitrida
>   **Family:** Accipitridae
>   Subfamily: Pandioninae (osprey)
>   Subfamily: Accipitrinae (kites, eagles, Old World vultures, harriers, hawks and buzzards)
>   **Family:** Sagittariidae (secretary bird)
>   **Parvorder:** Falconida
>   **Family:** Falconidae
>   **Infraorder:** Ciconiides
>   **Parvorder:** Ciconiida
>   **Family:** Ciconiidae
>   Subfamily: Cathartidae (New World vultures)
>   Subfamily: Ciconiinae (storks)

In this system, the infraorder Falconides corresponds to what was previously called the order Falconiformes, although without including the New World vultures. These have been grouped with the storks in the subfamily Ciconiinae. Wink (1995) is very skeptical of this close relationship between New World vultures and storks, suggesting instead, that they both split from a common ancestor approximately 30 to 35 million years ago.

Falconers still use the term hierofalcons (*Falco hierofalco*) coined in 1901. Kleinschmidt included gyrfalcons, saher falcons, lanner falcons, and laggar falcons in this group because of their many similarities, contrasting these "hunting falcons" with the peregrine falcon. Baumgart (1992) even suspects that hierofalcons could be considered a single polymorphic species, if their close genetic relationship were demonstrated. One year later, Heidenreich et al. (1993) proved with breeding experiments that hybrids within the hierofalcon group are fertile and can reproduce indefinitely within that group. The definition of a species as an isolated reproductive entity thus does not apply to these falcons, and Baumgart's assertion that hierofalcons are a single species with geographical variations is supported. On the other hand, Wink (1995) was able to find distinctive differences between these falcons on the basis of DNA-sequence analyses. His data places the saker falcon in a special position with genetic relationships to both gyrfalcons and peregrine falcons.

Many further questions regarding the relatedness among birds of prey remain open. For example, is there a relationship between osprey and eagles or between Bonelli's eagle and other eagles? Can the species distinctions be maintained between the Iberian and the Eastern imperial eagle, or between the peregrine falcon and the barbary falcon? Preliminary answers to these questions are being provided by DNA sequencing analyses being performed by Seibold (1994).

Despite the uncertain phylogenetic position of the New World vultures, they have been included in this book. Their requirements in captivity are similar to those of other birds of prey and they are often grouped together in zoos and bird parks.

References and literature of further interest

AMADON, D. and J. BULL (1988):
Hawks and Owls of the world.
Proc. West. Found. Vert. Zool. **3**, 295-357

BAUMGART, W. (1992):
Der Beitrag der Greifvogelforschung zur Formierung der funktionellen Arttheorie.
Greifvögel und Falknerei 94-101
Verlag Neumann-Neudamm, Morschen-Heina

GARROD, A.H. (1873):
On certain muscles of the tigh of birds and their value in classification.
Proc. Zool. Soc. London 1873, 626-644

HEIDENREICH, M., KÜSPERT, H., KÜSPERT, H.J. and R. HUSSONG (1993):
Falkenhybriden. Deren Zucht, zum Verwandtschaftsgrad verschiedener Falkenarten, sowie zum Thema Faunenverfälschung durch Hybridfalken.
Beitr. Vogelkd. **39**, 205-226

KLEINSCHMIDT, O. (1901):
Der Formenkreis Falco Hierofalco und die Stellung des ungarischen Würgfalken in demselben.
Aquila **8**, 1-49

KÖNIG, C. (1982):
Zur systematischen Stellung der Neuweltgeier (Cathartidae).
J. Ornitol. **123**, 259-267

SEIBOLD, I. (1994):
Untersuchungen zur molekularen Phylogenie der Greifvögel anhand von DNA-Sequenzen des mitochondriellen Cytochrom b-Gens.
Hartung-Gorre-Verlag, Konstanz

SIBLEY, C.G. and J.E. AHLQUIST (1990):
Phylogeny and classification of birds. A study in molecular evolution.
University Press, Yale

WEICK, F. (1980):
Die Greifvögel der Welt.
Verlag Paul Parey, Hamburg und Berlin

WINK, M. (1995):
personal communication

3 Management of raptors in captivity

3.1 Reasons for maintaining raptors in captivity

Raptors are kept in captivity by a wide variety of people and organizations and for many different reasons.

Zoological parks and public aviaries
These public facilities often display birds of prey together with many other types of animals. They are exhibited for purposes of education and to foster a better understanding of zoological and conservation issues. The public's physical proximity to the animals and the resulting awareness that develops cannot be replaced by media coverage. In addition, several raptor species, especially the larger, quieter ones, have been successfully reproducing in zoos for many years. Zoos and public aviaries almost always exhibit birds of prey in large wire mesh enclosures where they are easily observed.

Public centers for falconry and birds of prey
These private or community-supported facilities limit themselves to the keeping and display of birds of prey and owls. In most of them, the raptors are also exhibited in free flight demonstrations. These demonstrations are often accompanied by lectures and displays intended to discuss issues pertaining to the natural history or training of the birds. Well-managed facilities of this kind certainly fulfill a similar role as do zoos, and can even surpass them in terms of specific educational goals. Since such raptor centers are usually managed by experts in the field who have many years of experience, they are frequently more successful in breeding rare or unusual species than are zoos.

The facilities for housing birds of prey at such raptor centers may vary considerably. Flight cages are often available for breeding birds, while the hawks flown daily in demonstrations are more commonly maintained on blocks, ring perches or perch-and-wire arrangements. Regrettably, some birds are permanently kept on blocks or ring perches – a practice that should be discouraged for reasons of animal rights.

Raptor rehabilitation centers
These federally approved facilities are run privately or by conservation groups and serve to treat and rehabilitate orphaned, sick or injured birds of prey. Their goal is to reintroduce the birds into the wild after recovery. In surprising contrast to the extensive training required of other people who deal with raptors, these rehabilitation centers can be staffed by people who have no special schooling in this field. Although the care of injured birds of prey requires a large degree of knowledge and skill, the situation is such that any interested lay person can end up responsible for the bird's fate and can proceed as he or she sees fit. A rudimentary knowledge base combined with an excessive zeal for animal protection frequently lead to inhumane situations where

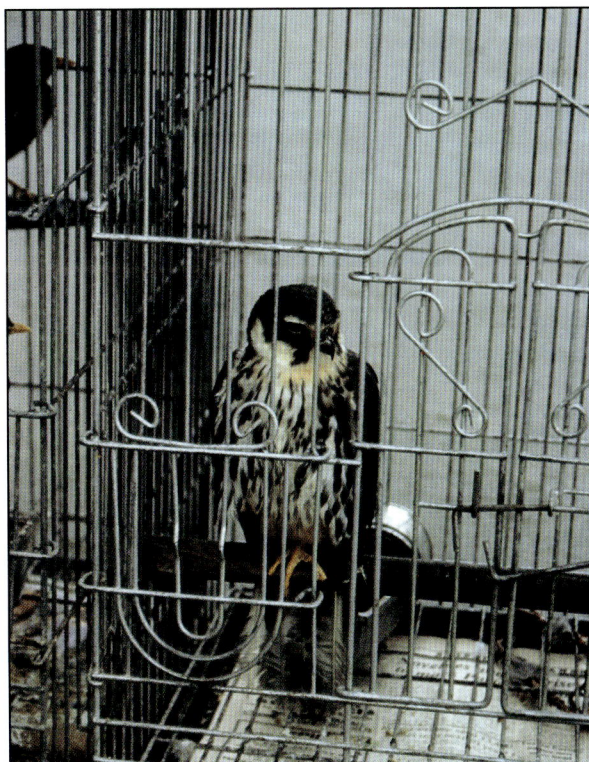

Fig. 3.1: This wild European hobby (*Falco subbuteo*) was confined to a wire cage for weeks. His plumage was soon completely frayed and a successful release thus out of the question. This is an example of the unacceptable conditions in some government-approved "raptor rehabilitation centers". (Photo: Lierz)

raptors may be kept in parrot cages (Fig. 3.1) or permanently crippled birds spend years in crowded aviaries instead of being painlessly euthanized.

Birds at such centers are kept primarily in flight cages, although falconry techniques for maintaining them would often be better. Such methods, however, are often rejected for purely political reasons or because there is a lack of understanding of their advantages.

The existence of such publicly supported facilities is hardly justified and succeeds only in demonstrating some sense of concern and care for wild raptors. The true goal of rehabilitating these birds and returning them successfully to nature is rarely realized. This problem was clearly pointed out by O'Brien in 1992 when he wrote:

"An injured or orphaned bird of prey usually becomes a dead bird of prey and the release of such birds, though exhilarating to the rehabilitator, is simply an execution. Birds of prey are fragile. They have evolved so that only the very best survive. The very best are not orphaned; they do not break wings. The very best are perfect and don't need anything that a human can give them except a decent environment. The system that has evolved in nature for the raising and selection of birds of prey is complicated and, in human terms, cruel and severe. The idea that we can improve this system is a classic case of hubris."

Falconry and hunting
The hunting of animals with the help of birds of prey is an ancient art. The hawk's natural instincts are channeled in such a way that they can be used in the capture of game for the hunter.

Falconry is practiced almost all over the world, and the type of bird used varies with the local fauna and geography. The northern goshawk (*Accipiter gentilis*), the European sparrowhawk (*Accipiter nisus*), the peregrine falcon (*Falco peregrinus*), the merlin (*Falco columbarius*) and occasionally the golden eagle (*Aquila chrysaetos*) are commonly used in central Europe. North American falconers also hunt with gyrfalcons (*Falco rusticolus*), prairie falcons (*Falco mexicanus*), red-tailed hawks (*Buteo jamaicensis*), Harris' hawks (*Parabuteo unicinctus*) and Cooper's hawks (*Accipiter cooperi*). Falconry in the Mongolian steppes and Kirghizia is practiced almost exclusively with golden eagles, while in the deserts of the Near East, various falcons are popular, primarily saker falcons (*Falco cherrug*) and peregrine falcons. Most of these falcons are wild-caught passagers obtained during fall migration according to ancient Bedouin tradition.

Hunting hawks are almost always kept in traditional falconry style, tied to blocks or perches. Since the majority of questions and problems relating to raptor management are directly associated with falconry issues, a short introduction to falconry, including training methods for hunting hawks, is important.

Historical overview: Nothing certain is known about the origins and early development of falconry. The beginnings of this sport lie so far in the distant past that the cultures involved can be considered prehistoric. They had no form of writing, but did leave behind sculptures, relief carvings and paintings of people carrying birds of prey on the fist. These by themselves are not proof of the existence of falconry at that time, as the rulers of these early cultures were often simply accompanied by raptors and other large carnivores as symbols of power.

Most historians believe that the steppes of central Asia harbored the origin of true falconry (Voegele, 1931). The oldest work of art which seems to represent a falconer is a bas-relief from Khorsabad dating to about 700 B.C. Falconry appears to have spread from there, accompanying human migrations to the east and west and adapting to local landscapes and cultures over time. Further distribution of the art of falconry occurred thanks to Islamic culture and its contact with Western societies via the European Crusades. Frederick II of Hohenstaufen (1194–1250), ruler of the German and Roman empires, King of Sicily and of Jerusalem, and an ardent student of natural history, became the most prominent ancient author of writings about animals after Aristotle. He discussed falconry with the most prominent Eastern experts of the time. His extensive book entitled "De arte venandi cum avibus" (On the art of hunting with birds) excels not only on the topic of falconry, but also in its recognition and description of biological processes and ecological associations. Many of his ideas were revolutionary for that time. Much of his falconry knowledge was acquired through his close contacts with Arab culture and Eastern rulers. It is certain that the use of hoods became common in Europe only after his crusade of 1229. The Arabs were also more advanced in medicine then, and it is not surprising that they themselves published an extensive treatise on the diseases of birds of prey as early as the 8th Century. Falconry flowered in Europe in the Middle Ages and was practiced with great fanfare by all the nobility. The most prominent falconer in France was King Louis XIII, who is said to have spent day and night with his hunting hawks. The Kings of Denmark sent a so-called "falcon ship" to Iceland every year to capture the highly desirable gyrfalcons found there. In 1764 the Danish king imported over 200 falcons, of which he gave 30 to the German Emperor, 50 to the King of France, 60 to the King of Portugal and 20 to the Earl of Hessen. Frederick the Great, who did not engage in falconry, gave away a falcon he had received as a gift. The Prussians were never given a falcon again.

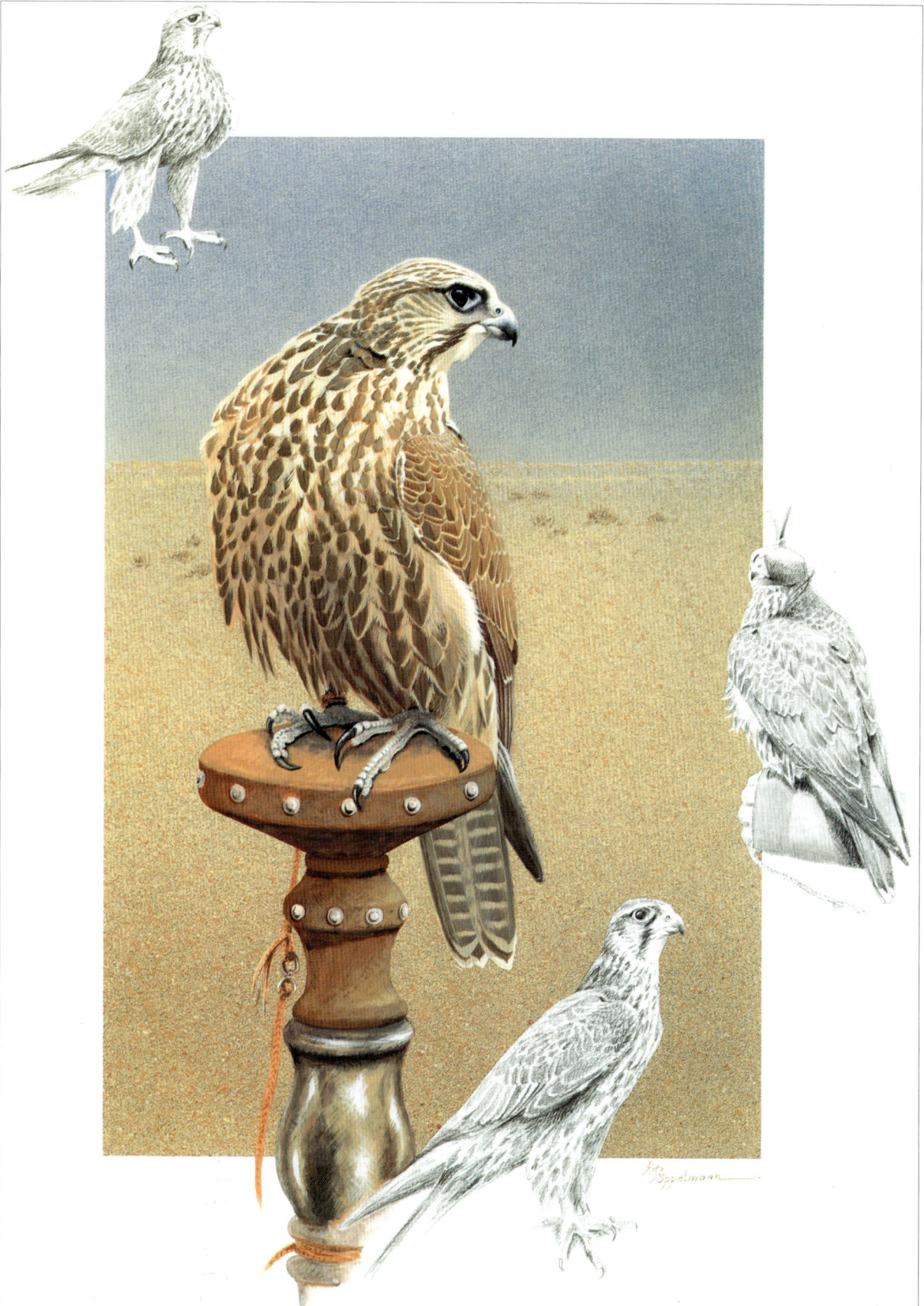

The incredible effort that nobles and kings invested in falconry during the Middle Ages and beyond became part of the reason that the rights of the upper classes were eliminated during the French Revolution. Today, falconry is practiced in almost all European countries, North America and eastern Asia. The number of people who are willing to put in the effort involved in training and hunting with hawks, however, is small. Only in some of the wealthy Arab countries is falconry still practiced with the intensity and pomp it once enjoyed in the Middle Ages.

Manning and training a hawk: Birds of prey to be trained for hunting can be taken from the nest (eyas or nestling), captured after fledging in their first year of life (passagers), or less commonly, captured as wild adults (haggards). Primarily captive-bred hawks are used in the West, in part due to the strict and very important laws protecting endangered and threatened species. The Arabs still prefer wild-caught birds.

The goal of manning and training a hawk is to teach it to lose its fear of man while at the same time retaining its hunting instinct and also returning to the falconer after free flight. A large amount of patience and sensitivity are required to achieve this. Falconry critics often claim that the birds are induced to perform by hunger alone. A certain desire for food is certainly necessary. Even a wild bird will not hunt if not hungry. The basis of a hawk's training, however, lies primarily in the utilization of natural, inborn behaviors and in an understanding of their application to the purposes of man.

All training begins with the taming or "manning" of the hawk. A shy or frightened bird will fly away instead of returning to the falconer. The first phase of manning is accomplished by establishing an association between food and man. Initially, the bird is fed on the falconer's gauntlet, later from the lure or dummy. During the first few days, the bird is kept on a leash or creance (long line) for safety until it reliably returns to the fist. Thereafter it can be flown free. For inexperienced young birds there now follows a period of flight training to condition the muscles of flight and hone the hunting skills. The northern goshawk can be flown in "free pursuit" during this time, following the falconer from tree to tree and receiving an occasional reward of a small piece of meat. Falcons, on the other hand, will fly to a moving lure as to prey. If the lure is repeatedly pulled away as the bird approaches, it will continue turning and stooping until it is exhausted. Well-trained falcons can stoop to the lure up to 200 times, which corresponds to approximately 45 minutes of actual flying time.

Only after the birds have been adequately trained and brought into good physical condition, can they be-gin to fly at live game. Wild-caught birds do not usually require any special schooling, since they have acquired enough experience hunting in the wild prior to capture. Captive-bred birds need to be introduced to the intended game animal. It is up to the falconer to motivate the hawk by making its initial attempts to capture the animal easy and successful. Once the bird has succeeded in capturing its prey, it will not return to the falconer with the animal, as is often assumed. On the contrary, the falconer must take the captured animal away by inducing the bird to step onto the gauntlet with a piece of meat offered there.

Depending on the type of hawk and game, different techniques are applied in the hunt. Goshawks, European sparrowhawks and eagles fly directly from the fist when they spot prey. Falcons can also be hunted in this manner. More commonly, the falcon is trained to climb high and then wait-on overhead while the game is flushed. Once the falcon spots the animal, it stoops in free fall to strike the pheasant or grouse.

Well-trained hawks recognize man as a "helper" in their effort to obtain food and require only a good appetite every day to hunt in much the same manner as their wild counterparts. This is also the goal of good falconry – to experience the fascination of a raptor hunting in free flight in a way that is rarely observed in nature. A falconer and his hawk are not judged by the number of animals they capture, but on whether they have mastered "the art of hunting with birds".

Various interest groups that consider themselves conservationists or animal protectionists try, with sometimes absurd arguments, to malign falconry and to have it banned. They have already succeeded in several European countries. Falconry is not permitted in any of the Scandinavian countries and Spain has outlawed game hawking in several regions of the country. What is forgotten in all this, is that few relationships between man and beast permit such a deep understanding of the nature of these birds. It is no coincidence that falconers around the world were the first to succeed in the captive propagation of birds of prey, thereby contributing immeasurably to the preservation of numerous endangered species. Horst Stern, a German journalist and author of various television documentaries and books on the topic of human-animal interactions, described falconry as follows:

"The game with the lure. It is the bird's preparation for the hunt. The bond between falcon and falconer, which once was the basis for this form of hunting, has become a useless art which merely provides aesthetic pictures that bring great pleasure. Centuries of human patience lie behind this game with one of the freest animals on earth. Those who want to forbid this have only a superficial understanding of the cultural treasure that falconry represents. A ban would be useless in any case. There will always be men who devote them-

selves passionately to this most difficult of arts: To bind a living creature to oneself by giving it its freedom again and again."

Rearing birds of prey
Anybody who fulfills the established legal requirements can breed birds of prey, even without a particular interest such as falconry. Raptor breeding can be done purely for the enjoyment of it. It is done almost exclusively in aviaries that have been specially constructed according to designs developed by falconers. They are the ones who have been successfully breeding their own hunting hawks since the early 1970's. These efforts have naturally emphasized the propagation of species commonly used in falconry.

Birds of prey are maintained in captivity and used for various purposes. This, in turn, determines the various forms of housing and maintaining them, as described below.

3.2   Aviaries

3.2.1   Aviaries for display

Aviaries are flight cages that are used primarily in zoological parks and bird parks for the display of birds. These occasionally very large enclosures are typically made of wire mesh in order to allow an unobstructed view (Fig. 3.2). Because of the close contact with visitors, these enclosures should be used only for the larger and more quiet species such as vultures and eagles. These large birds are generally more popular than the smaller raptors anyway. In addition, the smaller and more agile species are not usually suited for display in wire-enclosed flight cages because they can achieve rapid flight speeds in only short distances and thus become vulnerable to wire mesh injuries.

As a matter of principle, display aviaries should be constructed with sufficient height to permit the birds to perch above the passing spectators, where they feel safer. Protection from the elements in the form of partial roofing or windproof indoor housing is essential.

It is frequently difficult to achieve a functional compromise between the desire to exhibit a bird and its species-specific requirements within the constraints of these aviaries. The highest priority should always be the well-being of the bird.

3.2.2   Breeding aviaries

These enclosures are designed specifically for breeding birds of prey. The emphasis is on minimizing visual disturbances to the inhabitants of the aviary. For this reason, the structure, often called a chamber, is completely enclosed on all four sides and covered one

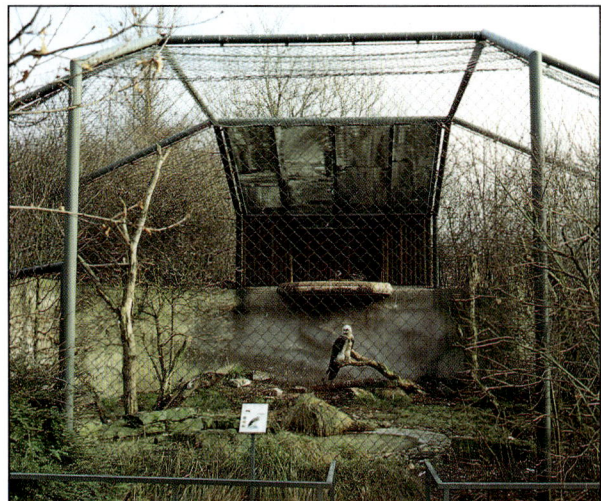

Fig 3.2: An aviary for a bearded vulture (*Gypaetus barbatus*) at the Hannover Zoo.   (Photo: Heidenreich)

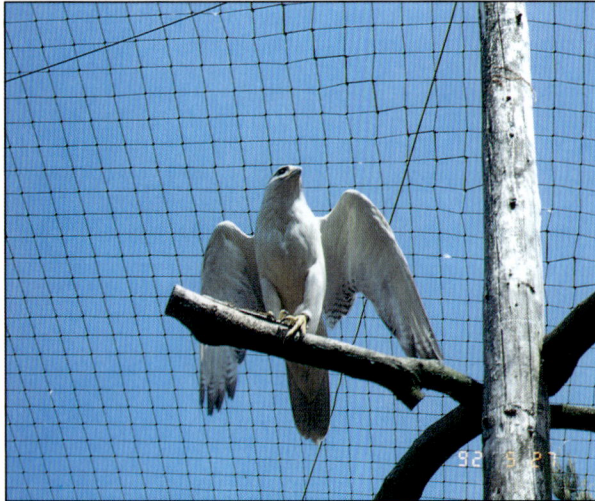

3.3 △   3.4 ▽

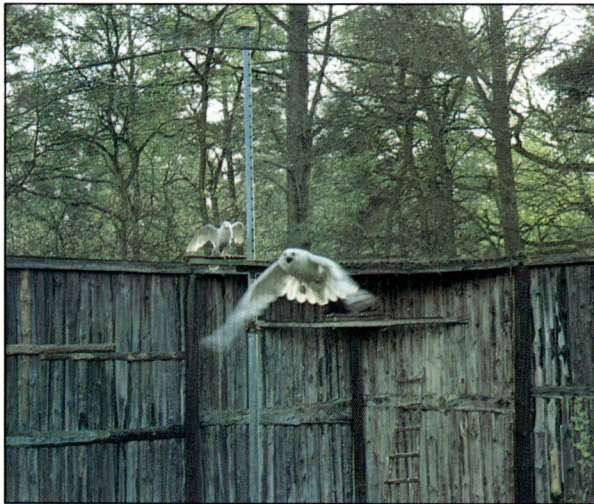

Fig 3.3: An aviary covered with netting is preferable to wire mesh. In either case, the mesh size should be small enough to prevent the birds from being able to put their heads through. One disadvantage of netting is the accumulation of snow in winter.
(Photo: Heidenreich)

Fig. 3.4: For larger falcons, a circular breeding chamber has proven very effective. The birds can fly in endless circles. Such exercise benefits the metabolism and health of the breeding birds.
(Photo: Heidenreich)

quarter to one third of the way with a roof. The remaining opening is secured with wire mesh or, preferably, strong netting. If the breeding chamber is spacious enough, the occupants may even be free to fly within it (Fig. 3.4). The breeding birds are observed only through peepholes or via video camera. Food and

water are supplied through trap doors and pipelines or hoses.

In such an isolated environment, even normally very shy raptors will remain calm, avoid injury and engage in undisturbed breeding activity (Figures 3.5 and 3.6).

3.2.3   Moulting chambers

These enclosures, also called mews, were designed for the hunting hawk, as housing during the moulting period or between hunting seasons (Fig. 3.7). They are completely enclosed on three sides with flat walls, and only the front is made of wood or metal bars. At least two thirds of the roof should be constructed of translucent material. The primary goal of keeping the bird in this chamber is the prevention of injury to the developing feathers. Only perfect plumage will permit the bird to hunt successfully the next season.

3.2.4   Minimum sizes
for raptor aviaries

Every raptor species has special requirements in terms of the aviary in which it is to be kept. Strict guidelines that rely simply on the size of the bird are not good enough. Construction of an optimal enclosure requires empathy and observational skills. Frequently, very large aviaries are encouraged. The larger-is-better concept may not apply to all birds of prey, however. As previously mentioned, the smaller and more nervous species such as goshawks, sparrowhawks, small falcons and harriers can achieve rapid flight speeds in relatively short distances. This puts them at risk of serious injury in the event of impact with the walls or wire mesh of larger enclosures.

Individual differences must also be taken into account. A goshawk can be very nervous in an aviary and risk injuring itself, for example, and yet remain calm and quiet tethered to a perch with a flight wire.

The dimensions given in Table 3.1 are therefore only guidelines. Animal safety cannot be measured with a yardstick! The most important principle aside from meeting the bird's needs for exercise and space is always prevention of injury!

Some birds of prey, especially those found in zoos, are not native species and have special temperature requirements. Appropriate cold weather shelters must thus be included in the construction of aviaries for these species. The dimensions given in Table 3.1 are based on the recommendations of the German Ministry of Nutrition, Agriculture and Forestry's expert panel for "humane captive management of birds", January 10, 1995.

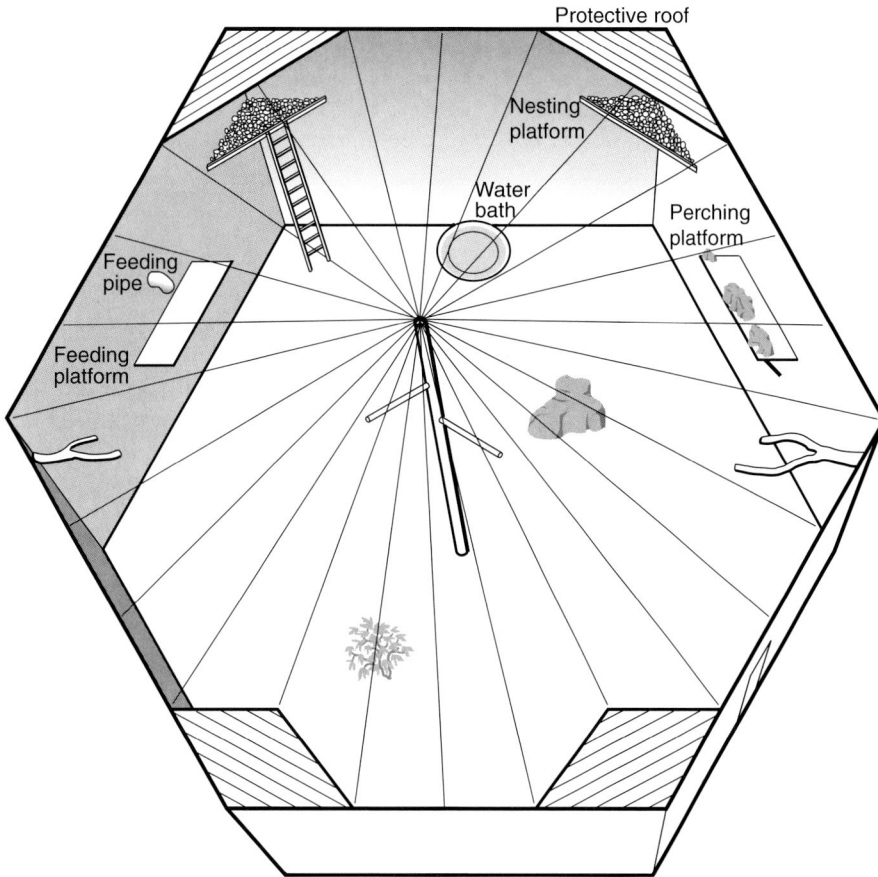

Fig 3.5: The so-called "circular falcon aviary" based on a design by Müller, who successfully bred gyrfalcons in such a chamber in 1973. These aviaries have a diameter of more than 20 meters and permit a large degree of freedom of movement for the inhabitants. The structure can be up to 6 meters high. It is therefore wise to place a ladder in the aviary on a permanent basis, allowing the birds to get accustomed to its appearance and use. (Illustration: R. Gattung-Petith and A. Gattung)

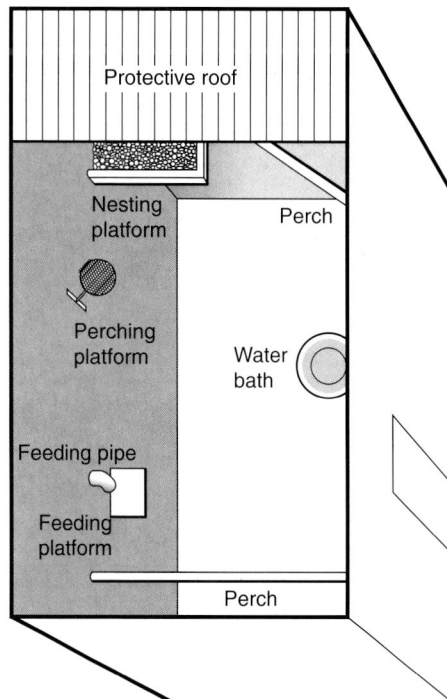

Fig. 3.6: The more traditional breeding chamber for birds of prey is usually significantly smaller than the circular aviary, but can be used successfully as long as the minimum dimensions for breeding are upheld. (Illustration: R. Gattung-Petith and A. Gattung)

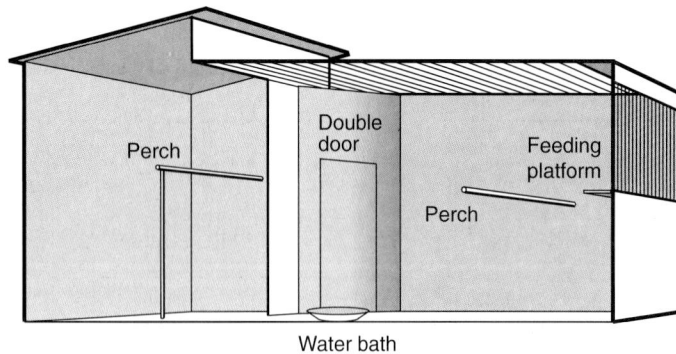

Fig. 3.7: The moulting chamber (mews) serves to house a hunting hawk during the off season when it is not being flown. (Illustration: R. Gattung-Petith and A. Gattung)

Categories of minimum size requirements for raptor enclosures (given per animal; young birds are not included until they gain independence)

A. Aviary: outdoor area 2m², width 1m, height 2m.
Each additional animal: 1m² added to outdoor area, and 1m² shelter area
If kept exclusively in heated indoor chamber: area 2m², height 1m,
each additional animal 1m² more.

B. Aviary: outdoor area 5 m², width 2m, height 2m.
Each additional animal 1m² added to outdoor area, and shelter, if necessary: 1.5 m², height 2m, width 1m.

C. Aviary: outdoor area 7.5 m², width 2m, height 2.5 m.
Each additional animal: 3m² added to outdoor area, and shelter, if necessary: 2m², height 2m, width 1m.

D. Aviary: outdoor area 12m², width 2m, height 2.5m.
Each additional animal: 6m² added to outdoor area, and shelter, if necessary: 4m², height 2m, width 2m.

E. Aviary: outdoor area 18m², width 3m, height 2.5m.
Each additional animal: 6m² added to outdoor area, and shelter, if necessary: 4m², height 2m, width 2m.

F. Aviary: outdoor area 24m², width 3m, height 3m.
Each additional animal: 10m² added to outdoor area, and shelter, if necessary: 4m², height 2m, width 2m.

G. Outdoor aviary for a pair of birds at least 100m².

Categories of temperature requirements

I. Hardy in winter, requires only protection from rain and wind.

II. Sensitive to very cold temperatures, requires an unheated enclosure or chamber.

III. Sensitive to moderately cold temperatures, requires indoor room protected from frost and drafts.

IV. Not tolerant of cold temperatures, requires heated indoor chamber kept at temperatures above + 15⁰ C.

Table 3.1: Aviary size and temperature requirements for birds of prey

Family	Species	Category of aviary size requirement	Category of temperature requirement
New World Vultures *Catharthidae*	Black vulture *Catharthes atratus*	D	III
	Turkey vulture *Cathartes aura*	D	IV
	King vulture *Sarcoramphus papa*	D	IV (very sensitive to frost)
	Andean condor *Vultur gryphus*	F	I
Osprey *Pandionidae*	Osprey *Pandion haliaetus*	D	II
Secretary Birds *Sagittariidae*	Secretary bird *Sagittarius serpentarius*	G because they are ground birds, can also be maintained with unilaterally trimmed flight feathers	IV
Hawks *Accipitridae* G. Elanus	Black-shouldered kite *Elanus caeruleus*	C	IV
G. Milvus	Black kite *Milvus migrans*	D	I–II Consider origin*
	Red kite *Milvus milvus*	D	I
	Brahminy kite *Haliastur indus*	D	IV
G. Ichthyophaga	Gray-headed fishing eagle *Ichtyophaga ichthyaetus*	D	IV
G. Haliaeetus	White-tailed sea eagle *Haliaeetus albicilla*	F	I
	Bald eagle *Haliaeetus leucocephalus*	F	I
	White-bellied sea eagle *Haliaeetus leucogaster*	D	IV
	Pallas' sea eagle *Haliaeetus leucoryphus*	D	I
	Steller's sea eagle *Haliaeetus pelagicus*	F	I
	African fish eagle *Haliaeetus vocifer*	D	IV
G. Gypaetus	Bearded vulture *Gypaetus barbatus*	F	I
G. Aegypius	European black vulture *Aegypius monachus*	F	I
G. Gypohierax	Palm nut vulture *Gypohierax angolensis*	D	IV
G. Neophron	Egyptian vulture *Neophron percnopterus*	D	II–III Consider origin*
G. Necrosyrtes	Hooded vulture *Necrosyrtes monachus*	D	IV
G. Sarcogyps	Indian black (King) vulture *Sarcogyps calvus*	F	IV
G. Torgos	Lappet-faced vulture *Torgos tracheliotus*	F	IV
G. Trigonoceps	White-headed vulture *Trigonoceps occipitalis*	F	III
G. Gyps	Griffon vulture *Gyps fulvus*	F	I
	Himalayan griffon *Gyps himalayensis*	F	I
	Rüppell's griffon *Gyps rueppellii*	F	III
G. Pseudogyps	Indian white-backed vulture *Pseudogyps bengalensis*	D	
	African white-backed vulture *Pseugogyps africanus*	D	III
G. Circaetus	Brown harrier (Snake) eagle *Circaetus cinereus*	D	IV
	Short-toed (Serpent) eagle *Circaetus gallicus*	D	IV
G. Terathopius	Bateleur eagle *Therathopius ecaudatus*	D	IV
G. Spilornis	Crested serpent eagle *Spilornis cheela*	D	IV
G. Circus	Marsh harrier *Circus aeruginosus*	D	II
	Hen harrier *Circus cyaneus*	D	I
G. Melierax	Pale chanting goshawk *Melierax canorus*	D	IV
G. Polyboroides	African harrier hawk *Polyboroides typus*	D	IV
G. Accipiter	Northern goshawk *Accipiter gentilis*	D	I
	European sparrowhawk *Accipiter nisus*	C	I

Family	Species	Category of aviary size requirement	Category of temperature requirement
G. Kaupifalco	Lizard buzzard *Kaupifalco monogrammicus*	C	IV
G. Geranoaetus	Grey eagle-buzzard *Geranoaetus melanoleucus*	D	II
G. Buteo	Common buzzard *Buteo buteo*	C**	I
	Red-tailed hawk *Buteo jamaicensis*	C**	I–II Consider origin*
	Rough-legged buzzard *Buteo lagopus*	D	I
	Red-backed buzzard *Buteo polyosoma*	D	II
	Ferruginous hawk *Buteo regalis*	D	I
	Jackal (Augur) buzzard *Buteo rutofunus*	D	III
	Long-legged buzzard *Buteo rufofuscus*	D	I
G. Pernis	Honey buzzard *Pernis apivorus*	C**	III
G. Harpia	Harpy eagle *Harpia harpyija*	F	III
G. Morphnus	Guiana crested eagle *Morphnus guianensis*	F	III
G. Pithecophaga	Philippine monkey-eating eagle *Pithecophaga jefferyi*	F	IV
G. Polemaetus	Martial eagle *Polemaetus bellicosus*	F	III
G. Stephanoaetus	Crowned eagle *Stephanoaetus coronatus*	F	IV
G. Lophaetus	Long-crested eagle *Lophaetus occipitalis*	D	IV
G. Hieraaetus	Bonelli's eagle *Hieraaetus fasciatus*	D	I–II Consider origin*
G. Spizaetus	Ornate hawk eagle *Spizaetus ornatus*	D	IV
G. Aquila	Wedge-tailed eagle *Aquila audax*	F	I
	Greater spotted eagle *Aquila clanga*	D	II
	Golden eagle *Aquila chrysaetos*	F	I
	Imperial eagle *Aquila heliacea*	F	I
	Lesser spotted eagle *Aquila pomarina*	D	II
	Tawny (Steppe) eagle *Aquila rapax*	E	I–II Consider origin*
	Verreaux's (Black) eagle *Aquila verreauxii*	F	III
Falcons Falconidae	Chimango *Milvago chiachima*	C	III
G. Milvago	Yellow-headed caracara *Milvago chiachima*	C	III
G. Phalcoboenus	Forster's caracara *Phalcoboenus australis*	D	I
	Mountain caracara *Phalcoboenus megalopterus*	D	II
G. Polyborus	Common caracara *Polyborus plancus*	D	II
G. Poliherax	African pygmy falcon *Polyhierax semitorquatus*	B	IV
G. Microhierax	Red-legged falconet *Microhierax caerulescens*	A	IV
G. Falco	Lanner falcon *Falco biarmicus*	D	I–II Consider origin*
	Saker falcon *Falco cherrug*	D	I–III Consider origin*
	Merlin *Falco columbarius*	C	I
	Eleonora's falcon *Falco eleonorae*	D	III
	Laggar falcon *Falco jugger*	D	II
	Prairie falcon *Falco mexicanus*	D	I
	Peregrine falcon *Falco peregrinus*	D	I
	Gyrfalcon *Falco rusticolus*	D	I
	American kestrel *Falco sparverius*	B	II–III Consider origin*
	European hobby *Falco subbuteo*	C**	III
	Common kestrel *Falco tinnunculus*	B	I
	Red-footed falcon *Falco vespertinus*	B	III

* Consider origin: Temperature requirements will vary with regional geographic origin. Other categories may be more appropriate.
** Individually-housed birds require the same space as pairs do, 10.5 m^2

3.2.5 Aviary accessories

The majority of space inside a flight cage should be free of perches and obstructions in order to maximize the opportunities for flight. Perches should be mounted on the wall or near the ground in such a way that the birds cannot defecate into the bath or drinking water. Variously shaped and textured materials are recommended for the surfaces of platforms and perches (bark, cork, coco mats, artificial turf).

Two nesting platforms should be available for selection by breeding pairs.

3.2.6 Aviary hygiene

3.2.6.1 Aviary floors

The primary rule in protecting the health of raptors confined to an aviary or mews is the prevention of contact with their own wastes. The floor of the enclosure always presents a problem in this regard, since the feces will accumulate there over time. This is especially true in breeding chambers, which cannot be entered for the duration of the breeding period for fear of disrupting mating activity. Therefore, large aviaries appear to do best if planted with grass and small bushes or trees. A wire mesh ceiling will allow natural rain and sunshine to enter and promote biodegradation of wastes in the soil. The removal of surface dirt under the perches several times a year will suffice to keep such aviaries relatively clean.

For smaller aviaries, a floor covered with a thick layer of sand or fine gravel is recommended. This will permit adequate drainage of water and keep the surface relatively dry. The use of bark chips or mulch is not advised. Although they may provide the appearance of cleanliness, these organic materials decay quickly, retain moisture and may foster a dangerous buildup of microorganisms. Fungal infections are a particular risk with such organic substrates (see Ch. 9.3).

3.2.6.2 Drinking water and baths

Even though some raptor species almost never drink water, every aviary must have fresh water available at all times. Diseases accompanied by diarrhea or vomiting will lead to dehydration, which in turn brings about rapid death unless the animal has access to water. Even the barbary falcon, a desert species, will drink water occasionally in captivity. Sometimes the confined environment inside an aviary can get hotter in the summer than the open air ever does.

Water containers should be made of easily cleaned, smooth materials such as plastic or stainless steel. This will facilitate their daily cleaning. Many raptors like to

bathe, and not only in water. Gyrfalcons will take baths in snow. Small falcons as well as lanner falcons and peregrines enjoy an occasional dust bath too. Bearded vultures derive the reddish color of their plumage from bathing in red dust.

3.3 Maintaining tethered raptors

The keeping of birds of prey tied to blocks or perches is absolutely necessary in the practice of falconry. The

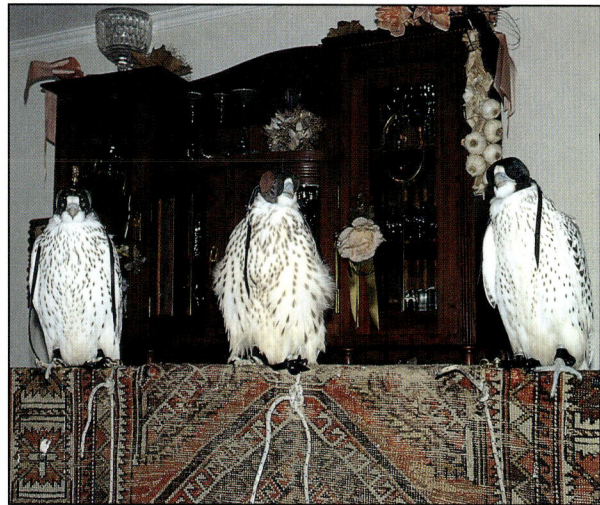

Fig. 3.8: Gyrfalcons (*Falco rusticolus*) spending the night on a perch inside the house. Only falcons can be kept this way without a hood.
(Photo: Heidenreich)

various forms of this ancient practice are described below. If applied correctly, hawks do not suffer, endure pain, or sustain physical damage under such conditions. Despite, or maybe thanks to, a certain limitation in freedom of movement involved with tethering, some birds will do better with that system than in spacious flight cages.

All falconry birds kept tied to blocks or perches must be fitted with jesses, a swivel and a leash.

Jesses: Jesses are 10 to 15 cm long leather straps that are attached to each leg just above the foot. Only very strong, yet pliable leather such as kangaroo or cowhide should be used. The jesses are fastened by means of a special knot that cannot tighten around and thereby injure the leg.

In recent years, Aylmeri jesses have become widely used. These consist of a set of anklets attached to each leg with a grommet through which the jesses are pul-

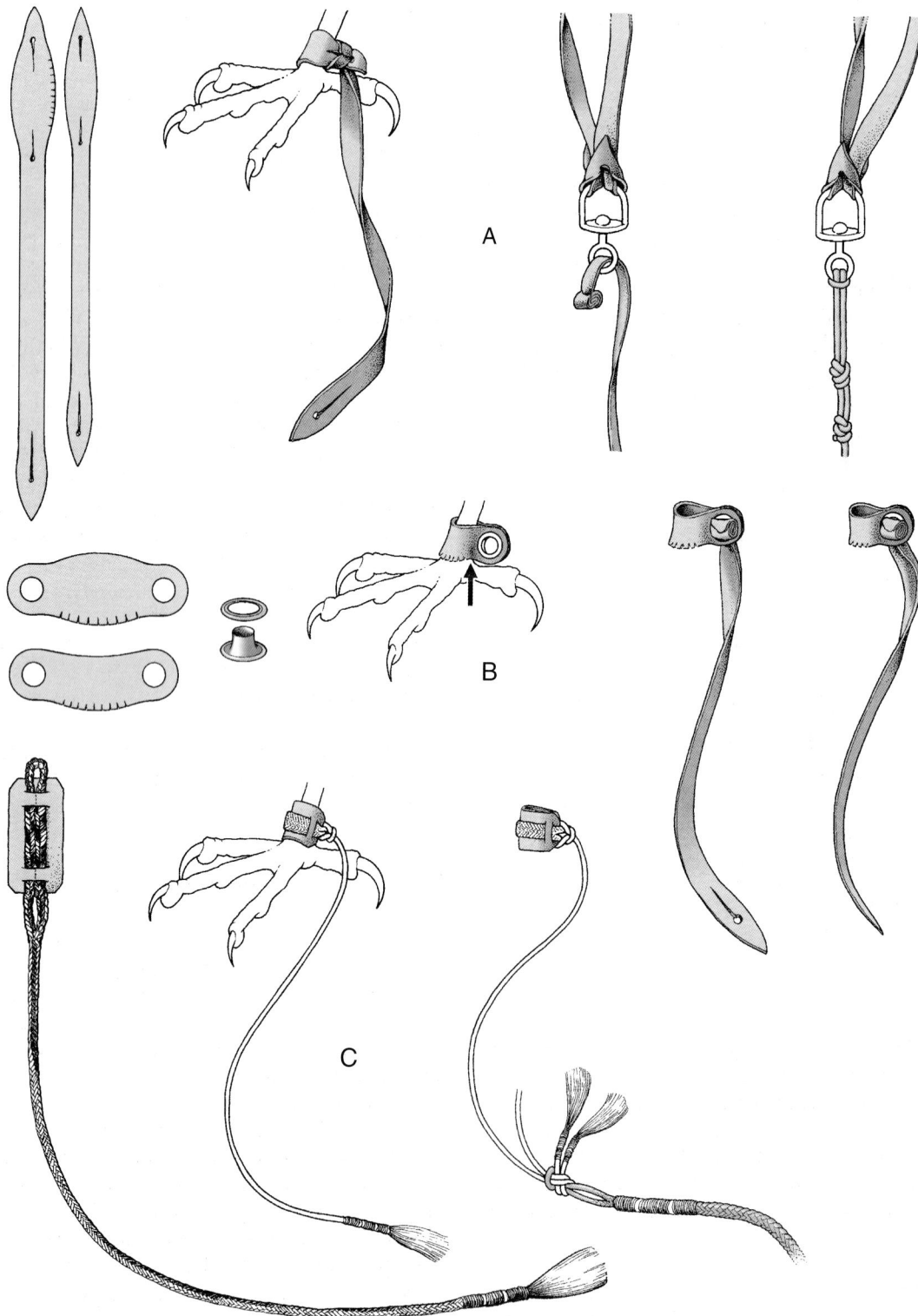

Fig. 3.9: Various systems for tying a hawk:

A: The traditional European jesses have the drawback that they can become entangled when the bird turns around.

B: Aylmeri jesses have an additional center of rotation at the grommet. During free flight, the jesses can be removed or replaced by lighter hunting jesses that do not have a slit in the end. This allows the bird to fly unencumbered and avoid getting caught in branches or other obstructions.

C: Arabic jesses are made of fine braided cords that weigh very little and can remain on the bird during flight.

(Illustrations: R. Gattung-Petith and A. Gattung)

led. This method has the advantage that the jesses cannot become twisted around the bird's legs.

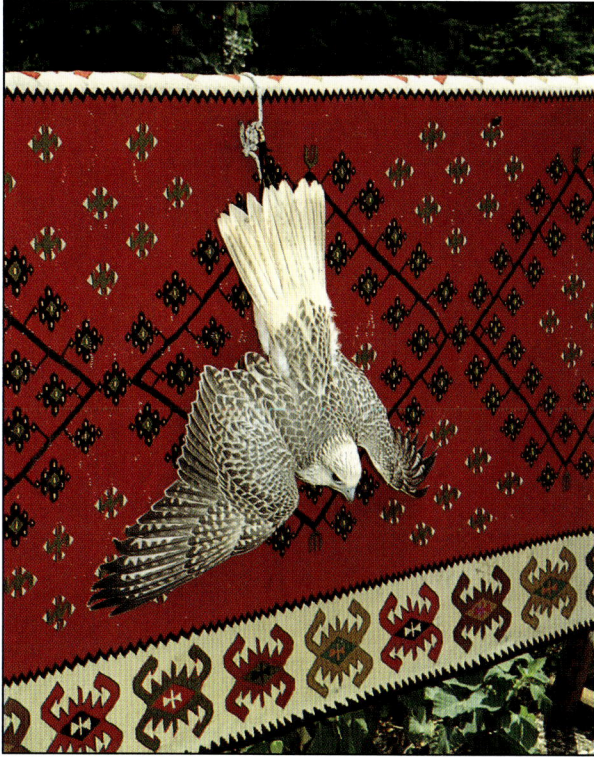

Fig. 3.10: Only a hawk that has proven it can remount a screen perch should be kept on one. Otherwise, deaths can occur, especially in birds with a full crop. (Photo: Heidenreich)

Swivel: The swivel is composed of two attached rings that swivel freely with respect to each other. It is usually made of a light metal such as brass or stainless steel. Both jesses are attached to one ring of the swivel, and the leash is attached to the other. This device has to be very strong and reliable to prevent the inadvertent escape of a hawk with its jesses still tied to the broken swivel.

Leash: The leash is a 1 to 1.5 m long unbreakable leather strap or nylon cord. One end is attached to the swivel and the other is tied to the block or perch.

3.3.1 Screen perches

A screen perch is a horizontal perch to which the hawk is tied with the leash (Fig. 3.9). It should be mounted such that the bird sits at approximately chest-level to the falconer. The perch must be wide enough that the bird cannot reach the ends with its wings when jumping off. This will prevent injury to the flight feathers.

It is absolutely necessary to attach a screen to the bottom of the screen perch. This sheet of material is stretched between the perch and the wall to prevent the bird from remounting on the wrong side. Entanglement of the leash around the perch is thus avoided. The leash is fastened to the perch with a special knot.

Due to the limited mobility permitted a bird tied to a screen perch, its use should be limited to special situations and short periods of time. For example, an unmanned wild bird can be kept this way for a little while to prevent escape maneuvers. This will speed up the taming process, but such training should be limited to a few days at the beginning of the manning period.

Another practical use for the screen perch involves putting trained hawks on them at night or in inclement weather when they need to be kept indoors. Such birds quickly learn to appreciate these protected sleeping arrangements and don't even need to be tied.

Only birds that have learned to remount the screen perch after bating or jumping off should be left tied to such structures.

3.3.2 Block and bow perches

Birds of prey (commonly eagles, falcons or vultures) are tied to blocks or bow perches by means of the leash and a movable metal ring attached to the perch. To avoid damaging the feet, the surface must be made of appropriate materials such as astroturf or rough cork. The ideal block has a surface that can be exchanged, so that a variety of different materials can be used. The diameter of the block should be such that the jesses of the bird cannot slide over the top and bind the bird's legs to the perch. A revolving block can also prevent the inadvertent entanglement of a tied bird.

Bow perches or ring perches are most often used with goshawks, sparrowhawks and eagles. They require similar care in the selection of surface material. Easily gripped surfaces such as leather, cork or sisal rope are suitable. In addition, the circumference of the perch should be large enough that the talons of the standing bird do not touch underneath.

Blocks or bow perches should be set up on a lawn or gravel area surrounded by enough space that the hawk will not damage its plumage while tied to them (Fig. 3.11). The bath and drinking water are placed such that they will not be contaminated by mutes. If the bird is to remain on the perch unsupervised for longer periods of time, a small shed to provide protection from wind and rain and shelter for sleeping should be available as well.

Maintaining falconry birds tethered to such perches is a practice thousands of years old. It is appropriate only for birds of prey which are adequately trained and which are flown at least several times a week. Because freedom of movement is markedly reduced with such methods, they should not be used on a long term or permanent basis.

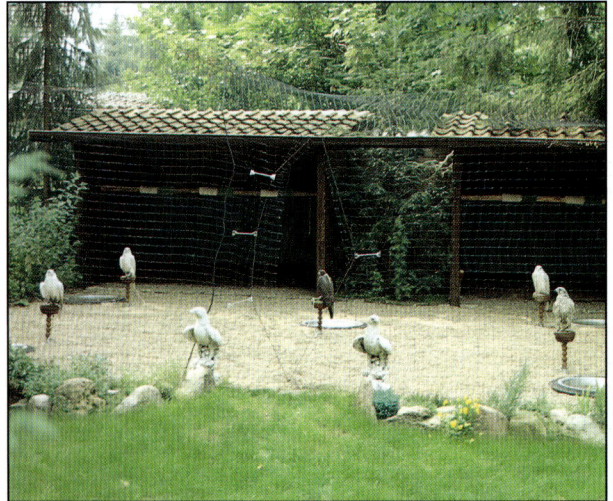

Fig. 3.11: The author's facility for housing five hunting hawks. The blocks are placed in a 20 cm thick base of gravel that is easily cleaned. In the background are sheltered perches for use at night. In principle, all such facilities should be protected from wild raptors by wire mesh or netting.
(Photo: Heidenreich)

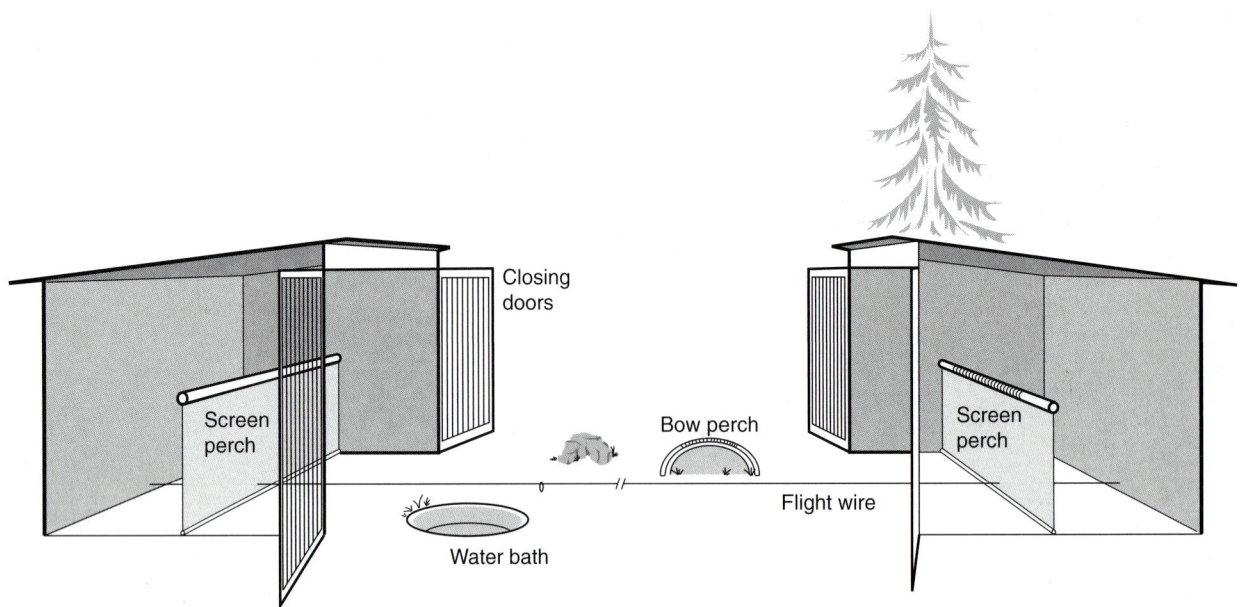

Fig. 3.12: A well-designed wire-and-perch arrangement gives the bird substantial freedom to fly and protects the plumage from damage better than an aviary. It is a humane alternative for maintaining trained birds of prey.
In contrast to birds in mews, those on the perch-and-wire can be easily observed and monitored for illness.
The shelter doors can be closed at night to protect the hawk from predators.
(Illustration: R. Gattung-Petith and A. Gattung)

3.3.3 Wire-and-perch flight arrangement

The arrangement of two widely spaced perches with a taut wire between them represents a method of tying hawks that permits substantial freedom of movement. The flight distance thus available to a bird can be larger than that provided in an aviary (Fig. 3.12). One of the perches can be under cover for protection from the weather. The freedom to fly allows the bird to choose different locations for a bath or sunning. Some birds such as goshawks and sparrowhawks can gain speed rapidly over relatively short distances. Therefore, the wire should be no longer than 15 m and each end should be clearly marked by a wall or a wooden blind.

The advantages of this setup lie in the relatively large degree of mobility available to the bird. The freedom of movement may equal or even exceed that available in the mews. If properly constructed, it can therefore serve as a very acceptable way to maintain a captive hawk, even long term during the molt.

3.4 Maintenance under special circumstances

Veterinarians are often forced to keep an injured or ill bird of prey until recovery. To promote healing, and primarily to protect the plumage, such birds must sometimes be confined in a small, dark cage. Wild birds or birds of prey from aviaries that are unaccustomed to man often act very nervous and restless in traditional open-front cages and should not be kept in them. Sturdy cardboard boxes supplied with ventilation holes have proven very functional. Only enough light to allow the bird to find its food enters through the holes. When the box becomes soiled, it can easily be replaced. If the bird is to be kept in the box for a longer period, the floor can be covered with some type of absorbent material. The use of sawdust, peat moss or other dusty materials should be avoided. Hay and straw are also not recommended, as they can promote

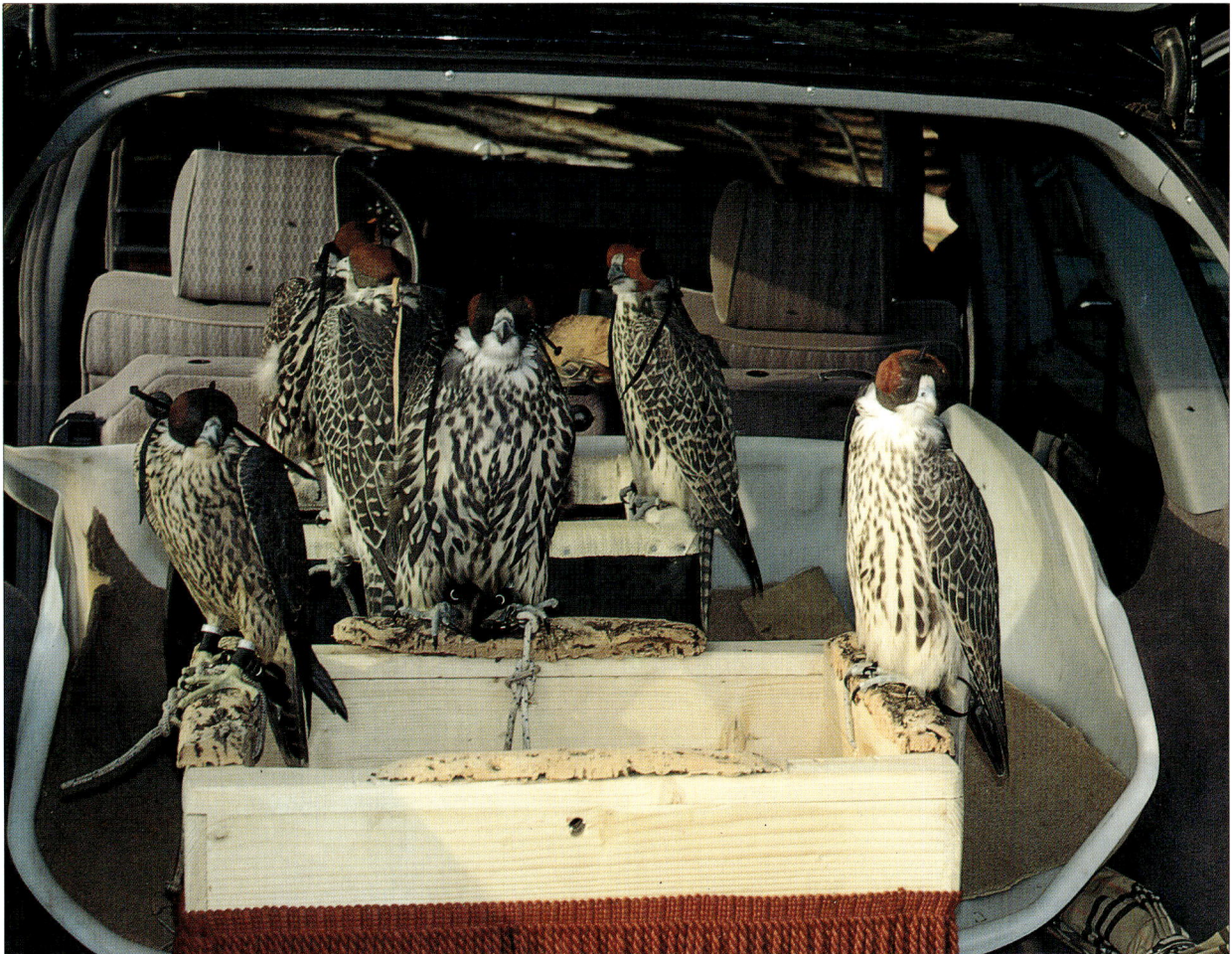

Fig. 3.13: If accustomed to it, falcons can easily be transported openly on a cadge in the car. (Photo: Heidenreich)

the growth of mold or mildew that can lead to illness in the bird. This type of confinement should be limited to the time absolutely necessary and used only by veterinarians or under veterinary supervision.

3.5   Transporting raptors

The most important principle in transporting and shipping birds of prey is the health and well-being of the animal.

3.5.1   Supervised transport

Well-trained birds that are accustomed to being handled, as well as hand-raised, i.e., tame and calm animals, can travel freely perched in the car. Some may not even require a hood (Fig. 3.13).

A hood is a hand-made leather cap fitted to the individual bird. It covers the eyes and the beak but leaves the nostrils open. If accustomed to it, the bird will tolerate the hood easily and remain calm in the darkness thus created.

Nervous birds should be transported in sturdy boxes. Transport boxes are usually made of lightweight material with a tightly-closing door and sufficient ventilation holes. They should be dark inside in order to keep the traveling bird calm. The size of the box should be adequate to give the perched bird enough head and tail room to turn around easily. Problems can arise if the transport box is not kept meticulously clean. Dried mutes and castings can easily create dust inside the box. This will be inhaled by the bird, particularly if it is restless. In addition, odor can become a problem during longer transports. Based on the suggestion of Vogt (1990), Richter (1993) therefore recommends the ventilation of such boxes with a small mechanical ventilator. This device should remove dust and odors from the bottom while allowing fresh air to enter at the top.

Trained hawks should be transported with the leash attached and partly exiting the box so that they can be safely brought onto the fist upon opening the container.

3.5.2   Unsupervised transport

The transport of raptors on trains or airplanes, where intervention in case of a problem is not possible, requires special safety precautions. The transport box should be very strong and have smooth walls supplied with plenty of ventilation holes. The outside of the container should be outfitted with bars or blocks that prevent it from being packed so tightly that air circula-

tion would be impaired. It should be big enough to permit the hawk to stand upright and turn comfortably. A perch should not be used since the bird will certainly not remain sitting on it and might damage its plumage during travel. The floor is best covered with firmly attached carpeting that gives the talons something to grasp without getting caught in it.

Aggressive birds like raptors should always be shipped individually!

Because the bird will move and turn during transport, the jesses, if present, should be left free. Attaching the swivel or leash carries too high a risk of entanglement.

To further calm the bird, a hood can be used. This is especially helpful with falcons. Very nervous birds can be sprayed with a fine mist of water before closing the box (Fig. 3.14). Plant sprayers work well for this purpose. The advantage is that the moist bird will be much calmer. In addition, the plumage becomes more pliable and thus less vulnerable to bending or breaking.

The tail can also be wrapped with easily-removed tape (Tesacrepp®) to prevent damage.

When shipping by airplane, the sender often has to deal with the requirements for animal transport established by the IATA. They prescribe a transport box like those typically used for small mammals (jet box) or, more recently, a special container for raptors that must have a double wall of wire mesh. Such containers are completely unsuitable for transporting birds of prey and can lead to serious injury for the occupants. The

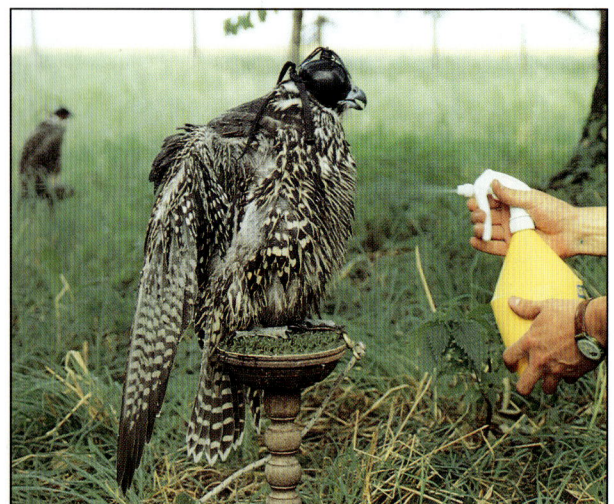

Fig. 3.14: Nervous or restless birds can be calmed and prevented from jumping around prior to transport by moistening the plumage. In addition, moist feathers are more flexible and thus less vulnerable to damage. (Photo: Heidenreich)

requirement that food and water dishes be available is also not applicable to raptors. The birds do not need food or water as long as they travel less than 24 hours in the case of smaller species, or 48 hours for larger ones. In addition, feather damage is certain to occur if the dishes are present inside the box.

The IATA would be well advised to consult a raptor expert in the development of such travel regulations if it wants to avoid injury to the animals!

If the airport or airline authorities insist on following IATA regulations, the local veterinary officials responsible may be able to help.

Before booking the flight, it is advisable to consult with the airline regarding its policy on transporting endangered species. Some airlines refuse to carry such animals.

3.6   Behavior problems

Many wild animals, and domestic animals too, can develop abnormal behavior in captivity. The stereotypical pacing of a large cat in a cage or featherpicking in pet parrots are well-known examples of such problems. Raptors, too, may occasionally develop unnatural behavior patterns in captivity despite optimal conditions and the most humane circumstances.

3.6.1   Aggression

Many birds of prey are predators and thus naturally demonstrate aggressive tendencies that are normally channeled and dissipated in the capture of prey. In captivity, such birds kept in pairs or groups may occasionally demonstrate misdirected aggression that can lead to problems.

3.6.1.1 Intraspecific aggression

If aggressive birds of prey are placed in group situations, be they community aviaries or attempts at pairing, there is always the possibility that they will not get along. In the confinement of a flight cage there is no possibility for evasion or escape. The less aggressive bird may fly against the wire mesh and become entangled, thereby stimulating the hunting instinct of the other bird.

The significant size differential between the sexes in most raptorial species encourages such behavior (Fig. 3.15). In most cases, the smaller male bird is attacked or even killed by the stronger female. Such "accidents" are known to occur among goshawks and in some other species such as merlins (see Ch. 5.1.4.2).

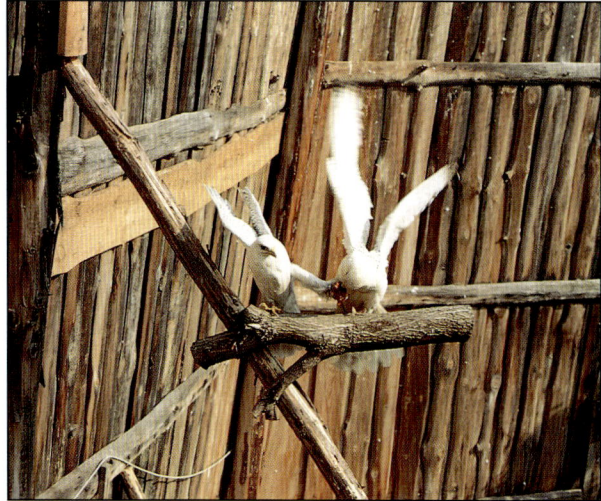

Fig. 3.15: Even normally harmonious pairs (here *F. rusticolus*) can occasionally fight about food and cause injuries. Especially talon injuries can be dangerous in birds of prey (see Ch. 9.2.2.2). (Photo: Heidenreich)

It may be helpful to place the tiercel in the breeding chamber a few weeks before adding the female. The male thus has the advantage of establishing his territory first and improving his chances of escape in a familiar environment once the female is added. Some goshawk breeders trim the flight feathers of the female to impair her ability to pursue the tiercel.

3.6.1.2 Aggression between nestlings

The killing of siblings (cainism) has been described in several raptor species, primarily among eagles (Meyburg and Pielowski, 1991). This usually involves the killing of one or several fellow nestlings by the strongest chick in the clutch. Such behavior is common in the wild also and serves as a brutal form of selection pressure. This type of behavior is promoted by the fact that one chick always hatches before the others. The resulting size differences among the chicks make it difficult for the younger and smaller ones to defend themselves against their stronger sibling's attacks. Even at only a few days of age, the stronger chick will incessantly try to pick or bite at the smaller ones. In a short time the head and back of the victim will be covered with blood. The injured nestling becomes less successful at obtaining food from the parents and eventually dies. The adults permit this to happen without reacting.

Once the chicks have reached a certain size and grown some feathers, this phenomenon is no longer observed. This knowledge has led to the practice of removing the smaller, otherwise doomed chick from the nests of wild Spanish imperial eagles (*Aquila heliaca adalberti*) and greater spotted eagles (*Aquila clanga*), and then later replacing it when the nestlings have matured sufficiently to eliminate the risk of aggression (Meyburg and Garzon Heydt, 1978).

Interestingly, this behavior may occur in captivity among species that do not demonstrate it in nature. The author has observed aggression between nestlings in common buzzard chicks (*Buteo buteo*) and attributes this to the fact that the birds were being kept under a heat lamp in the open air instead of being brooded by a parent bird. Rothman(1994) observed similar behavior among the chicks of red-tail hawks (*Buteo jamaicensis*) and long-legged buzzards (*Buteo rufinus*).

3.6.1.3 Aggression in trained hawks

Trained hunting hawks, especially those imprinted on humans, may display inappropriate aggressive behavior in some situations. Goshawks, for example, may fly at and attack the falconer or his dog if no game has been successfully flushed during a day of hunting. It seems as if the accumulated aggressions have to be released somehow. In trained eagles, this can become such a serious problem that the falconer can no longer fly them free for fear that they will attack and seriously injure dogs or even humans. Hawks that are regularly successful at the hunt tend to remain tractable and tame towards the owner and other people.

3.6.2   Behavior problems during the rearing of young

Under natural conditions, the parenting duties of a pair of raptors are well-defined. The female incubates the eggs most of the time while the male goes hunting, supplies food and occasionally briefly takes a turn at sitting on the nest. After hatching occurs, the female also bears the primary responsibility for feeding the young.

In captivity there is always adequate food available and the tiercel's responsibilities are eliminated. This frequently leads to competitive behavior between the two adult birds. A pair of captive white-tailed sea eagles attempting to fulfill their nesting instincts put the entire clutch at risk with their frustrated efforts to push each other off the nest and the eggs. Later they displayed great jealousy in feeding the chicks, each trying to push away the other in the process. Such competitiveness can endanger the welfare of the young.

3.6.3   Feather picking

The problem of feather picking is well-known in parrots and parakeets housed alone in captivity. The bird will destroy and pluck its body feathers in certain areas and can eventually appear completely naked. Only the head will remain normal because those feathers cannot be reached with the beak.

The reasons for such abnormal behavior usually are psychological ones. Lack of stimulation, as well as various frustrations and fears, among others, can precipitate feather picking. If the problem is discovered and eliminated, such self-destructive activity can often be stopped.

Birds of prey can show very similar behavioral pathologies, albeit more rarely. A laggar falcon (*Falco jugger*) was seen ripping out all the feathers on its inner thighs, until even the skin was bleeding. This falcon was kept tied to a block for many years without anything to do. When he began removing his breast feathers as well, the bird was put into training and the problem resolved. Within a few weeks his feathers had all regrown.

Similar behavior problems are observed in the "more intelligent" birds of prey. Especially eagles have a tendency to engage in mating behavior toward humans if they are imprinted. When the human partner fails to respond with the appropriate behavior in turn, the sexually frustrated bird may compensate by feather picking.

References and literature of further interest

BEYERBACH, U. (1978):
Gutachten über art- und verhaltensgerechte Unterbringung und Gefangenschaftshaltung von Taggreifvögeln.
Prakt. Tierarzt **59**, 680-684

GERLACH, C. (1980):
Hygiene in Greifvogel-Haltungen.
Voliere **3**, 107-108

HAMMER, W. (1974):
Die Bedeutung des neuen Tierschutzgesetzes für die Falknerei.
Jb. Dtsch. Falkenorden 54-57

HAMMER, W., HEIDENREICH, M., TROMMER, G. and J. KÖSTERS (1989):
Empfehlungen zur tierschutzgerechten Haltung von Greifvögeln und Eulen.
Tierärztl. Praxis **17**, 59-70

HAVELKA, P. (1981):
Zur Problematik der »art- und verhaltensgerechten« Unterbringung von Greifvögeln (*Falconiformes*).
Vogel und Umwelt **1**, 307-311

HEIDENREICH, M. (1988):
Tierschutzrechtliche Aspekte in der Falknerei.
Dtsch. Tierärztl. Wschr. **95**, 56-58

HUSSONG, H.K. (1992):
Falknerprüfung. Leitfaden zur Vorbereitung
Eigenverlag, 90768 Fürth, Oberführberger Straße 91

KIEL, H. (1988):
Gibt es tierschutzrelevante Probleme bei der Haltung von Beiz- bzw. Greifvögeln?
DVG, VI. Tagung, Verhandl. Ber. 311-315

KÖSTERS, J. (1974):
Haltungsbedingte Krankheiten bei Greifvögeln.
Prakt. Tierarzt **55**, Supplement 31-33

KRUSE, D. (1988):
Überschnabel bei Lannerfalken und die Folgen.
Greifvögel und Falknerei 77-79
Verlag Neumann-Neudamm, Morschen-Heina

KÜSPERT, H., HEIDENREICH, M. and H.J. KÜSPERT (1993):
Falkenzucht Teil 1: Haltungstechniken
Voliere **16**, Sonderheft

MEYBURG, B.U. and J. GARZON HEYDT (1978):
Sobre la protección del Aguila imperial (*Aquila heliaca adalberti*) aminorando artificialmente la mortandad juvenil.
Ardeola **19**, 105-128

MEYBURG, B.U. and Z. PIELOWSKI (1991):
Cainism in the greater spotted eagle (*Aquila clanga*).
Bull. Birds of Prey **4**, 143-148

O'BRIEN, D. (1992):
The Rites of Autumn. A Falconer's Journey Across the American West.
Doubleday, N.Y., 6-7

PILS, H. (1986):
Richtlinien für sachgemäße Greifvogelhaltung.
Der Falkner **35**, 12-14

RICHTER, T. (1993):
Luftikus, der belüftete Transportbehälter.
Falknerei und Greifvögel 99-100
Verlag Neumann-Neudamm, Morschen-Heina

RICHTER, T. (1994):
Mindestanforderungen an die Haltung von Greifvögeln.
Broschüre Tierärztl. Vereinigung Tierschutz, Hamburg

RUEMPLER, G. (1984):
Grundsätzliche Erwägungen zur Haltung von Greifvögeln in menschlicher Obhut.
Zschr. Kölner Zoo **27**, 143-147

ROTHMANN, F. (1994):
personal communication

SCHULZ, T.A. (1990):
Raptor restraint, handling, and transport methods.
in : Ludwig, D.R. (1990): Wildlife rehabilitation 97–115
Sartell, MN. Ithaca, USA

VÖGELE, H.H. (1931):
Die Falknerei.
Verlag Neumann-Neudamm, Melsungen

VOGT, G. (1990):
personal communication

WÖLFING, P. (1983):
Erfahrungen in einer Vogelauffangstation – eine kritische Bilanz aus Sicht der Veterinärmedizin, des Natur- und Tierschutzes.
Vogel und Umwelt **2**, 247–252

4 Feeding

Published information regarding the feeding of birds of prey in captivity is scarce. Brown and Amadon (1968) discuss daily food requirements, stating that they may vary from 25% of body weight in small raptors to 4% of body weight in large vultures. To maintain normal body weight, a small falcon of 100 grams required 25 grams of food a day and a sparrow-hawk twice that weight needed 53 grams daily. A 683 gram peregrine falcon consumed an average of 104 grams of food per day, approximately 15% of its body weight, while a red-tailed hawk weighing 1200 grams took in 127 grams of food and a golden eagle of over 4 kilograms consumed only 251 grams daily, 10.7 and 6.25% of their body weight respectively. A white-tailed eagle from the London Zoo had a body weight of 7030 grams and ingested barely 240 grams or 3.55% of his body weight in food per day.

Naturally, the daily food requirements will also vary depending on environmental temperature and physical activity level. Unlike with poultry, there is no detailed information regarding food requirements for raptors under circumstances of variable temperature or activity. On the one hand, this may not be necessary, since special demands such as rapid weight gain or continuous egg-laying are not required of birds of prey. On the other hand, hunting with trained hawks requires that the bird be in the exact physical condition that permits prolonged hunting flights while at the same time retaining the incentive to return to the falconer. During the breeding of birds of prey, one must also pay close attention to a balanced diet, since mating behavior, fertility and egg quality are all directly dependent on the nutritional status of the breeding pair. Raptor breeders, who value high fertility and hatching rates have long known that a varied diet is an essential part thereof.

Regrettably, the diet of raptors in captivity is often determined by the availability and cost of food animals, too often resulting in the exclusive feeding of day-old chicks which are easily and inexpensively obtained from poultry hatcheries. Although there are many reports of birds, especially small falcons, maintained and even successfully bred on such a diet, Klosters and Meister (1982) suspect a chronic iron deficiency anemia in birds fed only day-old chicks. The peak performance required of trained hawks daily during hunting season can hardly be achieved if they are kept on a monotonous diet of such questionable quality.

Table 4.1: Protein, fat, metabolizable energy and mineral content of various food animals (from HORN, 1990 and REDIG, 1993).

Food source	Total protein (g/kg DM*)	Total fat (g/kg DM)	Calcium (g/kg DM)	Phosphorus (g/kg DM)	Energy (kcal/kg)
Hare	199	71	31,0	16,2	1243
Pigeon	181	76	37,0	16,6	1228
Rat	216	75	20,6	14,8	1926
Beef	207	57	0,3	6,6	1149
Washed beef**	144	42	0,4	4,9	819
Day-old chicks (chicken)	151	43	15,5	14,9	850
Day-old chicks (turkey)	147	79	12,8	11,3	1145

* Dry matter (DM)   ** Soaked for 24 hours, with three changes of water

Diet and nutrition are thus very important in the maintenance of health and peak performance in captive birds of prey. In general, the feeding of birds of prey, still considered wild animals despite many generations of captive breeding in some cases, is best based on their natural diet in the wild. As a matter of principle, whole animals with all internal organs should be offered in order to prevent the development of such nutritional deficiencies as are often the result of feeding only parts of larger animals.

Table 4.1 summarizes the nutritional content of various common food animals used for captive birds of prey. With the exception of beef, all are listed as whole animals with only the digestive tract removed.

4.1 Feeding breeding birds

Special demands in terms of reproductive performance are placed on breeding birds. Frequently breeding success is increased by the removal of a clutch so that second or even third clutches are encouraged and often laid. The egg-pulling method (see Chapter 5.4.2.2) can result in the laying of up to 20 eggs or more by a female bird and requires optimal nutrition for the laying female. Every breeder has a special recipe for feeding breeding birds and guards it like a secret. Trommer (1974) gave his male breeding birds only male prey animals in order to stimulate the bird's hormonal condition. Others use a vitamin/mineral supplement formulated specifically for birds of prey. This is of questionable value since the nutrient requirements for birds of prey are not well-known and it is difficult to produce such a supplement and use it appropriately if the nutritional content of the intended food animals is not known either.

Supplementation with vitamin E, a so-called fertility vitamin, remains entrenched among breeders despite the fact that the fertility-promoting qualities of this vitamin have until now been proven only in rats. Additionally, indiscriminate supplementation with this fat-soluble vitamin is unwise, just as with vitamins A, D and K , since overdosing is possible and can lead to disease. Manika et. al. (1994) measured normal values for this vitamin in a raptor (*Buteo swainsoni*) and recommend supplementation with 15 mg vitamin E per kg of body weight in cases of deficiency.

More important than such experimentations is the feeding of a varied diet of preferably fresh-killed, whole prey animals and, above all, a special feeding schedule for breeding pairs or individuals. A pair of birds can be stimulated to initiate mating behavior more quickly if the tiercel gets frequent opportunities throughout the day to offer prey items to the female, similar to what occurs in the wild. This requires the frequent feeding of small portions that can be easily carried by the male.

Individually maintained female birds, which are usually imprinted on humans and kept for artificial insemination, are also stimulated by more frequent daily visits accompanied by small gifts of food.

When the breeding pair is raising young, the demand for quality food is increased again. The growing youngsters should receive only the freshest and best quality foodstuff from their parents. A precisely measured and frequently offered daily ration is especially important to prevent hoarding of food by the parent birds, which could result in the feeding of spoiled meat to the young. For the same reasons, it is preferable to feed whole animals such as rats with the skin left intact, avoiding the rapid drying which can happen to exposed meat. In order to prevent contamination of the food, it should be offered on platforms specifically designed for that purpose. These can be made of easily cleaned plastic screens (Fig. 4.1) and constructed such that injuries to the talons during landing and takeoff are prevented. The advantage of offering food in this way is that it is kept off the ground and thus avoids contamination with fecal material and aviary substrate. Especially if a diet low in fibrous casting materials such as feathers and fur is offered, there is a risk of excessive uptake of sand or gravel with food from the ground, posing a health risk to the bird (see Chapter 13.8.3.1.).

During the breeding and rearing of young, caution is indicated in the feeding of poultry or pigeons. The risk of transmitting disease to birds of prey in this way is always present, and young raptors are particularly vulnerable. For example, the feeding of inexpensive, frozen quail imported from England to Germany during

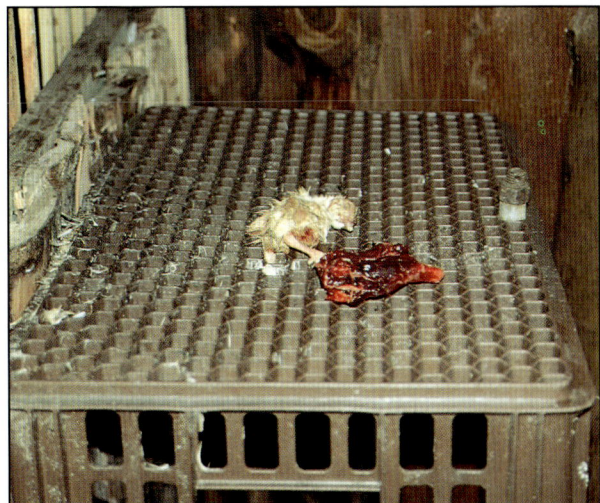

Fig. 4.1: Offering food on feeding platforms prevents contamination with ground materials and excretions.
(Photo: Heidenreich)

the 1994 breeding season resulted in the complete loss of some breeder's young birds to Pasteurellosis. It is hard to imagine that a savings of pennies can be of importance when captive-bred falcons can be sold for such handsome sums.

4.2   Hand rearing young birds

Raptor chicks will gape or beg for food only a few hours after hatching. Nevertheless they should be kept in the hatching incubator until their down is completely dry. Thereafter food should be offered six times a day. Since the amounts required will vary with each individual, hand-raising raptor chicks requires a large amount patience, endurance, sensitivity and skill (Fig. 4.2).

In order to save time, some breeders feed a prepared, mashed diet using a pastry squeeze bag, thus filling the

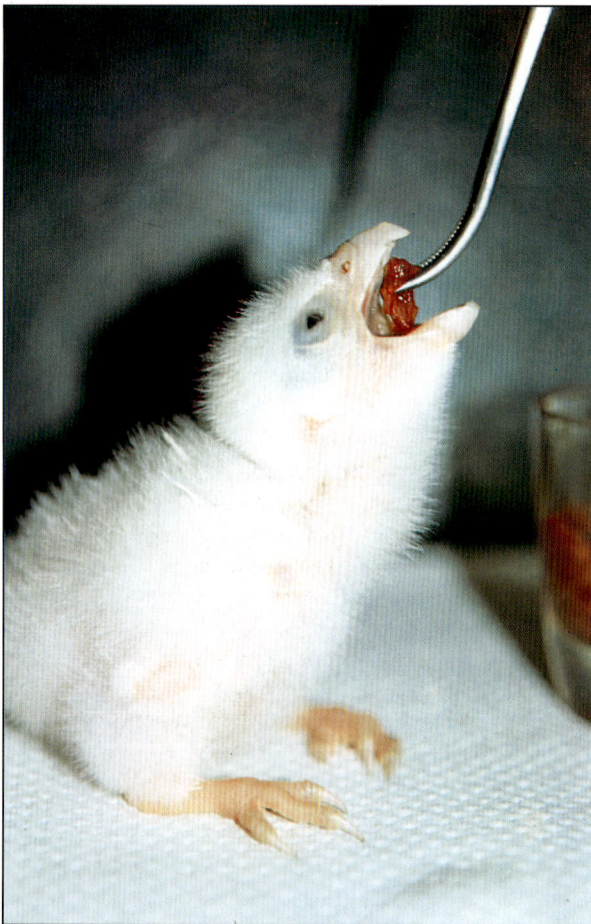

Fig. 4.3: At only a few days of age, the chicks are already begging actively. At this stage they are fed at least six times a day.
(Photo: Heidenreich)

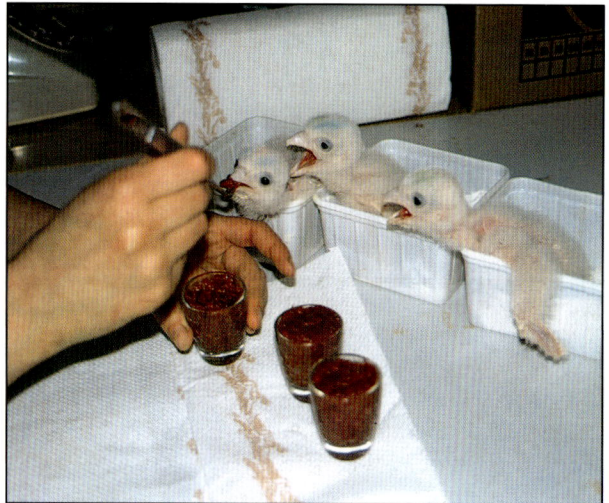

Fig. 4.2: Chicks (here falcon chicks) begin gaping and are ready to be fed only a few hours after hatching.
(Photo: Heidenreich)

chicks' crops more quickly. Such methods should be strongly discouraged, since only slow, piece by piece feeding ensures adequate coating of the food morsels with saliva and appropriate digestion. Even with this method, convenience should not replace efforts to feed the chicks in the most natural manner possible. The feeding of ground food with its larger surface area promotes rapid spoilage and can lead to contamination with Clostridial toxins that pose a risk to the entire crop of young birds (see Ch. 9.2.2.1).

It is therefore recommended that raptor chicks be reared exclusively on freshly prepared parts of just-killed and still warm food animals. Mice or young rats work well for the first few days after hatching. The rodents should be SPF (specific pathogen free) animals that can be obtained from research animal suppliers. SPF animals are free of certain disease-causing organisms that could otherwise be a source of infection for the vulnerable young birds. The rodents are killed by cervical dislocation, skinned and the feet are removed. Then they are immediately fed to the chicks. Storage of food should be avoided at all costs, since the chopped meat can quickly spoil and thus pose a risk to the birds' health.

Because the risk of rickets is great (see Ch. 11.2.1.1), the diet should include finely ground bones, chopped mouse tails or mineral supplements (such as Osspulvit®) from the second day of life on. Raptor saliva contains a large amount of calcium. The food morsels offered by raptor parents to their young are thus sufficiently fortified with minerals and deficiencies are avoided even though they may feed only clean meat. In addition, their saliva contains enzymes that assist the chicks in digestion. For these reasons some breeders mix the first few days' food with human saliva (caution smokers!). For the same reason, some people recommend the use of digestive enzyme supplements (such as Enzynorm®). One tablet of this product is dissolved in 100 ml of lukewarm water and every fifth morsel of food is dipped in this solution prior to feeding. In this way, the rates of weight gain and fledging success are substantially improved.

Often the feeder means too well and tries to feed the chicks too frequently. The result can be prolonged storage of food in the esophagus or stomach, causing fermentation that can lead to rapid death in the young bird (Fig. 4.4). In this context, the regular passing of mutes can be an important indicator of digestive activity. Short periods of fasting, similar to what occurs under natural circumstances, are better for the chick than excessive amounts of food.

Special attention should also be paid to the chicks' vocalizations. Healthy chicks are quiet or chirp softly.

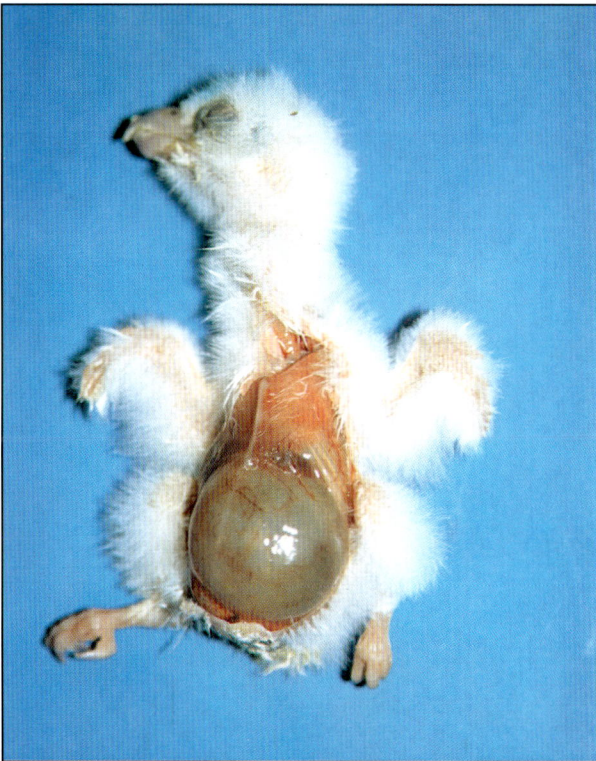

Fig. 4.4: This falcon chick succumbed to a maldigestive stomach disorder in the first few days of life. The reasons for this can include inadequate warmth with a resultant slowing of the digestive process, dehydration due to water loss under excessively warm conditions, or contaminated, pathogen-laden food. A bottom heater that warms the bird's abdomen and thus stimulates digestion has proven more effective in the rearing of chicks than an overhead heater whose warmth is unable to penetrate the lower body parts.
(Photo: Heidenreich)

The slightest discomfort is announced by a prolonged "complaint". The caretaker does well to pay attention to these sounds, as they may permit the timely intervention and correction of problems.

As soon as the chicks are standing and tearing their own food, eating should be left completely to them. This encourages muscular development.

4.2.1   Rearing vulture chicks

Although all vulture species can be fed meat in adulthood, the hand-rearing of chicks in some species differs markedly from the method described above. Most vulture chicks require a specially prepared diet during the first few weeks of life. Parent birds normally predigest the food in their stomach, then regurgitate this material and feed it to their young. Unprocessed meat is therefore not digestible for vulture chicks during the first three weeks of life. The exceptions are the Egyptian vulture and the bearded vulture, which don't feed their young with regurgitated food, but rather with food directly from the beak like other birds of prey (Baumgart 1991). The recipe in Table 4.2 has proven successful in raising several vulture species.

4.3   Feeding hunting hawks

At least at the beginning of the season, birds of prey used for the hunt have to be kept in a condition that encourages voluntary hunting and maintains the desire to return to the falconer. This is initially achieved by reducing the bird's weight, since a fat hawk with no appetite will not be interested in hunting. To achieve this, many birds are kept on an excessively restricted diet causing unnecessary hunger and poor performance when flown. Some even die. During simple starvation, the energy reserves of the body, fat and protein, are metabolized. Since fat reserves are mobilized more slowly, the starving body will initially draw its energy requirements from the protein available in muscle and blood. This soon leads to a loss of rapid energy resources and impairs the body's ability to function optimally. Many hawks at hunting weight have not only reduced breast muscle mass, but also decreases in plasma protein levels. Redig (1994) lists normal serum protein levels in wild birds of prey between 3.6 and 4.6 g per 100 ml of blood. Most trained hawks being flown by falconers, in contrast, have levels between 3.2 and 3.4 g/100 ml, in extreme cases even falling below 3.0 g/100 ml. The consequences are not only a marked reduction in flight performance resulting from a lack of rapidly mobilized energy reserves, but also an anemia due to the lack of protein. While healthy raptors generally have a hematocrit (the volume percentage of red blood cells in whole blood) between 42 and 45%, even up to 50% in large falcons, clinically ill animals may fall below 30%! Since this type of anemia occurs primarily during the winter months in trained hawks, this decrease in performance ability has also been called "midwinter anemia" by Redig.

Simply starving a bird can therefore not be the appropriate method to obtain an effective hunting hawk. Rather, the falconer should strive to reduce the fat reserves while maintaining the protein reserves and muscle mass, or even increasing them. This can be achieved only with a high quality diet and sufficient training to permit the buildup of muscle, just as in human athletes.

It is popular among falconers to use a scale to determine the appropriate hunting weight of a trained hawk. However, a simple body weight measurement is not a reliable indicator of optimal hunting condition. Large fat deposits and little muscle mass may weigh the same as few fat deposits and well-developed musculature, but flight performance will differ greatly.

The restricted feeding of a trained hawk should not be viewed as a form of starvation that infringes on animal rights, but rather as a skilled form of training involving food rewards and utilization of the natural hunting instincts of the particular bird involved.

4.4 Force-feeding

For veterinary purposes, raptors sometimes have to be force-fed when they refuse to eat voluntarily. This can occur in cases of illness, but also in wild birds that find themselves suddenly in captivity and refuse to take food, putting themselves at risk of serious weight loss.

Excessive loss of body weight due to disease involving diarrhea or other severe illnesses accompanied by decreased food intake, as well as improper weight reduction, can lead to pronounced protein deficiencies. When accompanied by dehydration, proper digestion of the food being offered is often no longer possible.

One must caution strongly against the administration of laxatives such as sugar or salts (for example ammonium nitrate), to make the hawk eager to hunt! Such treatments can also easily lead to the syndrome of "digestive inefficiency":

The bird will become lethargic and emaciated, with a pronounced keel. Its eyes sink into their sockets and the eyelids narrow to almond-shaped slits. The plumage is fluffed, especially around the head and on the

back between the wings and the legs. The animal will refuse food despite its emaciated condition, or it may regurgitate what it ingests. Any regurgitated material will have a strong odor of decay. Birds like this often die of generalized debilitation or secondary gastrointestinal bacterial infections only a few days after showing the first symptoms.

Diagnosis
The clinical presentation and emaciation together with the regurgitation of food are sufficient indications for immediate medical intervention.

Necropsy findings
The most obvious necropsy finding will be an extreme state of emaciation, especially noticeable in the pronounced atrophy of the flight muscles of the pectoral area (Fig. 4.5). In advanced cases, all fat reserves of the body, including those in the subcutaneous and cloacal areas, will be absent. Complete reabsorption of the coronary fat, utilized by the body as a last resort, leaves behind a clear, gelatin-like mass on the heart that is pathognomonic for starvation. The gastrointestinal

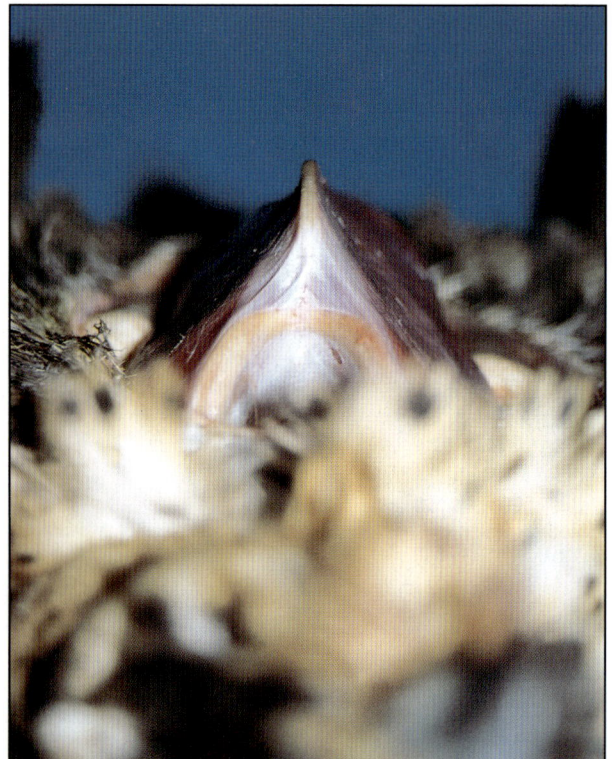

Fig. 4.5: A picture of the pectoral muscles of a peregrine falcon *(Falco peregrinus)* that died of starvation. These muscles that normally come off the keel in a convex shape are now atrophied and concave. At this stage of emaciation, the keel is prominent and palpable even in the living bird. (Photo: Heidenreich)

tract is either completely empty or contains the putrid remnants of undigested meat. If this decaying material has led to sepsis, the liver, spleen and kidneys may be swollen.

Treatment and Prevention
At the first signs, or even the suspicion, that a bird has reached a body weight low enough to pose a health risk, its weight must be brought back up. Training or hunting must be discontinued and the animal should be placed in a warm, dry room. It is best to keep the hawk hooded or the room relatively dark. If it will still accept food without regurgitating it, only small amounts of high quality food rich in moisture should be offered. It is particularly important to pay attention to fluid intake, since raptors that are not eating enough will die of dehydration before they starve. The feeding of ground, freshly killed pigeon breast mixed with egg yolk or fresh pigeon blood but no fibrous casting material has proven effective. Since the rate of digestion is markedly slowed with this condition, the amount should be limited to that which can just barely be palpated at the thoracic inlet after feeding. A second feeding of equal volume should be given two or three hours later, but only after the patient has passed mutes from the first meal and the initial mixture can no longer be palpated in the crop, indicating adequate digestive activity. Usually the bird will recover sufficiently in one day that self-feeding can be resumed. Nevertheless, casting material should be kept out of the diet until a normal body weight has been regained.

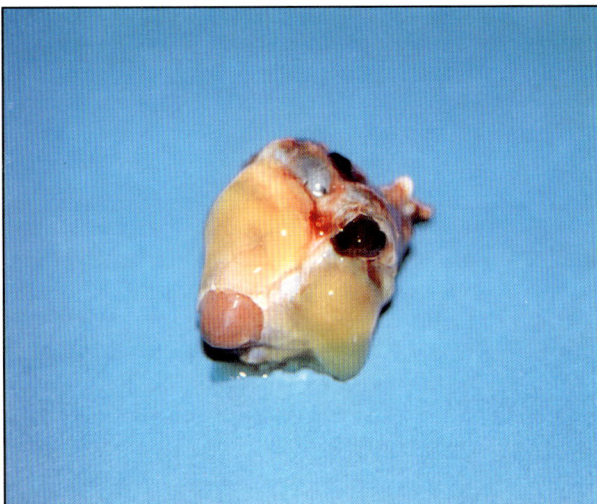

Fig. 4.6: The heart of a falcon that starved to death shows the characteristic serous atrophy, or absence, of fat in the coronary groove.
(Photo: Heidenreich)

If the hawk will no longer accept food, or shows evidence of digestive trouble and decaying crop and stomach contents, the undigested material must be removed. Although the procedure can be very stressful to the bird, it cannot be avoided, since the continuing process of decay may otherwise lead to sepsis.

The process of emptying is begun by inserting a thin, flexible stomach tube attached to a syringe and administering an appropriate amount of warm physiological saline as far as possible past the esophagus into the proventriculus. During this procedure, the patient should be held upside down to prevent aspiration of the stomach contents being flushed out. Gentle massaging motions are used to propel the food from the thoracic inlet toward the head manually. If necessary, this procedure can be repeated several times. Thereafter the bird should be kept absolutely quiet for approximately an hour. Then several ml of warm physiological saline should be administered using a deeply placed stomach tube. Once the fluids result in watery urates, more caloric fluids can be given. Beef serum has proven effective for this purpose, and is available commercially as Boviserin®. A broad spectrum antibiotic (such as Terramycin-Hen® from Pfizer at a dose of 100 mg/kg body weight per day) is added to the serum.

If one begins with small quantities of fluids (5 ml hourly for a bird weighing 1000 g) and they are well-tolerated, the quantities can be doubled within the first 24 hours. If no bovine serum is available, fresh blood or egg yolk can be tried. Once these fluids are absorbed and tolerated by the bird, one can begin to add small quantities of pureed fresh lean meat on the following day.

Administration of antibiotics should also continue for at least 5 days, even if the patient appears to have recovered, in order to prevent the development of resistant pathogens.

In severe cases, even oral fluids may no longer be tolerated by the hawk. They will be regurgitated after administration. These animals require intravenous administration of fluids such as lactated Ringer's solution at a rate of 15 ml per kg body weight initially to replenish body fluids.

The process of recovery may take several days, depending on the initial condition and response of the bird. Treatment should be discontinued only after plasma protein has reached levels of at least 4.0 g/dl and the hematocrit is between 45 and 50 percent.

Prevention
In order to avoid illness, the falconer must make sure that his bird does not fall below a certain body weight. This limit lies at a maximum of 15% below its molting weight or approximately 10% below the capture weight of a wild falcon. Weight losses exceeding these

limits are a risk to the bird's health and can easily be avoided by daily weighing. Palpation of the breast muscles as a sole indicator of body condition is not sufficient! Inexperienced falconers often try to raise their hawk's readiness to hunt only by weight reduction while neglecting the proper manning and psychological conditioning. Besides the fact that such a bird is unable to perform at its best, these falconers don't seem to understand that an excessively hungry hawk will behave similarly to one who is not hungry at all. It will be uninterested in its prey and fly unpredictably. If the weight reduction is pursued further, the animal will rapidly succumb to the syndrome described above. Wild-caught birds have an especially active metabolism and rapid digestive process. They tolerate several days of fasting only poorly and quickly become lethargic. Birds like this require plenty of food daily during the manning period.

4.5 Evaluating the quality of various food sources

There is a variety of meat and animal sources available for the feeding of raptors, and one should take advantage of them in the interests of a varied and species-appropriate diet. However, some of the available sources of meat may pose risks in terms of contamination or animal health. Therefore, food selection should be based on the following criteria of quality.

4.5.1 Day-old chicks

The poultry industry produces huge quantities of chicks that are sorted out and killed shortly after hatching. In the egg-laying industry, for example, the male chicks are collected in large containers and killed by carbon dioxide gassing. Since these chicks hatch from relatively sterile eggs, and are sacrificed immediately, before contamination can occur, they can be considered very safe from the standpoint of potential pathogens. Storage and transport of the bodies must be done in such a way as to maintain this condition. Overheating of the chicks, which are frequently stored in large bags or containers, can be prevented by spreading and cooling the carcasses prior to freezing them. Smaller portions allow more rapid freezing.

It cannot be denied that many birds of prey remain perfectly healthy and even breed and raise their young on a diet consisting exclusively of day-old chicks. However, the soft nature of this food source can frequently lead to overgrown beaks (see Ch. 13.3.1), a result of

insufficient wear on the upper beak. Day-old chicks are generally well-accepted and raptors accustomed to them may be reluctant to take other sources of food. Chicken or turkey chicks provide a good basic diet, but should be supplemented with other meat sources occasionally.

4.5.2 Pigeons

Pigeon meat is an excellent, energy-rich food source for birds of prey, both in terms of acceptance and nutritional value. This type of high quality nourishment is especially valuable in the rehabilitation of weakened or sick birds. The peak performances required of trained hawks during hunting season are difficult to achieve without the supplementation of pigeon meat. Nevertheless, the feeding of pigeons is not without risk. Several of the diseases carried by rock doves can be transmitted to birds of prey. This certainly includes tuberculosis (see Ch. 9.2.2) and paramyxoviruses (see Ch. 9.1.1), and possibly herpesviruses as well (see Ch. 9.1.3). An early or latent infection in these food animals is often not recognized. Infected birds may appear healthy and one should not feed purchased pigeons unless the breeder is known to have high standards of quality. It is wiser in any case to raise rock doves oneself, thus making health control and evaluation of the birds easier. On principle, pigeons should always be fed immediately after killing. Death by decapitation should be avoided in order to prevent bleeding out of the carcass. Blood is a valuable source of nutrients that should be available to the hawk. Under natural conditions, killed prey animals also do not bleed out. Falcons, which kill their victims by biting through the cervical spine, enjoy drinking the blood that collects under the skin of the neck.

Pigeons can be humanely killed by flinging the body back-first against a hard surface. This results in a rapid and painless death.

Before being offered as food, the pigeon should be only partly plucked, leaving a portion of the feathers to provide roughage for casting. The coelomic cavity should be opened to remove the digestive tract and permit a brief inspection of the other internal organs for abnormalities. Punctate liver lesions or masses along the intestine or in the abdominal cavity are reason enough not to utilize the carcass as food. Many falconers also remove the entire head and neck, including crop, to prevent transmission of trichomonads (see Ch. 10.1.2). Pigeons thus constitute a good source of food if certain precautions are taken.

4.5.3   Quail

Quail are commercially raised in large quantities for human consumption. In contrast to day-old poultry chicks, which are sacrificed shortly after hatching, quail are usually older birds that have been culled from the commercial flocks for various reasons. Regrettably, a common reason for culling is disease, a frequent problem under conditions of intensive production.

It can therefore occur that a commercial producer will foresee an epidemic after losing a few early animals, and decide to sacrifice the remainder of the flock immediately. This will permit him to minimize his losses by selling the quail as animal feed. The result can be disease or even death in the birds of prey which consume them.

In general, older fowl of any kind are potentially risky to the health of raptors. If they come from the commercial poultry industry, it is certain that they contain an additional burden of various drugs, usually antibiotics and coccidiostats. Exposure to these medications can create resistant strains of microorganisms in the raptors, thus potentially complicating future medical therapy for them.

4.5.4   Poultry processing byproducts

The least expensive, but also the most dangerous food for birds of prey is the meat discarded from poultry slaughtering plants processing chickens, turkeys or ducks. Since the innards and legs are immediately discarded, only the head and a short section of neck can potentially be used as food.

Normally the animals to be slaughtered are suspended upside down on a moving conveyer belt. The head is then submerged in a water bath where the animal is stunned by a strong electric shock. The water in this bath quickly becomes a concentrated source of bacterial contamination. The agonal breaths of the dying birds draw this dirty material into the upper airways, thus seriously contaminating the head and neck that will potentially be a food source for birds of prey.

In addition, a variety of potential raptor pathogens such as *Chlamydia* and *Pasteurella* species (see Ch. 9.2.5 and 9.2.6) are often latently present in poultry sinuses and so easily transmitted by consumption of this material.

The byproducts of poultry meat processing thus present a significant risk and should not be used as a food source for raptors!

4.5.5   Small rodents (rats, mice, hamsters and guinea pigs)

These animals are obtained from research laboratories or are raised by the falconer himself. In the former situation, it is important to confirm that the animals come only from untreated control groups and not from the potentially risky experimental ones.

The feeding of rodents from relatively pathogen-free sources has the advantage that there are currently no known diseases that they can transmit to raptors. In addition, the feeding of whole animals with all their internal organs is the most balanced and natural diet possible. Older rats and guinea pigs may have a disadvantage in that their skin is thick and difficult for smaller birds of prey to penetrate.

Small rodents can be humanely killed by cervical dislocation or by sharply striking their upper skull against a hard surface such as the edge of a table. Bleeding out should be avoided in these animals also.

4.5.6   Rabbits and hares

These two animals differ substantially in nutritional value. The dark red meat of hares is richer in calories than the pale meat of rabbits, especially that of rabbits raised in captivity. The larger size of rabbits and hares means that smaller birds of prey can consume only parts of the carcass. The drawback is that the bird will not benefit from the complete set of nutrients available in the body as a whole. Lagomorphs are best suited for larger raptors such as eagles or vultures, however. The feeding of wild animals killed with shotguns is to be avoided due to the risk of lead poisoning (see Ch. 12.1).

4.5.7   Muskrats

The muskrat is an aquatic, vegetarian rodent that inhabits waterways and ponds. It is extensively trapped in Europe because of the damage done by its burrowing in dams and embankments. They are usually captured in underwater traps.

Muskrats have dark red, tender and very nutritious meat and are therefore popular as a food source for birds of prey. The drawback is that the animals die while submerged under water, which results in contamination of the lungs with water and ingesta. Bacteria may be distributed throughout the body during the agonal phase. Although the traps are checked frequently, the muskrat bodies may remain submerged for hours. This accelerates the process of decay. After collection, the animals are skinned and then distributed to the user. Two days may thus pass before the carcass, usually still containing the intestines, is utilized as food.

The high level of bacterial contamination quickly leads to decay. The usually bright red muskrat meat may turn brown and greasy and the abdominal wall will be stained green. Even if the carcasses are frozen relatively quickly, the process of decay only slows down and resumes rapidly during thawing. Thus the quality of muskrat meat is directly dependent on the degree of freshness and a continuous process of refrigeration.

4.5.8 Mink

Occasionally the skinned bodies of mink from fur farms are utilized as food for birds of prey. This practice has proven extremely risky. Mink are killed in various ways. They are supposed to be humanely euthanized using injectable solutions such as T 61[®] or Eutha 77[®]. These rapidly acting poisons distribute themselves throughout the body and may cause death or unconsciousness also in the raptors consuming them (see Ch. 12.3).

For reasons of convenience, mink are also sometimes killed in large numbers by pumping vehicle exhaust fumes into closed rooms containing stacks of caged animals. The resulting meat is certainly safer, but such inhumane practices should not be supported by the purchase of these carcasses.

In principle, the use of mink meat as food for raptors must be strongly discouraged. In addition, the birds often don't like the flesh of these mustelids due to the strong odor imparted by their anal gland secretions.

4.5.9 Large animal meat

The byproducts of large animal slaughterhouses can be considered as food only for vultures. Horse meat is reported to promote gout in birds of prey (see Ch. 11.2.2). The exclusive feeding of mutton to falcons is sometimes done in Arabic countries. Saker falcons seem to tolerate this relatively well. A more varied diet would nevertheless be preferred even in this species if the trained falcon is expected to remain healthy and perform well.

4.5.10 Fish

It may be justified to add fish to the regular diet of some species such as sea eagles and fishing eagles. It must be remembered, however, that fish are especially prone to rapid decay and therefore freshness is of the utmost importance. Even the thawing of frozen fish must be done with special care. Buckets or bowls can quickly become filled with a protein-rich mixture of slime and water which acts as an ideal medium for the proliferation of pathogenic clostridial bacteria. The deadly toxins produced be these bacteria can then contaminate the food. Since these bacteria have special temperature requirements and prefer anaerobic conditions, the thawing of fish is best done on open grates or in cold running water. Ocean fish contain the enzyme thiaminase, which inactivates the B vitamin thiamine within the body. Excessive feeding of ocean fish can thus lead to clinical thiamine deficiency (see Ch. 11.12).

4.5.11 Natural prey

The game caught during a hunt is often fed to the hawk completely or in part. Since birds of prey are selective hunters, often killing weakened and therefore also sick animals, many falconers worry that their birds could become infected or ill after consuming their prey. This is very unlikely if the hawk consumes a wild mammal. Wild birds, on the other hand, can definitely transmit diseases to the hawks that consume them. Therefore the bird's carcass should always be opened and inspected before feeding to the hawk, especially in the case of captured crows and gulls. The body cavity of the killed bird can easily be opened and the internal organs examined without disturbance to the hawk as it plucks the feathers off its prey. Tuberculous granulomas of the liver (see Ch. 9.2.3) and gastrointestinal tract are not uncommon in these prey species (Giering 1992). If disease is suspected in the prey animal, it can easily be exchanged for a safer food item.

The risk of disease transmission by prey animals should not be overrated. Wild caught animals usually pose less of a risk of infection and contamination than birds raised under conditions of overcrowding and stress in commercial ventures. A healthy and immunocompetent hawk is unlikely to become a victim of its prey while fulfilling its evolutionary role as a regulator of weakened wildlife.

4.5.12 Commercial diets

The Hill's Company of Kansas, U.S.A., has been manufacturing a commercial diet for birds of prey for several years. "Zupreem Birds of Prey Diet" is based on horse meat, chicken, liver, fish and dried egg with added minerals and vitamins. The nutritional composition is 18% total protein, 5% total fat, 0.5% total fiber and a total of 40% dry matter and 60% moisture.

There is little information regarding the suitability of this diet. It is questionable whether it makes sense to feed all species with commercial diets. The consumption of this food by birds of prey cannot replace the eating of freshly killed, blood-warm animals and should be rejected as unnatural.

Table 4.2: Sample feeding schedule and diet for hand-rearing vultures using a European black vulture (*Aegypius monachus*) chick as an example.

Age in days (weight in grams)	Diet
1–3 (163 g on day 3)	4 day-old chicks (with head, legs, down and yolk sac removed) plus $1/3$ of the above quantity cleaned rabbit meat are mashed well in a blender, then poured into a glass and covered with water. Crush 2 tablets Enzynorm® (Nordmark) digestive enzymes and mix into the mash. Incubate for 2 hours at 37° C before feeding to the chick.
4–6 (243 g on day 12)	Same recipe as above, with the addition of 1 tablet Osspulvit® calcium supplement per day
7–12 (600 g on day 12)	Same recipe, with the addition of predigested mouse meat and 2 tablets of Osspulvit®
13–19	Same recipe as on days 7–12, 4 tablets Osspulvit®
20–34 (2000 g on day 20) (3000 g on day 34)	Half of the diet may now consist of undigested food (day-old chicks), 6 tablets Osspulvit®
35–40	Predigested food is no longer necessary, 8 tablets Osspulvit®
40 +	The nestling is eating independently, add Nutria meat and 1 teaspoon yogurt, 8 tablets Osspulvit®
61	The nestling can stand up
110 (7000 g)	The bird fledges

References and literature of further interest

BAUMGART, W. (1991):
Über die Geier Bulgariens. A. Der Schmutzgeier (*Neophron percnopterus*).
BEITR. VOGELKD. **37**, 1-48

BROWN, L. and D. AMADON (1968):
Eagles, Hawks and Falcons of the world.
Country Life Books, Hamlyn House, Feltham, Middlesex, England

DUKE, G.E., JEGERS, A.A., LOFF, G.U. and O.A. EVANSON (1975):
Gastric digestion in some raptors.
Comp. Biochem. Physiol. **50**, 649–656

GIERING, R. (1992):
Ein mecklenburgischer Sommer mit meinem Falken.
Greifvögel und Falknerei 114–118
Verlag Neumann-Neudamm, Morschen-Heina

HORN, W. (1990):
Ergebnisse von Atzungsanalysen - ein Beitrag zur optimalen Ernährung unserer Beizvögel.
Greifvögel und Falknerei, Neumann-Neudamm, Morschen-Heina

KÖSTERS, J. and B. MEISTER (1982):
Hämatokrit- und Hämoglobinwerte bei einigen einheimischen Greifvögeln und Eulen.
Prakt. Tierarzt **63**, 444-448

MAINKA, S.A., DIERENFELD, E.S., COOPER, R.M. and S.R. BLACK (1994)
Circulating alpha-tocopherol following intramuscular or oral vitamin E administration in Swainson's hawks (*Buteo swainsonii*).
J. Zoo Wildl. Med. **25**, 229–232

REDIG, P.T. (1988):
Midwinter anemia: a new look and a new name for an old problem.
Hawk Chalk **27**, 45

REDIG, P.T. (1993):
Raptor nutrition and feeding.
Medical management of birds of prey. 61–72
Raptor Center, Minnesota

REDIG, P.T. (1994):
More bang for the buck with trained raptors.
Hawk Chalk **33**, 44–47

TROMMER, G. (1974):
Erfolgreiche Lannerfalkenzucht 1973/74.
Jb. Dtsch. Falkenorden 26–28

5　Captive Breeding

Decades ago, the captive breeding of birds of prey was occasionally successful among private breeders and in zoos. Most of these successes were unplanned and coincidental. Efforts to propagate these birds in captivity gained momentum after the public became aware of the need to protect declining wildlife populations. In addition, national and international laws made it difficult or impossible to take wild raptors into captivity. Falconers, in particular, began systematic efforts at breeding falcons and other birds of prey. Initial successes occurred in the United States in the 1960's under T. J. Cade. Shortly thereafter, in the early 1970's,

C. Saar was successfully breeding large falcons in Europe as well.

5.1　Maintaining paired raptors

The most natural way to breed hawks is to maintain reproductively active pairs (Fig. 5.1). Several important conditions must be met to ensure success in such situations (Fig. 5.2).

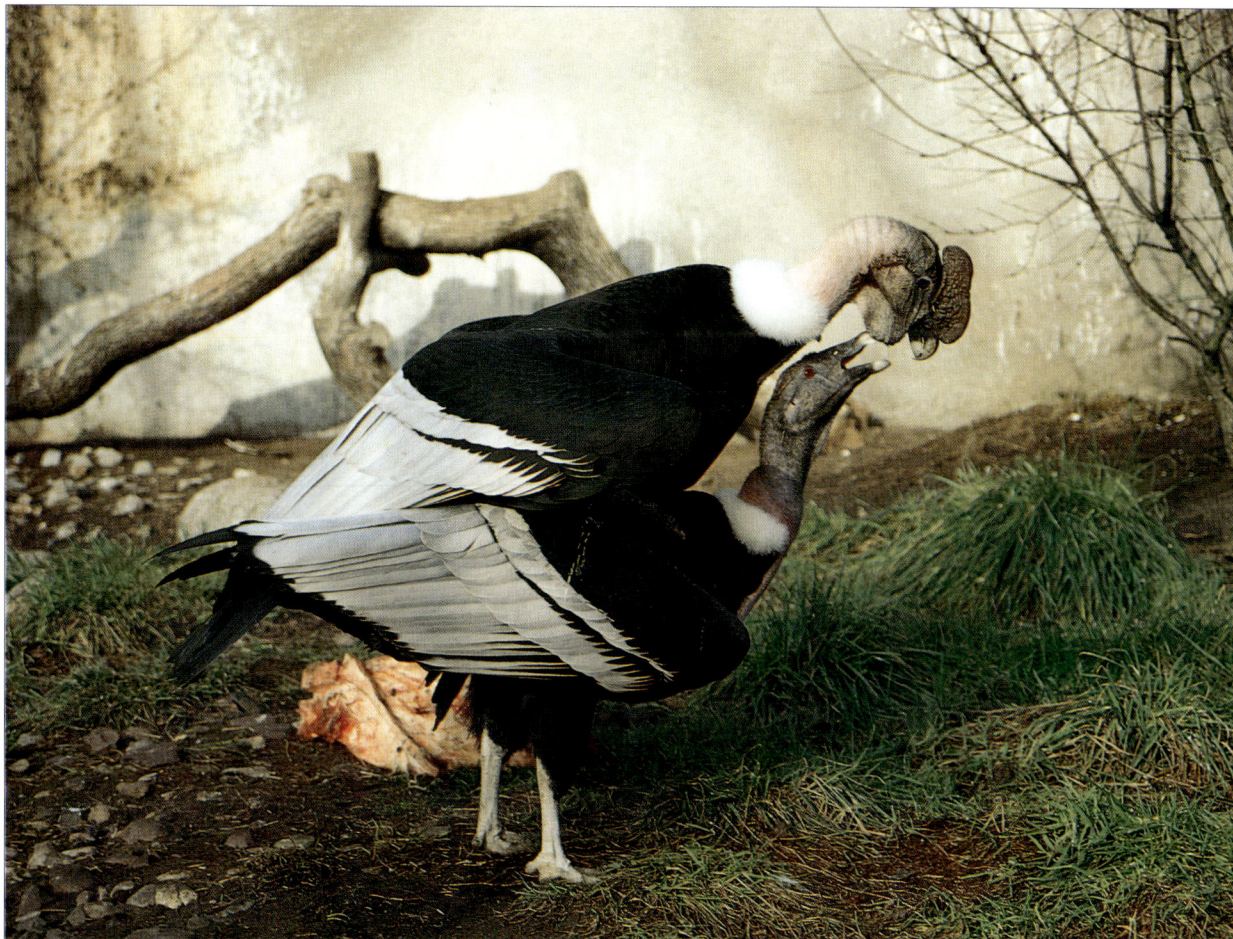

Fig. 5.1: A pair of Andean condors (*Vultur gryphus*) copulating at the Hannover Zoo. (Photo: Heidenreich)

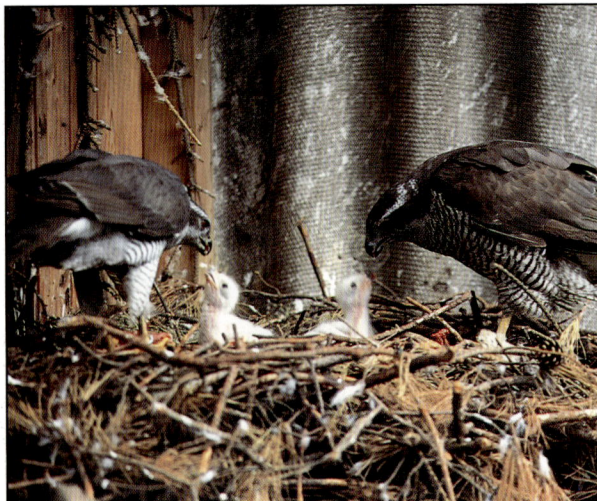

Fig. 5.2: A captive pair of goshawks feeding their young. (Photo: Poeppelman)

5.1.1 Imprinting

It is especially important that the paired birds be correctly imprinted on their own kind and not on humans. This is absolutely necessary, since otherwise normal mating behavior will not take place. In the early years of captive breeding efforts, this was the primary reason for lack of success. Breeding was being conducted primarily with birds that had been removed from the nest at an early stage and kept individually, thus imprinting them on man. Even today there are occasional breeding pairs whose lack of success one can attribute to incorrect imprinting. As long as human beings are absent, such birds behave relatively normally, tolerating their assigned partner but never fully accepting him or her as a mate.

It is important, therefore, to recognize such birds as unsuitable for natural breeding purposes. Such recognition involves manning the birds, or at least keeping them in close proximity to humans for a period of time. Their behavior will then reveal whether they are attracted to man as a partner. If they mantle over their food, vocalize, beg when hungry, or make mating sounds and bowing movements during feeding, one can assume they have been human-imprinted. Such birds are not useless for breeding purposes. They can be employed successfully in reproductive efforts involving artificial insemination.

5.1.2 Avoiding stress

The second important condition for breeding success in naturally paired birds is a breeding aviary or chamber that permits undisturbed mating and nesting activity. The inhabitants of the chamber will only feel secure if external sources of disturbance and stress are eliminated. Visual disturbances are less well-tolerated than disruptive noises. Even just the caretaker's daily appearance to monitor the birds and supply food and fresh water can cause shy birds to panic or fail to breed. Experience has shown that naturally calmer species also breed in captivity more successfully than shy or nervous ones. Trained hunting hawks are familiar with people and make better candidates for breeding efforts than unmanned birds. Wild-caught birds have a limited usefulness in reproductive efforts, as they require a relatively long period to become accustomed to captivity.

5.1.3 Pair bonding and mating behavior

Not only psychological well-being, but also the mutually correct timing of mating behavior, are important to the success of breeding efforts. Although some species that normally mate in the fall in their country of origin are known to do so in the spring in Europe, even slight misalignments in timing between a pair of birds can lead to failure. The timing of breeding behavior is often genetically determined. If, for example, a peregrine falcon of a southern European subspecies (*F. peregrinus brookei*) which lays early in the year, is paired with a northern European tiercel who begins breeding activity somewhat later, the first clutch of eggs will frequently be infertile. One must therefore pay attention to geographic origin in the selection of breeding pairs as well.

Once these conditions have been met, there is still no guarantee that the two birds will bond. Birds of prey can show likes or dislikes for other individuals of the same species. Some pairs may cohabitate in a breeding chamber for years without ever mating. If a new partner is then suddenly placed in the aviary, obvious acceptance and willingness to bond may be evident by the birds' vocalizations within minutes. It can also be helpful to put a young, inexperienced female with an experienced and avid tiercel. Such a male may encourage her to successfully mate and care for their young. Stronger bonding is also often observed after the temporary separation of a breeding pair.

Frequently, the tiercel's restraint or even fearfulness toward the naturally larger, more dominant female is the reason for a lack of harmony between the two birds. It is therefore particularly important that the tiercel be relatively self-confident. This can be achieved by allowing him to inhabit the breeding chamber first, thus establishing his territory and becoming familiar with the environment before the female is added. Trained hawks that are successful hunters are also less likely to be intimidated by a larger female.

Less dominant tiercels, or those who have had bad experiences with other females and are therefore reluctant to try again, can be stimulated with hormones. Administration of male hormones (see Ch. 13.9.3) will result in increased confidence and breeding activity within a few days. Such measures do not increase fertility, serving only to encourage pair bonding and mating activity.

While experienced breeding pairs will need no further help, fussier pairs may benefit from special feeding techniques. In nature, it is the male's responsibility to woo the female with frequent offerings of small prey items. Such gifts of food are an important part of the mating ritual. Tiercels in captivity should be given the opportunity to bring such offerings as well. If the birds are fed their daily ration once a day, the female will satisfy her hunger at once and show little interest in the tidbits brought by the male for the remainder of the day. It makes more sense to supply the male frequently with small amounts of food. He can then offer these to his partner. This also allows the tiercel to fulfill his role as provider and gain a higher dominance ranking than he would otherwise have.

5.1.4 Special concerns in selected species

While natural pair bonding in the form of permanent cohabitation is a successful system for most birds of prey, some species require special conditions without which reproductive success is unlikely or impossible.

5.1.4.1 Northern goshawk (*Accipiter gentilis*)

Only rarely is it possible to house paired northern goshawks together year-round without risk. Frequently, the markedly smaller males are injured or killed by the female in the aviary. The reasons for this may lie in the natural aggressiveness of this species, and in the fact that the wild tiercel remains near the female only briefly, spending most of his time hunting and providing food.

Goshawk breeding chambers are therefore designed differently than those for other birds of prey. They consist of two chambers separated by a window or wire

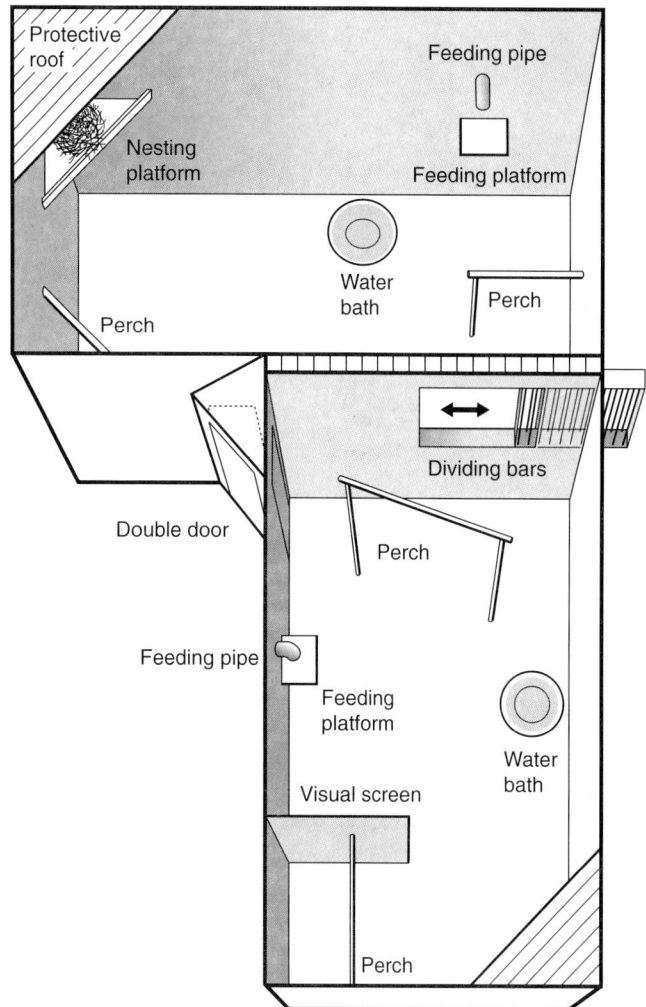

Fig. 5.3: A breeding chamber for goshawks. (Illustration: R. Gattung-Petith and A. Gattung)

mesh (Fig. 5.3). Only after both partners show obvious mating behavior and readiness to copulate, should the birds be permitted to come together. If necessary, they can be immediately separated afterwards. Recognizing the correct time to allow them to join each other requires a fair amount of experience and a thorough knowledge of the individual birds. Definite signs of mating readiness include offerings of food by the tiercel and copulatory posturing on the part of the female. The female's vocalizations also help pinpoint the correct timing. When her the vocalizations become softer and quieter, she is most likely to tolerate copulation and it is safe to introduce her partner (Fig. 5.4).

Despite all precautions and observational efforts on part of the breeder, incidents resulting in injury to the male can occur.

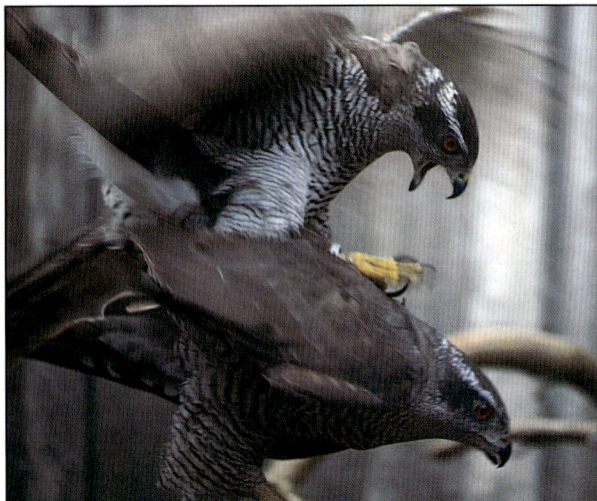

Fig. 5.4: A pair of northern goshawks copulating. (Photo: Pöppelmann)

5.1.4.2 Merlin (*Falco columbarius*)

There are several reports of the female injuring the tiercel among merlins as well (Pöppelmann, 1995). The male is considered especially vulnerable and frequently attacked by his partner right after he has bathed. It is known that merlins in the wild have only a seasonal relationship. In other words, they share a territory during the breeding period and then separate for the rest of the year, meeting again the next year in the same territory to resume the relationship and raise young (Fig. 5.5). Housing a pair of merlins together year-round thus appears to contradict their natural behavioral tendencies and could be the reason for occasional disagreements between the two birds. In order to avoid such risks, it is advisable to separate merlins

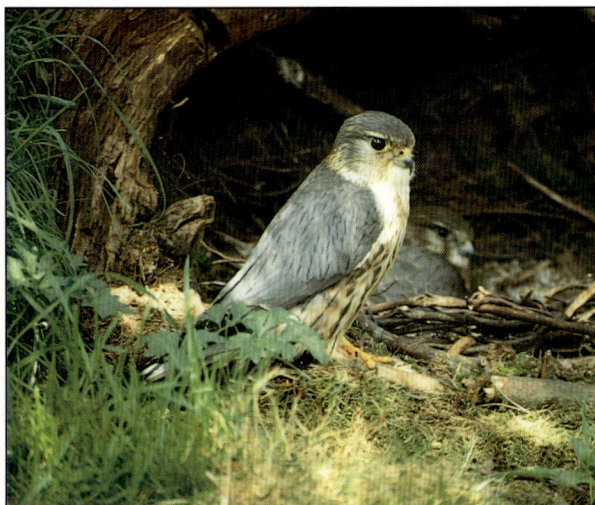

Fig. 5.5: A pair of merlins during incubation. (Photo: Pöppelmann)

after they have raised their young and to reunite them again the next spring.

5.1.4.3 Bateleur eagle (*Terathopius ecaudatus*)

According to Cade (1988), the bateleur eagle is a species that requires special attention from breeders. Their wild populations in southern Africa have been drastically and mysteriously reduced in recent decades.

Captive propagation of these birds is extremely difficult and has succeeded only rarely thus far. This may be attributed to the fact that this tropical species can be reproductively active year round in its natural habitat, thus giving it no fixed biological breeding season. In addition, wild bateleur eagles have been observed engaging in certain behaviors that are not taken into account or made possible in captive situations. For example, it was discovered that in the wild, a single, usually male bird frequently joins the breeding pair. He is permitted to remain near the nest without being directly involved in building it or raising the young. This type of arrangement has been described by Davygora (1993) in other birds of prey as well. He calls these solitary birds "brood assistants". This type of three-way relationship is not well understood, but may be of importance for reproductive success in captivity as well.

5.1.4.4 Harris' hawk (*Parabuteo unicinctus*)

The Harris' hawk shows exactly the opposite behavior from the goshawk. Wild Harris' hawks hunt and breed in groups. Sometimes a male may even mate with more than one female. This social behavior is very conducive to captive propagation. Several birds may even be housed together, since monogamous relationships are not formed. Haigh (1991) goes so far as to suggest that these birds even enjoy the association with humans, not simply tolerating it the way other raptors do. Since the above traits guarantee a stress-free situation for these birds in captivity, breeding them is easy.

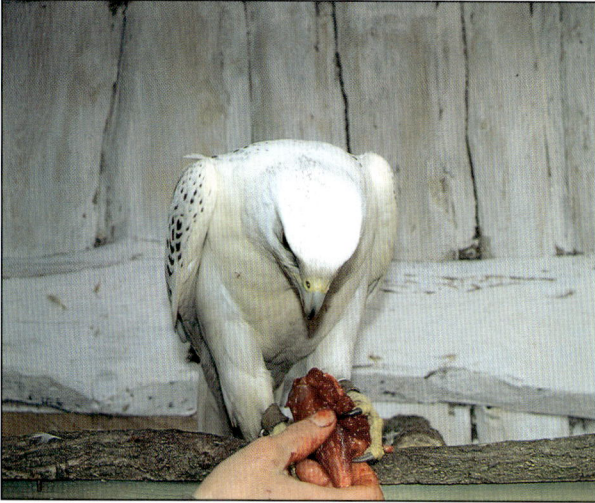

Fig. 5.6

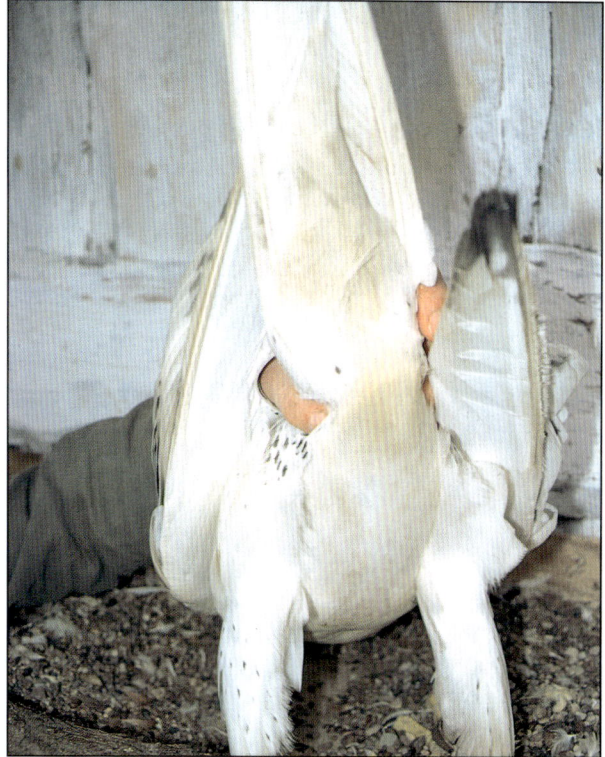

Fig. 5.8

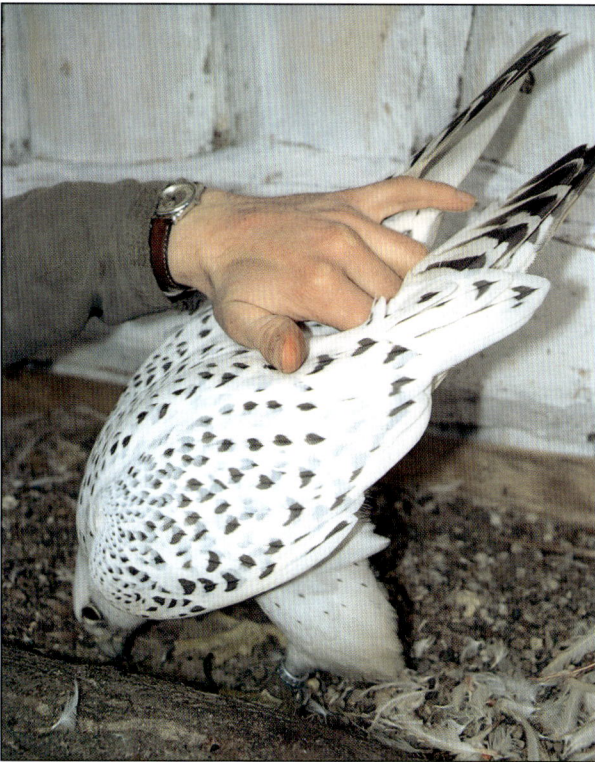

Fig. 5.7

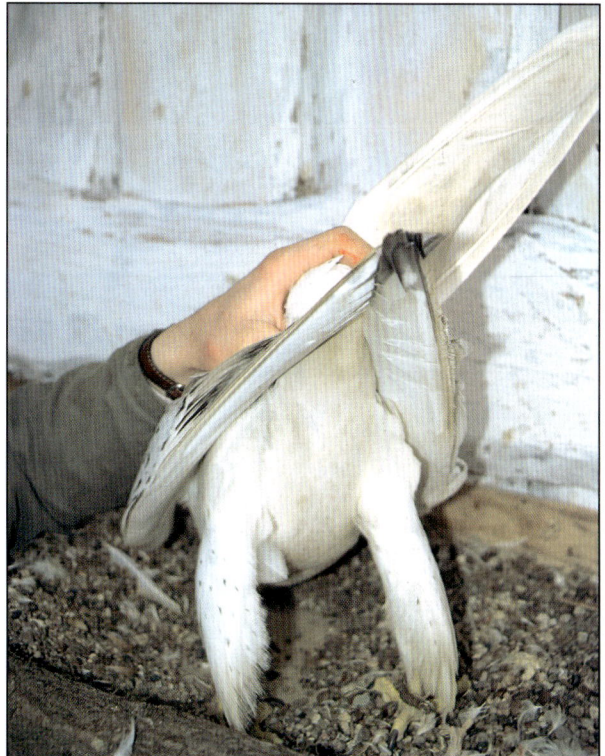

Fig. 5.9

Figs. 5.6, 5.7, 5.8, 5.9: Frequent offerings of food during the mating period simulate the normal pattern of male behavior and stimulate egg-laying in the imprinted female [here a white gyrfalcon (*F. rusticolus*)] (5.6).
An imprinted female offers herself to a human partner (5.7), permitting cloacal manipulations (5.8) and inviting copulation by tilting her tail sideways (5.9).
(Photos: Heidenreich)

5.2   Maintaining single raptors

Breeding birds are housed individually only if they are intended for artificial insemination. In almost all cases, these are birds that have been imprinted on humans. Not only does such imprinting make a natural pairing impossible, but it greatly facilitates the manipulations required to collect semen from or inseminate the bird.

5.2.1   Stimulating mating behavior in females

Imprinted birds are very tolerant of humans and perceive them as their intended mating partners. It is thus necessary for someone to assume the tiercel's role in stimulating the appropriate breeding and egg-laying behavior in isolated, imprinted females. This involves frequent daily hand-feeding to resemble the food offerings of a male. Gentle stroking of the feathers of the back and contact with the cloacal region are also tolerated and even solicited (Fig. 5.6 - 5.9). Human imitation of breeding noises will increase the female's willingness to mate. Such close contact between the breeder and the bird permits an exact determination of the correct time to inseminate, especially if an enlarging abdomen can be clearly palpated.

5.2.2   Stimulating mating behavior in males

As with females, imprinted males intended as semen donors have to be appropriately "handled" to produce adequate sperm and show a willingness to mate. Frequent small meals fed by hand are helpful in this situation as well. Since semen donors sometimes have to be collected daily during the egg-laying period, keeping them tied to a perch in falconry style is useful. This allows the breeder to handle the bird without having to put it through a potentially stressful capture procedure.

5.3   Artificial insemination

Artificial insemination techniques became necessary in the early stages of captive breeding efforts. Most of the birds available at that time were imprinted on man and thus incapable of reproducing naturally. Today, many breeders produce hybrid falcons (see Ch. 17.3.2). This would also not be possible without artificial insemination techniques. Differences in mating behavior between species normally prevent hybridization in nature or in a breeding chamber.

Artificial insemination was first widely used in mammals and in the commercial poultry industry. It was logical that hawk breeders initially applied the techniques developed for poultry to their attempts at propagation in raptors.

Beyerbach and Maatsch (1973) were the first Germans to succeed in artificially inseminating birds of prey, using peregrine falcons (*Falco peregrinus*). In the years that followed, a number of publications describing the methods to be used became available. This resulted in a substantial improvement in the rates of success. Today we seem to have solved all the problems associated with artificial insemination in raptors, and the technique is well-established. While initially

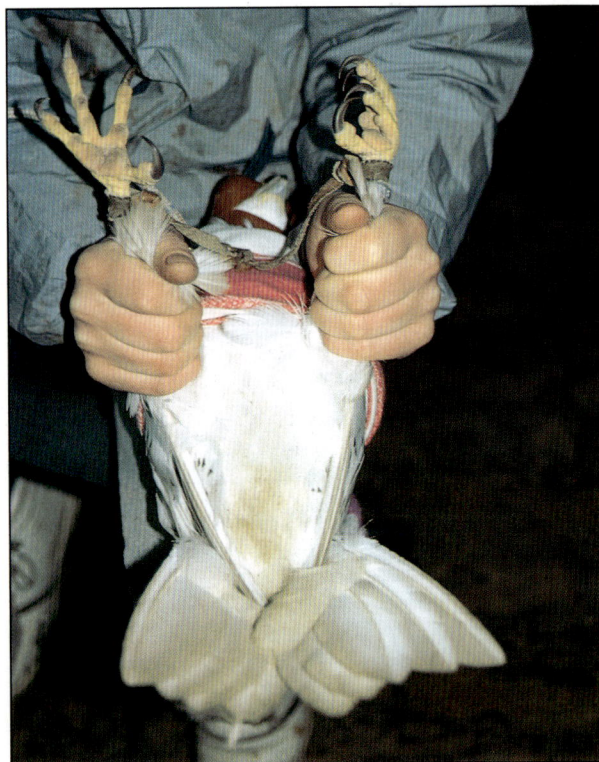

Fig. 5.10: To collect semen by the massage method, the bird must be firmly restrained. It is hooded and wrapped securely in a towel, taking care not to interfere with respiration.
(Photo: Heidenreich)

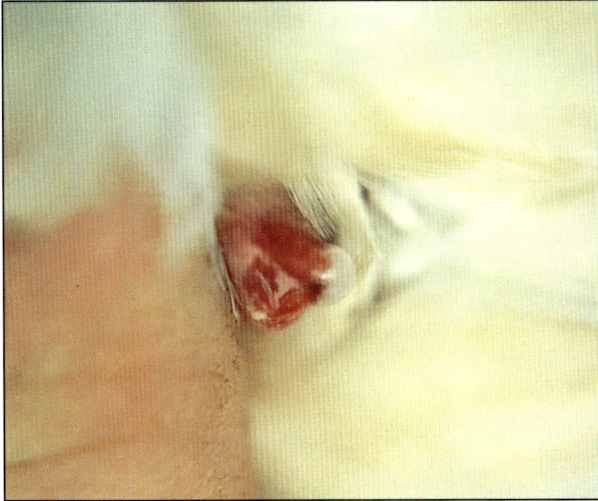

Fig. 5.11: Very gentle pressure on the seminal glomus is often sufficient to release the semen. (Photo: Heidenreich)

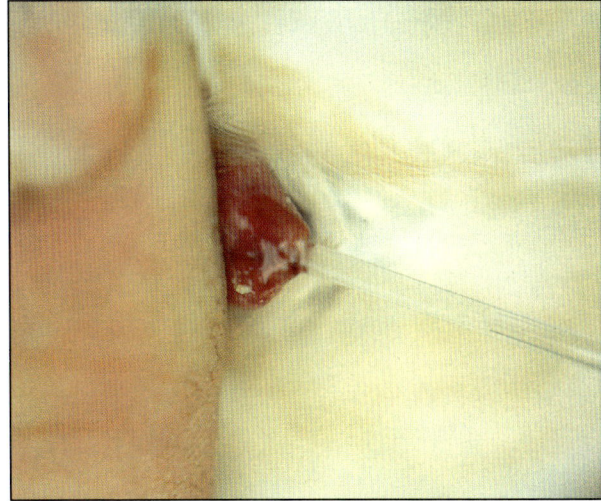

Fig. 5.12: Semen can be collected in variously calibrated microliter pipettes, depending on the quantity produced. (Photo: Heidenreich)

performed primarily by veterinarians and scientists, artificial insemination now lies in the realm of every breeder's capabilities.

5.3.1   Semen collection

There are several different methods of obtaining semen from birds.

5.3.1.1 Massage collection

The massage method involves manually obtaining semen from the seminal glomus located on either side of the tiercel's cloaca. The bird must be restrained on its back for this procedure. To prevent struggling, the animal may be wrapped in a towel (Fig. 5.10). Because this is an involuntary activity for the hawk, it helps if he is very tame or human-imprinted and accustomed to such manipulations. Otherwise, the bird may be too tense to release the semen. Hooding eagles and falcons will further calm such birds. If the tiercel is unaccustomed to being hooded, the head can be left free. The extensive massaging of back and abdomen used in this collection technique with domestic poultry is not necessary in birds of prey. Gentle massaging motions using a finger to stroke a few centimeters from abdomen towards cloaca usually suffice for passive emptying of the seminal glomus on either side.

Birds that are accustomed to this procedure hardly need to be massaged and may even spontaneously ejaculate. Quick reactions are required in such cases to catch the semen and avoid its contamination.

The expressed semen will appear at the vent as a milky liquid (Fig. 5.11) that should be immediately collected by suction with a pipette or venous catheter (Fig. 5.12).

Occasionally, inappropriate massage or pressure may result in the expression of urates or feces. To avoid this, the bird should be allowed to defecate prior to massage collection. Contamination of the ejaculate with foreign material or germs is to be strictly avoided.

5.3.1.2 Cooperative collection

Birds of prey imprinted on humans choose them as mating partners and will try to copulate with them. It will become rapidly obvious which human body part (head, back, shoulder, shoe, etc.) the bird prefers to mount. Boyd and Schwartz (1981) describe a hat designed for semen collection in cases where the tiercel chooses to copulate with a person's head. The ejaculate can be collected from this hat with a syringe after it has been deposited. Such methods carry the risk of sample contamination and can potentially lead to infection of the oviduct in the inseminated female. They are therefore not recommended.

5.3.1.3 Semen evaluation

The evaluation of semen samples and their separation based on sperm quality is possible only in large breeding facilities. Such facilities will have several tiercels available to donate sperm at the same time.

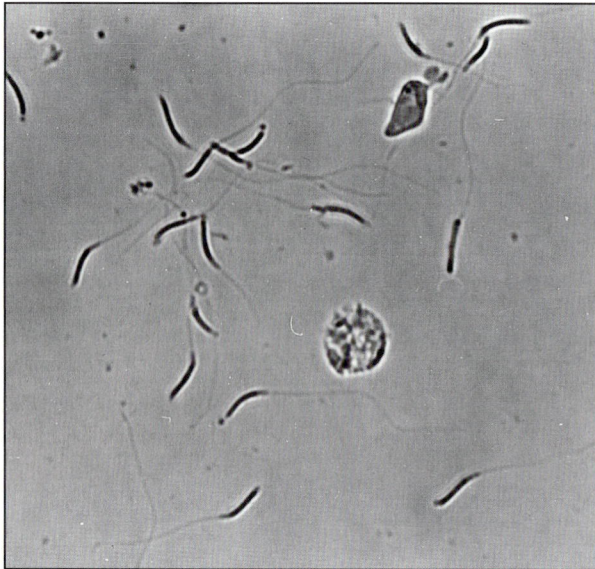

Fig. 5.13: Goshawk sperm seen under a microscope. (Photo: Brüning)

bility at temperatures of 4° C for up to 24 hours. Raptor semen has been successfully transported this way over several hundred kilometers on the ground or over entire continents by airplane.

The volume of semen normally obtained from a single bird is quite small. Therefore, each valuable microliter used for microscopic examination is lost for insemination purposes. To avoid this, the sample is often examined directly in the glass pipette in which it was collected, allowing an estimate of the percentage of living, motile sperm present (Fig. 5.13). More exact measurements of semen quality, as used in mammals, have so far not been developed for birds of prey. This is due in part to the small volume of ejaculate obtained from birds. Every sample is needed for insemination.

5.3.1.4 Semen storage

The older literature (Corten, 1975) claimed that raptor semen should be mixed with an extender or diluent in order to permit short-term preservation, as is done in the commercial poultry industry. These attempts all failed and such techniques are not applied to semen from birds of prey today. Long-term storage using cryopreservation methods similar to those utilized with other domestic animals has also proven fruitless. Brock (1986) and Parks (1986) diluted falcon semen with cryoprotectants (glycerol or dimethylsulfoxide) and had some degree of success. However, dialysis is required to remove the glycerol from the sample before insemination.

The storage and transport of freshly obtained, undiluted semen over a limited time-span is certainly feasible. The sample should be protected from evaporation and kept cool. Microliter pipettes that have been stoppered at each end work well and will retain sperm via-

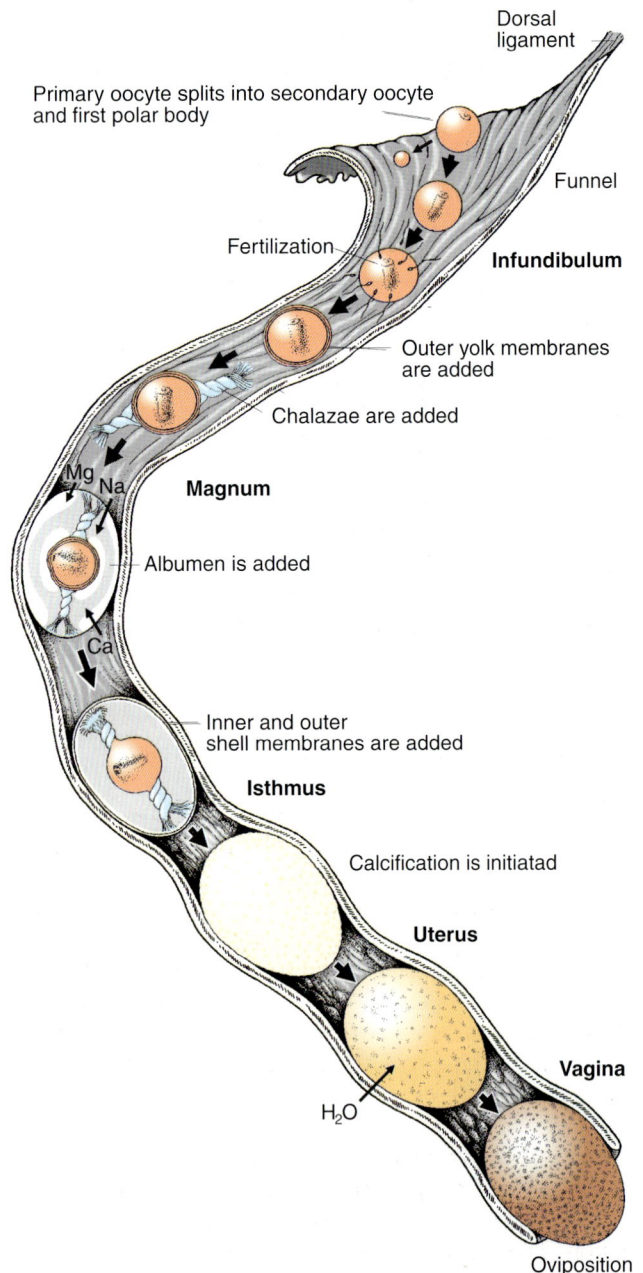

Fig. 5.14: The development of an egg in the oviduct. (Illustration: R. Gattung-Petith and A. Gattung)

5.3.2 Insemination

The best time to inseminate a female is largely determined by her laying activity. An overview of egg
production is given in illustration 5.14. Because sperm
have only a limited survival time in the oviduct of the
female, repeated inseminations are required for a
single clutch. The procedure is typically performed
with a micropipette or a small catheter.

Some raptor species lay only one or two eggs. The
determination of the optimum insemination time is
especially problematic in these cases and requires an
exact knowledge of the anticipated laying date. Insemination is then carried out several days before egg-
laying is to occur, thus permitting fertilization of the
eggs within the oviduct. The laying date may be anticipated by the development an enlarged abdomen with
thickened skin or because the bird lays her eggs on the
same date every year. In any case, insemination must
take place at least 52 hours before the egg is laid if fertilization is to succeed. It should not be performed too
early either, since sperm remain viable in the oviduct
for an average of only six days. There is a report by
Rosenkranz (1995) of a fertile falcon egg resulting
from an insemination performed twelve days earlier.
Regardless of such extreme instances, inseminations
prior to the laying of the first egg should be performed
at three day intervals. Thereafter, insemination should
be repeated immediately after each egg is laid. In falcons, the second egg is usually produced within 48
hours, indicating that it is fertilized before the last insemination takes place.

Two different methods of insemination are used in
raptor breeding. Both can be successful and each has
different advantages and disadvantages.

5.3.2.1 Cloacal insemination

Natural copulation in birds always involves cloacal
contact between the partners. The female will invite
copulation by bending forward, spreading the vent
feathers, displacing the tail feathers laterally and
presenting her open cloaca. At mating readiness, the
cloaca is engorged, allowing the inner mucus membranes to be everted to receive the male's sperm.
After deposition of the semen, but before copulation is
completed, the cloacal tissues are retracted back into
place and the semen is directed toward the vaginal
opening.

Human-imprinted birds of prey perform the same
mating behaviors in the presence of a person and will
tolerate manipulations of their cloaca to simulate copulation. The previously obtained semen can then easily
be deposited in the cloaca. The advantage of this method lies in the fact that the procedure is relatively stress-

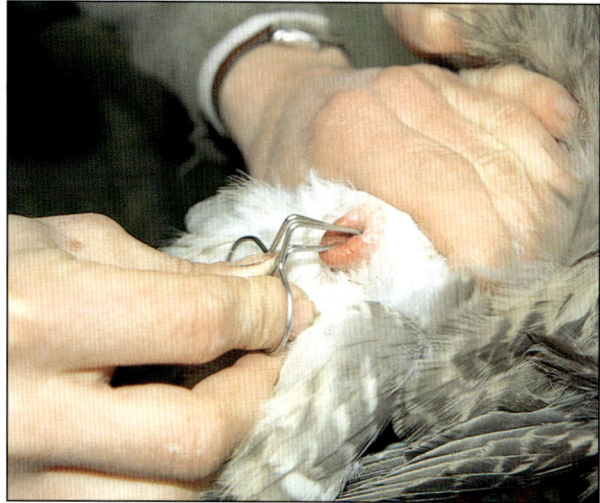

5.15

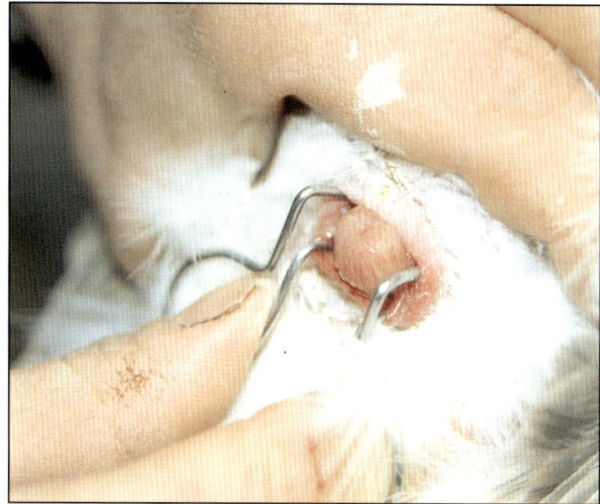

△ 5.16   ▽ 5.17

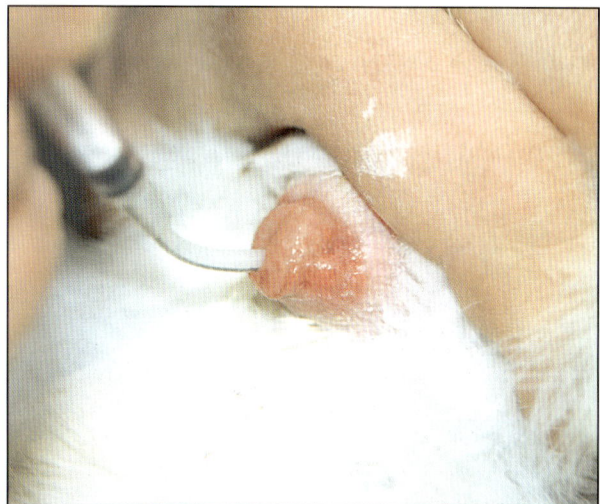

Figs. 5.15, 5.16, 5.17: Using a specially-made speculum,
the cloaca is carefully opened (5.15). Gentle pressure on
the abdomen then allows exposure of the oviductal
opening (5.16). The pipette is then inserted a few
centimeters into the vagina to deposit the semen (5.17).
(Photo: Heidenreich)

free and well-tolerated by the unrestrained female. The disadvantage is that fertilization rates may be somewhat lower. Natural copulations take place multiple times a day, a frequency usually not possible with manual methods.

5.3.2.2 Oviductal insemination

The second method involves depositing semen directly in the distal oviduct, also called the vagina. This method can be used in birds that are not imprinted on humans. Because these birds will be less tame, physical restraint is unavoidable. The bird is captured, wrapped in a towel and placed on its back. An assistant can hold the hawk and gently spread her legs. A special speculum is used to open the cloaca (Fig. 5.15) and gentle pressure is used to visualize the vaginal opening (Fig. 5.16). The pipette is then carefully inserted a few centimeters into the lumen of the cone-shaped vagina and the semen is deposited (Fig. 5.17). The pipette is gently withdrawn, the oviduct is released and the cloaca allowed to close. With enough experience, this procedure should not take more than a minute.

This method of insemination has the advantage that fertilization rates are generally higher because the sperm are deposited accurately within the oviduct. The disadvantage lies in the fact that the stress of the unaccustomed manipulations may cause the female to interrupt egg-laying or put it off altogether. If eggs are already present in the oviduct, they may develop shell defects that can interfere with successful incubation or hatching. In her distress, the female may even drop the egg from the perch rather than laying it in the nest.

Older females who are familiar with this procedure and have successfully hatched and raised young in the past will possess stronger brooding instincts and be less stressed. They will usually tolerate oviductal insemination well.

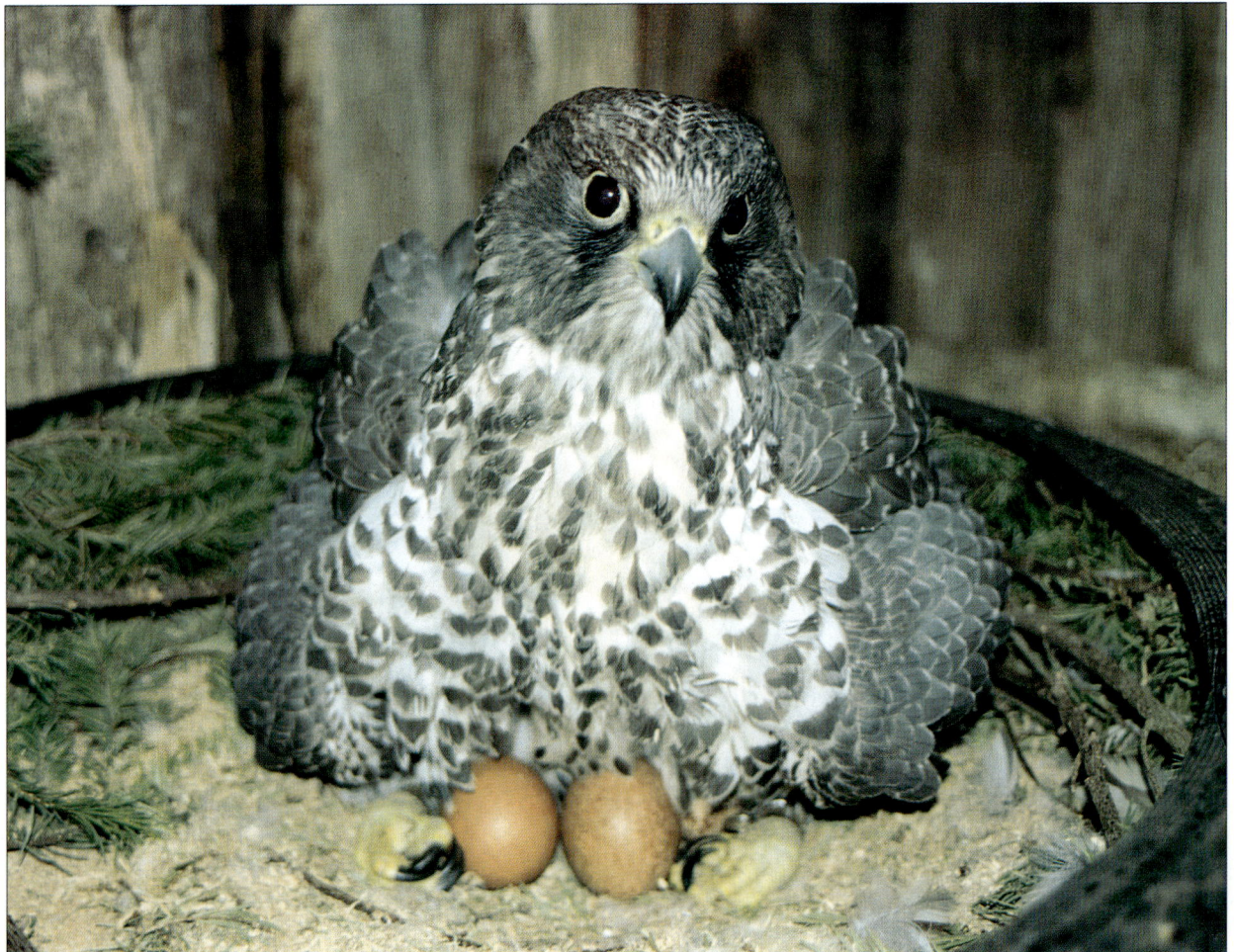

Fig. 5.18: Birds of prey (in this case a gray gyrfalcon) incubating on a nest carefully close their taloned feet to protect the delicate eggs. Not only gyrfalcons, but also other raptor species, often have a "dreamy, mothering facial expression" while brooding.
(Photo: Heidenreich)

An additional risk with this method involves potential infection of the oviduct. This can occur if strict standards of cleanliness are not observed, the instruments are not sterilized or the semen has been contaminated with fecal material from the donor.

5.4   Incubation

There are various options for incubating raptor eggs. Experienced pairs can incubate their own eggs and raise the chicks (natural incubation). Alternatively, the eggs can be removed from the nest immediately after being laid or after several days of natural incubation to be placed in an incubator for the remainder of the incubation period. Each method has advantages and disadvantages that will be discussed below.

5.4.1   Natural incubation

In captivity, completely natural incubation and parent-raising of chicks should be entrusted only to experienced and well-bonded pairs (Fig. 5.18). Too many unknowns could otherwise impair success. For example, the eggs may be damaged or broken, incubation could be abandoned due to disturbances, or the newly hatched chicks might be killed by the adult birds. To test a pair of inexperienced breeding birds, the real eggs can be removed and replaced by artificial ones. If they proceed to incubate them responsibly and carefully, it can be assumed that they will do so with their own clutch in subsequent years as well. The pair's chick-raising skills can be evaluated in a similar manner by giving them fertilized eggs of a less valuable species to hatch and raise.

An alternative to incubation by the parents themselves is natural incubation by other birds, also known as foster parenting. In chicken and duck breeding, this method is frequently used and is often preferred to artificial incubation because of better hatching rates. It is important that the foster parent be of approximately the same size as the female hawk. Thus the eggs of a small falcon should not be incubated by a chicken hen and eagle eggs will not do well under a pigeon. In general, chickens are not well-suited for incubating raptor eggs because of their prominent keel. Various pigeon breeds do well with falcon eggs and ducks are suited for the eggs of larger birds of prey. Since both these foster parent species normally have a much shorter incubation period than hawks do, a second foster parent should always be available to take over if the first one abandons the clutch. Many falconers opt to avoid the risk involved in foster parenting and use artificial incubation methods instead.

5.4.2   Artificial incubation

Artificial incubation of eggs as it is practiced on a large scale in the modern poultry industry is not a modern technique. Such practices were already established, albeit on a smaller scale, during the time the Egyptians were building the pyramids. Brown (1979) describes these ancient fire-heated Egyptian incubators. The temperature was measured by holding the egg to one's eyelid and the fire was then accordingly stoked or reduced. Humidity was assessed by rolling two eggs against each other in the palm of the hand and listening for the quality of the sound produced. Despite these primitive methods, the hatch rate was greater than 70%.

The Chinese, in 1000 B.C., incubated eggs in manure and Aristotle describes a similar technique among the Greeks around 400 B.C. Particularly fascinating are the many historical references to egg incubation using human body warmth. Ancient Roman women believed that they would be able to foretell the gender of their unborn child if they hatched an egg under their breasts.

Mechanical incubators were developed in the West by 1749. The first commercial brooder, marketed in 1895, utilized hot water and held up to 20,000 duck eggs at a time. In 1922 the first fully automatic, electric incubator became available. Today, poultry production without the use of incubators has become unthinkable. Modern breeding efforts with wild birds also rely heavily on artificial incubation. With proper management, this technology has permitted a substantial increase in reproductive rates as compared to natural methods.

Proper incubation techniques alone are not enough, however. Many other factors play a role in the successful rearing of young raptors.

5.4.2.1 Clutch removal

An entire clutch may be removed from the nest for various reasons. It might be safer to remove the eggs from the adult birds. If done correctly, egg removal may also induce the pair to double or triple clutch. Many species of birds are capable of laying again if their first clutch is somehow destroyed. Frequently the second clutch contains fewer eggs than the first. However, there are cases among peregrines and saker falcons where three consecutive clutches of four eggs each have been produced.

In order to increase production successfully this way, it is necessary to time the removal just right. If the female incubates her eggs beyond a certain time, hormonal changes that prevent repetition of mating and egg-laying that same season will take place. In birds of prey one therefore waits only two or three days beyond the laying of the last egg before removing the entire clutch. The nest should be moderately disturbed or disorganized at this time without completely destroying it. Otherwise there is a risk that the female will continue to brood on it and not lay again. In addition, nest building is often a stimulating component of breeding behavior.

The readiness to repeat egg-laying varies among individuals and is directly related to the broodiness of the female. Falcons have been observed carrying large pebbles to their nest after the removal of their clutch (Behrens, 1994). These particular birds continued to incubate the stones and failed to lay again.

Most smaller birds of prey lay the first egg of the second clutch approximately two weeks after the removal of the first clutch. Eagles may take substantially longer. Among nine pairs of bald eagles (*Haliaeetus leucocephalus*) the average time until the second clutch was laid averaged 32 (range 22–57) days.

Multiple clutching will definitely increase the reproductive rate for a pair. However, artificial incubation or foster parenting is absolutely necessary if such methods are used.

The ability to increase production this way in captivity has led to attempts to apply similar techniques to wild-living endangered species. The first clutch can be removed from the nest, artificially incubated and hacked out, allowing the original pair to raise a further set of offspring. In this way initial successes have been achieved with bald eagles in the U.S. and with bearded vultures in Spain.

5.4.2.2 Egg-pulling

Egg-pulling is also designed to increase production and consists of the immediate removal of each egg as it is laid. In particular those species that lay several eggs will persist in trying to achieve a certain number of eggs to complete their clutch. They will often continue laying as the eggs are removed. Some species of falcons can produce up to 24 eggs in a row this way.

Critics of this practice fear that it imposes too severe a burden on the female and therefore discourage its use. On the other hand, it can be argued that egg-laying is a particularly sensitive indicator of a bird's well-being. The slightest physical or psychological stress to the animal will usually result in cessation of laying activity.

When forcing increased egg production, especially with the egg-pulling method, special attention must be paid to a balanced, high-quality diet and adequate availability of calcium for egg shell production. The

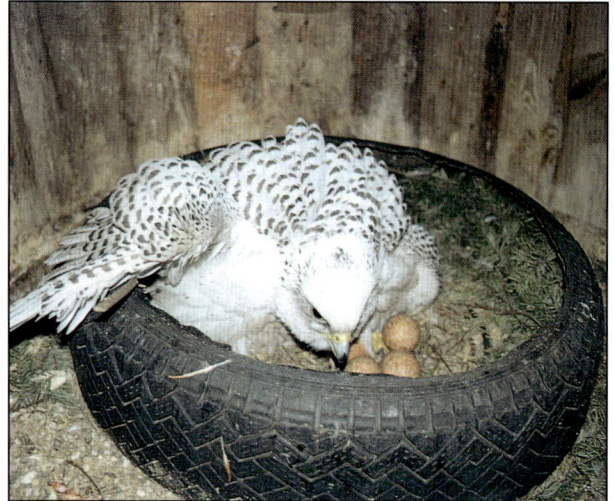

Fig. 5.19: While it is relatively easy to remove the eggs from the nest of a human-imprinted bird, wilder hawks will sometimes defend their clutch so aggressively that the eggs are in danger.
(Photo: Heidenreich)

chicks will require an appropriate balance of nutrients and a strong egg in order to develop and hatch successfully.

5.4.2.3 Egg transport

Removing a clutch from the nest is not always an easy task. Some birds will vigorously defend their eggs (Fig. 5.19). Especially defensive species such as eagles can only be robbed of their eggs with the protection of a padded suit and helmet. Aggressive encounters in the nest should be avoided as much as possible to prevent damaging the eggs during removal.

The method of transport is important to the success of artificial incubation. The eggs should be shaken or disturbed as little as possible. Placing them immediately in a small box lined with foam rubber has proven safe and convenient (Fig. 5.20).

Even if the eggs were being incubated already, the reduction in temperature that occurs during transport is usually not a problem. Cooling to room temperature can be tolerated by the egg for up to 24 hours without risk. Shaking or jarring, on the other hand, is lethal to the developing embryo. Experience with the eggs of other species has shown that motionless storage for 24 hours before placement in the incubator can improve the hatch rate of previously disturbed or shaken eggs.

If incubated eggs need to be shipped over larger distances, a larger box filled with heat-sterilized wheat kernels can be used. This type of packaging allows for

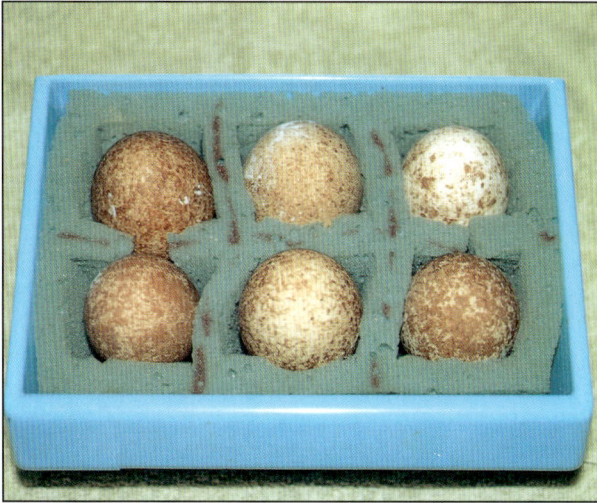

Fig. 5.20: Safe short-distance transport of eggs can be accomplished in a specially-constructed foam box. Travel over longer distances requires packing the eggs in a container that allows free air exchange. (Photo: Heidenreich)

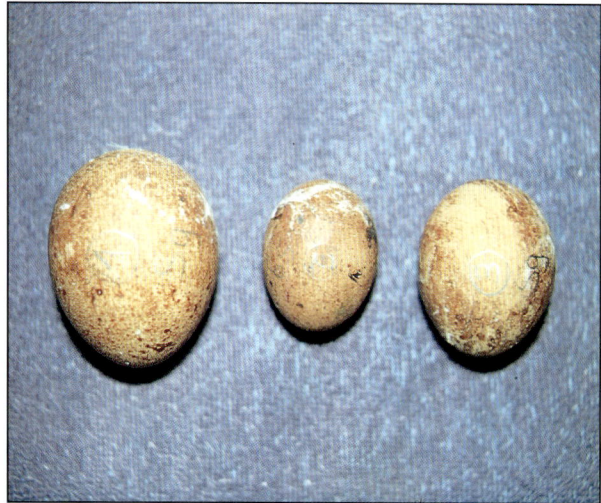

Fig. 5.22: The complete clutch of a red-naped shaheen X gyrfalcon hybrid shows three completely different sized eggs. The left egg is gyrfalcon-sized, the middle egg is obviously too small, and on the right is an egg of normal shaheen size. Whether the falcon's hybrid status is responsible for these differences is not known. (Photo: Heidenreich)

adequate gas exchange. The grain also acts as a good insulator and protects the eggs from impact.

5.4.2.4 Egg abnormalities

In the captive propagation of raptors, especially if artificial insemination is employed, defects in egg shell production are occasionally seen. Such egg abnormali-

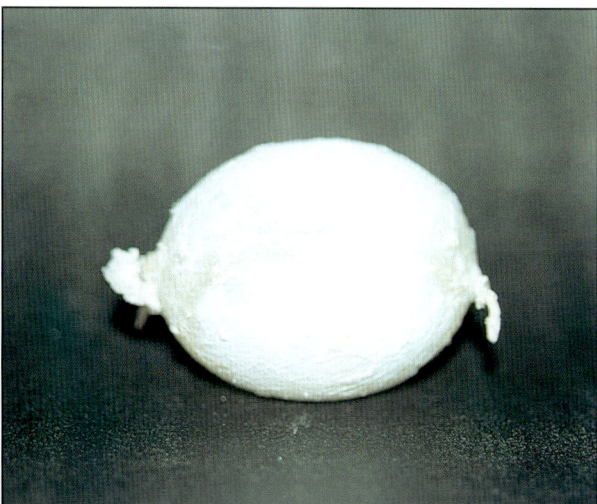

Fig. 5.21: A typical so-called "wind" or "snake" egg, which lacks a calcium shell. One can clearly see the polar chalazae which normally stabilize the yolk inside the egg. (Photo: Heidenreich)

ties can make embryo development difficult or impossible. The most extreme cases are the so-called, "wind" or ,"snake" eggs (Fig. 5.21), in which the almost fully developed egg lacks a calcium shell. The cause of this defect may be related to inadequate perfusion of the uterine shell gland. Stress during artificial insemination procedures or ascending oviductal infections could also be involved. Incubating such abnormal eggs is useless.

All other kinds of egg abnormalities are possible as well, including malformations involving size, shape and shell composition (Fig. 5.22). For genetic reasons alone, malformed eggs should never be incubated.

If the quality of the egg shell is poor, or if the egg is mistreated or damaged, cracks or dents may occur in the shell. If such defects are immediately treated, and contamination of the egg is avoided, these eggs can easily be incubated and hatched in a normal manner. Commercially available glue, wax and liquid bandaging material from a spray can have all been successfully used.

One may attempt to incubate any defective egg, but it should be recognized that such eggs may pose a danger to the others in the incubator if they become contaminated with infectious agents.

5.4.2.5 Incubation hygiene

The prevention of bacterial contamination of the eggs is of fundamental importance to the success of artificial incubation. The warm and humid environment of an incubator is an ideal place for microbial growth. This can pose a serious risk to the developing eggs. Therefore, the incubator should be thoroughly sterilized before placing eggs in it. The eggs themselves should be cleaned before incubation. The worst dirt can be gently removed from the shell by brushing. Washing should be avoided as this may damage the cuticle on the egg surface and promote infection.

Formaldehyde works well for the disinfection of both incubator and eggs. A 40% aqueous solution of formaldehyde is called formalin and can be used for disinfection according to the following directions:

1.35 ml of formalin are added to 0.84 g of potassium permanganate ($KMnO_4$) in a large, heat-resistant container. A strong exothermic reaction is produced by the mixture and formaldehyde gas will be released. The volumes above will suffice to disinfect an area 30 liters in size, excluding the space taken up by the eggs themselves. Gassing should take place at 21 °C for 30 minutes. A higher concentration can be used for the initial disinfection of the incubator without the eggs, as long as everything is aired well afterwards. Normally, an initial disinfection will suffice for the entire incubation period. If necessary, this procedure can be repeated later during incubation. The formalin concentration should be reduced to 0.5 ml formalin in 0.2 g $KMnO_4$ in such cases to avoid damaging the developing embryos. Formaldehyde gassing should not be performed in the first four days of incubation or after the embryos begin to breathe from the air cell!

The concentrations described above have proven effective for the eggs of various birds of prey. However, there are cases where there is some suspicion that this method has injured the embryos. A risk-free alternative to formaldehyde gassing involves treating the eggs with ultraviolet light. Both sides of each egg should be irradiated for 20 minutes from a 30 Watt ultraviolet light bulb from a distance of 20 cm. To protect the eyes of the handler, this procedure should be performed in an opaque chamber or box.

5.4.2.6 The incubation environment

Storing eggs outside the incubator

Even outside the incubator, especially during temporary storage, environmental factors play an important role in the health and eventual survival of the freshly laid egg. At the time of laying, development of the embryo has already progressed to the blastula stage. If the egg is cooled, this development is temporarily interrupted. The embryo can remain in this arrested state for some time without suffering harm. Once the egg temperature again rises above 21°C, development is resumed but not successfully completed unless the proper incubation temperature is reached. Continued exposure to such intermediate temperatures will result in death of the embryo.

The humidity level to which the egg is exposed during storage also affects hatch rates. If the environment is too dry, excessive evaporation will occur from the egg. Under excessively humid conditions, condensation on the egg surface can lead to microbial contamination. The optimal humidity during storage for all eggs is between 75% and 85%. Temperature should be maintained around 13°C. If the eggs are stored properly, they do not need to be turned during this time. Maintaining eggs this way for longer than a week reduces hatchability and is usually not necessary if sufficient incubators are available.

Brown (1979) reports on some interesting observations regarding hatchability in previously stored eggs. He found that warming the eggs to 26°C before putting them in the incubator improved hatch rates. Good results were also obtained if the stored eggs were warmed this way every day. This effect may be due to the fact that such temperature fluctuations simulate natural conditions. The female will briefly incubate the eggs already present each time a new one is laid, and begins truly incubating them only after the last one arrives.

Egg incubation

Temperature: After the eggs are placed in the incubator, temperature, humidity, air flow (gas exchange) and egg turning are the most important factors involved in successful incubation. The most important of these is temperature, since embryo development is directly dependent upon it. All raptor eggs seem to do well at a temperature of about 37.2°C. If the temperature is a little higher, the chicks will hatch a bit earlier. Slightly lower temperatures will delay hatching somewhat. Some breeders (Pedersen, 1995) raise the temperature to 37.8 °C towards the end of the incubation period to increase the chicks' strength and activity during hatching.

Almost as important as the temperature inside the incubator is the room temperature outside it. Strong temperature fluctuations in the room itself can sometimes affect temperatures inside the incubator as well!

In the early days of artificial incubation for raptors, some breeders recommended that the eggs be allowed to cool occasionally. The eggs were removed from the incubator and left at room temperature for several hours. Such measures have not only proven unnecessary, they may actually pose a risk to the embryos. Sudden cooling causes the egg contents to contract and potentially draw microorganisms present on the egg surface in through the shell pores. Bacterial infections commonly result. The argument that the incubating female will occasionally leave her nest under natural conditions, thus allowing the eggs to cool briefly, is not relevant. A natural antibacterial substance called lysozyme is present in the oil on avian feathers. During natural incubation, the eggs are coated and protected by this substance – an advantage that artificially incubated eggs lack.

Egg turning: Turning the eggs during incubation is important in preventing the shell membranes from adhering and to promote nutrient exchange. Under natural conditions, the adult bird will turn her eggs in short intervals, almost hourly. Regular turning has a great influence on hatchability and it should be done frequently during artificial incubation as well, especially in the early stages. A good turning rate is every three hours, and this should be discontinued only after the embryo has turned itself in the egg and assumed the pipping position shortly before hatching.

Humidity: Breeder's recommendations regarding relative humidity in the incubator vary considerably. One may be successful with 60%, while another recommends only 20%. These large differences may in part be due to the variety of incubators available, and to differing rates of air exchange. The most important thing is that the incubated egg lose the appropriate amount of weight due to evaporation. Establishing a fixed recommendation for relative humidity is impossible.

To achieve a certain humidity, water must be present in the incubating chamber. Such containers of water present a large risk of infection, as they can rapidly develop a metallic, glistening surface film of dust and bacterial growth in the warm atmosphere of the incubator. The ventilator then distributes the bacteria throughout the incubator and deposits them on the egg surfaces. This can easily lead to fatal infections in the embryo. If the addition of water to the incubation environment cannot be avoided, a few drops of an iodine solution added as a disinfectant will help prevent bacterial growth.

Egg weight reduction: The amount of weight that should be lost by a normal egg between laying and hatching is estimated at 12% for most bird species. For birds of prey, this value is certainly too low. Best results with raptors have been obtained with a weight loss between 15–18 %. Fifteen percent of the initial weight should have been lost by pipping, and 18% by the time the chick hatches (Rahn and Ar, 1974).

Since weight loss of the egg is based solely on evaporation, it can be represented by a linear relationship on a graph. One must know the initial egg weight and the expected incubation period, by the end of which the egg should have lost 15% of its weight. With these three values, an individual graph can be created for each egg. While the desired weight loss and the incubation period are fixed quantities, the fresh weight of the egg might need to be estimated in cases where the egg has been naturally incubated or stored for a few days after being laid. Thompson (1990) gives a mathematical formula which permits determination of the egg's initial weight:

$$(A^2 \times B) \times C = F$$

where A = the width of the egg (in mm),
B = the length of the egg (in mm),
C = the coefficient for that species, and
F = the fresh weight of the egg.

The correction coefficient C is different for each bird species. For example, for the peregrine falcon (*Falco peregrinus*) C is 0.0005474, while for a Harris' hawk (*Parabuteo unicinctus*) its value is 0.0005499. Since the species differences are very small and vary only at the sixth decimal, the peregrine falcon value can be used for other raptors as well.

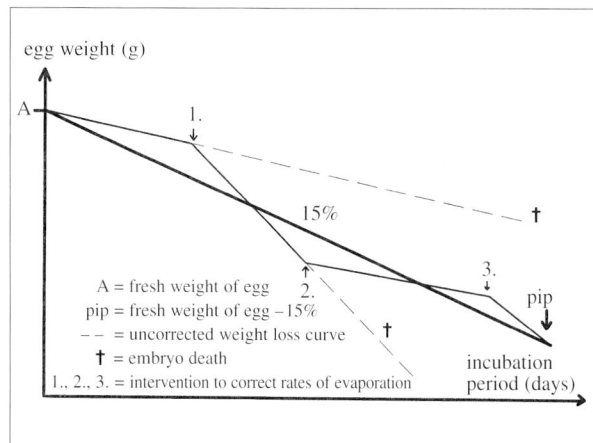

Fig. 5.23: The effect of egg weight loss on chick hatchability in birds of prey.

Sample calculation:
With a caliper, the egg is determined to have a width of 40 mm and a length of 50 mm. Plugging these values into the formula:

$$(40^2 \times 50) \times 0.0005474 = 43.79 \text{ grams}$$

Another, simpler but less accurate calculation of the egg's fresh weight can be performed by determining the average weight loss for the first few days before incubation.

Sample calculation:
An egg has been naturally incubated for 6 days and is removed from the nest with a weight of 42.0 grams. In the incubator, it loses 0.22 grams per day.

$$6 \text{ days} \times 0.22 \text{ g per day} = 1.32 \text{ grams lost before artificial incubation}$$

The egg thus weighed approximately 43.32 grams when it was laid.

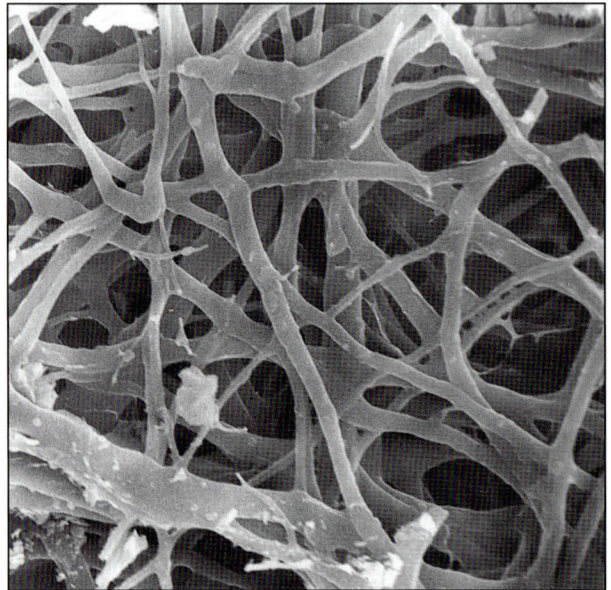

Fig. 5.25: Excessive egg shell sanding can expose the inner shell membranes (shown here magnified 2000 X by an electron microscope). The barrier of protection provided by the shell is disrupted, leaving the egg at greater risk of infections.
(Photo: Hussong)

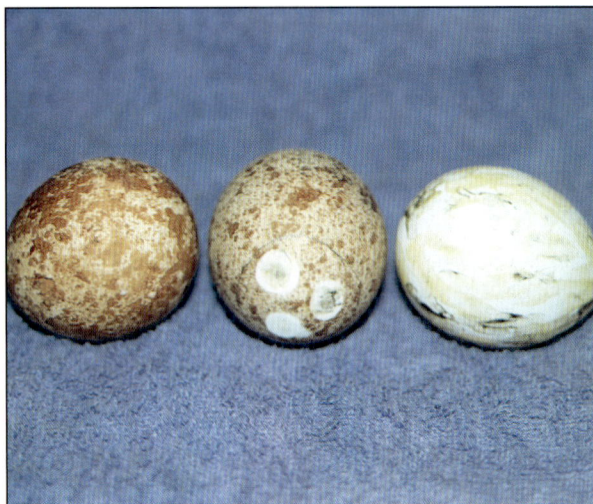

Fig. 5.24: Egg shell treatments can alter the evaporative rate so that the desired 15% weight loss is achieved by the time of pipping. On the left is an egg that was losing weight at the correct rate and therefore remained untreated. The middle egg was not losing enough weight, so sandpaper was used to thin the shell over the air cell (rounded end) and increase the rate of evaporation.
The egg on the right was not only unpigmented, it also lost too much water as a result of abnormal egg shell porosity. If that egg had not been partially coated with waterproof substances, the embryo would surely have died.
(Photo: Heidenreich)

With the three values now determined, an incubation graph can be created for each egg. Based on the requirement that an egg weighing, for example, 43.79 grams needs to lose 15% of its weight at the end of an incubation period of 32 days, we can calculate that it will weigh 36.79 grams at hatching. A line can now be drawn between these two points of weight. Frequent weighing of the egg during incubation will reveal whether weight loss is following the line established on the graph. Weight measurements performed every few days are sufficient to allow humidity adjustments to be made as needed.

Figure 5.23 shows an idealized sample curve for 15% weight loss, as well as plots resulting from weight loss due to insufficient or excessive evaporation of moisture from the egg (dotted lines).

The potential reasons for inappropriate weight loss during incubation are many. Egg shell quality, especially pore size, may play a role, as does the humidity level inside the incubator. By altering these two factors, the weight loss curve for an egg can easily be corrected.

Adjusting relative humidity: If the egg's weight remains above the desired curve for several days, it is not losing enough weight. Reducing the humidity in the incubator can correct this. If measurable weight loss and a closer approximation to the desired curve are not achieved, the water reservoir in the incubator can be removed entirely, or desiccants (such as Blaugel) may even be added. Desiccants are strongly hydrophilic chemicals such as silica that absorb environmental moisture. Gyrfalcon eggs are usually incubated without placing water in the incubator at all (PEDERSEN, 1995).

Correcting egg shell factors: If humidity adjustments alone are not successful, the egg itself must be treated. Gentle sanding over the air cell area (rounded end) using fine sand paper (Fig. 5.24) will raise evaporation rates substantially. This process removes the outer layer of the shell, exposing the secondary pores or even the shell membranes (Fig. 5.25). If excessive weight loss makes it obvious a few days later that too much of the shell was removed, a portion of the exposed shell area can be closed again. Liquid beeswax, paraffin or liquid bandage material work well for this purpose. The same repair methods can also be tried for cracks or other defects of the shell (Fig. 5.26). In the latter case, microorganisms have usually already succeeded in penetrating the egg and the chick often dies of infection.

Bednarek (1987) claims that sanding the eggs is not necessary if they are sprayed several times a day with distilled water. This method may seem counterintuitive since its purpose is to promote weight loss. The egg

will initially absorb moisture instead of losing it. Presumably, however, the distilled water dissolves calcium structures around the pores, enlarging the pore size and thus eventually promoting evaporation. Frequent weighing is always necessary to determine the effectiveness of the measures implemented.

Egg shell abrasions that permit increased evaporation through the pores take place in nature as well. Naturally incubated eggs are constantly rubbing against each other and against the rough surface of the nest, especially when subjected to frequent turnings by the female. This explains why natural incubation is more successful, even at higher humidity levels, than is artificial incubation.

5.4.2.7 Egg candling

Candling an egg is the process of shining a bright light through it in order to visualize the contents. One can thus identify unfertilized eggs or those in which the embryo has died. Embryo development can also be monitored this way. The size and shape of the air cell as observed during candling can indicate when pip is about to occur.

Candling is done with commercially available lamps sold for this purpose. Very bright mercury vapor lamps have proven especially useful. Because these strong light sources also produce much heat, the egg should be transilluminated only briefly. This prevents heating the shell and damaging the embryo. The fiberoptic light source of an endoscope can also be used for candling without the risk of heat.

Whether an egg is fertile or not can be determined after about three days. In some species, egg shell pigmentation and markings can make this a little more difficult. Very large, thick-shelled eggs like those of eagles must be evaluated somewhat later than those of smaller species.

Towards the end of the incubation period, the size and shape of the air cell help indicate when hatching will occur. When the chick breaks into the air cell with its egg tooth, the air pocket will collapse and appear asymmetric when candled. Two to three days will pass from this point until pipping and then hatching occur.

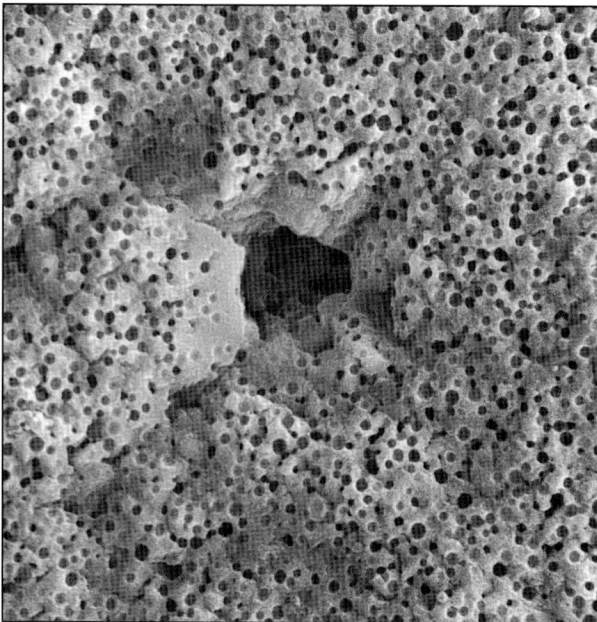

Fig. 5.26: This electron micrograph shows the surface of a peregrine falcon egg magnified 3000 times. The shell structure is abnormally loose. In the center is a breathing pore in whose depths the so-called secondary pores are visible. Eggs like this lose too much moisture during incubation and require egg shell coatings or higher levels of humidity during incubation.
(Photo: Hussong)

5.4.2.8 Incubation periods

Knowledge of incubation periods is very important. The various species of birds of prey vary significantly in this regard. Table 5.1 gives an overview of incubation periods. It should be noted that these are average values only. Incubation factors can shift the time periods in either direction.

Table 5.1: Incubation periods for various birds of prey

Species	Incubation period (days)
Bearded vulture (*Gypaetus barbatus*)	53–58
European black vulture (*Aegypius monachus*)	50–55
Griffon vulture (*Gyps fulvus*)	48–54
Egyptian vulture (*Neophron percnopterus*)	42
White-tailed sea eagle (*Haliaeetus albicilla*)	38–40
Pallas' sea eagle (*Haliaeetus leucoryphus*)	38
Osprey (*Pandion haliaeetus*)	35–38
Peregrine falcon (*Falco peregrinus*)	31–33
Gyrfalcon (*Falco rusticolus*)	30–34
Saker falcon (*Falco cherrug*)	31–33
Lanner falcon (*Falco biarmicus*)	32
European hobby (*Falco subbuteo*)	(28) 31–33
Common kestrel (*Falco tinnunculus*)	28–30
Merlin (*Falco columbarius*)	28–30
Eleonora's falcon (*Falco eleonorae*)	28–30
Northern goshawk (*Accipiter gentilis*)	32–34 (39)
European sparrowhawk (*Accipiter nisus*)	32–34
Common buzzard (*Buteo buteo*)	31–33
Rough-legged buzzard (*Buteo lagopus*)	31–34
Long-legged buzzard (*Buteo rufinus*)	33–35
Golden eagle (*Aquila chrysaetus*)	43–45
Imperial eagle (*Aquila heliaca*)	43
Tawny or steppe eagle (*Aquila rapax*)	35
Lesser spotted eagle (*Aquila pomarina*)	38–41
Greater spotted eagle (*Aquila clanga*)	42–44
Bonelli's eagle (*Hieraaetus fasciatus*)	37–39
Booted eagle (*Hieraaetus penatus*)	35–38
Red and black kites (*Milvus milvus* and *Milvus migrans*)	30–32
Marsh harrier (*Circus aeruginosus*)	33–35
Montagu's harrier (*Circus pygargus*)	28–30

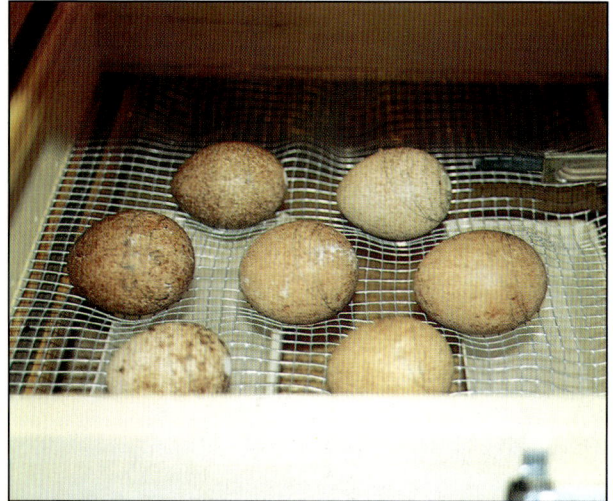

Fig. 5.27: Shallow depressions in the hatcher keep the pipped eggs stable and aid the chick's hatching efforts. The egg is prevented from rolling around during the hatching process, which conserves energy for the hatchling.
(Photo: Heidenreich)

prevents the egg membranes from sticking to the chick's downy feathers and impeding hatching.

It is helpful to place the eggs in a small depression in the hatcher to help stabilize them (Fig. 5.27). The eggs could otherwise roll around during hatching, slowing the process and weakening the chick. Once the chick has begun breaking a circular opening into the egg shell with its egg tooth, the hatching process will be completed in only a few minutes.

The hatchling should be left inside the hatcher for a few hours until the down has dried completely. Thereafter, it can be transferred to a warmed brooder (Figs. 5.28–5.33).

5.4.2.9 Hatching

The hatching of a raptor chick is an exciting event, even for the experienced breeder. Small chirping sounds can be heard a few days beforehand. Once pipping has occurred, one may have to wait up to two more days until the chick begins breaking out of the shell.

Pipped eggs should be removed from the incubator and placed in a hatcher. Hatchers are kept at a somewhat warmer temperature (37.8 °C) and have a higher humidity than the incubator. The increase in humidity

Figs. 5.28, 5.29, 5.30, 5.31, 5.32, 5.33:
The hatching of a raptor chick is a fascinating process. One or two days after pipping, the shell is sawed open in a circular pattern using the egg tooth (5.28). The chick stretches its body inside the egg in order to enlarge the resulting crack, eventually pushing one half of the shell away with its feet (5.29). The two halves of the egg fall apart (5.30) and the exhausted hatchling opens its eyes to a new world (5.31). The down feathers are allowed to dry (5.32) before removing the chick from the hatcher. For the next two days the vulnerable chick is kept warm in an incubator or brooder at approximately 35 °C (5.33).
(Photos: Heidenreich)

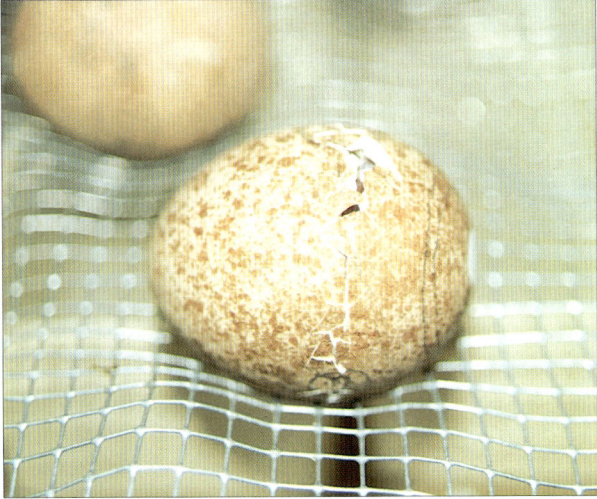

5.28

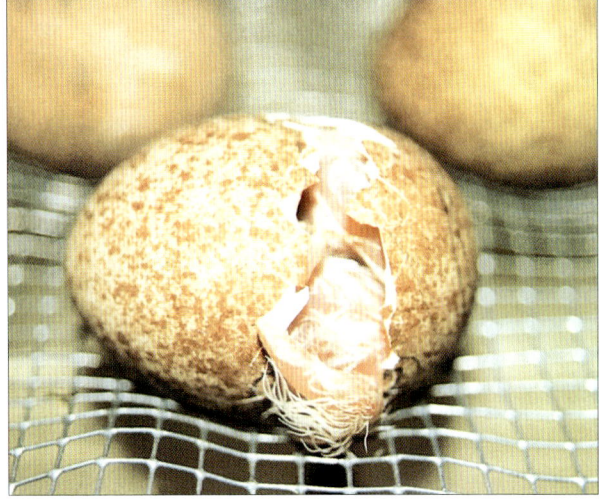

5.29

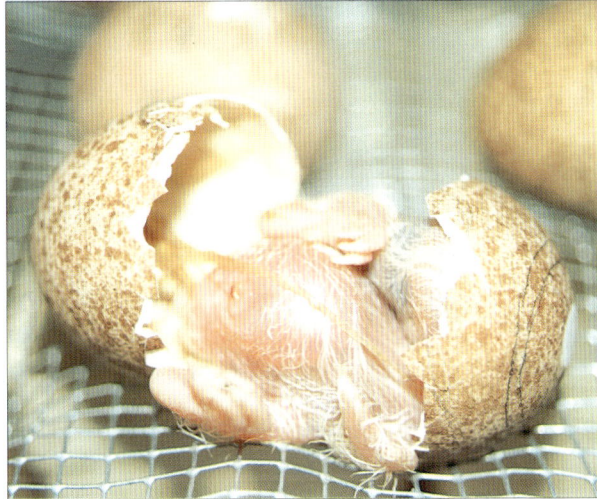

5.30

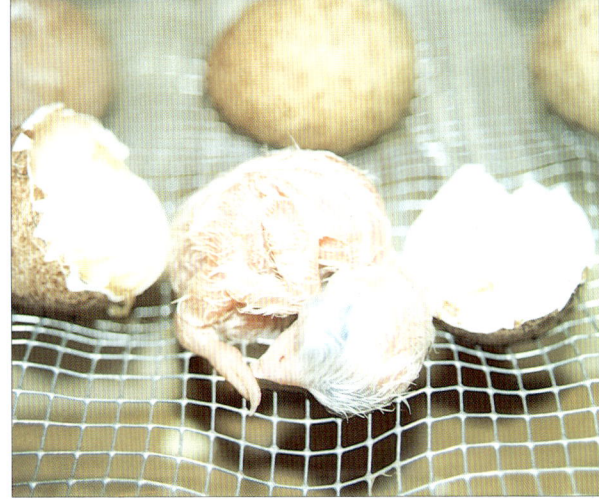

5.31

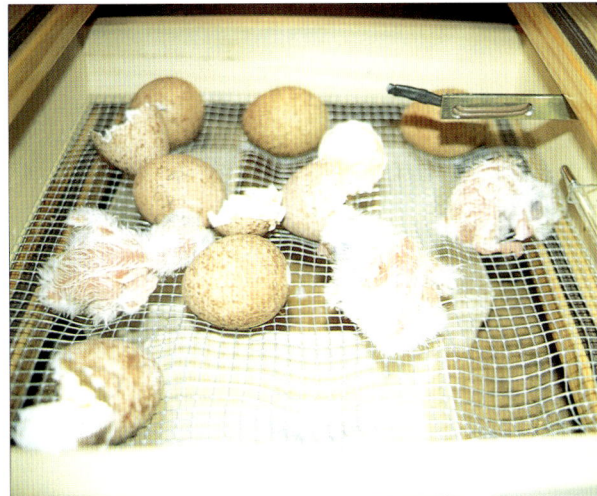

5.32

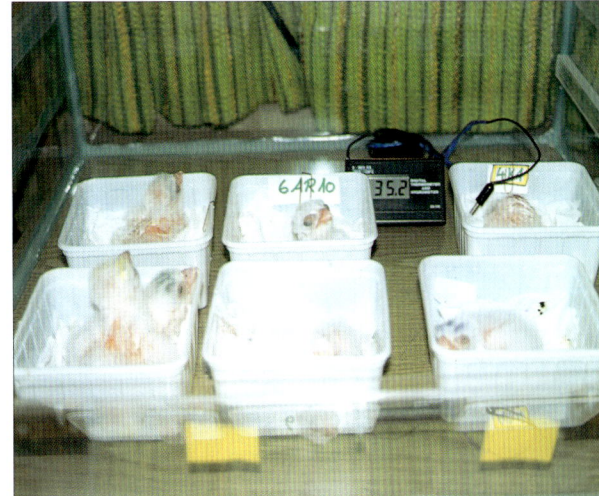

5.33

Table 5.2: Incubation problems and their possible causes [Based on Brown (1979), Siegmann (1992) and Joyner (1994)]

Finding	Possible causes
Infertile eggs	Parent birds too old, extreme temperatures, poor nutrition, interrupted mating, hybridization, asynchronous breeding behavior, apparent infertility due to improper storage
Early embryonic death (1st week)	Environmental temperatures too hot or too cold even before eggs are collected, eggs too warm during storage or stored too long or without turning, inadequate disinfection, jarring of eggs, incubation temperature too high, insufficient turning
Embryonic death (2nd and 3rd week)	Overheating during candling, all the problems listed above can also result in later embryonic death, fluctuating temperatures, excessive humidity, insufficient air exchange, insufficient turning, infections
Late embryonic death (just before hatching)	Jarring during transfer to hatcher, weakened chicks due to malnutrition of parent birds, excessive humidity
Death during hatching	Insufficient humidity resulting in adhesion of egg shell membranes, malpositioning inside the egg, excessive humidity earlier in incubation resulting in edema of the chicks and preventing pipping
moist, sticky, edematous chicks	Incubation temperature too low, humidity too high
unabsorbed yolk sac	hatching temperature too low, humidity too high in the hatcher
umbilical infections	poor hygiene, temperatures too high
weak, lethargic chicks	temperature too high, humidity too low
difficulty breathing	Incubated with excessive humidity, insufficient humidity during hatching, hatching temperature too high and insufficient air circulation
curly toes	temperature too high, substrate too soft in hatcher
bent neck	hatching took too long because temperatures or humidity were too low
prolonged hatching time	temperature too low, shell membranes too dry

5.4.3   Incubation problems

Some eggs will always fail to hatch in spite of all the care put into incubating them. Even under natural, parent-raised conditions, hatch rates of 100% are not always achieved.

The reasons for decreased hatchability under artificial conditions are often lumped together as "incubation problems". More commonly, however, these problems are due to mistakes in the process of egg production (improper feeding of the breeding pair) or insufficient hygiene, and not to incubation factors. Research with other types of bird eggs has shown that approximately 20% of the problems with hatchability are due to pre-incubation storage, 20% are due to improper incubation environments and another 20% result from insufficient egg turning. All other possible causes of poor hatchability, such as genetic factors, in-

fertility, nutrition, incubator environment, infections or lack of expertise are less important. The eggs of wild birds lack a so-called "incubator tolerance". This term denotes the decades of selection which domestic fowl eggs have undergone to increase their tolerance of artificial incubation techniques. Generations of artificially incubated poultry chicks have all been derived from parents who themselves hatched in incubators. This type of selection pressure has not yet been brought to bear on birds of prey, which have been captive-bred for only six generations.

Head at the pointed end of the egg
This malposition is not necessarily lethal, although the air cell is located at the blunt end of the egg. Approximately 50 % of chicks that end up in this position will hatch. To be safe, a small breathing hole should be made in the shell over the chick's beak when chirping

sounds become audible. This particular problem is more common in eggs that have been incubated at low temperatures or those that haven't been turned frequently enough.

The head is under the left wing

Normally the chick's head lies tucked under the right wing inside the egg. It will rotate its head counter clockwise while chipping out of the egg shell. If the head is positioned on the left, it rotates clockwise and the chick is unable to hatch.

The feet lie over the head

The feet normally help break open the egg shell by pushing it away. If they are malpositioned, this becomes impossible and the chick is unable to hatch.

The embryo lies transversely in the egg

This can occur if the egg is rounded in shape and the embryo is small. The chick is unable to hatch from this position.

Most of these malpositions are promoted by incubation problems, especially insufficient turning, poor temperature control or rough handling. Occasionally, genetic factors may be involved (Figs. 5.34 – 5.39).

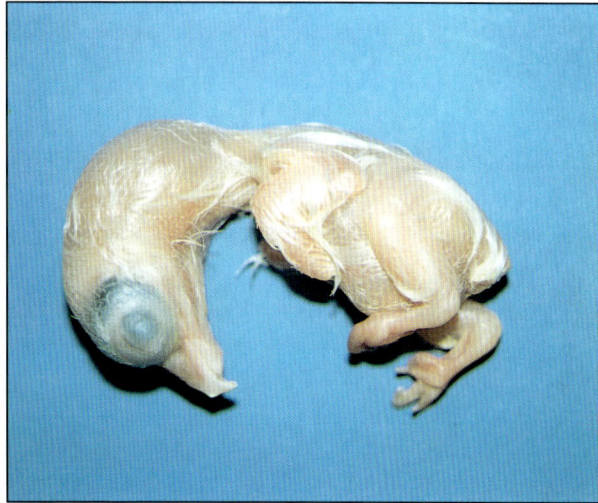

5.34

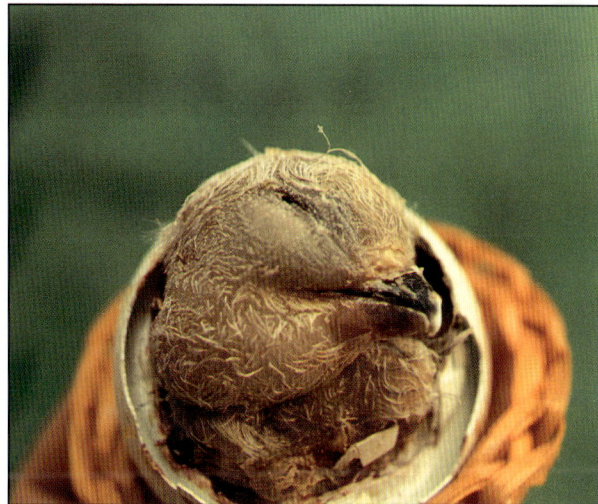

5.35

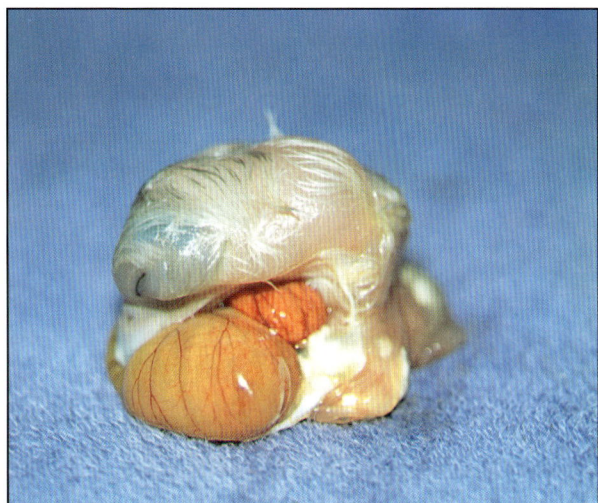

5.36

Figs. 5.34, 5.35, 5.36: The most common problem during artificial incubation is excessive humidity. It results in inadequate weight loss due to insufficient evaporation from the eggs. The subsequent accumulation of fluids in the body (edema) occurs primarily in the nape of the bird's neck (5.34) and interferes with mobility. The chick is unable to crack the egg open and dies fully developed and ready to hatch. A bald eagle chick (*Haliaeetus leucocephalus*) that died due to insufficient fluid loss is seen in Fig. 5.35. The embryo is distended with water and died several days before it was due to hatch, drowning in the fluids accumulated in its air sacs and lungs. The yolk sac is normally absorbed shortly before hatching. Its presence indicates an immature chick (5.36).
(Photos: Heidenreich)

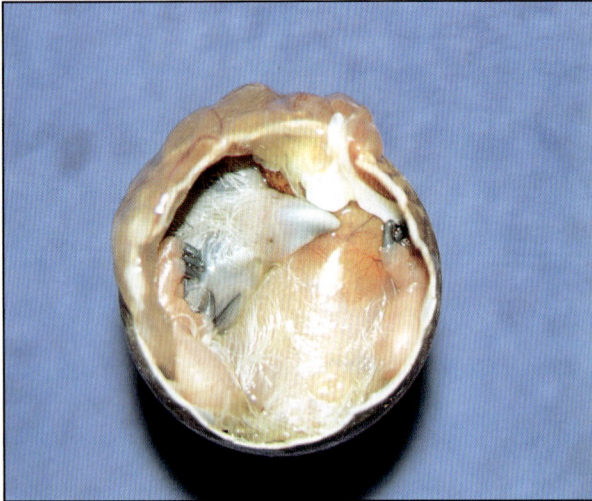

5.37

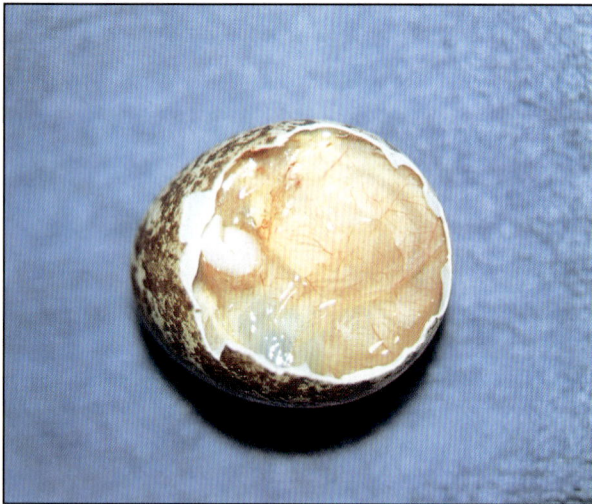

5.38

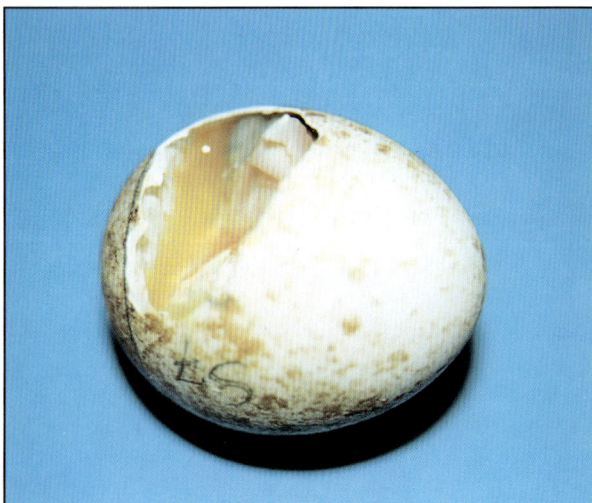

5.39

5.4.4   Assisted hatching

Every breeder will try to save his chicks, even if they require assistance during hatching. In many cases, however, such chicks are weak or otherwise compromised already and die within a few days. For reasons of selective breeding and fitness, such animals should not be raised in any case. If every chick is valuable, as for instance with certain rare species, hatching assistance may be appropriate. The period between external pip and hatching in birds of prey generally lies between 36 and 48 hours. Time periods of less than 24 hours or long ones of up to 80 hours indicate a deviation from the norm and usually require intervention. Chicks that have already opened a quarter to one half of their shell, then pause for a prolonged period of time or begin chipping away at the same spot all over again may also need help.

In many cases it is sufficient to open the air cell so that the chick can breathe more easily. The whitish, paper-like air cell inner membrane will be exposed. A small hole in it usually reveals the embryo's beak tip and egg tooth. Before proceeding further, one should check for blood vessels. This can be done by moistening the membrane with a few drops of physiologic saline. It will become transparent, making the blood vessels visible. If they are still perfused, the egg should be returned to the incubator. Only after the vessels turn blackish-brown will they not bleed when broken. Further parts of the shell can then be removed.

Once the chick has been given enough mobility and breathing space, it should be left in the remaining shell. It will usually take several more hours for yolk sac absorption to occur. Since evaporation will be greatly increased by the large hole present in the egg, the chick should be maintained at high ambient humidity with adequate air circulation. A few drops of physiologic saline placed between the chick and the egg shell membranes will help prevent unwanted adhesions.

Figs. 5.37, 5.38, 5.39: Malpositioning inside the egg:
Fig. 5.37 shows a chick with its feet over its head. Normal hatching is impossible because the egg tooth cannot be employed to crack the shell. The embryo dies fully developed.
If the head is located in the small end of the egg, opposite the air cell (5.38),death often occurs unless one intervenes in time. This malposition is often a result of infrequent egg turning.
The chick in Fig. 5.39 is positioned correctly, but a tear in the inner shell membranes resulted in the embryo's drowning in the egg fluids. The tear was caused by rough handling of the egg.
(Photos: Heidenreich)

After hatching, the umbilical area of all chicks should be disinfected with iodine solution or some other suitable disinfectant (Fig. 5.40).

5.4.5 Persistent yolk sac

One incubation problem that is occasionally seen involves chicks that hatch with or without assistance and have not fully absorbed the yolk sac. If one can see that the yolk sac is still exposed while extracting an embryo, the animal should be gently returned to the shell and left there for a few more hours.

After hatching, the umbilicus closes rapidly, making it impossible to retract the yolk sac further. In such cases, the yolk sac remnant must be amputated. This is done be tying a sterile ligature of absorbable suture material (6-0 catgut) around the sac at the umbilicus. The sac is then cut off close to the ligature. The umbilical stump will be retracted within a few minutes. A moistened cotton swab can be used to assist this process. The umbilical area should be disinfected with iodine. Despite all precautions, most of the chicks treated this way succumb to a lack of important yolk sac nutrients within the first few days of life.

5.5 Chick rearing

After they have hatched and their down has been allowed to dry, the chicks are transferred from the hatcher to an appropriately warmed brooder. In the first few days of life, raptor hatchlings are unable to maintain their body temperature. They depend on external heat sources to keep warm. Therefore the brooder

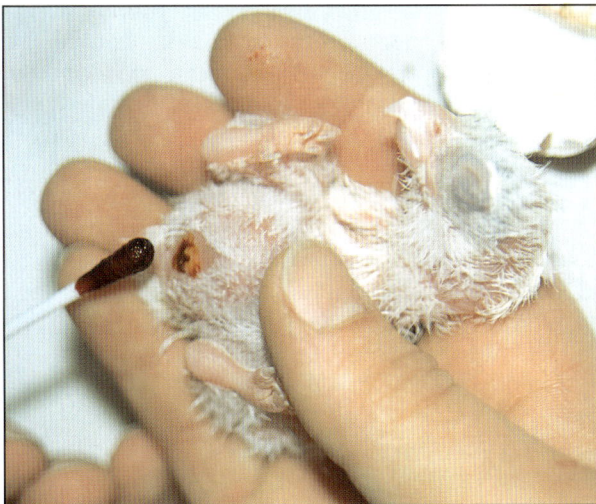

Fig. 5.40: The umbilicus of a newly-hatched chick should always be disinfected with an iodine solution.
(Photo: Heidenreich)

should be kept at around 35 °C for the first three days of life, then at 33 °C until the fifth day, around 30 °C between days six and eight and at 27 °C from the ninth to eleventh days. Fifty percent relative humidity is recommended for this entire period of time. Thereafter the chicks can be kept at room temperature. The values given above are general guidelines and may vary, especially for the smaller birds of prey.

Heat is usually supplied by infrared lamps that are mounted a certain distance above the chicks. Direct infrared exposure should be avoided in the first few days because it may result in excessive fluid loss. Wrinkled, gray feet may be the first sign of dehydration. It is better to cover the chicks with a cloth, similar to the way they would be protected by the plumage of their parent. Bottom heaters that keep the chicks' abdominal area warm and promote digestion have also proven quite successful (Pedersen, 1995).

A clear indicator of correct brooding temperatures is the "contentedness" of the chicks. They will be mostly quiet and sit comfortably positioned. Hunched-up nestlings are probably too cold, while those that lie stretched out may be indicating that they are too warm.

Raptor hatchlings can be placed on a substrate of shredded, absorbent paper towels inside a small nesting container for the first few days. A smooth surface or large enclosure can easily lead to splayed legs. After a few days, the chicks may be transferred to larger containers. At this stage, a substrate of fine pea gravel has proven effective. The rough texture of this material prevents the legs from splaying while the excretions sink to the bottom, keeping the nestlings clean and dry.

Now is the time to decide how the birds are to be raised and socialized because this is the age at which imprinting on their own kind or on humans will occur.

5.5.1 Isolated rearing (imprinting on humans)

If, for purposes of future breeding using semen collection or artificial insemination, the bird is to be imprinted on humans, it should be isolated and exposed only to humans immediately. In altricial birds such as raptors, the imprinting period is significantly longer than in precocial birds, which imprint for life in the first few hours after hatching.

Large falcons react impartially until their 14th day of life. In other words, they will beg from humans as well as from birds. After this point, they become imprinted on the person or bird feeding them. If the chicks are returned to their parents after this critical phase of life, they will react with fear towards the unaccustomed adult birds.

The critical turning point occurs later with eagles and vultures, generally between four and five weeks of age. It is interesting that these birds will still respond to their own species even after this time. If, for example, an eagle chick is removed from the nest at four weeks of age and placed in human hands, it will refuse to eat for the first few days and react fearfully in the presence of man. On the other hand, an eagle chick of the same age taken from a situation where it was hand-raised and placed suddenly in a nest with adult eagles, will immediately accept and beg from the new parents. Knowledge of these critical periods can be very useful when reintroducing captive-bred birds of prey to the wild.

5.5.2 Rearing with siblings (double imprinting)

In cases where human-imprinting is not desired, but foster parents are not available, the clutch can be raised together. This will allow the birds to imprint on each other and avoid an excessive fixation on humans. Such birds should be transferred to a closed aviary as soon as they are capable of feeding themselves. The discontinuation of all visual and physical contact with humans will promote their further estrangement from man.

Nevertheless, birds raised in this way will often be "double imprinted". This means that they behave normally towards their own kind only as long as there are

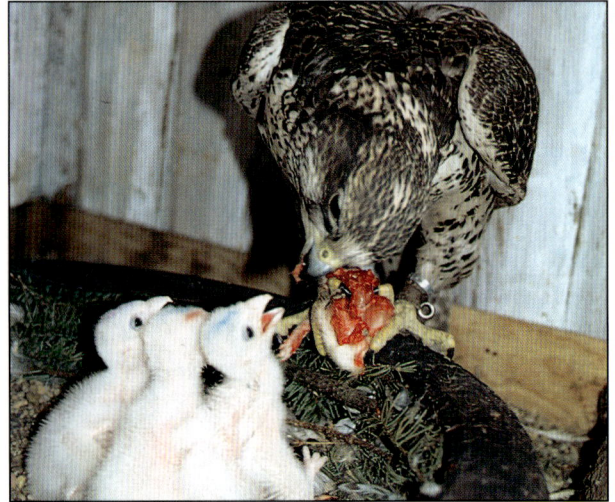

Fig. 5.42: Only a few minutes after being placed in the nest, the hand-raised chicks are begging from an adult of their own species. The falcon responds by providing them with food.
(Photo: Heidenreich)

no people around. With renewed close human contact they will revert to displaying the behavior typical of human-imprinted birds.

5.5.3 Foster parenting

In order to raise birds that are properly imprinted on their own species, it is necessary to place them with an appropriate set of foster parents before the critical window of time has been closed. However, one cannot place a clutch of chicks with just any individual bird or pair for adoption, whenever the need arises. The foster mother must have previous experience in laying, and, preferably, also in raising chicks successfully. Occasionally, adult birds with no previous experience also make good adoptive parents. The parenting instincts of such birds are so strongly developed that they will immediately begin to feed the hungry young chicks placed in their care.

It is recommended that the intended adoptive mother be allowed to incubate artificial eggs for the normal incubation period. At the end of this time, the eggs can be removed and the chicks to be fostered put in their place (Fig. 5.41). Although ten-day old chicks are distinctly larger than hatchlings would be, they are usually accepted without trouble and immediately fed (Fig 5.42).

Adoption techniques are one way to increase wild populations of threatened species of birds. This usually involves placing one or two captive-bred chicks of the same species into a wild pair's nest. There they will be accepted and raised with the adult birds' own clutch.

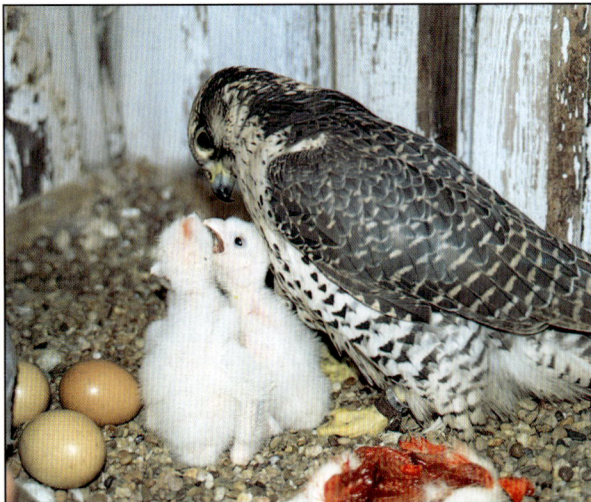

Fig. 5.41: This falcon had been incubating artificial eggs (seen on the left) for the normal incubation period. The eggs were then replaced by 10-day old chicks. Despite the chicks' large size, they were immediately accepted. The food item at the bottom of the picture served to distract the adult from the procedure. This bird was given food whenever a person entered the aviary.
(Photo: Heidenreich)

5.6 Inbreeding

The captive breeding of birds of prey is often limited by a restricted set of founder birds. Inbreeding becomes inevitable to some degree and this raises concerns about genetic diversity and inbreeding problems. Returning such animals to nature could be dangerous, as it would permit the reintroduction of captive-bred birds with potential genetic defects. This type of change in the population has been called inbreeding depression. Radler (1988) and others claim that it results in higher rates of nestling death. Similar effects are seen in nature among small, isolated populations of birds, however, and are thus not only a problem of captive breeding efforts. Radler (1990) also feels that many changes observed in captive-bred birds are not genetic in origin, and will thus not be passed on to their wild offspring. According to him, genetic "contamination" of wild populations is not really an issue.

If decreased rates of nestling survival are truly an indication of inbreeding depression, then this is not a serious problem with most captive-bred raptor species. On the contrary, many breeders have observed increasingly better survival rates among their breeding birds from year to year and from generation to generation (Küspert, 1994).

Captive-bred populations of Harris' hawks, however, may already be showing signs of inbreeding. Haigh (1991) claims that commercial breeders are producing unusually small birds with defects affecting the musculoskeletal system, the internal organs or behavioral traits. Such birds are derogatively called "clones" in the U.S.

All conscientious breeders should refrain from raising weak chicks or those with obvious physical or behavioral abnormalities. Such birds should also never be used for breeding purposes.

References and literature of further interest

BARNARD, P. (1989):
Faecal bacteria in unhatched eggs of box-nesting kestrels (*Falco sparverius*).
Proc. Symp. XIX World Conf. Int. Council for Bird Preservation
Queens University, Kingston, Ontario, Canada 135–139

BEDNAREK, W. (1978):
Der Einfluß unterschiedlicher Lichtprogramme auf die Eiablage bei Rotkopffalken (*Falco chiquera chiquera*).
Jb. Dtsch. Falkenorden 30–32

BEDNAREK, W. (1978a):
Beziehungen zwischen Eiablage, Mauserbeginn und Tageslänge bei Rotkopffalken (*Falco chiquera chiquera*)
Jb. Dtsch. Falkenorden 32–33

BEDNAREK, W. (1987):
Die Greifvogelzucht: Ergebnisse, Methoden, Techniken
Jb. Dtsch. Falkenorden 15–22

BEHRENS, P. (1994):
personal communication

BERRY, R.B. (1972):
Reproduction by artificial insemination in captive American goshawks.
J. Wildl. Management **36**, 1283–1288

BEYERBACH, U. and I. MAATSCH (1973):
Samengewinnung und -Übertragung bei Zuchtfalken.
Jb. Dtsch. Falkenorden 25–26

BOYD, L., BOYD, N.S. and F.C. DOBLER (1977):
Reproduction of prairie falcons by artificial insemination.
J. Wildl. Management **41**, 266–271

BOYD, L.L. (1978):
Artificial insemination of falcons.
Symp. Zool. Soc. London **43**, 73–80

BOYD, L.L. and C.H. SCHWARTZ (1981):
Training imprinted semen donors.
North. Amer. Falc. Ass. 65–69

BRESINSKI, W., PIELOWSKI, Z. and M. SZOTT (1978):
Habichtszucht in Polen.
Jb. Dtsch. Falkenorden 19–22

BROCK, M.K. (1984):
Cryogenic preservation of spermatozoa of the American kestrel.
Int. Zoo Yearb. **23**, 67–71

BROWN, A.A.F. (1979):
The incubation book.
WPSA, England

BRÜNING, H., HEBBELER, J. and B. PÖPPELMANN (1978):
Erfolgreiche künstliche Besamung beim Habicht.
Jb. Dtsch. Falkenorden 23–25

CADE, T.J. (1988):
Vermehrung von Taggreifen in Gefangenschaft.
Greifvögel und Falknerei 17–30
Verlag Neumann-Neudamm, Morschen-Heina

CAMPELL, J. and R. FLOOD (1981):
Artificial incubation of Merlin eggs.
J. North. Am. Falc. Ass. 76–83

COOPER, J.E. (1988):
Reproductive disorders in birds of prey.
Vet. Annual **28**, 129–135

COOPER, J.E. (1987):
Investigation of mortality in embryos and newly hatched
chicks.
in: Hill, D.J. (1987):
Breeding and management in birds of prey. 63–70
Proc. Conf. University of Bristol

CORTEN, P. (1974):
Die künstliche Besamung bei Greifvögeln.
Jb. Dtsch. Falkenorden, 35–40

DAVYGORA, A.V. (1993):
Geschlechstrieb bei Greifvögeln.
Falknerei und Greifvögel. 95–98
Verlag Neumann-Neudamm, Morschen-Heina

DIETZEN, W. and A. SCHREYER (1975):
Sperberzucht - auf dem richtigen Weg?
Jb. Dtsch. Falkenorden 41–42

FORBES, N.A. (1987):
Diagnosis and treatment of diseases commonly occurring in
breeding aviaries of raptors.
in: HILL, D.J. (1987):
Breeding and management in birds of prey. 71–80
Proc. Conf. University of Bristol

GRIER, J.W., BERRY R.B. and S.A. TEMPLE (1972):
Artificial insemination with imprinted raptors.
J. North Amer. Falc. Ass. **11**, 45–55

HAIGH, R. (1990):
Raptor incubation - some intriguing observations and
figures.
Int. Hatchery-Practice **4**, 5, 7

HAIGH, R. (1991):
Allgemeines über Haltung und Zucht des Harris-Hawk.
Jb. Dtsch. Falkenorden 21–22

HEIDENREICH, M. (1978):
Kunstbrut und Bruthygiene bei der Vermehrung von Greif-
vögeln in Gefangenschaft.
Der Falkner **25/26**, 18–21

HEIDENREICH, M. and H. KÜSPERT (1992):
Métodos de la reproducción en cautividad de las diferentes es-
pecies de halcones. El problema de los híbridos.
Congr. Nacional Cría Aves Rapaces, Madrid **1**, 15–17

HUSSONG, R. (1995):
Speziesspezifische Unterschiede von Eischalenmerkmalen bei
Falken.
Vet. Med. Diss. München, in Vorbereitung

JOYNER, K.L. (1994):
Theriogenology
in: RITCHIE, B.W. et al.:
Avian medicine: principles and application
Wingers Publishing, Lake Worth, Florida

KOLLINGER, D. (1974):
Sechzehnjähriger Sakerfalke legt erstmals Eier.
Jb. Dtsch. Falkenorden 47

KOLLINGER, D. (1992):
Einiges über ein Habichtszuchtpaar und dessen Nachwuchs.
Greifvögel und Falknerei 33-35
Verlag Neumann-Neudamm, Morschen-Heina

KÜSPERT, H., HEIDENREICH, M. and H.J. KÜSPERT (1993):
Falkenzucht.
Die Voliere **16**, 9, 10–11

KÜSPERT, H. (1994):
personal communication

PARKS, J.E. (1986):
Cryopreservation of peregrine falcon semen and post-thaw
dialysis to remove glycerol.
Raptor Res. **20**, 16–20

PEDERSEN, A. (1995):
personal communication

PÖPPELMANN, B. (1978):
Mögliche Voraussetzungen für eine erfolgreiche Sperberzucht.
Jb. Dtsch. Falkenorden 25–29

PÖPPELMANN, B. (1987):
Sperberzucht und Auswilderung.
Jb. Dtsch. Falkenorden 34–35

PÖPPELMANN, B. (1988):
Merlinzucht und Wildflug.
Greifvögel und Falknerei 34–36

PÖPPELMANN, B. (1995):
personal communication

RADLER, K. (1990):
Zur Diskussion über genetische Aspekte bei Artenhilfsmaß-
nahmen.
Greifvögel und Falknerei 19–20
Verlag Neumann-Neudamm, Morschen Heina

RAHN, H. and A. AR (1974):
The avian egg: incubation time, water loss and nest
humidity.
Condor **76**, 147-152

ROSENKRANZ, D. (1995):
personal communication

SAAR, C. and R. WEINSHEIMER (1974):
Wanderfalkenzucht in Berlin 1974.
Jb. Dtsch. Falkenorden 19–22

SAAR, C., GERRIETS, D., PAASCH, B and C. SPAETER (1983):
Die künstliche Besamung beim Wanderfalken (*Falco peregrinus*). Ein Beitrag zur Rettung einer vom Aussterben bedrohten Art.
Kleintierpraxis **28**, 163–176

SAAR, C. (1992):
Ein Beitrag zur Methodik der Zucht von Habichten.
Greifvögel und Falknerei 30–33
Verlag Neumann-Neudamm, Morschen-Heina

SALZGER, A. (1976):
Erste gelungene Zucht von Präriefalken in Österreich.
Der Falkner **25/26,** 33–34

SIEGMANN, O. (1992):
Kompendium der Geflügelkrankheiten.
5. Auflage, Verlag Paul Parey, Berlin und Hamburg

SIGL, G. (1980):
Erste Habichtszuchterfolge in Österreich.
Der Falkner **29/30,** 4–5

TEMPLE, S.A. (1972):
Artificial insemination with imprinted birds of prey.
Nature **237**, 287–288

THOMPSON, K. (1990):
Determining fresh egg weight in Harris' hawks.
Hawk Chalk **24**, 61–63

TROMMER, G. (1974):
Erfolgreiche Lannerfalkenzucht 1973/74.
Jb. Dtsch. Falkenorden

WILKENS, W.M. (1987):
Veterinary care of wild raptors.
in: HILL, D.J. (1987):
Breeding and management in birds of prey.153–166
Proc. Conf. University of Bristol

6 Marking and identification

Marking birds with leg bands or rings is an important part of ornithological research, especially in the study of migration patterns.

Raptor breeders utilize leg bands to identify every bird they produce, recording parentage for each and using this information in future breeding efforts. Colored bands help others keep track of birds of prey that are released back into the wild.

In cases of theft or other loss, positive identification of a particular bird can sometimes be important. National and international laws require endangered species to be clearly and permanently identified. This rule includes birds of prey and serves to regulate trade

in these species as well as to hinder illegal commerce in endangered animals.

Various methods of raptor identification have been tested over the years. No single one has proven ideal. Problems with health risks to the animal, unsuitability for certain species or possibilities of falsification plague them all.

Until now, the most common form of raptor identification has involved leg banding. In hunting hawks, the ring should always be placed above the jesses. Otherwise, it will be pressed against the base of the foot by the leather straps whenever the bird jumps. If a bird's legs swell due to illness or trauma, the band can easily impair blood flow to the leg, sometimes even leading to necrosis of the surrounding tissues or the entire foot. In cases like this, the ring should be immediately removed to prevent further damage to the extremity. Even if it is an official or governmental band and removal constitutes an illegal act, the bird's welfare should take first priority. A witness or a veterinarian's statement indicating the need for removal and recording the relevant information should suffice to protect the owner from inquiries by the authorities.

Several methods of identification are used in raptors today.

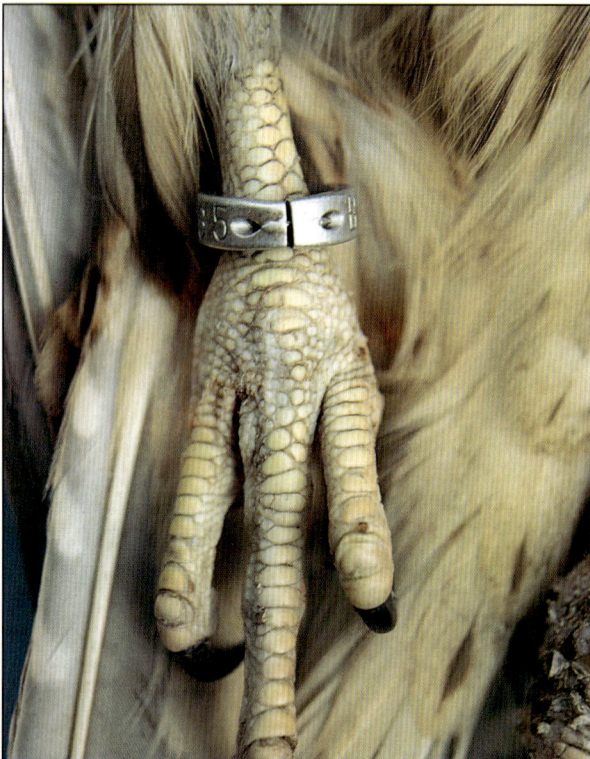

Fig. 6.1: The open rings available in Europe close with a pin and are made of a relatively soft aluminum alloy. They are easily removed and reapplied to the leg of another bird using the same pin. The legal requirement of being impossible to falsify is certainly not fulfilled!
(Photo: Heidenreich)

6.1 Open bands

In member countries of the EU, official open bands are used to identify birds of prey. These aluminum rings are applied to the bird's leg with a special pair of pliers and then closed with a pin (Fig. 6.1). The rings are engraved with the country of origin and a sequential number. The use of open bands cannot be avoided since they are usually placed on adult birds or on young birds of sufficient size to rule out sliding a closed band over the foot.

Disadvantages of open banding

a. Because the aluminum alloy rings are relatively soft, the engraved markings wear off or become unrecognizable after a few years.

b. Birds banded in adulthood often perceive the ring as a foreign object and attempt to remove it using their beak. Eagles and vultures are particularly good at this, often succeeding in removing the ring (Fig. 6.2) or seriously injuring themselves in the attempt.

c. Although supposedly impossible to falsify, these bands can easily be opened with the appropriate tools and placed on another bird using the same pin.

d. The ring from a deceased bird can easily be slipped onto the leg of a nestling.

6.2   Closed bands

Closed bands or rings can be applied only to nestlings while they are still small enough to permit sliding it over their foot. This form of identification is often used by raptor breeders because it helps prove that their animals were captive-bred. Larger falcons are usually banded this way at an age of 13 days (Fig. 6.3). If the

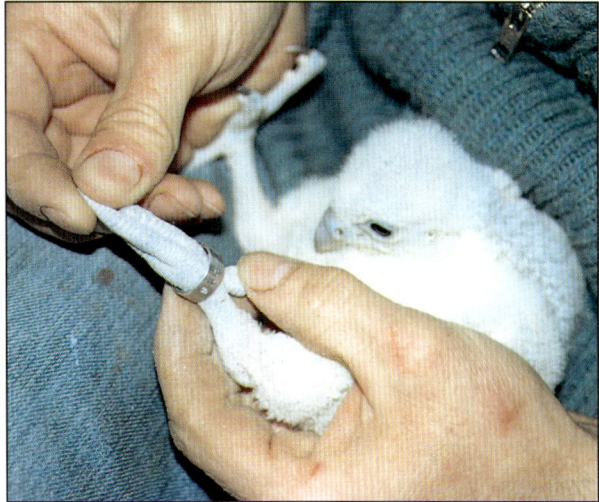

Fig. 6.3: Closed rings that are applied to the leg of a nestling provide a reliable form of identification. Their removal requires destroying the ring. (Photo: Heidenreich)

chicks are younger than this, the ring might easily fall off the leg and get lost. Only a few days after banding, the chick's rapid growth has made removal of the closed band without injuring the foot relatively difficult.

Since this procedure is done at an age at which the birds still tolerate foreign objects, the band is usually well-accepted and attempts to remove it at a later time are rare.

6.3   Tattoos

Ink markings placed in the skin of birds have not proven to be a good method of identification. This is partly due to the very thin skin that birds have. The ink easily spreads to the subcutaneous tissues and makes detailed markings unreadable. It is also difficult to find featherless tracts suitable for tattooing in birds of prey. Even areas devoid of contour feathers are covered by down. Reading a tattoo would require parting or removing the feathers.

6.4   Pedigrams

The pattern of horny scales on the upper or dorsal aspect of a hawk's digits is different for each individual bird. They can therefore be used for identification purposes much like a fingerprint. A dye is applied to the digits and then partially removed, allowing easy photographic documentation of the patterns (Figs. 6.4 and 6.5). Long-term studies have shown that an indivi-

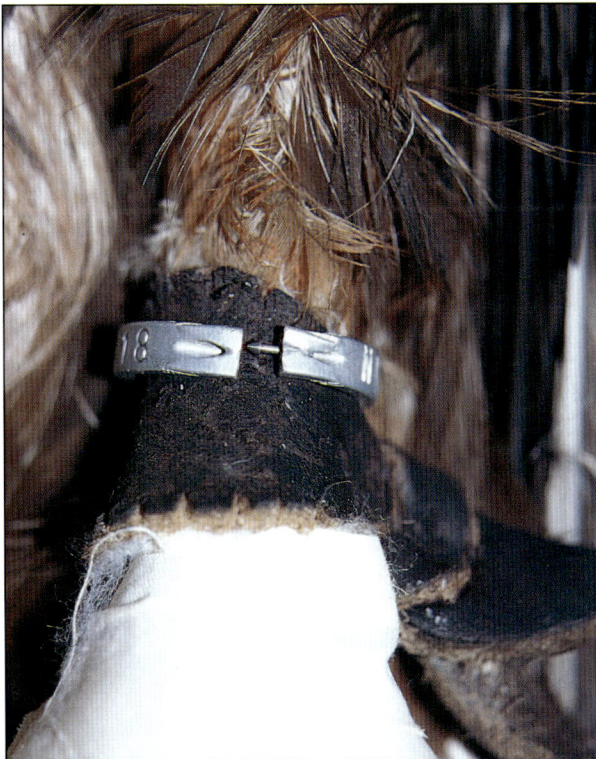

Fig. 6.2: Large raptor species such as eagles and vultures can open leg bands with their powerful beaks, occasionally injuring themselves in the process. (Photo: Heidenreich)

dual's pattern of digital scales remains unchanged for life (Stauber, 1984, 1985).

The drawback with this technique is that injuries or disease can alter the pattern of scales on a bird's foot. In addition, removal of the scales or alteration of their patterns by surgical intervention can interfere with identification.

6.5   Address tags

All hunting hawks being flown in the field carry an address tag in addition to their leg band, jesses, bells and sometimes a transmitter. This tag bears the name and telephone number of the owner. Identifying marks have been used by falconers since the earliest times, when special patterns were cut into the plumage on a hawk's back. Such techniques are still used in Arab countries today. These forms of identification are also easily falsified. Usually the reward for return of a bird is so high, however, that the finder is happy to return the animal to its rightful owner.

6.6   Microchips

The most recent innovation in animal identification consists of a microchip and a small antenna encased in a narrow (2.2 X 11 mm) tube. This nonreactive device, also called a transponder, is injected under the skin or into the muscle of an animal to provide a permanent identification number. The microchip encodes a unique ten-digit combination of numbers and letters which can be read by use of an appropriate receiver device. The hand-held reader emits a radio frequency which allows it to receive and display the microchip's code number.

German authorities now recommend the use of microchip transponders in the pectoral muscle of birds of prey in order to minimize the risk of false identification. Radiographs can be used to establish the presence and location of such a device.

Disadvantages
a. There are currently five different manufacturers for these transponders, and they are not mutually compatible. Thus the receiver of one company cannot read the microchip of another.
b. Injection into the pectoral muscles of hunting hawks, which actively use those muscles for flight, can result in dangerous migration of the chip to other body areas (Heidenreich and Küspert, 1994).

△ **6.4**   **6.5** ▽

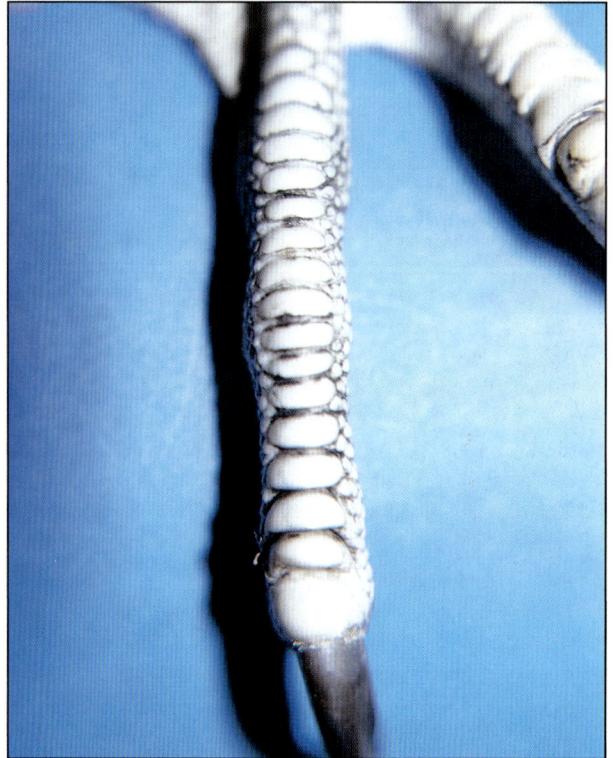

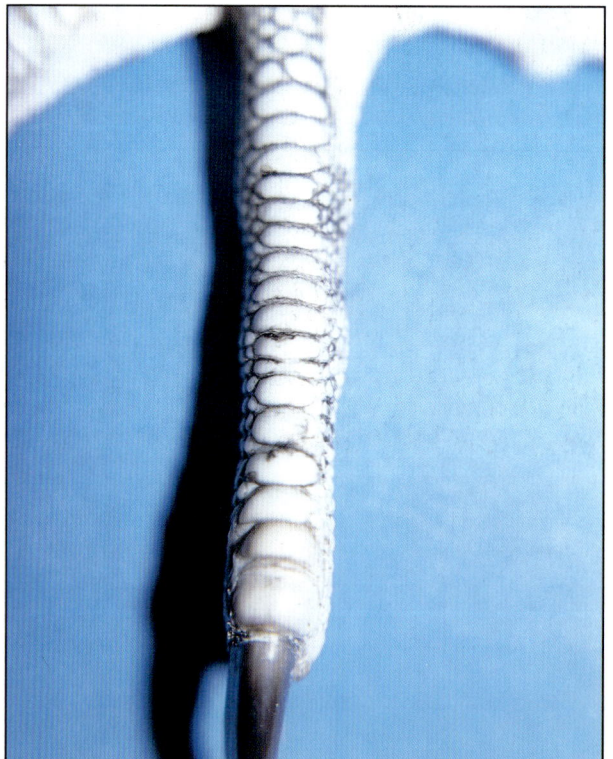

Figs. 6.4 and 6.5: These pictures show the pattern of scales on the middle digit of two different gyrfalcon X saker falcon hybrids.
(Photos: Heidenreich)

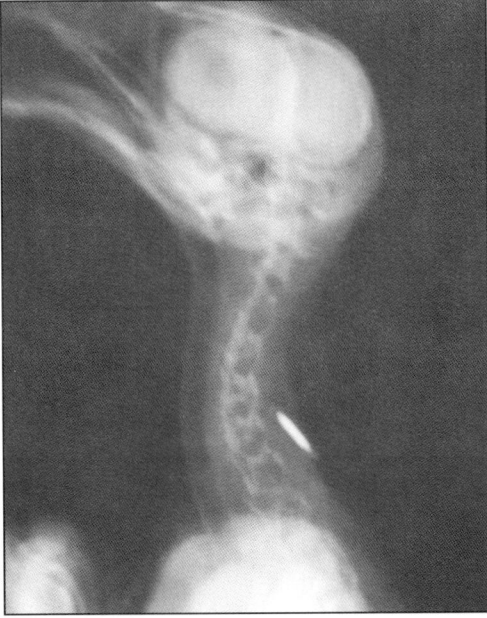

6.6

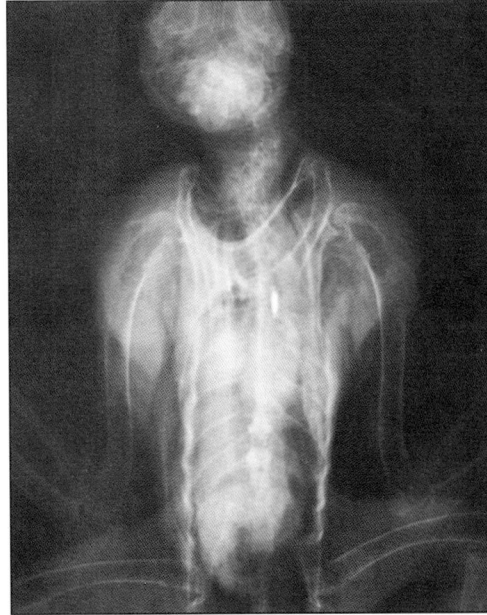

6.7

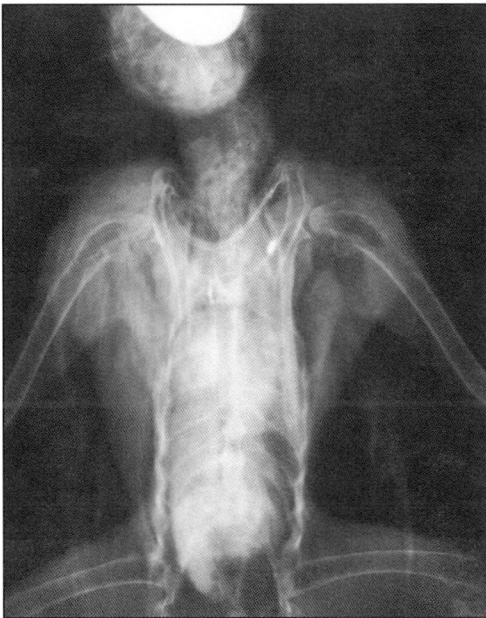

6.8

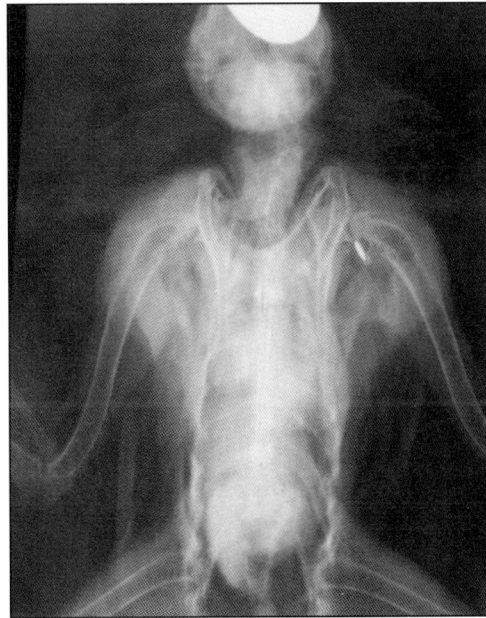

6.9

c. Subcutaneous placement of a microchip is safest in terms of the animal's health. However, the microchip is then identifiable by palpation, making it potentially easy to remove and transfer to another bird (Fig. 6.6–6.11).

Figs. **6.6, 6.7, 6.8, 6.9, 6.10, 6.11:** The least dangerous location for transponder implantation is under the loose skin in the nape of the neck (6.6). 6.7, 6.8, 6.9: These radiographs show a transponder located in the pectoral muscles (6.7) of a hunting falcon (*F. peregrinus*) that migrated towards the shoulder (6.8 and 6.9) in only a few weeks.
The same phenomenon was observed with a microchip located in the thigh muscles of a bird (6.10). The device migrated within the muscle belly to the tendinous insertion near the joint (6.11).
(Radiographs and photos: Heidenreich)

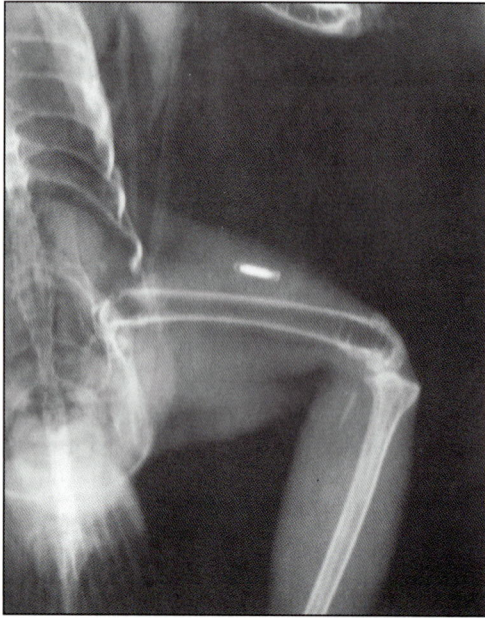

6.10

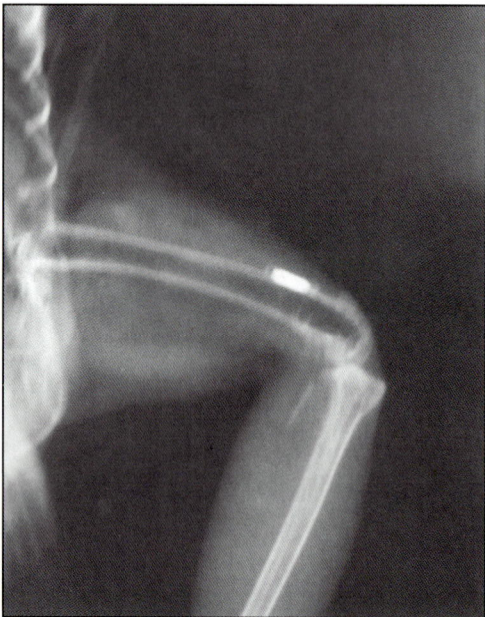

6.11

6.8   Color marking of chicks

Chicks that are being hand-raised are often kept in groups to facilitate imprinting on their own kind and promote socialization skills. Such chicks must nevertheless be individually identifiable. Before they are leg-banded, the animals can be marked with permanent marker on the downy feathers of the head (Fig 6.12). These markings will be lost as adult plumage replaces the down.

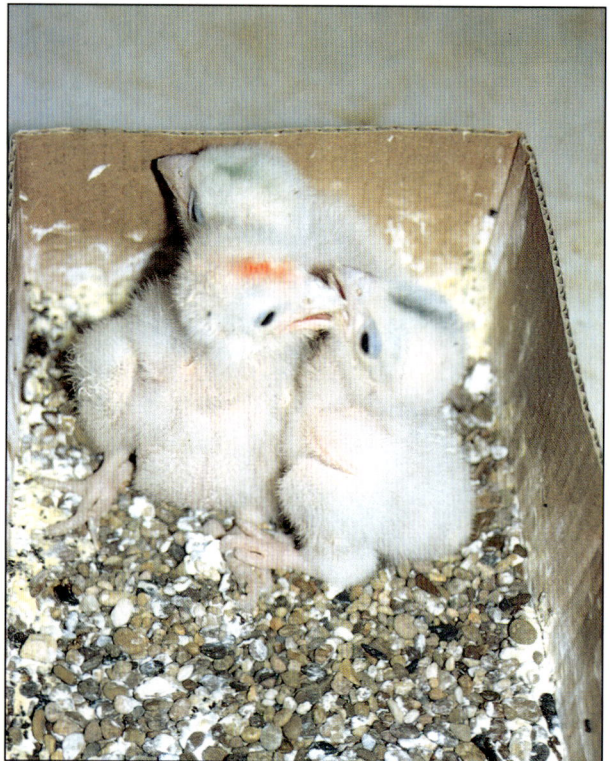

Abb. 6.12:

Fig. 6.12: In order to keep track of individual chicks before they are banded, the downy feathers of the head can be marked with a permanent marking pen. (Photo: Heidenreich)

6.7   Egg marking

When breeding raptors, the positive identification of eggs can be very important. Frequently, several clutches will be artificially incubated simultaneously, but the parentage of each needs to be known and recorded. Eggs can easily be labeled with non-toxic graphite pencils. Care must be taken to separate the eggs prior to hatching so that each chick can be identified by the egg shell it came from.

6.9   DNA fingerprinting

Gene technology, too, has become a part of raptor management in recent years. There are two areas where this technology has proven particularly useful. Genetic relationships between various species can be explored using DNA analysis (Seibold, 1994) and familial relationships can be established in this way as well. The latter can be of special use to authorities seeking to investigate false breeding claims.

Another use for this technology lies in confirming the identity of escaped or stolen birds. A DNA sample can be stored in advance for any bird. The genetic fingerprint is unique for each individual and can be checked at any time. If necessary, the previously stored sample can later be compared to that of a recovered bird in order to prove its identity. Blood or tissue samples usually contain ample nuclear material for this procedure. In raptors, a mere 0.2 ml of blood are required for DNA sampling.

DNA fingerprinting methods

The DNA molecule is a double-stranded helix composed of four different building blocks, called nucleotides. The nucleotide sequence encodes for genes that in turn contain the information required by the cell to build proteins. Complex interactions within this system determine the function and appearance of an organism. The exact DNA sequence varies slightly for each individual animal, and these small differences are utilized in the process of DNA fingerprinting (Fig. 6.13).

In a laboratory, special procedures permit extraction of the DNA from cell nuclei. Restriction enzymes are then used to cut the long DNA strands at certain locations bearing a specific nucleotide sequence. The result is a mixture of countless DNA segments of variable size. The mixture of DNA fragments will be different for each individual, because each genome is different.

The DNA fragments are applied to one end of an agar gel and then subjected to an electric current that pulls them through the thick material. Naturally, smaller fragments will travel faster than larger ones. This results in a separation of the fragments based on size along the gel. Special labeled probes that attach to cer-

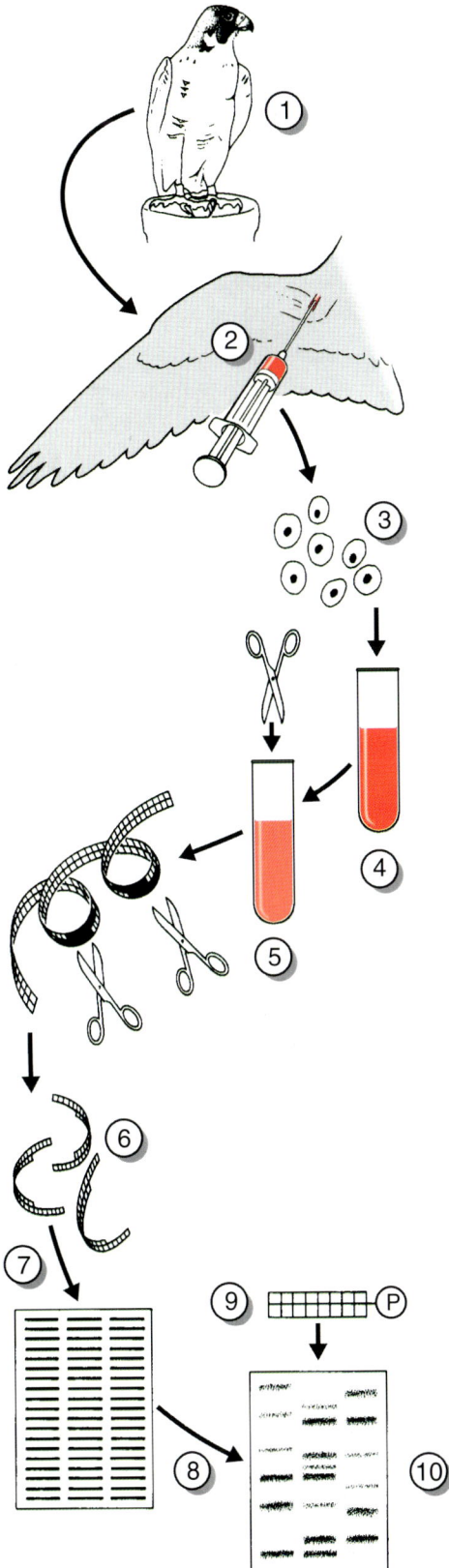

Fig. 6.13: A blood sample (2) is easily obtained for purposes of DNA fingerprinting. Avian red blood cells are nucleated (3) and contain ample DNA (4). This is broken down in a laboratory by restriction enzymes (scissors, 5) that cut the DNA double helix at certain nucleotide sequences. A large number of DNA fragments of different lengths (6) are produced and separated by gel electrophoresis (7). After the fragments are split into single strands (denatured), they are hybridized (bonded) with special DNA probes designed to complement certain DNA sequences (8). The probes (9) are labeled such that they allow visualization of the DNA fragments to which they bind in the form of bars when combined with special dyes or exposed to X-ray film (10).
(Illustration: R. Gattung-Petith and A. Gattung)

tain DNA fragments are then applied to produce a distinct pattern of visible bands.

The band pattern of an individual should be a combination of the parent's patterns, since one half of the genetic code is inherited from each (Fig. 6.14). More distantly related individuals will still have certain patterns in common. Only identical twins, highly inbred populations or DNA from the same individual will show identical band sequences. This is the basis of DNA fingerprinting. A very good introduction into this subject is given by Lubjuhn et al. (1994).

This technology has been used in court in Germany in a case involving false raptor breeding claims. Since then, both the authorities and breeders have demonstrated increasing interest in such technology.

Studies have shown that DNA fingerprinting itself is remarkably independent of the laboratory methods used. This does not imply that such procedures can be performed by just anyone. Only well-established laboratories should be used if reliable results are to be obtained. Some people have criticized the statistical analyses employed in establishing paternity by these methods. However, so far such results have always agreed with paternity determinations obtained by other methods.

DNA fingerprinting is available very reliably in Germany through EBW DNA-Analytik, Institut für molekulargenetische Diagnostik GmbH, Universitätsstrasse 142, 44799 Bochum. They will provide an information sheet, submission forms and the required sample tubes upon request. Results usually take two to three weeks. The cost per individual bird is DM 150.00. Proof of paternity costs DM 450.00, since three DNA samples are required, one from each parent and one from the offspring. Further offspring for the same pair cost only DM 150.00.

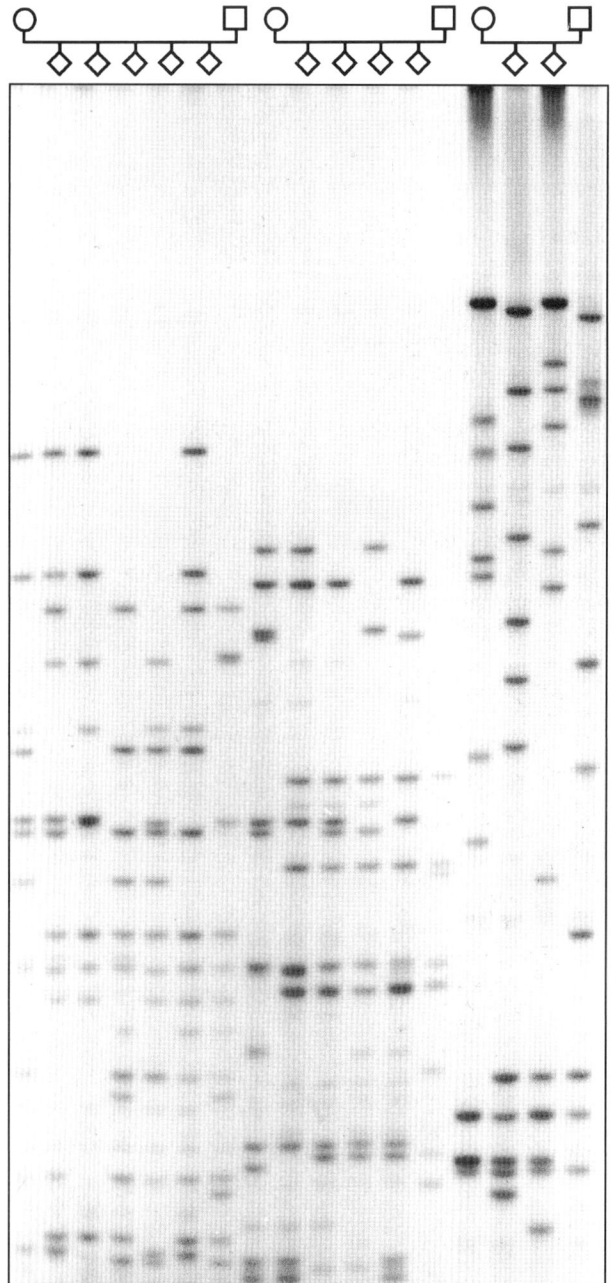

Fig. 6.14: Three families (parents designated as ○ and □) were investigated using DNA fingerprinting technology. The offspring of the families on the left and in the middle all show a banding pattern that is a combination of that displayed by their parents. On the basis of the number of bands examined, there is 99.9% certainty that the paternity is correct as shown. The offspring of the family on the right display some bands that are not present in the DNA fingerprint of their supposed parents. This clearly indicates that they are not derived from the pair shown.
(These figures were kindly provided by Dr. V. Wagner, EBW DNA-Analytik, Bochum)

References and literature of further interest

BEDNAREK, W. (1990):
Greifvogelzucht und DNA-Fingerprinting.
Greifvögel und Falknerei 15–19
Verlag Neumann-Neudamm, Morschen-Heina

BEYERBACH, U. (1980):
Kennzeichnung und Identifikation von Greifvögeln.
Prakt. Tierarzt **61**, 936, 938, 940

HEIDENREICH, M. and H. KÜSPERT (1994):
Zum Einsatz von Transpondern bei Falken.
Zool. Garten **64**, 124–136

KÜSPERT, H., HEIDENREICH, M. and H.J. KÜSPERT (1993):
Falkenzucht Teil 3: Verwaltung und tierärztliche Betreuung
Voliere **16**, 330– 335

LUBJUHN, T., SCHARTL, M. and J.T. EPPLEN (1994):
Methodik und Anwendungsgebiete des genetischen Finger-
abdruckverfahrens.
Biologie **24**, 9–14

RICHTER, T. (1990):
Der kleine Unterschied.
Greifvögel und Falknerei 21-23
Verlag Neumann-Neudamm, Morschen-Heina

RYCHLIK, I., KUBICEK, O., HOLCAK, V., BARTA, and I.J. PAVLIK
(1994):
DNA fingerprinting in Falconidae.
Vet. Med. **39**, 111–116

SEIBOLD, I. (1994):
Untersuchungen zur molekularen Phylogenie der Greifvögel
anhand von DNA-Sequenzen des mitochondriellen Cytochrom
b-Gens.
Diss., Heidelberg, Hartung Gorre-Verlag, Konstanz

STAUBER, E.H. (1984):
Footprinting of raptors for identification.
Raptor Res.**18**, 67–71

STAUBER, E.H. (1985):
Greifvogel-Identifikation mit Hilfe fotografischer Analyse der
Zehenschilder.
Jb. Dtsch. Falkenorden 37–39

WOLFES, R., MATHE, J. and A. SEITZ (1991):
Forensics of birds of prey by DNA fingerprinting with
33P-labeled oligonucleotide probes.
Electrophoresis.**12**, 175–180

WINK, M., SWATSCHEK, I., FELDMANN, F., SCHARLAU, W.
and D. RISTOW (1990):
Untersuchungen von Verwandtschaftsbeziehungen in Vogel-
populationen mittels DNA-Fingerprint.
Vogelwelt **111**, 86–95

WINK, M. (1993):
Molekulare Methoden in der Greifvogelforschung.
Greifvögel und Falknerei 17–28,
Verlag Neumann-Neudamm, Morschen-Heina

7 Clinical examination

7.1 Capture

While the handling and transport of trained hawks is usually not difficult, capturing birds of prey housed in aviaries generally poses some problems. Aviary birds are often shy and react with panic to capture, sometimes injuring themselves in reckless attempts to escape. This is when a properly designed aviary pays off. The first requirement is a large capture net made of lightweight material. The rim should be flexible, at least on one side, and the netting strong and tight enough that neither head nor wings can get caught in it. Capture should involve trapping or pushing the hawk down on the ground rather than entangling it in the net. Once in the net, both the raptor's legs should be restrained in one hand while its neck is firmly grasped below the head in the other. Covering the eyes with a hood or a towel will calm the bird and reduce struggling. Care must be taken to ensure that the animal can still breathe freely (Fig. 7.1).

Birds that kill their prey by grasping, such as eagles and goshawks, threaten the handler primarily with their talons, although some of them have learned to employ the beak in defense as well. Falcons kill by biting and will therefore readily use their sharp beak as well as their feet. Large vultures can bite very hard, producing serious wounds if handled carelessly.

Occasionally, injured or sick wild raptors or escaped captive birds must be captured. This can be difficult and requires a thorough knowledge of the animal's behavior and biology. Baited traps or sedative-laced bait are often employed in these cases.

The type of trap used varies with the kind of bird to be captured. Below is a brief list of possible capture methods.

Goshawk cage trap
This trap consists of a wire basket outfitted with two large, netted, spring-activated bows on top that close over the bird after being sprung. Live pigeons typically serve as bait in the basket, remaining visible but separate underneath the actual trap. The bait animals should be left there only during the day and should be supplied with food and water. An additional door

opens once the trap has been sprung, releasing the pigeons. This avoids the stress of having a predator trapped above them. If homing pigeons are used, the added advantage is that their return signals the falconer that the trap has been sprung. The catcher can often wait within sight of the trap if the bird to be trapped was previously captive and is therefore less shy.

These commercially available devices are suitable only for goshawks or smaller birds of prey. The trap doors can sometimes cause injuries if they close directly on a bird. Padding them can help, or one can choose to use a different capture technique.

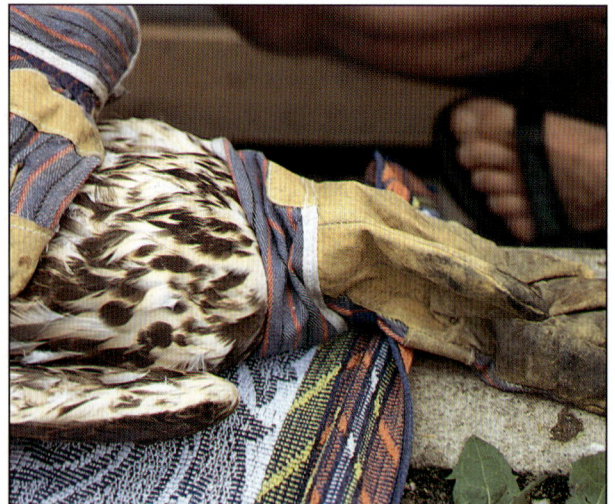

Fig. 7.1: Inexperienced people assigned to draw blood from this falcon (*F. cherrug*) placed its head inside a work glove to protect themselves from being bitten. This type of treatment is to be strongly discouraged. There is no guarantee that the excited bird is receiving enough oxygen.
(Photo: Heidenreich)

Bal-Chatri noose trap

This capture device is easy to make using a wire cage outfitted with many strong nooses of nylon fishing line all around. The nooses should have a diameter twice as large as the foot span of the bird to be caught. Depending on the raptor to be captured, small birds, mice, rats or pigeons can be used as bait. The wire mesh should be fine enough to prevent the occupant of the cage from pulling a noose inside and becoming entangled. This type of trap should be used only under constant supervision, since the nooses can get wound around a bird's neck as well as its feet, requiring immediate intervention. Although any kind of raptor can be trapped with such a device, the cage should be chosen heavy enough that the entangled bird cannot fly away with it (Bednarek, 1992).

Snare harness

Very shy hawks that cannot be captured with other types of traps can often be caught using a snare harness. This device consists of a wire or leather harness with a number of nooses attached (Fig. 7.2). The harness is attached to the bait animal such that the nooses lie on its back without interfering with its mobility. The bait animal with its harness is tied to a long string. When released near the hawk to be captured, it will lure the bird down and entangle it in the nooses on the harness.

This technique is used very successfully in Arab countries to capture wild falcons.

Winding up

A bird that will come to a lure but not permit a person to approach or pick it up may be captured by "winding up". A lure or bait is placed on the ground and tied to a line, one end of which is fastened next to it with a peg in the ground. Once the hawk is on the lure and eating, the catcher begins to walk around the bird carefully, keeping the line relatively taut and so winding it around the bird's legs a few times until it is unable to escape.

Anesthetics

If nothing else works, anesthetics can be employed to catch a wild or escaped bird. This method carries a much greater risk, since the birds may be able to fly quite a distance after administration of the drug and may then be difficult to find. Orally administered anesthetics have the slowest absorption time and should therefore be avoided. Other methods of administration are justified only under special circumstances.

If a larger raptor can be approached closely, an injection with a dart from a blow pipe into the breast muscles may be possible. This method requires experience and accuracy. The main drawback is the resulting panic and escape on the part of the bird. Parenterally administered drugs take effect relatively rapidly, and the distances covered by the escaping animal are usually small.

7.2 Transport to veterinarian

The principles of raptor transport were discussed in Chapter 3. When taking a bird of prey to a veterinarian, it is wise to bring along all the accessories the bird may need if it is to stay there for a while. This generally includes a gauntlet, a hood and a perch of some sort. A recent sample of the animal's mutes can also be useful, especially since most birds travel better on an empty crop and stomach or may be anorexic due to illness.

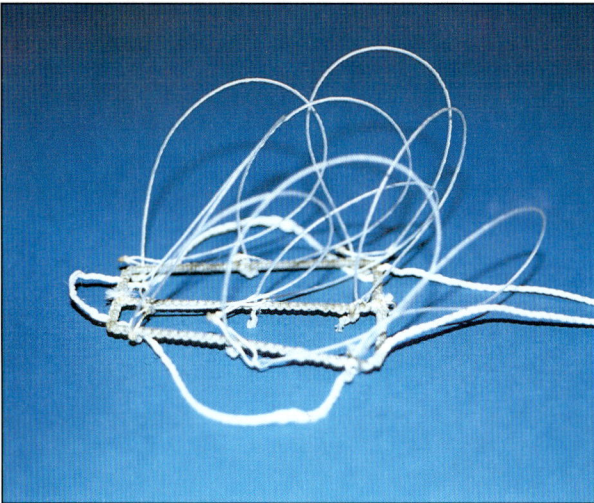

Fig. 7.2: The snare harness is placed on a living pigeon and reliably used by Arabs to capture falcons.
(Photo: Heidenreich)

7.3   The examination process

7.3.1   Clinical history

The animal's history as reported by the owner is of great importance in making a diagnosis. Most falconers and animal caretakers know their animal very well and will pick up on subtle changes in attitude or behavior. In addition, they have the opportunity to observe the bird during eating, mating, flight and other activities which are not possible in the veterinary clinic. In fact, many sick birds will pull themselves together and appear brighter and more alert in unfamiliar surroundings.

Wild animals are also capable of hiding minor illnesses until they have progressed to the point where it is impossible to conceal them anymore. This is a survival strategy, as the appearance of illness makes any wild animal vulnerable to predation. The early stages of disease are thus easily overlooked in birds of prey.

7.3.2   Observation from a distance

Valuable information is obtained if the bird can be evaluated from a distance in its normal environment. Ideally, the animal is unaware of being observed and is acting completely naturally. Sometimes examination of its surroundings can also provide clues or information regarding the patient's problem.

Table 7.1 gives some guidelines for determining when a bird of prey is ill.

7.3.3   Restraint

Uncooperative raptors need to be firmly restrained for physical examination. This prevents injury to both the bird and the examiner. Raptors that kill with their talons tend to defend themselves with their feet, sometimes throwing themselves on their back and viciously grasping at anything that comes near. Those that kill by biting rely more on their beak for defense,

Table 7.1: Behavioral differences between healthy and sick birds of prey

Behavior	Healthy bird	Sick bird
Involvement and responsiveness	Alert, reacts to visual and auditory stimuli	Sleepy, unresponsive
Activity level	Flies around in aviary except after eating or bathing	Motionless for hours
Confined flight (in aviary)	Typical flight for species	Flies "crooked", tail feathers spread, unstable landing
Free flight (trained hawk)	Typical flight for species	Rests frequently, low endurance, hawk may refuse to leave falconer or fly away altogether
Posture at rest	One leg tucked up, wings folded comfortably along body	Stands on two legs, frequently shifting from one to the other, may lie down, wings droop
Posture during sleep	Head tucked into feathers on back	Eyes closed, head retracted
Eating	Consumes food rapidly and ravenously	Eats slowly with frequent pauses, may fling bits of food away
Defecation	Lifts tail to expel mutes	Feces may run out involuntarily, bird may not defecate at all, or may strain excessively
Breathing	Quiet, regular breaths with beak closed, respirations barely visible	Works hard to breathe, open mouth, irregular breaths, tail bobbing, abdominal breathing noticeable

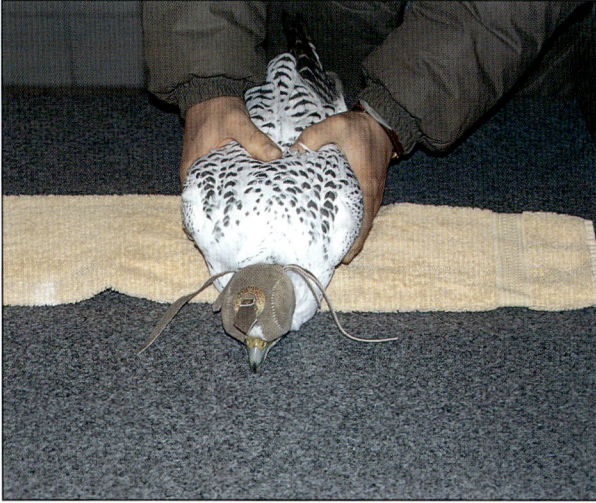

7.3

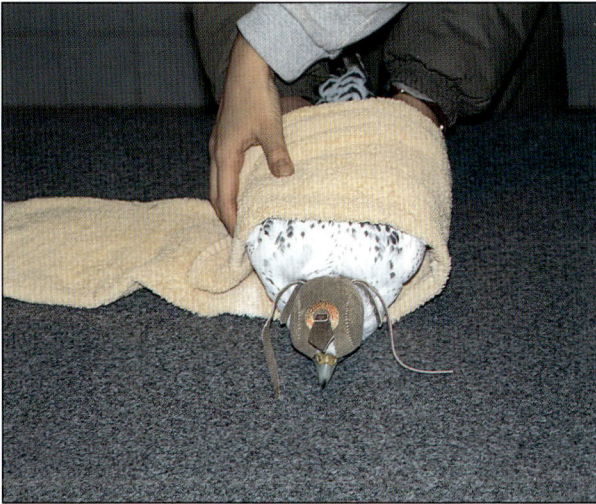

7.4

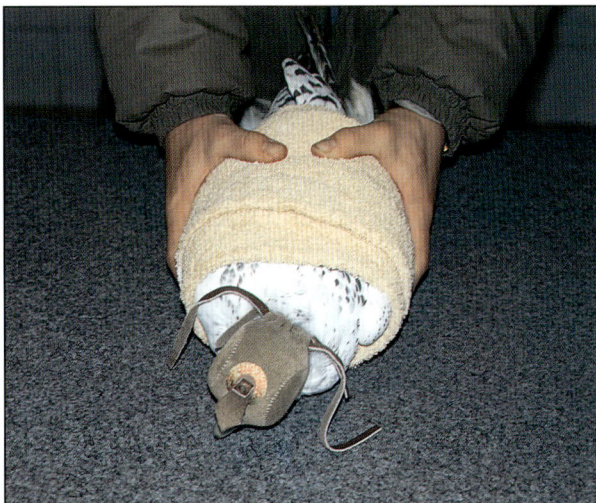

7.5

but will employ their talons as well if given the opportunity.

It is best to grasp both legs of such birds firmly between the hock and foot in one gloved hand, making sure to keep one finger between the two legs. The animal can then be supported upright with its back against the handler's chest.

Wrapping the bird in a towel can help reduce struggling and protect the plumage (Fig 7.3–7.5). A slightly damp towel is best. The animal should be wrapped tightly enough that it can't fight or free itself, yet breathing should be unimpaired. This type of restraint should be limited to a few minutes only. Never transport a bird wrapped this way, since hyperventilation and hyperthermia can rapidly lead to death under such circumstances. A large number of falcons were killed this way in Spain in 1992. The environmental authorities had confiscated them and wrapped them in paper towels secured with adhesive tape for several hours of transport. Many of the birds succumbed to hyperthermia and stress or suffocated on their own saliva!

The grasping of legs, tail and flight feathers together in one hand, as is sometimes suggested, should be avoided as well. It may damage the plumage and does not provide adequate restraint.

Any examination of a wild bird entails significant stress. If there are no medical contraindications, short-term anesthesia may permit an examination to be performed with less strain on both the bird and the veterinarian.

7.3.4   Physical examination

7.3.4.1 Body condition and body weight

Body condition and weight are usually directly correlated, that is, a bird in good body condition typically has an adequate body weight for its species and sex. Body weight is determined with a scale while body condition is evaluated by manual palpation of the breast muscles.

Exceptions to this correlation can occur under certain circumstances. Birds that do not fly much and

Figs. 7.3, 7.4, and 7.5: This white gyrfalcon (*Falco rusticolus*) is grasped with both hands over the back and placed in sternal recumbency on a folded towel (7.3). The shorter end of the towel is brought snugly across the back and tucked in under the keel (7.4). The other end is brought across the bird's body in such a way that the wings are firmly restrained against the body while the abdomen remains free (7.5).
(Photos: Heidenreich)

spend most of their time sitting on a perch may be in poor physical condition and fat. Their body weight will be in the normal range, but palpation of the pectoral muscles reveals severe atrophy and a prominent keel. Active hunting hawks, on the other hand, often weigh less than expected and yet show well-developed breast musculature. They have no fat deposits and a lean, athletic body.

7.3.4.2 Examination of individual organs

The same pattern should be followed for every examination. This helps to avoid forgetting an organ system. A useful rule of thumb is: from front to back and from outside to inside. Table 7.2 gives a suggested order of examination and lists some possible abnormalities that may be encountered.

7.4   Laboratory diagnostics

Frequently, a thorough physical exam will not suffice to make an accurate diagnosis. Further diagnostics are required.

7.4.1   Fecal examination

An examination of a fecal sample is simple and can provide a great deal of information. Fecal parasite checks should be done every six months in hunting hawks. Parasite burdens can become a special problem during training due to the stress associated with such activity. Stress impairs immune function, and thus a latent parasitic infection that would otherwise not be noticed can flare up and cause problems.

Table 7.2: Suggested physical examination sequence and possible abnormal findings

Organ system	Abnormal findings
Plumage	Feathers dull or soiled, no powder down, patchy plumage or alopecia, broken or moth-eaten feathers, water fails to bead on surface
Skin	Scaly, crusty (parasitism), wounds, pruritus, swollen or discolored lesions (pox, etc.)
Eyes	Corneal opacities due to injury, cataracts (old age), fundic lesions (retinal detachments with head trauma), proptosis (tumors) or enophthalmos, abnormalities in pupillary size or response
Eyelids	Crusty or watering, swollen, torn, lesions of the third eyelid (nictitans)
Infraorbital sinus	Swelling between eye and cere, "owl's head" appearance
Ear canal	Crusty or sticky exudate with otitis, growths, foreign bodies
Beak	Cracked or crusty (mites, nutritional deficiencies), misshapen (rickets or trauma), overgrown, soiled (fractures of the basihyoid bone)
Oral cavity	Mucosal lesions with parasitic or fungal infections, abscesses after injuries, swelling of the glottis, tongue infections, choanae, atypical odor
Nares	Discharge, crusting, fractured operculum
Cere	Injuries, discoloration
Thorax	Asymmetry of pectoral musculature (indicates disuse of one wing), sternal fractures, misshapen sternum with rickets
Abdomen	Distention with egg binding, tumors and fractures, edema of abdominal skin (normal prior to egg-laying)
Cloaca	Soiling, prolapse, tears after dystocia
Wings	Fractures, luxations, joint swelling; necrosis and sticky feathers – wing tip edema
Legs and feet	Deformities, fractures, paresis, ruptured extensor tendons, neurological disorders, leg band injuries, pododermatitis, talon deformities, necrosis or gangrene after frostbite, roughened epidermal scales
Tail	Paresis with neurological disorders or fractures of the pygostyle, broken feathers due to poor management
Uropygial gland	Impaction, swelling, injuries (usually self-inflicted)

Breeding birds confined to aviaries can also be exposed to a mounting parasite burden within their small home. Regular parasite control and occasional replacement of the aviary substrate can help minimize such risks.

Obtaining feces

A teaspoon's worth of feces (about 10 g) is sufficient for a parasite examination. It is best obtained by spreading plastic wrap, wax paper or aluminum foil under the bird's perch in an aviary or around a block or bow perch. The fecal material will thus not be contaminated by the substrate. In the clinic, one may have to wait for a bird to defecate. Hooded birds frequently do so right after removal of the hood. Placing a small amount of water in a bird's mouth with a syringe may also induce it to defecate. The excitement of being in an unfamiliar place stimulates more frequent excretion, so obtaining feces is not usually a problem. If necessary, a moistened cotton swab can be used to obtain a sample directly from the cloaca.

Mailing fecal samples

Fecal samples should be mailed to a veterinarian for examination in a stable, unbreakable container such as a plastic film canister and shipped well-packaged. Regular letters are run through a stamping machine by the postal service and are therefore unsuitable for submitting samples.

Visual inspection of feces

Close evaluation of the fecal sample with the naked eye can provide valuable information. Form and color will vary substantially depending on the type of diet, the fullness of the GI tract and other factors (see Figs. 7.6–7.11). Occasionally, simply washing the sample with tap water and then passing it through a sieve will reveal abnormal materials such as sand, grass or fibrinous pseudomembranes.

Microscopic examination

Two methods can be employed in the search for fecal parasite ova (eggs):

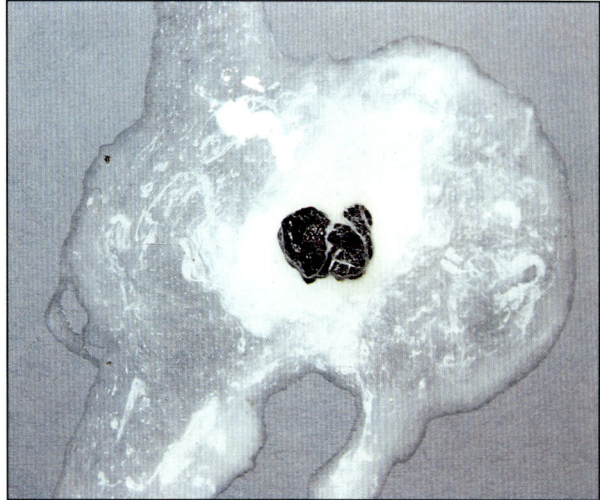

7.6

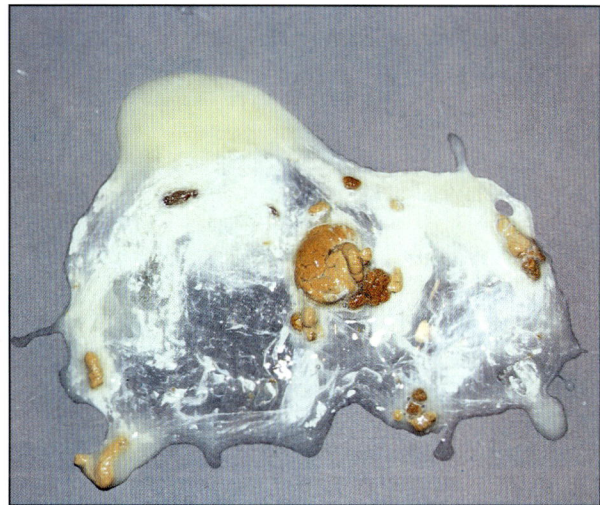

7.7

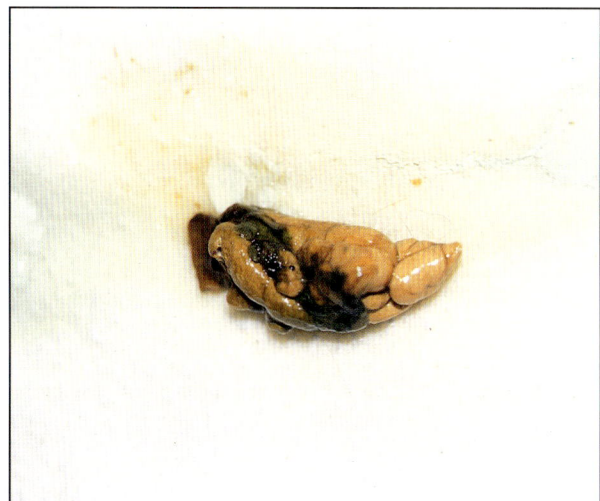

Figs. 7.6, 7.7 and 7.8: Mutes from healthy raptors: The fecal material is formed and black in color due to the normal digestion of red meat (7.6). The fecal material can also appear yellowish and granular if white, fatty meat has been consumed (7.7). If the bird is eating day-old chicks, which have little down, the sausage-like pellet may be excreted with the feces rather than being cast (7.8). (Photos: Heidenreich)

7.8

Fecal flotation: The fecal material is suspended in a salt or sugar solution with a high specific gravity. The parasite ova will be less dense than the solution and float to the surface, where they can easily be removed for examination. Different ova have different densities (nematode eggs are lighter than trematode eggs), therefore one should use a solution with the highest possible specific gravity. Saturated sugar or salt (NaCl) solutions may fail to float some of the heavier eggs. The best solution is therefore made using zinc chloride and salt (25.7g $ZnCl_2$ + 26.3 g NaCl in 100 ml of water).

Several grams of fecal material are suspended in approximately 10 ml of flotation solution and then filtered through a sieve into a centrifuge tube. The mixture is centrifuged for three minutes at 300 G, then a few droplets from the surface of the tube are applied to a slide and scanned at low power.

Sedimentation: The eggs of cestodes and acanthocephalans are particularly heavy and will not float using the techniques described above. To find them, the sediment in the centrifuge tube must also be examined. This involves decanting the solution from the tube and then resuspending the pellet found at the bottom in a small amount of water. Microscopic examination of this suspension in a petri dish will reveal any eggs that failed to float.

Figures 7.12–7.23 show some of the more common parasite ova or oocysts found in birds of prey.

Evaluating the results

Finding and identifying parasite ova in a fecal sample makes the diagnosis obvious and easy. However, failure to find such eggs does not always indicate that the bird is free of parasites. All endoparasites have a prepatent period between the time of initial infection and the detectable presence of ova in the host's feces. This period of time can last up to several weeks, during which the host is infected and possibly suffering from

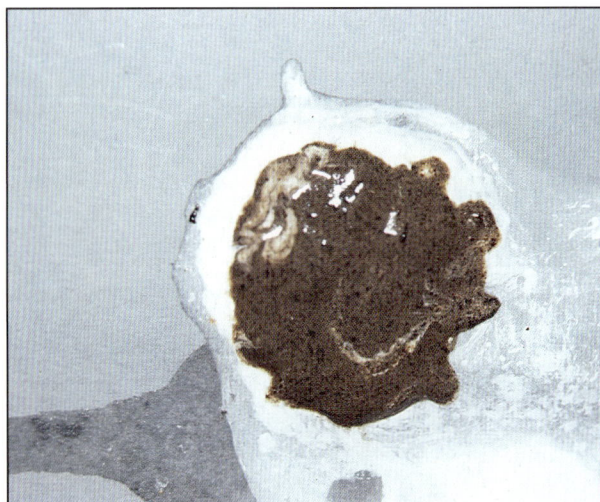

7.9

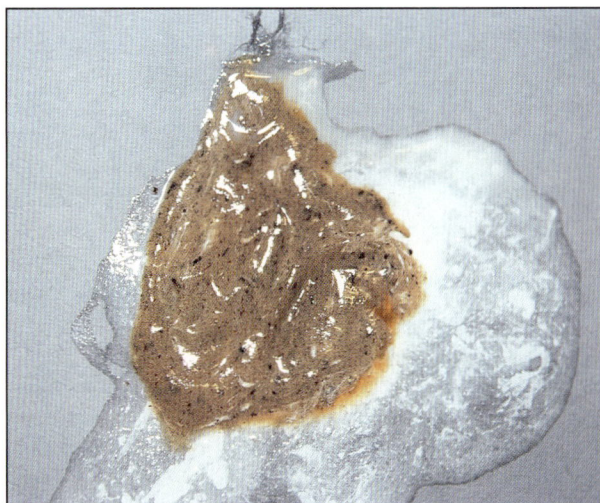

7.10

Figs. 7.9, 7.10 and 7.11:
Mutes from diseased raptors:
A bird with coccidiosis excreted this soft, pasty fecal material (7.9). Two days later, the same bird produced feces that are beginning to show traces of blood (7.10).
Characteristic pastel-green urates are seen a few days before death in cases of severe disease involving liver and kidneys. The green color derives from biliverdin produced in the liver and verdiglobin produced from the breakdown of hemoglobin in the kidneys after renal hemorrhage (7.11).
(Photos: Heidenreich)

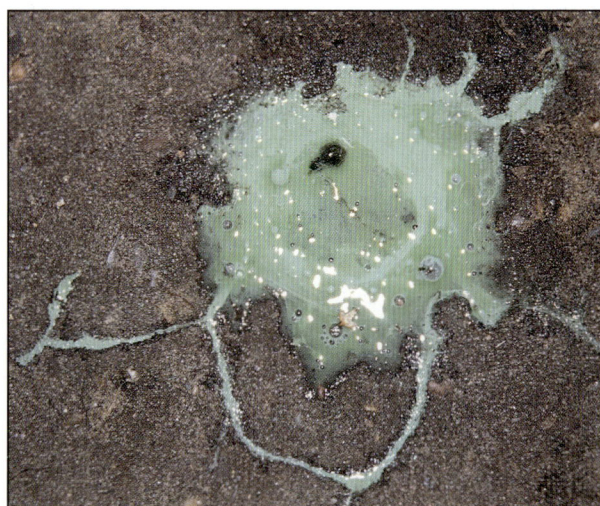

7.11

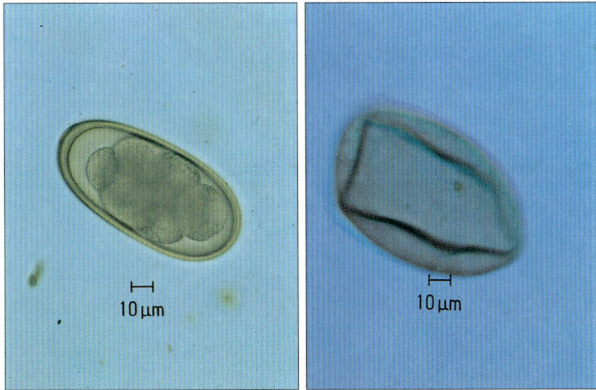

7.12

7.13

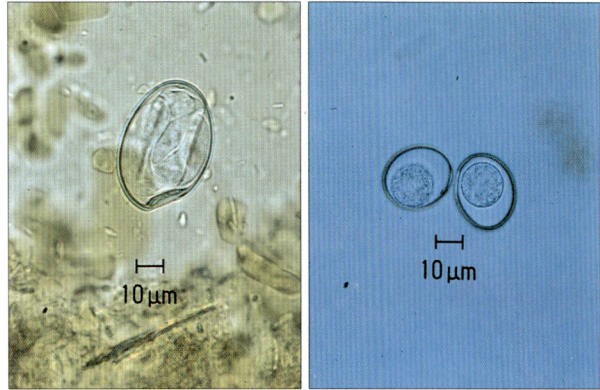

7.14

7.15

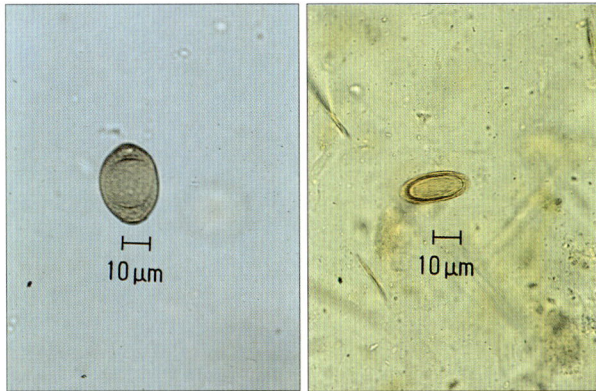

7.16

7.17

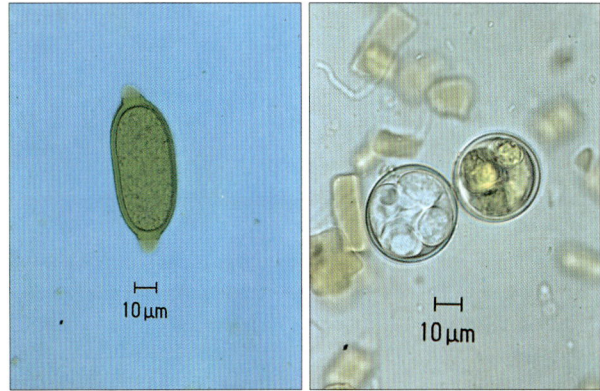

7.18

7.19

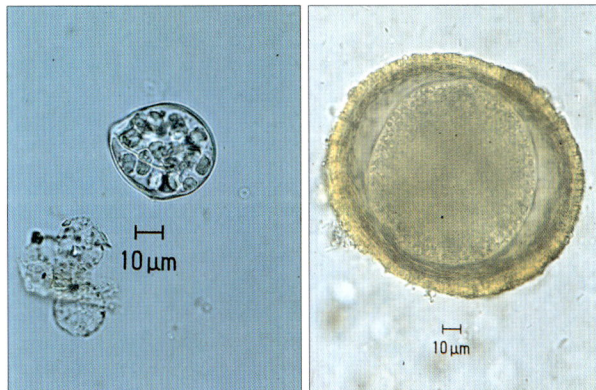

7.20

7.21

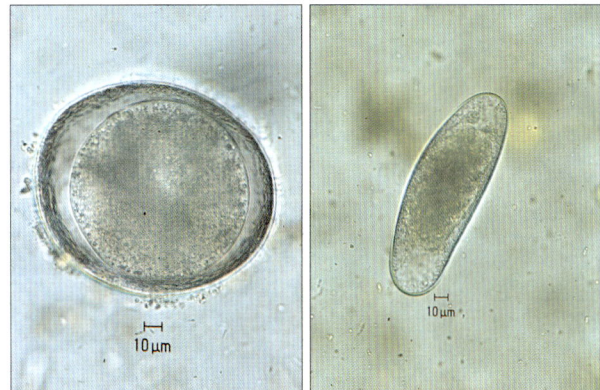

7.22

7.23

Fig. 7.12: A gapeworm (*Syngamus sp.)* egg.
Fig. 7.13: A tapeworm egg from a raptor
Fig. 7.14: The embryonated egg of an air sac nematode
(*Serratospiculum* sp.*).
Fig. 7.15: Coccidial oocysts (*Caryospora* sp.*).
Fig. 7.16: A trematode (fluke) egg.
Fig. 7.17: An acanthocephalan egg.
Fig. 7.18: *Capillaria sp.* egg showing the typical bipolar
plugs.

Fig. 7.19: An incidental finding of a sporulated coccidial
oocyst (*Eimeria* sp.). The parasite probably
stems from a bird ingested by the raptor.
Fig. 7.20: An unidentified parasite egg.
Fig. 7.21: An ascarid egg (*Porrocaecum* sp.*).
Fig. 7.22: An ascarid egg (*Porrocaecum* sp.*).
Fig. 7.23: The egg of an ectoparasite.
(Photos: Lierz, with kind assistance from B. Nothelfer
(Central Veterinary Research Laboratory, U.A.E.)

the effects of the parasite without one's being able to make a diagnosis. It is therefore wise to reevaluate a second sample from a previously negative bird after several weeks.

The identification of parasitic infections in raptors requires a thorough knowledge of the parasites common in these species and their eggs. Even so, one often encounters parasites that are not readily identifiable, especially in wild birds.

Additionally, parasites from a prey animal that has been consumed can pass unchanged into the feces of raptors, adding to the challenge of making a diagnosis. Fecal samples from hunting goshawks, for example, often contain large quantities of rabbit bile duct coccidia. Not infrequently, capillaria or ascarid ova found in a sample from a raptor actually come from the poultry used as a food source for the bird. An occasional louse or mite egg (Fig. 7.23) can be swallowed during preening and add to the confusion. Their chitinous shell protects them from digestion during their passage through the GI tract.

Frequently, a well-intentioned raptor owner will also request that a bacterial culture be performed on a fecal sample. Apart from the remote possibility of detecting potential tuberculosis, chlamydia or salmonella organisms, fecal cultures are of limited usefulness in otherwise healthy birds. The results are more likely to create unnecessary concern than to aid in making a diagnosis of disease. Normal fecal samples harbor a large variety of bacteria that make up the normal enteric flora of a carnivore and do not cause disease. If they are cultured and tested for antimicrobial sensitivities in order to place the bird on antibiotics, more harm than good will come of it.

As with parasites, bacterial cultures may reveal bacteria (such as *Salmonella* spp.) that were simply ingested and passed through with the food. Only repeated cultures after changing the diet can resolve the question of the importance of such a finding. It is probably wise to let go of the notion that every pathogenic organism isolated by culture indicates a disease process.

7.4.2 Swab samples

Samples of material from the mouth, nose, esophagus, trachea, or cloaca can be collected using a cotton swab or Q-tip® moistened with physiological saline. This technique is particularly effective at demonstrating trichomonads in birds with frounce. In such cases, the sample should be immediately evaluated under a microscope with phase contrast capabilities, since the tiny motile parasites quickly succumb at room temperature.

7.4.3 Skin scrapings and feather examinations

Skin lesions should be scraped with a scalpel blade until blood oozes. The sample thus obtained is mixed on a slide with 30% potassium hydroxide (KOH) and examined under the microscope after approximately 30 minutes. The potassium hydroxide will dissolve all protein-based connective tissue and cells, leaving the chitinous exoskeletons of skin parasites intact and easy to identify.

Feather examinations make sense only if the sample is obtained in the clinic and examined immediately. If feather mites are present in the shaft, they will quickly leave as the feather is removed from the body and cools off. If a feather sample needs to be mailed, it should immediately be placed in an airtight transparent plastic bag. Any parasites that were present may later be found in the corners of the bag.

7.4.4 Pellet examination

The pellet or casting regurgitated by a raptor after a meal consists of indigestible materials such as hair, feathers, claws, grains and even bones from the ingested animal. Evaluating these remains can provide valuable information regarding a bird's health and digestive activity. Normal castings are oval in shape, firm yet elastic, slightly damp and odorless. The surface may be coated with a thin layer of mucus. Un-

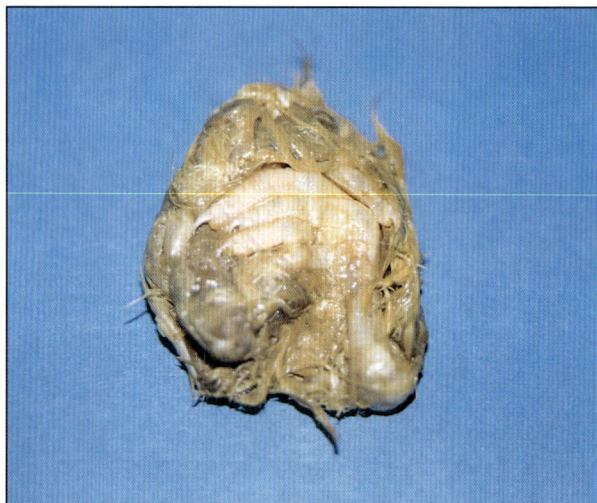

Fig. 7.24: Undigested pieces of food in the casting of a raptor indicate a serious digestive disorder.
(Photo: Heidenreich)

digested meat particles (Fig. 7.24) or a rotting odor indicate a digestive disorder or premature casting of the pellet (often due to stress). Blood stains on a pellet result from inflammatory processes or injuries in the esophagus or stomach. Pellet examinations are facilitated by the feeding of white laboratory rodents. The next casting will also be white and changes in color will be easier to detect.

In cases of oral and esophageal capillariasis, the typical bipolar eggs may also be found in a pellet.

7.4.5 Urate examination

A normal urinalysis is not possible in birds because they produce a relatively concentrated mixture of urates and feces. In cases of polyuria (watery urates), the urinary portion may be separated from the feces and evaluated to a limited degree. Microscopic amounts of blood can be detected using a special test strip (such as Combur®-Test). Because of possible fecal contamination, any abnormal results should be interpreted with caution.

More relevant in birds is the visual evaluation of urates. This requires a fair amount of experience. Even slight changes in color can indicate the presence of certain abnormalities or diseases. Any shade of green in the urates themselves is cause for concern. It typically indicates renal hemorrhage or severe liver abnormalities associated with serious disease. If the raptor's urates begin to appear truly pastel green (Fig. 7.11), death is probably not far away.

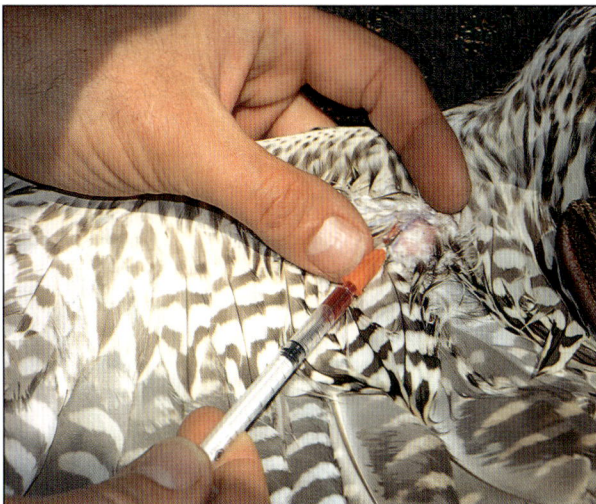

Fig. 7.25: Correct venipuncture technique using the cutaneous ulnar vein on the inside of the wing just above the elbow.
(Photo: Heidenreich)

7.4.6 Biopsies and washes

Tissue samples for histology can be obtained from almost any organ. For skin, the excision of a small piece from the affected area and simple closure of the resulting wound is all that is required. An endoscope allows access to and sampling of the air sac membranes (to diagnose aspergillosis for example). The diagnostic value and safety of tracheal, lung, and air sac washes is debatable.

7.4.7 Hematology

Bird blood differs from mammalian blood in many ways. All avian blood cells are nucleated, including erythrocytes and thrombocytes (equivalent to platelets). White blood cells tend to be less specialized and do not react to various types of insults as characteristically as mammalian leukocytes do.

Hematological and blood chemistry parameters vary significantly in birds depending on species, age, season, and even from one sample to the next in the same individual. Blood samples are therefore of limited value in raptors. Only obviously abnormal values that are obtained repeatedly and correspond with a suspected diagnosis can be considered significant.

The normal hematological values given in Tables 7.3 through 7.5 should be used only as general guidelines.

Venipuncture
Blood samples can be easily obtained from the wing vein (cutaneous ulnar vein, Fig. 7.25) or the leg vein (saphenous vein, Fig. 7.26). An assistant will be needed to restrain the bird. The feathers overlying the vessel are lightly moistened with water or alcohol to reveal the bluish vein underneath the wing in the elbow region or on the inner aspect of the lower thigh. Even in large raptors, samples should be obtained using a small needle (45 gauge, 13 mm), since the venous walls are thin and easily lacerated, resulting in large hematomas if carelessly penetrated. After the blood has been obtained, pressure should be applied to the venipuncture site for a few seconds before releasing the bird. With experience, blood sampling can be performed quickly and with minimal stress for the hawk. Regrettably, blood sampling ordered by the authorities, for paternity testing for example, is sometimes done by inexperienced people who end up causing much stress for the bird or even risking its health (Fig. 7.27).

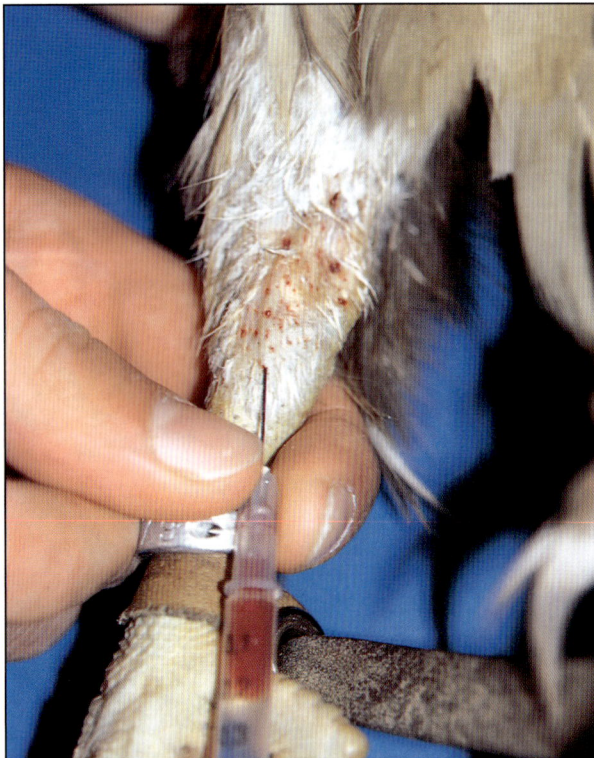

Fig. 7.26: Correct venipuncture technique using the saphenous vein on the inside of the hock. A few feathers have been removed to aid in visualization.
(Photo: Heidenreich)

7.4.7.2 Serum enzymes

Some serum enzyme values can be useful in raptor diagnostics. They are briefly described below.

Lactate dehydrogenase (LDH)
LDH values can be helpful in the diagnosis of diseases involving the liver, blood, skeletal muscle or tumors. Extremely high values are seen with toxicities such as organophosphate poisoning.

Aspartate aminotransferase (AST)
This enzyme is particularly useful in the diagnosis of liver disease or disorders involving the myocardium. Acute hepatitis will result in significantly elevated levels of AST. Serial monitoring of this enzyme can indicate how the disease is progressing.

Alanine aminotransferase (ALT)
Unlike in carnivores, ALT is found not only in the liver, but also in skeletal muscle and kidneys of birds. Elevated levels of this enzyme can therefore indicate problems with any of these organ systems. According to Gylstorff and Grimm (1987), elevated levels of ALT are seen with viral hepatitis and dieldrin toxicity.

7.4.7.1 Evaluating blood cells

The important parts of an avian hemogram include erythrocyte and leukocyte counts, determination of hemoglobin levels and the hematocrit. Anemias identified on the basis of red blood cell counts and the hematocrit can indicate blood loss or malnutrition, while white blood cell counts rise with inflammatory processes such as infections. Hemoglobin levels, when combined with other cell counts, can give information regarding iron deficiencies, chronic blood loss or toxicities (Kösters and Meister, 1982). The hematocrit is the percentage of red blood cells as a part of total blood volume. It will fall with anemias and rise in situations involving dehydration.

Table 7.3 gives some rough guidelines for normal raptor hematocrit values.

Redig (1993) lists normal hematocrits in wild raptors between 42% and 45%, even up to 50% in large falcons. Anything below that is considered an anemia.

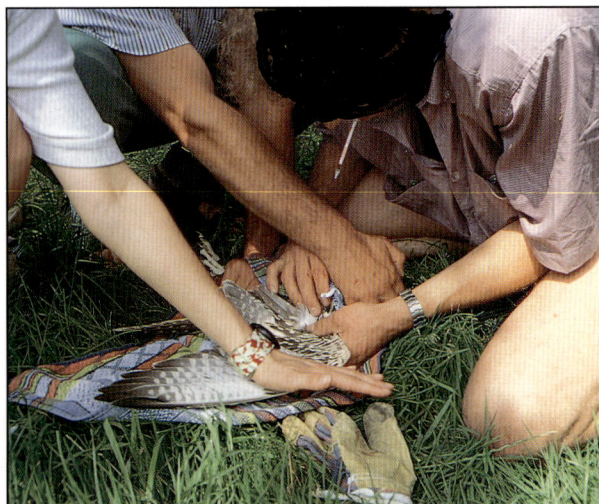

Fig. 7.27: Three people assigned by the state authorities incorrectly attempt venipuncture in a falcon.
(Photo: Heidenreich)

Table 7.3: Hematological values for selected raptor species
[from Gerlach (1977), Smith (1978), Gee et al. (1981), Rehder et al. (1982), Kösters and Meister (1982), Ferrer (1987), Gylstorff and Grimm (1987), Redig (1993) and Döttlinger (1995)]

Species	Leukocytes (WBC) [x 10^9/l]	Erythrocytes (RBC) [x 10^{12}/l]	Hematocrit [%]	Hemoglobin [g/l]*
Kites (*Milvus spp.*)	18.5	2.4	39.4–44.0	100–158
Harriers (*Circus spp.*)	13.7	2.8	42.1–49.5	138
Falcons in general (*Falco spp.*)	17.0	3.0	41.5	
Common kestrel (*F. tinnunculus*)	12.5–18.5	2.5–2.7	31.5–48.0	131–134
Peregrine falcon (*F. peregrinus*)	7.6–21.2	2.5–4.0	26.5–58.0	116–191
Gyrfalcon (*F. rusticolus*)	12.8–16		49	
Bonelli's eagle (*H. fasciatus*)		2.5	48	
Eagles in general (*Aquila spp.*)	15.0–19.0	2.7	32.6–48.5	
Bald eagle (*H. leucocephalus*)	12.85		44	
Imperial eagle (*A. heliaca*)	14.5–22.2	2.4–3.1	40.0–44.0	
Common buzzard (*Buteo buteo*)		2.1	37.7–44.7	146
Red-tailed hawk (*B. jamaicensis*)		2.45	39.4–44.6	
Northern goshawk (*Accipiter gentilis*)		1.5–3.1	32.0–45.0	160–216
Griffon vulture (*Gyps fulvus*)	13.8	2.3–2.9	43	137–142

* The International System of Units (SI) is used here. There is no change in any values except hemoglobin (divide by 10 to get g/dl) when converting to conventional American units.

Table 7.4: Serum enzymes of selected raptor species
[from Gerlach (1978), Gee (1981), Gylstorff and Grimm (1987) and Lavin et al. (1992)]

Species	LDH (U/l)	AST (U/l)	ALT (U/l)	AP (U/l)
Golden eagle (*A. chrysaetos*)	350–950	21–163	1–15	10–20
Imperial eagle (*A. heliaca*)	216–428	22–89	0–21	36–54
Greater spotted eagle (*A. clanga*)	86–283	52–101	13–28	24–45
Tawny or steppe eagle (*A. rapax*)	206–644	0–89	1–26	17–50
White-tailed sea eagle (*H. albicilla*)	270–420	30–160	0–30	7–76
Bonelli's eagle (*H. fasciatus*)	76–305	30	2–7	28–37
Northern goshawk (*A. gentilis*)	300–900	0–31	0–44	42–63
European sparrowhawk (*A. nisus*)	415	140–151	2.5–30.5	103–118
Red-tailed hawk (*B. jamaicensis*)	23–2286	152–303	8.9–32.5	47–160
Common buzzard (*B. buteo*)	168–446	0.5–27	0.5–58	35–86
Griffon vulture (*Gyps fulvus*)	160–240	90–140	39–47	9–50
Peregrine falcon (*F. peregrinus*)	575–1117	105–162		
Marsh harrier (*C. aeruginosus*)		140–440	18–58	

Alkaline phosphatase (AP)

Alkaline phosphatase is an enzyme found in almost all tissues of the body. It is associated particularly with the mucosa of the small intestine, the liver, kidneys and spleen, as well as bone and cartilage. Elevations in serum levels of AP can therefore indicate increased turnover or disease involving the skeletal system.

Gerlach (1978) described marked seasonal changes in the serum levels of these enzymes in birds of prey. He feels that they can still be valuable in the diagnosis of disease, as long as these fluctuations are taken into consideration. Table 7.4 lists some normal values for these enzymes in raptors. Again, the numbers should be used as general guidelines only.

7.4.7.3 Glucose, total protein, uric acid and cholesterol

Glucose

Normal blood glucose values in birds are more than twice as high as those of mammals. A reduction in food intake, seen sometimes in hunting hawks and commonly in injured wild birds, may cause pronounced hypoglycemia.

Total protein

Serum total protein levels can be a good indication of a bird's overall health status. Many problems including blood loss, malnutrition, severe liver disease, blood parasites and tumors can reduce total protein in the blood.

Table 7.5: Serum glucose, total protein, uric acid and cholesterol of selected raptor species [from O'Donell (1978), Gerlach (1978, 1979), Gee (1981), Ferrer (1987), Garcia Rodriguez (1987), Gylstorff and Grimm (1987), Lavin (1992) and Döttlinger (1995)]

Species	Glucose [mmol/l]	Total protein [g/l]	Uric acid [µmol/l]	Cholesterol [mmol/l]*
Common buzzard (*Buteo buteo*)	270–500	3.3–5.0	475–1314	3.5 –8.0
Red-tailed hawk (*B. jamaicensis*)	290–390		285–345	
Eagles in general	310–340	3.3	282–333	5.4
White-tailed sea eagle (*Haliaeetus albicilla*)		2.8–4.5		
Golden eagle (*Aquila chrysaetos*)	370	3.0–4.1		2.59–4.92
Bonelli's eagle (*Hieraetus fasciatus*)	305–390	3.8–4.7		5.0 –5.8
Booted eagle (*Hieraetus pennatus*)	275–305	2.8–4.2		3.4 –7.5
Northern goshawk (*Accipiter gentilis*)			267–324	
Common kestrel (*Falco tinnunculus*)	320–475			
Prairie falcon (*Falco mexicanus*)	415			
Peregrine falcon (*Falco peregrinus*)	290–366	2.7–4.1	128–1240	4.2 –21.0
Griffon vulture (*Gyps fulvus*)	230–320	3.0–5.5		3.4 –6.7
Montagu's harrier (*Circus cyaneus*)	370			
Marsh harrier (*C. aeruginosus*)	290–380	3.1–5.8	267–743	8.8 –20.0
Black kite (*Milvus migrans*)	260–420	3.0–4.1		5.7 –11.4

* The International System of Units is used here. The following conversion factors can be used to convert to conventional American Units: glucose – mmol/l X 18 = mg/dl, protein – g/l X 0.1 = g/dl, uric acid – µmol/l X 0.0168 = mg/dl, cholesterol – mmol/l X 38.7 = mg/dl

Uric acid

Uric acid is the primary end product for nitrogen, and therefore of proteins, in birds. Raptors, as primary carnivores, can have uric acid levels twice as high as other types of birds. Abnormal elevations in uric acid may indicate kidney damage or gout. Nevertheless, serum uric acid will change significantly only in advanced or severe cases of disease (Gylstorff and Grimm, 1987).

Cholesterol

Cholesterol is an important component of cell walls and is involved in many metabolic processes. Liver and kidney disease as well as high-fat diets can result in high serum levels of cholesterol. Whether cholesterol is associated with arteriosclerosis in birds is still under debate. Abnormally low cholesterol values are rarely seen. Table 7.5 lists some representative values for cholesterol in birds of prey.

7.4.7   Serum diagnostics

Serologic tests aimed at detecting antibodies or antigens are an important aspect of the diagnosis and monitoring of disease. Specialized private, state, or university-associated laboratories usually offer such services.

7.5   Radiography

Radiographic examinations play an important role in raptor diagnostics, providing information about the skeletal system and soft tissues. Two views (left-to-right lateral and ventrodorsal) are recommended for accurate interpretations (Figs. 7.28 through 7.31). Correct positioning, adequate restraint and high detail film-screen combinations are required to obtain quality images for interpretation. Anesthetics or sedatives may be of use with uncooperative birds.

Fractures or luxations of the long bones and joints are easy to diagnose radiographically. Changes in the shoulder and keel areas are more difficult to interpret and require absolutely symmetrical positioning. Metallic foreign bodies (shotgun pellets) are easily identified by their contrasting density (Fig 7.32). If made of soft lead, pellets may fragment upon impact with bone, leaving behind only small particles.

On a lateral view, the gastrointestinal system and lungs are well-visualized. The ventrodorsal view gives a better image of the heart, liver, and air sacs and outlines the kidneys. Large vessels near the base of the heart can sometimes be misinterpreted as tuberculous

granulomas or aspergillosis lesions when visualized end-on.

In patients suspected of respiratory disease, every effort should be made to obtain high detail images of the air sacs during the inspiratory phase. This may require several attempts.

Contrast procedures can be very useful in the evaluation of the gastrointestinal system (Figs. 7.33 and 7.34). A thick (yogurt consistency) suspension of barium sulfate is administered with a feeding tube. Radiographs obtained at appropriate intervals thereafter can help give information regarding transit time (delayed in cases of foreign body obstruction, for example), structural abnormalities (masses or perforations) and displacement (by tumors or organomegaly) of the digestive tract.

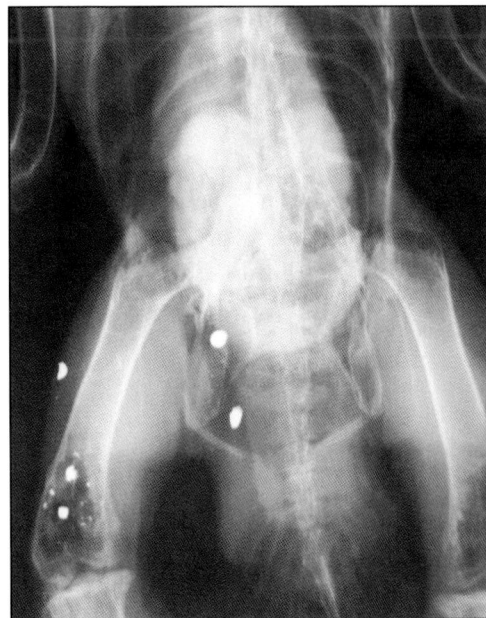

Fig. 7.28: Gunshot wounds can easily be identified by the shotgun pellets still present in the tissues. (Radiograph and photo: Heidenreich)

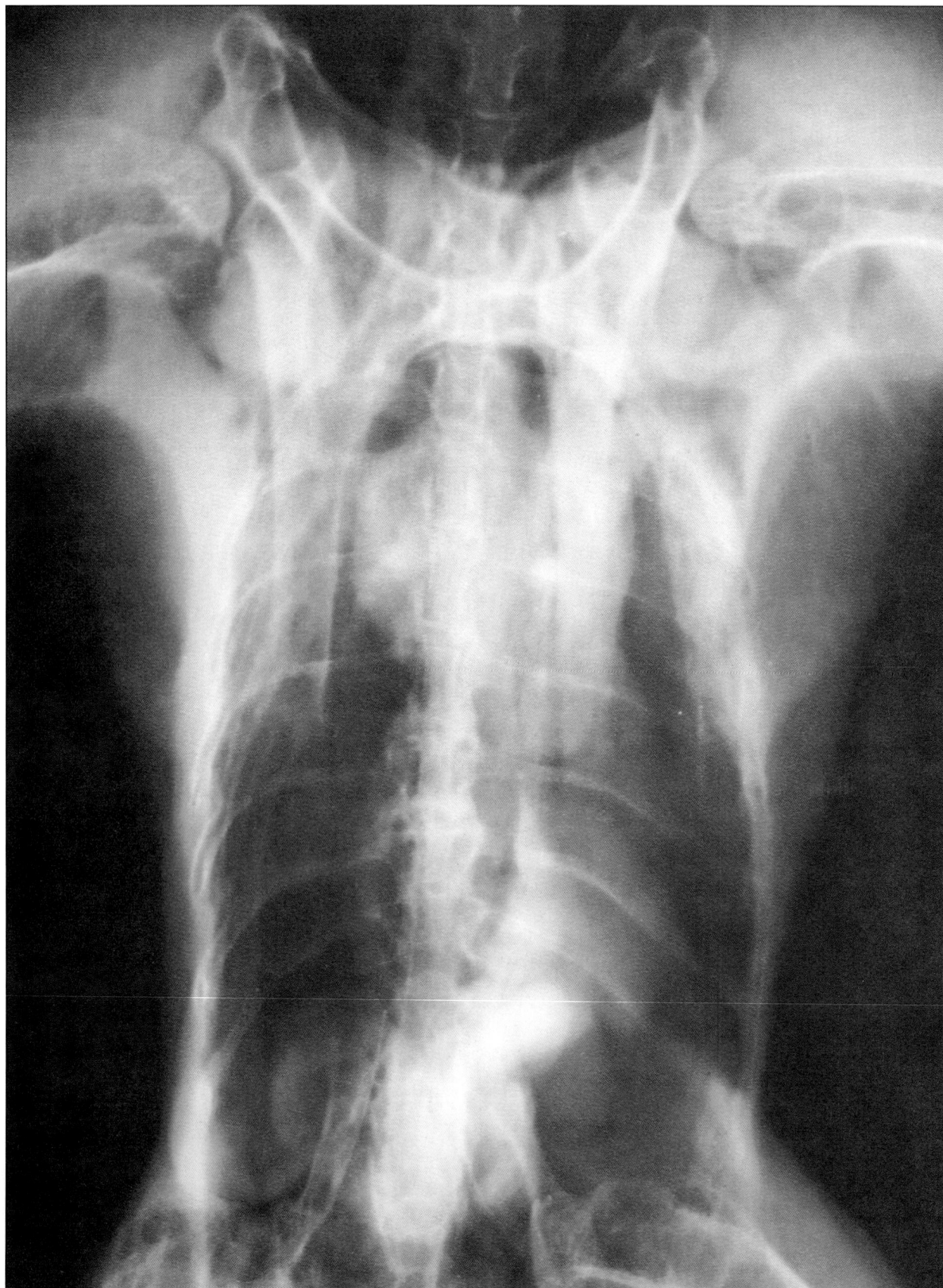

Fig. 7.29: A ventrodorsal radiograph of a normal golden eagle (*Aquila chrysaetos*).
(Radiograph and photo: Heidenreich)

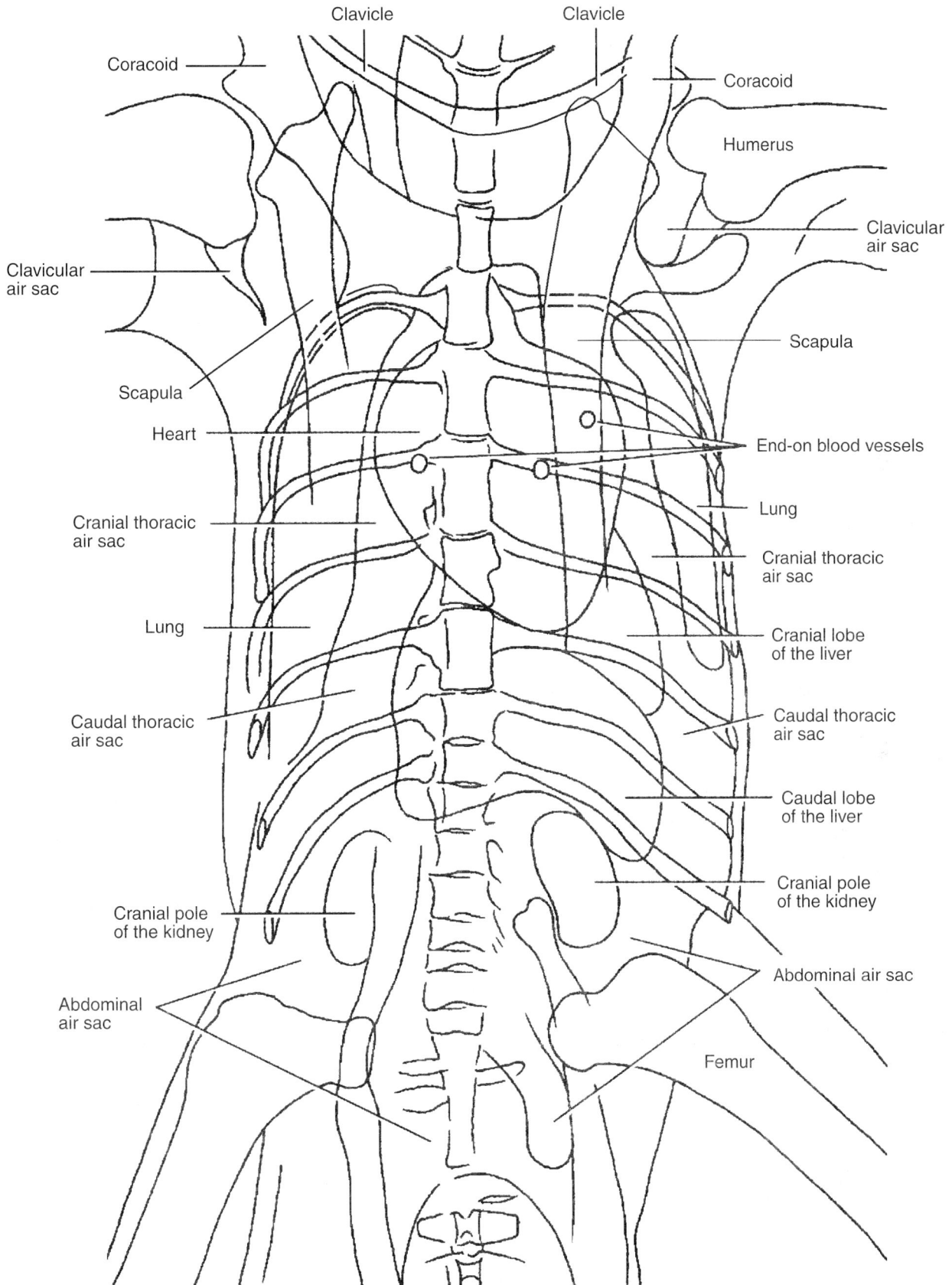

Fig. 7.30: Labeled illustration of the radiograph in Fig. 7.29.
(Illustration: R. Gattung-Petith and A. Gattung)

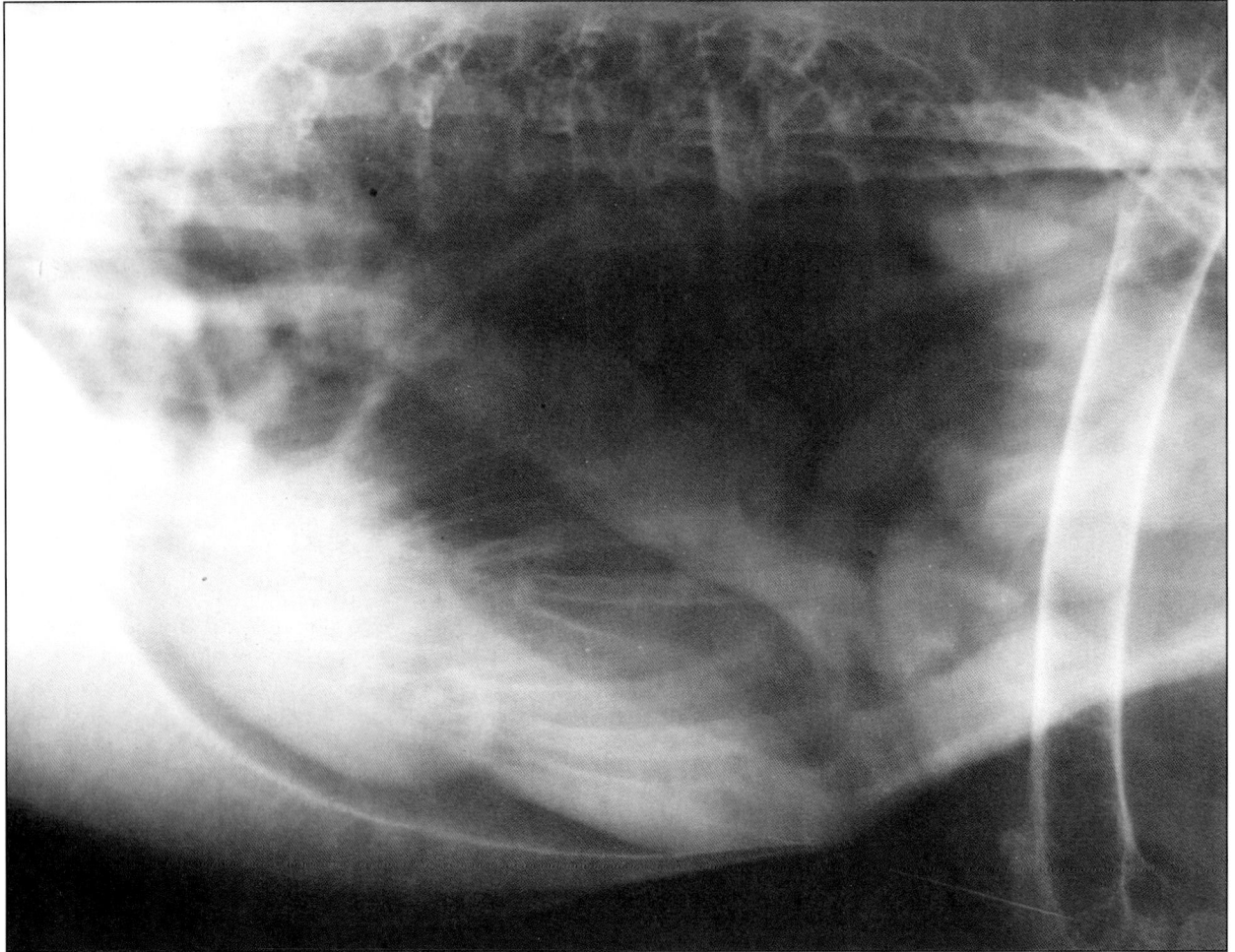

Fig. 7.31: A lateral radiograph of a normal golden eagle (*Aquila chrysaetos*). (Radiograph and photo: Heidenreich)

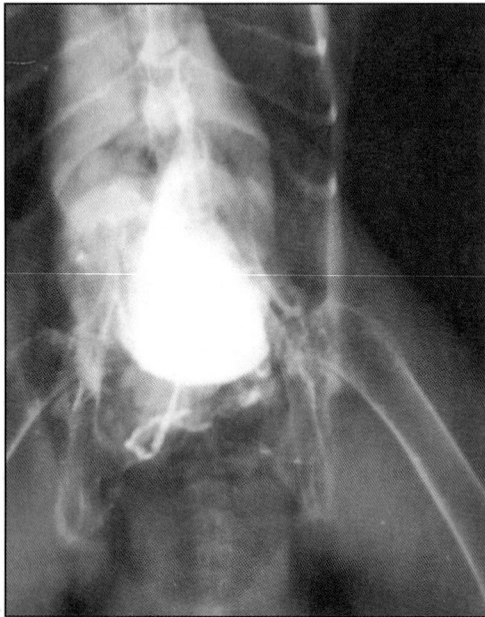

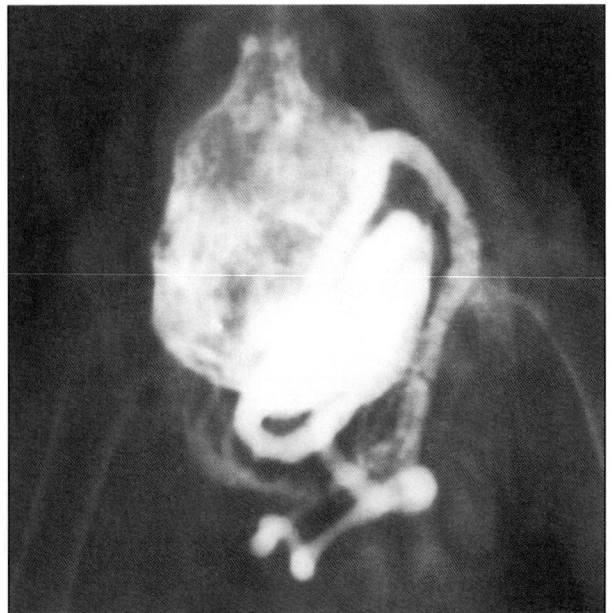

Figs. 7.33 and 7.34: Radiographic contrast studies are particularly useful in the diagnosis of diseases involving the gastrointestinal tract. Fig. 7.33 shows a bird with a ventricular sand impaction. The contrast material is held back by the impaction and only a small amount of barium manages to trickle through into the small intestine. Fig. 7.34 shows passage of contrast material through a normal ventriculus and small intestine.   (Radiographs and photos: Heidenreich)

Clavicular
air sac

Cranial thoracic
air sac

Caudal thoracic
air sac

Cranial pole
of the kidney

Lung

Spleen

Proventriculus

Heart

Liver

Small
intestine

Sternum

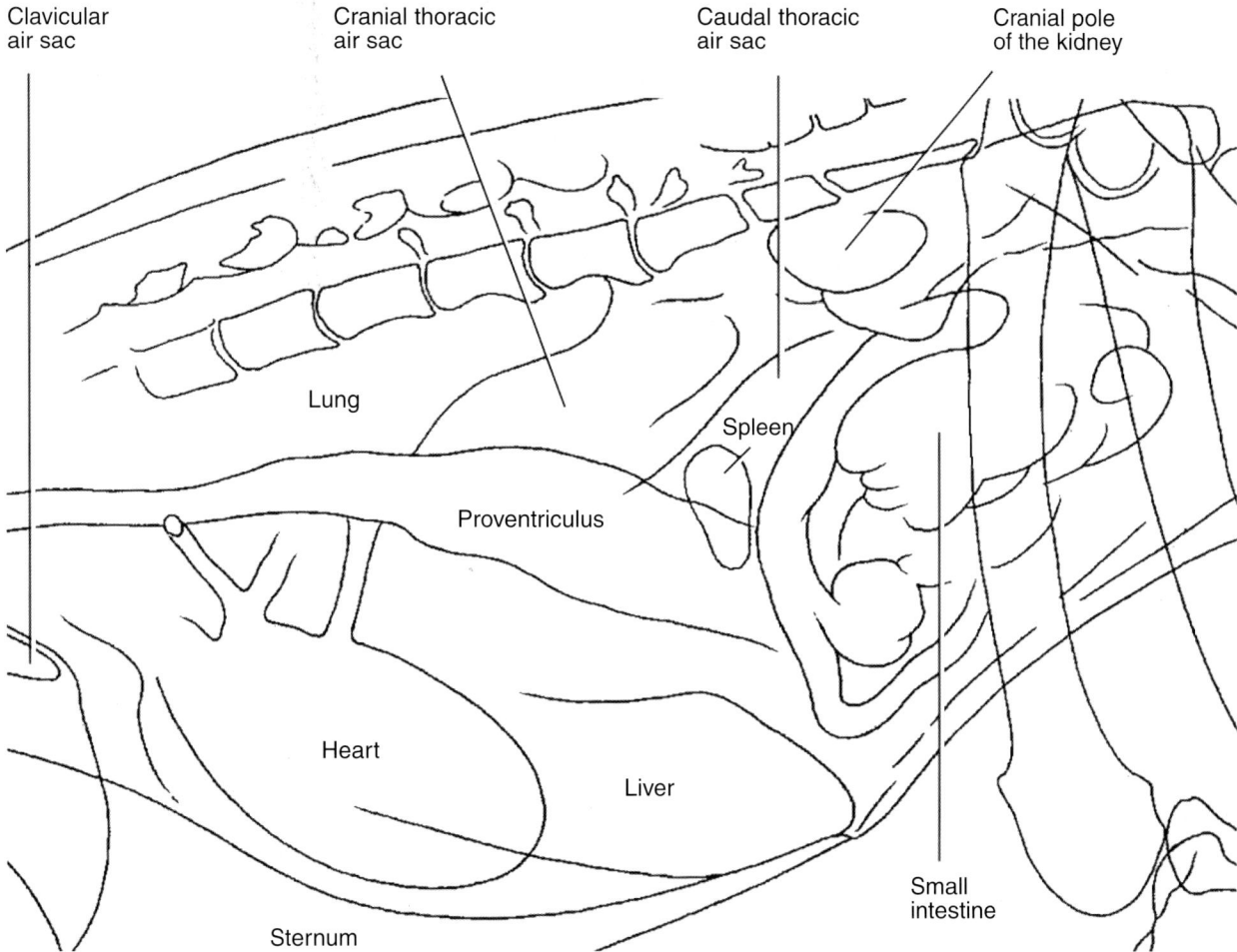

Fig. 7.32: Labeled illustration of the radiograph in Fig. 7.31 (Illustration: R. Gattung-Petith and A. Gattung)

7.6 Endoscopy

In 1978, both Harrison and Heidenreich independently developed the techniques for endoscopy in avian patients, primarily for determining gender in species that are not sexually dimorphic. The applications of endoscopy in birds have expanded since then, involving not only a wide range of diagnostic, but also surgical applications.

Instrumentation

Rigid rod-lens endoscopes useful in avian practice, sometimes sold as arthroscopes, are available in a variety of diameters between 1.9 and 5 mm. The smaller ones are more convenient but lack the light intensity available with the larger ones. The larger instruments can also be equipped with special lenses that help widen the field of view. In raptors, the 4 mm diameter endoscope has proven most useful.

A light source (at least 150 W) is attached to the en-

doscope by a flexible glass fiber cable. Endoscopic lens offset angles are available in $0°$ or $30°$ options. The $30°$ angle allows for rotation of the telescope and improved viewing in confined areas.

Applications

Safe and appropriate anesthetic techniques are a requirement for all endoscopic procedures (see Ch. 15.3).

Surgical sexing: Although the sex of most raptors can often be established by differences in body size and anatomic proportion, a definite determination can be difficult or impossible in some species. For breeding purposes, it is advantageous to identify a bird's gender as early as possible. Behavioral observations are unreliable for this purpose since birds of the same sex housed together can sometimes behave like a well-bonded, normal breeding pair. Laparoscopic sexing is a safe and reliable procedure that can be performed relatively quickly and easily by experienced veterinarians.

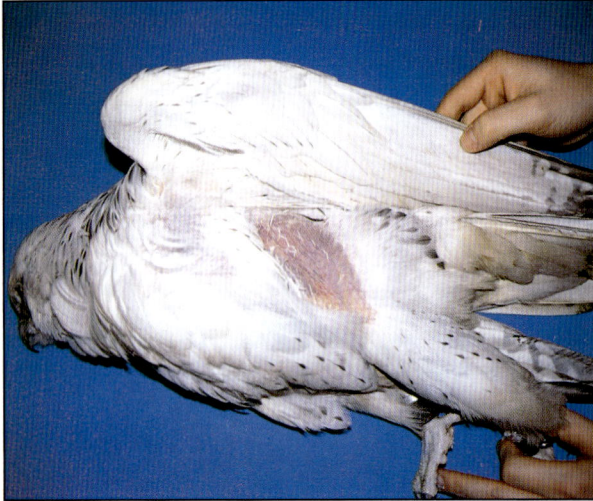

7.35

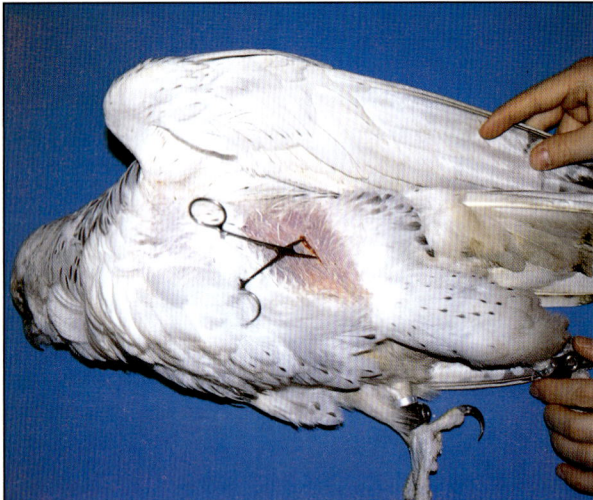

7.36

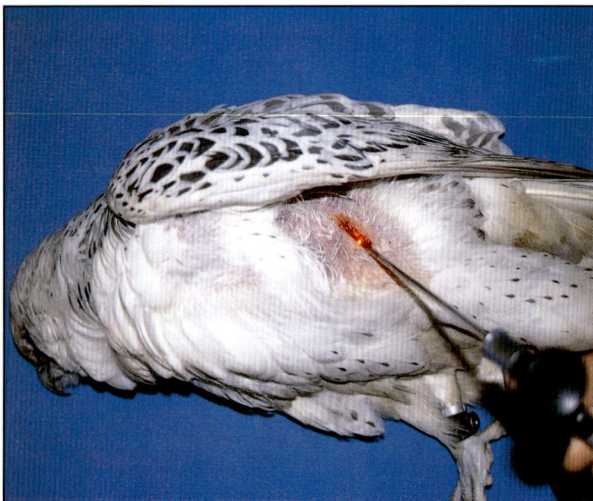

7.37

Female birds develop only the left ovary, so the avian patient is typically positioned in right lateral recumbency for this procedure. The entry point in the middle of the left flank (Fig. 7.35) is defined cranially by the last rib and caudally by the muscles of the upper thigh. A small incision is made at the point of entry. The sartorius muscle of the leg may overlie the last rib and can be pushed aside by lifting with curved hemostats and extending the leg caudally. Closed hemostats can now be used to pop through the body wall with a careful but sudden push. There should be an audible snap as the air sac is penetrated. If this sound is not heard or the hemostats are pushed in too slowly, the air sac membrane will simply be separated from the body wall, creating a hazy veil over the endoscopic field of view.

The hemostats can be used to enlarge the opening for passage of the endoscope (Fig. 7.36 and 7.37). The muscles will close around the endoscope after its insertion and prevent the entry of pathogens. A trocar is therefore not needed as a guide. With some experience, the gonads can be quickly identified. They are always found in the region bounded by the cranial pole of the kidney and the pink caudal edge of the lung. The small, yellowish-orange adrenal gland is usually located to one side of the ovary or testis.

The gonads are more easily identified in mature birds, although the ovary can be readily recognized in raptors only a few weeks old as a granular white structure. The testes are still tiny at this age, and lie on the caudal vena cava, making their identification much more difficult. In mature birds, surgical sexing can also provide information regarding the current state of gonadal activity, facilitating the prediction of reproductive status.

Fig. 7.35: Correct positioning and preparation of a white gyrfalcon (*Falco rusticolus*) for a left flank surgical approach.

Fig. 7.36: Opening the body cavity behind the last rib. This is facilitated by extending the leg on that side as far caudally as possible.

Fig. 7.37: The endoscope has been inserted into the body cavity. This approach is used not only for sexing or sterilization, but also for evaluating a number of internal organs.
(Photos: Heidenreich)

Diagnosis of disease: The same approach described above can be used to examine a variety of other internal organs including parts of the lung, air sacs, kidneys, adrenals, oviduct, epidydimis and ductus deferens, liver, and parts of the ventriculus and intestines. Other endoscopic approaches can expand the range even further.

Endoscopes are also used to examine the esophagus and proventriculus intraluminally. Similar examinations of the cloaca and distal oviduct are possible. If the instrument is narrow in diameter, it can even be used to explore the trachea. For prolonged examinations of the upper airway that may interfere with respiration, a large diameter catheter placed into the abdominal air sac will permit the bird to continue breathing freely.

7.7   Ultrasound

Ultrasound imaging has proven to be a valuable and non-invasive diagnostic modality in mammalian veterinary medicine. In birds, however, it is little used. The unique anatomic features of the avian family, including air sacs, subserosal fat deposits, extensive bony skeletons and compact viscera, often interfere with the penetration of high frequency sound waves, making it difficult to obtain quality images.

Hildebrandt et al. (1995) attempted ultrasound diagnostics in raptors using an 8 mm diameter transducer inserted into the cloaca. This technique was practical only in birds weighing more than 4 kg, but made it possible to visualize the gonads, liver, spleen, kidneys, proventriculus and ventriculus in golden eagles and vultures.

Despite these inherent limitations, the use of trans-intestinal ultrasound as an alternative to endoscopy for avian gender determination and evaluation of gonadal activity in raptors is to be encouraged. Its noninvasiveness is a distinct advantage, although a fair amount of experience is needed in the accurate interpretation of the images obtained. Overall, however, ultrasound does not yet seem to be a practical alternative to endoscopy.

References and literature of further interest

BALASCH, J., MUSQUERA, S., PALACIOS, L., JIMENEZ and J.M. PALOMEQUE (1976):
Comparative hematology of some falconiforms.
Condor. **78**, 258–259

BEDNAREK, W. (1992):
Beizjagd und Greifvögel in Südafrika.-Ein Reisebericht.
Greifvögel und Falknerei 62–76
Verlag Neumann-Neudamm, Morschen-Heina

BINI, P.P., FLORIS, B., NUVOLE, P., PAU, S. and M.T. ZEDDA (1989):
Caratteristiche ematologiche ed ematochimiche del gabbiano reale (*Larus argentatus*) e della poiana comune (*Buteo buteo*).
Boll. Soc. Ital. Biol. Speriment. **65**, 831–837

BÖTTCHER, M. (1980):
Endoskopie beim Greifvogel zu diagnostischen Zwecken mit endoskopischen Aufnahmen.
Prakt. Tierarzt. **61**, 942, 945–946

BÖTTCHER, M. (1982):
Endoskopische Diagnostik am erkrankten Vogel, unter Einsatz möglichst schonender Methoden der Schmerzausschaltung.
Kleintierpraxis. **27**, 305–308, 310

DÖTTLINGER, H.:
Influence of diet on haematological parameters in captive Peregrine Falcons (*Falco peregrinus*)
(in press)

ELLIOTT, R.H., SMITH, E. and M. BUSH (1974):
Preliminary report on hematology of birds of prey.
J. Zoo Anim. Med. **5**, 11–16

FERRER, M., GARCIA-RODRIGUEZ, T., CARRILLO, J.C. and
J. CASTROVIEJO (1987):
Hematocrit and blood chemistry values in captive raptors
(Gyps fulva, Buteo buteo, Milvus migrans, Aquila heliaca).
Comp. Biochem. Physiol. A **87**, 1123–1127

GARCIA-RODRIGUEZ, T., FERRER, M., RECIO, F. and
J. CASTROVIEJO (1987):
Circadian rhythms of determined blood chemistry values in
buzzards and eagle owls.
Comp. Biochem. Physiol **88**, 663–669

GEE, G.F., CARPENTER, J.W. and G.L. HENSLER (1981):
Species differences in hematological values of captive cranes,
geese, raptors, and quail.
J. Wildl. Manag. **45**, 463–483

GERLACH, C. (1978):
Grundlagen der Blutdiagnostik bei Greifvögeln.
Prakt. Tierarzt. **59**, 642–650

GERLACH, C. (1979):
Differentialblutbild und Plasmaenzymuntersuchungen bei
Greifvögeln im Verlaufe eines Jahres (Mai 1977 bis Mai 1978).
Prakt. Tierarzt. **60**, 673–674, 679–68

GERLACH, C., FUGGER, B. and C. ROTT (1984):
Blutdiagnostik bei Vögeln I. Jahreszeitliches Verhalten des
roten und weissen Blutbildes von Graureihern (*Ardea cinerea*),
Uhus (*Bubo bubo*) und Seeadlern (*Haliaeetus albicilla*).
Prakt. Tierarzt. **65**, 876–892

GYLSTORFF, I. and F. GRIMM (1987):
Vogelkrankheiten
Verlag Eugen Ulmer, Suttgart

HALLIWELL, W.H., IVINS, G., SCHMIDT, D.A. and G. WEDDLE (1975):
A preliminary report on the hematology and chemical profiles
in selected birds of prey.
Amer. Ass. Zoo Vet. 1975, 188–196

HALLIWELL, W.H. (1980):
Serum chemistry profiles in the health and disease of birds
of prey.
in: Recent advances in the study of raptor diseases. 111–112
Chiron Pub. Ltd., Keighley, West Yorkshire, England

HARRISON, G.J. (1978):
Endoscopic examination of avian gonadal tissue.
Vet. Med. Small Anim. Clin. **73**, 479–484

HEIDENREICH, M. (1978):
Geschlechtsbestimmung beim Vogel mittels Endoskopie.
Kleintierpraxis **23**, 193–198

HERNANDEZ, M. (1991):
Blood chemistry in raptors.
Proc. First Conf. Europ. Comm. Ass. Avian Vet., 411–419

HERNANDEZ, M. (1991):
Raptor clinical haematology.
Proc. First Conf. Europ. Comm. Ass. Avian Vet., 420–433

HILDEBRANDT, T., PITRA, C., SÖMMER, P. and M. PINKOWSKI
(1995):
Sex identification in birds of prey by ultrasonography.
J. Zoo Wildl. Med. **26**, 367–376

KÖSTERS, J. and B. MEISTER (1982):
Hamatokrit- und Hämoglobinwerte bei einigen einheimischen
Greifvögeln und Eulen.
Prakt. Tierarzt. **63**, 444–446, 448

LAVIN, S., CUENCA, R., MARCO, I., VELARDE, R. and
L. VINAS (1992):
Hematology and blood chemistry of the marsh harrier
(*Circus aeruginosus*).
Comp. Biochem. Physiol. **103**, 493–495

LIND, P.J., WOLFF, P.L., PETRINI, K.R., KEYLER, C.W., OLSON,
D.E. and P.T. REDIG (1990):
Morphology of the eosinophil in raptors.
J. Ass. Avian Vet. **4**, 33 38

O'DONNELL, J.A., GARBETT, R. and A. MORZENTI (1978):
Normal fasting plasma glucose levels in some birds of prey.
J. Wildl. Dis. **14**, 479–481

REDIG, P.T. (1993):
Medical management of birds of prey.
A collection of notes on selected topics. 147
Raptor Center, Minnesota

REHDER, N.B., BIRD, D.M., LAGUE, P.C. and C. MACKAY
(1982):
Variation in selected hematological parameters of captive
red-tailed hawks [*Buteo jamaicensis*].
J. Wildl. Dis. **18**, 105–119

SCHULZ, R., HERZOG, A. and H. HOHN (1980):
Zur Geschlechtsbestimmung bei Greifen.
Prakt. Tierarzt. **61**, 946, 948

SMITH, E.E. and M. BUSH (1978):
Haematologic parameters on various species of Strigiformes
and Falconiformes.
J. Wildl. Dis. **14**, 447–450

SNYDER, J.E., BIRD, D.M. and P.C. LAGUE (1980):
Variations in selected parameters in the blood of captive
American kestrels [*Falco sparvenus*].
in: Recent advances in the study of raptor diseases. 113–115
Chiron Pub. Ltd., Keighley, West Yorkshire, England

VEIL, K. (1978):
Feststellung von Blutwerten bei verschiedenen Vogelarten.
Vet. Med. Diss., München

8 Clinical therapy

The goal in treating any sick or injured wild bird is to help it regain the health it needs for life in the wild. If it is likely that this goal can not be achieved, euthanasia of the animal should be considered. Wild raptors are not suited to spending the rest of their lives as caged cripples in a rehabilitation center, living reminders of misguided animal rescue efforts. This goes for falconry birds as well, especially if they are unable to fly at all, unless permanent placement in an appropriate facility is available for them.

Therapeutics in this context include all measures employed in an effort to restore the animal to health. This can include plain cage rest, the correct feeding of malnourished birds or simple rehydration techniques. Usually, however, one will want to support such measures with the administration of appropriate medications. Even so, we should keep in mind that improvement with therapy is sometimes difficult to ascribe with certainty to the therapeutic measures used.

8.1 Administration of medication

Almost all drugs used in veterinary medicine are administered on the basis of body weight, making accurate dosing relatively easy. Medications used in human medicine, on the other hand, are often prescribed in dosages designed for adults or children, regardless of body weight. This can make the administration of human preparations in animals difficult. In calculating dosages for such drugs, it is helpful to know that the average adult is assumed to weigh 70 kg.

The regular monitoring of a patient's body weight is important not only for the administration of medications, but also because weight is a good indicator of the bird's ongoing response to therapy. Falconers often know their hawk's normal body weight exactly and should be asked for that information.

8.1.1 Topical administration

Medications for external use are usually supplied in the form of creams or ointments. This type of formulation quickly results in sticky, greasy feathers and its use should be restricted to the unfeathered areas of a bird's body. Care should be taken that the hawk cannot ingest such preparations during routine preening, as many of them are not intended for systemic use. Ointments can be rubbed into the skin until they disappear or the hawk should be fitted with a hood that prevents it from ingesting the ointment.

Some medications are combined with dimethylsulfoxide (DMSO) and are therefore absorbed into the systemic circulation after topical application. These are usually corticosteroids whose effect is not intended to be limited to the site of application.

Many preparations for the control of ectoparasites are supplied in spray or powder form. Care should be taken that the head is well-protected during the application of such products to prevent contact with the oral mucosa or eyes. The unfeathered parts of the legs should also be avoided.

Dirty or dusty birds can be gently sprayed with **cold** water from a plant mister. Warm water may be more effective, but will also remove the natural oils from the skin and plumage and make the feathers brittle. Birds contaminated with oil are an exception to this rule. They usually require repeated washing with warm soapy solutions to get clean.

8.1.2 Systemic administration

Oral (per os or PO)
Many medications are supplied in liquid or tablet form designed for oral administration. Most of them have an unpleasant taste and can be difficult to administer to raptors. They must therefore be placed deep in the pharynx or esophagus where the taste is no longer perceived and swallowing reflexes are initiated. Only very quiet hunting hawks will tolerate this without restraint. In order to avoid the aversive behavior acquired by birds that must be repeatedly caught and restrained, every effort should be made to hide the

medication in the animal's normal food. Tablets can be easily placed inside a chick head to be swallowed whole by larger birds of prey. One can also try wrapping them in a piece of meat or skin for hand-feeding. Liquids can be placed inside gelatin capsules and then administered like tablets quickly before the gelatin dissolves.

Intranasal or conjunctival

Diseases of the nose or eye are often treated locally. Liquids work best in the nose, penetrating more readily into the sinuses, while ointments are preferred for ocular use. Ointments will remain in the eye for a longer time and thus reduce the frequency of application required to maintain therapeutic levels. Because both the nose and eye tend to flush medications out relatively quickly, these areas should be treated at least four times a day.

Intradermal

Bird skin is very thin and intradermal injections are rarely performed. They can be done in raptors at the rim of the ear. Tuberculin tests, for example, can be performed there (see Ch. 9.2.3). Experiments with pox vaccines for falcons have been under way for several years. These may require intradermal administration. Pigeons are vaccinated against pox by plucking a few feathers from the leg and rubbing the vaccine into the follicles thus exposed.

Subcutaneous (SC)

Avian skin is loose enough for subcutaneous administration of medications in only a few places. Larger volumes can be given in the nape of the neck, whereby the skin is pulled up with the index finger and thumb of one hand while the injection is given into the tented area with the other. This site is also suited for the subcutaneous placement of transponders (see Ch. 6.6).

Intramuscular (IM)

The most common method of drug administration in birds is intramuscular injection. It should be performed with a small gauge needle in the breast muscles. The best site for injection lies in the thickest part of the muscle to one side of the keel and halfway between the thoracic inlet and the end of the sternum. The needle is inserted at a 45° angle. Very tame birds can be given injections as they stand on the fist. Touching their back may distract them so that penetration of the small needle is not even noticed.

Intravenous (IV)

Techniques for intravenous injection are the same as those for venipuncture. They are described in Ch. 7.4.7.

Inhalation (nebulization)

Infections involving the avian respiratory tract are often treated by inhalation therapy. This involves suspension of the desired medication in the form of an aerosol or gas so that it can be inhaled directly into the respiratory system. Droplet size in the aerosol should not exceed 5 µm to ensure adequate penetration to all parts of the lower respiratory tract and air sacs. Ultrasonic nebulizers fulfill this requirement (Gylstorff and Grimm, 1987), but the less expensive ones available commercially probably do not. Nebulization therapy is helpful in providing adequate drug concentration within the respiratory tract without necessarily resulting in systemic absorption of the drug.

Nebulization is usually performed in a closed chamber of limited size. This can be a drawback with some very nervous or large species of raptors. Hawks accustomed to being hooded can sometimes be treated using a hand-held face mask. Sick birds should be nebulized three to four times a day for at least several days. Table 8.1 provides an overview of the medications and dosages commonly used in inhalation therapy.

Table 8.1: Medications commonly used in nebulization therapy
(from Tully and Harrison, 1994)

Drug	Dosage
Amphotericin B	100 mg in 15 ml saline
Chloramphenicol	200 mg in 15 ml saline
Erythromycin	200 mg in 10 ml saline
Gentamycin	50 mg in 10 ml saline
Polymyxin B	333,000 IU in 5 ml saline
Spectinomycin	200 mg in 15 ml saline
Sulfadimethoxine	200 mg in 15 ml saline
Tylosin	100 mg in 10 ml saline, 1 g in 50 ml DMSO
Enrofloxacin	100 mg in 10 ml saline
Amikacin	50 mg in 10 ml saline

8.2 Drug therapy

The therapeutic use of drugs is intended to help the body overcome or manage a disease process without causing problems in other ways. Nevertheless, most medications have potential negative side effects in addition to their desired therapeutic actions.

We have a great deal of knowledge regarding the dosing, formulation, therapeutic levels, elimination rates and side effects of drugs in domestic animals. Medical recommendations in birds, on the other hand, are usually based on purely empirical information provided by a few specialists in the field. Even knowledge gained in the poultry industry is usually of only limited value in wild birds and raptors. As great as the variety of raptor species is, so varied are their responses to drug therapy. The therapeutic regimens and dosages provided here should therefore be used as rough guidelines only. Future research and further experience may change them.

The most important goal of any systemic therapy protocol is to achieve effective concentrations and durations of the drug in the bloodstream. These in turn, depend on the formulation and on the route of administration used. For economic reasons, the commercial poultry industry has developed oral forms of therapy involving medications administered to large groups of birds in the feed or water. Raptors have a greater inherent value to the owner or to society at large and are more commonly treated as individuals. Birds of prey are also very alert to unusual substances in their food and normally rarely drink water. For these reasons, intramuscular injections have proven the best method for administering medications reliably and accurately in these species.

8.2.1 Antibacterial therapy

Bacterial diseases are important in raptors and the careful selection and use of antibacterial drugs is critical to their successful treatment. The patient is often presented in advanced stages of the disease and a correct diagnosis and immediate therapy are required to save the bird. Nevertheless, diseases that are treated early are usually controlled more successfully.

The goal of antibacterial therapy is to reduce or eliminate the bacterial pathogen inside the host, thus assisting the animal's own immune system in its efforts to deal with the infection. As do other drugs, antibiotics can have undesirable side effects, not the least of which is a negative impact on the normal GI flora. Therefore, antibiotics should be used judiciously and only on a basis of evident need, not every time questionable bacteria are detected on a fecal culture (see

Ch. 7.4.1). Inadequate dosing or early termination of therapy can also result in incomplete elimination of the pathogen and lead to the development of resistance, making future treatment more difficult. Bacteria often develop cross-resistance, making a whole class of antibiotics unsuitable for use with that particular organism. The immediate adoption of newer products that come on the market is to be discouraged as long as effective alternatives are still available among established antibacterials. More resistances may develop from such actions, leaving the practitioner with few options in times of need.

8.2.1.1 Bacterial culture and sensitivity

In view of the risk of encountering resistant organisms, a bacterial culture and sensitivity screen is usually advantageous. This requires culture material obtained directly from the patient prior to the initiation of treatment. In cases where entire groups of birds are affected or if the animal has already died, sampling individual representatives of the population or obtaining postmortem cultures is possible. Since it may take several days to get results from a bacterial culture and sensitivity screen, the patient should be treated empirically until the results are received. Then antibacterial therapy can be adjusted as indicated.

The laboratory isolating the bacteria and testing them for antibacterial sensitivity initially has to separate the pathogens from the nonpathogenic bacteria in the submitted sample. The pathogens are then plated on an appropriate medium and exposed to small discs soaked in various antibiotics. The larger the zone of bacterial growth inhibition around the disc, the more effective that particular antibiotic is deemed to be. Each bacterium is then graded as very sensitive, moderately sensitive, or resistant to each drug tested.

The sensitivity results should not be the sole determinants of antibacterial therapy. Most drugs, as well as most pathogens, respond differently in the living patient than they do in a petri dish. Some medications may not be appropriate for an animal because of unacceptable side-effects or risks involved with their use. Sensitivity results, therefore, help primarily to indicate which antibacterials not to use.

Table 8.2 lists some antibacterial drugs and their dosages in raptors as determined by various authors and by personal experience. Although carefully selected, these are still primarily empirical dosages and they should be used carefully. Every veterinarian is ultimately responsible for the therapies he or she uses. The side effects listed are based in part on suspicions only and do not necessarily associate with that particular drug.

8.2.2 Antifungal therapy

Fungal infections are an important cause of disease in certain species of raptors. Birds from far northern climates such as gyrfalcons and merlins are particularly susceptible. It is possible that their immune systems have not evolved to handle certain pathogens that are normally not found in their natural habitat. Additional factors such as poor management and stress will also compromise a bird's immune system and can play an important role in the development of fungal disease. Any treatment plan for such infections must include the elimination of such predisposing factors, as well as direct medical therapy.

Treating avian fungal infections is often a long and expensive process. The intensity and duration of care involved can lead to further compromises in the pa-

tient's strength and resistance, creating a vicious circle that is hard to break. It is much easier to make every effort to prevent such diseases in the first place.

Table 8.3 lists some commonly used avian antifungal drugs with the dosages and routes of administration for birds of prey recommended by various authors.

8.2.3 Antiparasitic therapy

The treatment of internal parasites is relatively easy and effectively accomplished with any of a number of drugs. Follow-up fecal examinations should always be performed. If the parasite utilizes alternate or intermediate hosts, this should be addressed also. Management and sanitation practices can be reviewed and changed in order to prevent reinfection after treatment.

Table 8.2: Dosage, administration and possible side effects of various antibacterial drugs

Drug	Dosage	Administration	Comments
Amoxicillin	50–100 mg/kg	PO TID	IM route not well tolerated
Ampicillin	100–250 mg/kg 25–50 mg/kg	PO TID IM SID	Poorly absorbed PO
Chloramphenicol	50–100 mg/kg	IM or PO BID	Irritating to tissues May affect plumage
Chlortetracyclin	250 mg/kg 6–10 mg/kg	PO SID IM SID	May affect plumage
Cloxacillin	100–250 mg/kg	IM or PO SID	
Doxycyclin	75–100 mg/kg	IM every 5th day	USA product may be irritating to tissues
Enrofloxacin	10–15 mg/kg 5–15 mg/kg	IM SID PO SID to BID	May interfere with molt Do not use in growing birds
Gentamycin	4 mg/kg	IM every 8 hrs.	Risk of nephrotoxicity
Kanamycin	10–25 mg/kg	IM SID	May cause death!
Lincomycin	50–100 mg/kg 10–15 mg/kg	PO SID IM BID	
Neomycin	5–10 mg/kg	IM BID	Toxic if overdosed
Oxytetracyclin	250 mg/kg 35–50 mg/kg	PO SID IM SID	
Polymyxin B	10–15 mg/kg	IM SID	Not absorbed if given orally
Spiramycin	250 mg/kg 20 mg/kg	PO SID IM SID	Poorly absorbed
Streptomycin	15 mg/kg	PO SID	highly neurotoxic!
Trimethoprim/sulfa	50 mg/kg	IM or PO SID	Potentially nephrotoxic
Tylosin	250 mg/kg 15 mg/kg 5–10 mg/kg	PO SID IM SID – TID IM BID	

Table 8.4 lists some of the commonly used antiparasitic drugs and the dosages recommended for raptors.

8.2.4 Miscellaneous therapeutic agents

A variety of miscellaneous drugs used to treat birds of prey are listed in alphabetical order below. All dosages, indications and side-effects are based on the manufacturer's recommendations and reports, other publications, or personal experience. The pharmacokinetics of most of these drugs in birds of prey are not known and much of the information provided is empirical. In addition, many of these medications are approved only for use in humans or other domestic animals, even though they are frequently used in avian medicine. Every practitioner is therefore responsible for critically evaluating his or her therapeutic options and the possible side-effects thereof.

Alcohol is commonly used as a topical disinfectant prior to surgery or at venipuncture sites to aid in visualizing the vein. It evaporates very rapidly and should be used on small surface areas only. It may otherwise significantly cool the bird's body temperature and contribute to hypothermia, especially in the smaller species. Alcohol can also be absorbed through thin avian skin into the systemic circulation, leading to lethargy, incoordination and vomiting if used over larger areas.

Allopurinol is sometimes recommended for use in birds to treat gout. Raptors treated in this way have had anomalous reactions in which gout was actually caused by administration of this drug.

Aminoloid is supposed to induce a complete molt in raptors within two months. It is a diuretic and can result in severe dehydration. Its use is not recommended.

Table 8.3: Drugs commonly used to treat aspergillosis

Drug	Dosage	Reference
Ketoconazole	60 mg/kg PO BID	WAGNER et al. (1991)
Enilconazole	1 ml in 9 ml saline (nebulized)	BARONETZKY-MERCIER and SEIDEL (1995)
Itraconazole	<u>Prophylaxis:</u> 10 mg/kg SID PO x 10 days <u>Treatment:</u> 10 mg/kg PO BID	FORBES et al. (1992)
Fluconazole	10–25 mg/kg BID for 4 weeks	PARROTT (1991)
Miconazole	Nebulize TID for 15 min. x 10 days 10 mg/kg IM x 6–12 days	GYLSTORFF and GRIMM (1987) FURLEY and GREENWOOD (1982)
Flucytosine	40–50 mg/kg PO TID	REDIG (1981, 1993)
Rifampin	30 mg/kg PO TID	REDIG (1981, 1993)
Amphotericin B	Nebulize TID X 20 min. 1.5 mg/kg IV TID in conjunction with 1 mg/kg intratracheal BID, Air sac wash	FORBES et al. (1992) REDIG (1981, 1993) GYLSTORFF and GRIMM (1987)

Ammonium nitrate has been mentioned in medieval texts and is still used today in Arab countries. It is administered as a potent emetic to make falcons more eager to hunt. Such treatment is very dangerous and can lead to a bird's death in only minutes!

Anabolic steroids can sometimes be used to help rebuild muscle during convalescence after an illness. Regrettably, these steroids are now sometimes abused in the "doping" of falcons, aimed at achieving better performance or improving hunting success. The use of these substances is not without risk, since they can exacerbate preexisting liver or kidney problems and lead to death. Tiercels will be rendered infertile with prolonged use.

Ascorbic acid (vitamin C) can be given orally or intramuscularly to aid in the treatment of infectious diseases. Because it is a water-soluble vitamin, overdosing is virtually impossible.

Atropine is a parasympatholytic agent and the drug of choice in the treatment of organophosphate poisoning. It is not recommended in raptors otherwise, as it can cause cardiac arrhythmias and gastrointestinal stasis.

Barium sulfate is a powder that can be suspended in water and administered as a gastrointestinal contrast agent. It also acts to coat the GI mucosa and aids in the treatment of vomiting and enteritis.

Botulism anti-toxin (Schering) is sold for use in mink against *Cl. botulinum* Type C. One half the mink dose is suggested for birds.

Calcium is available as an aqueous solution for oral use or as an injectable solution (calcium gluconate). It can be administered in cases of egg binding, egg shell defects, hypocalcemic tetany or in the support of fracture repair.

Calcium EDTA is a chelating agent used in the treatment of lead poisoning. Long-term therapy can lead to chelation of other cations in the body. Intramuscular injection may result in localized necrosis.

Candy-sugar crystals have a potent osmotic effect in the GI tract, leading to diarrhea and loss of fluids. They were given to hawks in the past in order to make them more eager to hunt.

Table 8.4: Dosing, administration and side effects of selected antiparasitic drugs

Drug	Dose	Administration	Target Parasite/Comments
Amprolium	30 mg/kg	PO x 5 days	Coccidia, resistance may occur
Carnidazole	20 mg/kg	PO once	Trichomonads
Chloroquine	25 mg/kg 10 mg/kg	IM SID PO once	*Plasmodium, Leukocytozoon, Haemoproteus*
Clazuril	5–10 mg/kg	PO SID x 2 days	Coccidia
Fenbendazole	25–50 mg/kg 100 mg/kg	PO SID x 3–7 days PO once	Nematodes May be toxic to vultures
Haloxon	50–100 mg/kg	PO	Toxic!
Ivermectin	0,2–0,4 mg/kg	IM, PO or topically once	Most parasites, mites
Levamisole	15 mg/kg	PO or SC once	Nematodes
Mebendazole	25–50 mg/kg	PO once	Possibly toxic in some birds
Oxyfenbendazole	20 mg/kg	PO once	Nematodes
Praziquantel	10–50 mg/kg	PO or IM once	Cestodes and trematodes
Thiabendazole	100–200 mg/kg	PO BID x 10 days	Nematodes, may interfere with egg-laying
Toltrazuril	25 mg/kg	PO x 2 days	Coccidia, bitter taste

Cyanocobalamin (vitamin B12) can be given IM or SC. There is no risk of overdosing. The urates will appear yellow shortly after administration.

Dexamethasone is a glucocorticoid 20 times as potent as prednisolone. It is sometimes used in the treatment of shock, but can have immunosuppressive effects if used long-term. Birds treated with this drug will show marked increases in appetite and water consumption.

Diazepam is a sedative and tranquilizer used to keep birds calm during transport. The recommended dose is 1 mg/kg. Reactions to this drug can vary. Some birds may sleep for many hours.

Dimercaprol (BAL) is used like calcium EDTA to chelate heavy metals such as lead, arsenic and mercury. Intramuscular injections are very painful, but it can be administered orally as well. Dimercaprol is more effective and less toxic than Ca EDTA and is the drug of choice in cases of lead-related CNS disturbances.

Dimethylsulfoxide (DMSO) is used as a carrier to allow the percutaneous penetration of drugs after topical application. It also acts to reduce swelling and can be combined with corticosteroids in the treatment of pododermatitis. Personal experience indicates that this is not to be recommended. Birds will acquire a typical garlic odor with use of this drug.

Dimetridazole is an older drug used in the treatment of trichomoniasis, histomoniasis and hexamitiasis. It has been replaced by more effective medications such as carnidazole.

Doxapram is available as a 20 mg/ml solution for IV or SC administration. It is sometimes used as a respiratory stimulant for birds anesthetized with ketamine and xylazine or during anesthetic emergencies.

Enilconazole is available as a 13.8% solution. It is effective in the control of *Aspergillus* spores and can be used as a disinfectant in incubators. Caution – it is highly irritating to the eyes!

Glucose is used in the treatment of hypoglycemia. Only the 5% solution can be used parenterally. Intravenous administration should be done very slowly.

Haloxon is sometimes combined with piperazine to treat endoparasites in pigeons. It is poorly tolerated or even toxic in birds of prey.

Iron-III-chloride can be used for hemostasis in cases

of minor bleeding involving the beak or talons. Not for use in open wounds!

Iron dextran is administered intramuscularly as an aid to erythropoiesis in cases of anemia or hemorrhage.

Lactated Ringer's solution is the fluid of choice for volume replacement in cases of dehydration and fluid loss. With mild dehydration (5%) it can be given orally. Otherwise intravenous administration is preferred. Recommended volumes are approximately 50 ml/kg/day.

Levothyroxine sodium is a thyroid supplement. It can sometimes induce molt if given at very high doses (1 mg/kg) for 14 days, but can have negative side-effects at this level.

Manna is made from the sap of various types of trees and is mentioned in the older literature for use as a mild laxative to stimulate hunting activity in hawks.

Naloxone is administered intravenously as a narcotic antagonist.

Oxytocin stimulates oviductal contraction and is administered in cases of egg-binding. If egg passage is inhibited for mechanical reasons or by adhesions, it may cause uterine rupture!

Pancuronium bromide is sometimes used in birds to dilate the pupils for ophthalmic examination. Eagles may develop tachycardia, dyspnea and depression with this drug.

Penicillin G benzathine is a long-acting form of penicillin G that can be highly toxic in some species of raptors.

Mineral oil is not absorbed in the digestive tract and helps lubricate in cases of impaction or foreign body obstruction. Administration by gavage is recommended to prevent aspiration.

Multivitamin supplements are commercially available and are sometimes used indiscriminately by breeders to supplement the regular diet. Recommended daily allowances for nutrients in raptors have not been established and there is a risk of oversupplementation with vitamins A, D, E and K. A well-balanced, freshly-killed diet should make vitamin supplementation completely unnecessary.

Pancreatic enzymes are available for oral supplementation. They are used to predigest the food used in hand-raising vulture chicks.

Phenylbutazone is a non-steroidal anti-inflammatory drug that is not well-tolerated by raptors. Falcons and eagles may vomit or develop bloody diarrhea.

Prednisolone is a well-tolerated glucocorticoid for use in reducing swelling of the extremities in raptors. At a dose of 5 mg/kg it also acts to increase appetite and water consumption, thus promoting weight gain in anorexic birds.

Procaine penicillin G's procaine components are toxic in smaller species. This drug is not recommended for use in raptors.

Progesterone acetate is a female hormone used by some breeders to render female falcons infertile. At doses of 25 mg/kg, egg-laying was prevented, but the birds developed fatty livers and occasionally died after several weeks of treatment.

Prostaglandins increase the muscle tone in the oviduct and are sometimes used to treat egg-binding or to help expel material from the reproductive tract. Ruptures of the oviduct can occur if passage is obstructed.

Pyrethrins are derived from chrysanthemums and are used topically in the treatment of ectoparasites. The original pyrethrins are safe for use in birds. Newer pyrethroid derivatives should be used with caution, however.

Sodium sulfate is an osmotic cathartic that causes diarrhea and loss of fluids. It should be administered only in cases of suspected toxin ingestion and the affected bird should be given supplemental fluids.

Testosterone is a male reproductive hormone used to stimulate mating behavior in tiercels. It does not result in higher sperm counts and does not improve fertility.

Vitamin B complex is administered in cases of GI tract disease and after treatment for coccidia. Birds suffering from prolonged anorexia may also benefit. B vitamins are normally produced naturally in the intestinal mucosa.

Vitamin E is thought by some breeders to be a fertility vitamin and supplemented in the food before and during the breeding season. These are purely empirical measures, since neither the vitamin E requirements in raptors nor the quantities present in the food are well known.

8.3 Emergency treatment

A thorough clinical examination of a critically ill or injured bird of prey is usually too long and stressful and could pose additional risks to the animal's survival. In such cases, the primary goal is to stabilize the vital signs and once that is accomplished, to proceed with other relevant diagnostic and therapeutic measures.

Although each bird should be assessed and treated individually, there are some general rules of emergency therapy that apply to all. The first concern is always respiration. The depth and regularity of respiration can give initial indications as to the animal's overall status. Severe dyspnea may be seen with tracheal foreign bodies, severe blood loss or respiratory diseases such as aspergillosis. Dyspneic birds should be handled with great care, as they can easily die if stressed. Administration of oxygen by face mask or in a closed cage can be helpful. If an obstructive problem involving the trachea is suspected, an alternate airway can be created by inserting a large bore catheter or tube in the abdominal air sac behind the last rib.

Obtaining an accurate body weight is important for all further measures. If this involves too much stress, an attempt at estimating the animal's weight may be made. Most falconers are very familiar with their hawk's normal body weight and can help supply such information. Otherwise, the bird can be placed on a scale in a light cardboard box, and the weight of the box subtracted from the total.

Quisenberry and Hillyer (1994) recommend light anesthesia of emergency patients with isoflurane (see Ch. 15.3.2). This permits the rapid and relatively stress-free accomplishment of necessary diagnostic and therapeutic measures such as venipuncture, radiographs and fluid administration.

Fluid therapy

All chronically ill and many acutely injured raptors suffer from dehydration. Birds of prey derive most of their fluid requirements from the oxidative metabolism of their food and will become quickly dehydrated if they stop eating.

Skin turgor or elasticity is often used in mammals to assess the degree of dehydration present. Tented skin will return quickly to its normal position in well-hydrated animals. This return is slowed in the presence of fluid deficits. The thin skin of birds permits only limited interpretation of such tests. A more useful indicator of avian fluid status is the rate at which the ulnar vein underneath the wing refills after compression. If it takes longer than 2 seconds to refill, one can assume the bird is more than 7% dehydrated. More severely affected birds will have sunken eyes and dry mucus membranes. In dehydrated chicks, the skin of the toes will look dry and wrinkled instead of fleshy and moist.

Redig (1993) listed a variety of clinical parameters that can be used to assess the degree of dehydration in birds of prey (Table 8.5).

It is wise to assume that all emergency patients are at least 5% dehydrated and supplement with fluids accordingly.

The following formula is used to estimate the volume of replacement fluids needed:

approximate degree of dehydration (%) x body weight (g) = fluid deficit (ml)

Warmed (38–39 °C) lactated Ringer's solution is the replacement fluid of choice in birds. It can be given orally, subcutaneously or intravenously. Oral fluid therapy suffers from the drawback that it is rapidly excreted from the body and must be repeated hourly. In addition, the oral route should not be chosen in birds that are in shock or vomiting.

Subcutaneous fluid administered into the loose skin at the nape of the neck or under the wing is usually absorbed quite slowly from these poorly perfused areas. The fluids may accumulate in dependent areas and contribute to temporary protein loss from the plasma. However, subcutaneous administration may be the only option in very small birds such as chicks. A small gauge needle should be used to prevent the fluids from leaking back out through the injection site.

The best and most rapid response to fluid therapy is achieved via the intravenous route. The wing vein or even the jugular vein in the neck can be used. Butterfly catheters or small gauge intravenous catheters

should be placed in order to permit slow administration of intravenous fluids. Abou-Madi and Kollias recommend an administration rate of 10 ml/kg over a period of 5 to 7 minutes. Most intravenous catheters are not well tolerated by raptors, making their repeated use difficult.

Treatment of shock
Shock is always treated with immediate fluid therapy. The additional use of glucocorticoids in birds is debated. They are immunosuppressive, making the animal more vulnerable to bacterial or fungal infections. Their use should therefore probably be limited to cases in which steroids are clearly indicated. This includes injuries involving head or spinal cord trauma, in which swelling of the central nervous system within confined bony spaces can quickly lead to pressure and serious nerve damage. Corticosteroids can reduce such swelling if given soon after the traumatic event. Prednisolone at 1-2 mg/kg can be used for such cases.

Blood loss
The average blood volume in birds is slightly less than 10% of the total body weight. Healthy raptors are capable of tolerating a loss of up to 30% of their blood volume without showing significant clinical effects and can compensate for this loss within one or two days. Even severe blood loss of up to 70% can be safely treated with crystalloid fluid replacement alone.

The therapeutic value of blood transfusions in birds is debated. On the one hand, blood groups do not seem to be important in birds, making it possible to transfuse not only homologous, but even heterologous blood from donors of another species. Pigeon blood, for example, can be safely transfused into hawks at least once. On the other hand, even blood transfusions are unlikely to improve the survival of patients suffering from extreme blood loss or hypovolemic shock.

Head trauma
Wild raptors and free-flying hunting hawks are always in danger of sustaining head trauma in our complicated industrial landscapes. Collisions with cars or with reflective window panes are common causes of such injuries. Frequently, the initially stunned bird will recover after a short time. Because of the risk of cranial edema and the permanent CNS damage associated with it, the immediate administration of glucocorticoids is indicated in such cases. Fluid therapy should be put off unless there is evidence of hypotension. Again, the aim is to minimize intracranial pressure.

The injured bird should be kept as quiet as possible and placed in a dark cardboard box. If no improvement occurs in the hawk's condition over the first 24 hours,

Table 8.5: Estimated degree of dehydration based on clinical signs (from Redig, 1993)

Dehydration	Clinical signs
less than 5%	Not noticeable
7–10 %	Decreased elasticity ("tenting") of loose skin, eyes may appear dull, eyelids partly closed, tacky mucus membranes
10–12%	Tented skin remains standing, scales on feet darker than normal, dry mucus membranes, cool extremities, tachycardia, apathy
12–15%	Shock, agonal

the prognosis for full recovery is grave and permanent damage to the CNS may make euthanasia necessary.

Hyperthermia and heat stroke

The risk of hyperthermia exists when transporting birds in the car, brooding chicks under a heat lamp, or for hawks in completely enclosed aviaries during summer. Birds have no sweat glands in their skin and can reduce their body temperature only by panting or altering their posture. Hyperthermic chicks will spread their wings and legs and stretch out their neck, while when cold, they will do just the opposite and hunch up to minimize the body surface they expose.

Overheated birds should be placed with their feet in cold water. In advanced cases, they may have lost enough fluids by panting that fluid replacement therapy is indicated. Patients suffering from heat stroke should also be treated with corticosteroids to prevent cranial edema.

Emptying the stomach

In cases of toxin ingestion, immediate emptying of crop and stomach contents may be indicated. This procedure has already been described in Chapter 4.4 and must be performed if the bird is not vomiting or regurgitating on its own. Birds can be induced to vomit if they are alert and standing upright. This is accomplished by taking a rubber band and placing it over the bird's head and into the mouth like a bridle and bit on a horse. The hawk will try to remove this foreign body in its mouth by retching until vomiting occurs.

References and literature of further interest

ABOU-MADI, N. and G.V. KOLLIAS (1992):
Avian fluid therapy.
in: Kirk, R.W. u. J.D. Bonagura: Current veterinary therapy
1154–1159
W.B. Saunders, Philadelphia

BARONETZKY-MERCIER, A. and B. SEIDEL (1995):
in: GÖLTHENBOTH, R. u. H.G. KLÖS (1995):
Krankheiten der Zoo- und Wildtiere 462
Blackwell Wissenschafts-Verlag, Berlin

BIRD, J.E., MILLER, K.W., LARSON, A.A. and G.E. DUKE (1983):
Pharmacokinetics of gentamicin in birds of prey.
Amer. J. Vet. Res. **44**, 1245–1247

CLARK, C.H., THOMAS, J.E., MILTON, J.L. and W.D. GOOLSBY (1982):
Plasma concentrations of chloramphenicol in birds.
Amer. J. Vet. Res. **43**, 1249–1253

COOPER, J.E. (1974):
Trichlorphon as a safe insecticide for use on birds of prey.
Vet. Rec. **94**, 455

FERNANDEZ-REPOLLET, E., ROWLEY, J. and A. SCHWARTZ (1982):
Renal damage in gentamicin-treated Lanner falcons (*Falco biarmicus*).
J. Am. Vet., Med. Ass. **181**, 1392

FORBES, N.A., SIMPSON, G.N. and M.F. GOUDSWAARD (1992):
Diagnosis of avian aspergillosis and treatment with itraconazole.
Vet. Rec. **130**, 519–520

FURLEY, C.W. and A.G. GREENWOOD (1982):
Treatment of aspergillosis in raptors (Order Falconiformes) with miconazole.
Vet. Rec. **111**, 584–585

GYLSTORFF, I. and F. GRIMM (1987):
Vogelkrankheiten.
Verlag Eugen Ulmer, Stuttgart

JUREK, V. (1988):
Über Erfahrungen mit Ivomec bei Zoovögeln.
Int. Symp. Erkrank. Zootiere **30**, 343-347

KIRKWOOD, J.K. (1983):
Treatment [miconazole] of aspergillosis in raptors.
Vet. Rec. 112, 183

KLÜH, P.N. (1994):
Untersuchungen zur Therapie und Prophylaxe der *Caryospora*-Infektion der Falken (Falconiformes: Falconidae) mit Toltrazuril sowie die Beschreibung von zwei neuen *Caryospora*-Arten (*C. megafalconis* n. sp. und *C. boeri* n. sp.).
Vet. Med. Diss. Hannover

LAWRENCE, K. (1983):
Efficacy of fenbendazole against nematodes of captive birds.
Vet. Rec. **112**, 433-434

OETTLÉ, E. (1992):
Enrofloxacinbehandlung eines jungen Wanderfalken (*Falco peregrinus minor*).
Greifvögel und Falknerei 135–136
Verlag Neumann-Neudamm, Morschen-Heina

PARROTT, T. (1991):
Clinical treatment regimes with fluconazole.
Proc. Ann. Meeting Assoc. Avian Vet., Chicago 15–17

QUESENBERRY, K.E and E.V. HILLYER (1994):
Supportive care and emergency therapy.
in: Ritchie, W.B. et al.: Avian medicine: principles and application. 382–416
Wingers Publishing, Lake Worth, Florida

RAMISZ, A. and J. SKOTNICKI (1981):
Behandlung des Capillaria-Befalles bei Zoovogeln mit Fenbendazol.
Int. Symp. Erkr. Zootiere **23**, 237–241

REDIG, P.T. (1981):
The differential diagnosis and treatment of aspergillosis in birds.
Diss. Abstr. Int. 41B **7**, 2556–2557

REDIG, P.T. and G.E. DUKE (1985):
Comparative pharmacokinetics of antifungal drugs in domestic turkeys, red-tailed hawks, broad-winged hawks, and great horned owls.
Avian Dis. **29**, 649–661

REDIG, P.T. (1991):
A Formulary of Pharmacological Agents for Emergency Care of Raptors
Hawk Chalk **30**, 49–52

REDIG, P.T. (1993):
Medical management of birds of prey.
A collection of notes on selected topics 115–124
Raptor Center, Minnesota

SANTIAGO, C., MILLS, P.A. and C.E. KIRKPATRICK (1985):
Oral capillariasis in a red-tailed hawk: treatment with fenbendazole.
J. Am. Vet. Med. Ass. **187**, 1205–1206

SMITH, S.A. (1993)
Diagnosis and treatment of helminths in birds of prey.
in: Redig P.T. (1993)
Raptor Biomedicine, Chiron Pub. Ltd. Keighley, West Yorkshire, England

STEHLE, S. (1977):
Behandlung von Helminthosen bei Greifvögeln (Falconiformes) mit Fenbendazol (Panacur).
Kleintierpraxis **22**, 261–266

TULLY, N.T. and G.J. HARRISON (1994):
Pneumology
in: RITCHIE, B.W., HARRISON, G.J. and L.R. HARRISON (1994):
Avian medicine: principles and application
Wingers Publishing, Lake Worth, Florida

WAGNER, C., HOCHLEITHNER, M. and W.D. RAUSCH (1991):
Ketoconazole plasma levels in buzzards.
Proc. Conf. Europ. Com. Ass. Avian Vet., 333–340

*"Even when the physician's art cannot accomplish
that which is actually necessary, it would be foolish
to discard the limited benefits we can derive from it,
just as it would be foolish not to ride a donkey
when no horse is available."*

(RHAZES – Abū Bakr Muhammad b. Zakarīyā' ar-Rāzī, 865–925)

9 Infectious diseases

A large variety of infectious diseases are encountered in birds of prey. Frequently, they are transmitted by the bird's natural prey animals. In view of the important ecological role played by raptors in nature, this may seem maladaptive. Their tendency to cull ill or injured animals selectively is well-established and important. What sense would there be in a raptor's dying of the same disease as its victim?

This line of reasoning may hold for wild birds of prey, which are rarely exposed to high levels of infectious organisms and whose disease resistance remains strong under natural conditions. There is, however, a very fine balance between host and pathogen. This balance can be tilted to the raptor's disadvantage in captive situations. If there is, in addition, an unusually high level of exposure to disease-causing microorganisms, the bird's natural mechanisms of defense may be overwhelmed. An infection that would not normally cause disease in nature may thus lead to illness or death in captivity.

The primary rule of disease prevention in birds of prey should therefore involve optimizing the conditions in captivity to meet all the animal's natural requirements.

9.1 Viral diseases

Viral infections have always been an important cause of disease in birds of prey. Several raptor diseases have been traced to viruses only in recent years, thanks to in-depth research efforts and improved techniques for virus isolation and identification.

Large scale investigations involving raptor breeding facilities or populations of wild birds have found antibodies to or even isolates of numerous well-known viruses although none of the animals involved were suffering from clinical disease. Postmortem examinations of raptors have indicated that viral disease played a role in the animals' death approximately 14% of the time, while antibodies to various viruses were found in up to 30% of the cases (Heidenreich, 1976, Druener, 1978).

9.1.1 Newcastle disease

Newcastle disease is an acute viral disease with a high mortality rate that can affect almost all types of birds. It is of concern primarily in domestic poultry. Nevertheless there is a long list of wild birds that are also known to be susceptible. Because captive raptors often consume day-old chicks or poultry processing remnants, transmission of this virus to birds of prey is possible at any time. Several cases of Newcastle disease in wild raptors have been reported in the literature as well. Although the source of the virus in these cases is unknown, wild pheasants, crows, and especially pigeons are potentially capable of harboring and transmitting it to birds of prey in any number of ways.

Pathogen
Newcastle disease is caused by one of several different strains of avian paramyxoviruses that have been isolated worldwide. These strains vary considerably in their host specificity and virulence among birds. Strains that are less virulent in pigeons or poultry, causing only mild disease or resulting in latent infections, can cause serious disease and death when transmitted to birds of prey, especially falcons.

The virus is excreted in the urates and feces of infected animals, and is easily transmitted directly to other animals by ingestion or inhalation.

Clinical disease
Raptors that have been infected with Newcastle disease virus either naturally or experimentally are variably susceptible and show widely differing clinical pictures.

Silent infection: Attempts to infect vultures experimentally have been unsuccessful. Even vaccination does not result in measurable antibodies in this group of birds. Vultures are similarly resistant to other disease-producing microorganisms and even to toxins such as botulinum toxin. This phenomenon makes sense considering the many pathogens to which vultures are naturally exposed in their ecological role as scavengers.

Abortive disease course: Eagles and hawks can develop clinical disease after infection with Newcastle disease virus. Experimental infection by intramuscular injection resulted in development of the disease and death within 24 hours. Common buzzards showed clinical signs of Newcastle disease only two days after being inoculated conjunctivally. Ingestion of food containing the virus, on the other hand, resulted in illness after an incubation period of 7 to 9 days. Anorexia, fluffed plumage, somnolence, heavy flight, diarrhea, green urates and CNS disturbances were seen. Approximately one week after initial signs were noticed, the affected birds resumed eating, appearing almost normal a few days later. Some ataxia may remain and torticollis and tremors may persist for weeks or months. The significant weight loss incurred during the initial stages of the disease and the prolonged neurological disturbances make survival of affected wild raptors unlikely.

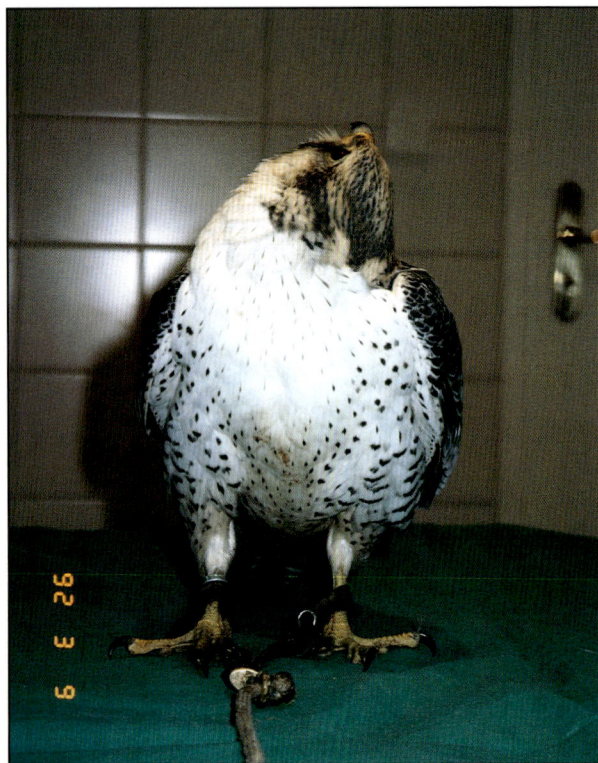

Fig. 9.1: This male red-naped shaheen (*F. pelegrinoides*) X gyrfalcon (*F. rusticolus*) hybrid was one of seven falcons that became infected with Newcastle disease virus by consuming chicken heads derived from a large poultry processing plant. Two days after showing initial signs of the disease (torticollis) this bird was dead. Newcastle disease virus was isolated from the brain, lung, spleen and kidneys.
(Photo: Heidenreich)

It is noteworthy that investigations involving wild birds of prey that succumbed due to accidents (Winteroll, 1976) found a high percentage of birds from whose organs this virus could be isolated. It is possible that these birds were more prone to injury as a result of Newcastle disease-related CNS disturbances.

Acute disease: In falcons, the ingestion of Newcastle disease virus usually results in severe illness and quickly leads to death. Common kestrels (*F. tinnunculus*), peregrine falcons (*F. peregrinus*), prairie falcons (*F. mexicanus*), saker falcons (*F. cherrug*) and gyrfalcons (*F. rusticolus*) will show initially mild neurological signs including gentle tremors within 4 to 12 days after infection. The falcons then become anorectic, develop severe ataxia and succumb to the disease within the following 48 hours (Fig. 9.1).

Pathology
Necropsy findings will vary considerably depending on the course and duration of the disease. Acute illness, as seen in falcons, may reveal only petechial hemorrhages in the coronary fat and gastric mucosa and larger hemorrhages in the brain. More chronic disease will result in inflammatory changes involving the liver, the pericardium and the entire gastrointestinal tract. Hemorrhages may occur in the heart, gastric mucosa and kidneys. Frequently, severe lung involvement with foamy exudate is evident even though no respiratory abnormalities were noted in the bird before death.

Diagnosis
Antemortem diagnosis of Newcastle disease virus is extremely difficult if not impossible. Multiple deaths in a group of falcons showing the typical clinical signs in conjunction with a history of feeding poultry products or sick pigeons will serve to raise the index of suspicion. Confirmation requires isolation of the virus or demonstration of antibody titers. Tissues obtained from the lung, liver, spleen, trachea or brain of dead birds are best for isolation attempts in chick embryos or cell cultures. Birds that survive the disease can be serologically tested for evidence of antibodies.

Treatment and prevention
Therapeutic measures initiated after a bird develops clinical disease are supportive at best. The majority of affected falcons will die despite treatment and the rest will have permanent CNS damage.

Chances of inadvertent exposure to Newcastle disease virus can be minimized by not feeding poultry or pigeons to captive birds of prey.

Vaccination can also be considered in attempts to prevent this disease. Hitchner B₁ and La Sota strain poultry vaccines intended for use in the drinking water are effective in raptors and can be administered intranasally or orally. Mild palpebral swelling and inflammation lasting a few days may be seen after vaccination. A booster vaccination three to four weeks after the initial dose is recommended. Immunity will last about six months.

9.1.2 Raptorpox

Diseases caused by poxviruses are seen in many different domestic and wild birds. In raptors, clinical infections with this virus have been reported in the broad-winged hawk (*Buteo platypterus*), rough-legged buzzard (*Buteo lagopus*), red-tailed hawk (*Buteo jamaicensis*), golden eagle (*Aquila chryseatos*), saker falcon (*F. cherrug*), laggar falcon (*F. jugger*), peregrine falcon (*F. peregrinus*), and gyrfalcon (*F. rusticolus*). The older literature sometimes refers to poxviral disease in raptors as diphtheria, diphtheroid or pox-diphtheria (Trommer, 1969). These vague terms merely describe pathologic findings and were actually used to describe a number of widely different diseases. They should therefore no longer be used.

Pathogen
Many different strains of poxviruses have been defined in the genus *Avipox*. They include fowlpox, turkeypox, pigeonpox, canarypox, quailpox, agapornispox and others. With the exception of canarypox, which has a somewhat broader host spectrum, most of these strains are species-specific. Raptors cannot be infected with the poxviruses listed above and even canarypox will merely cause a mild skin reaction at the site of infection.

Direct transmission of the virus from prey species to raptors is therefore not very likely. It is assumed, instead, that a separate strain of poxvirus, or maybe even several, exist for birds of prey.

It is known that gyrfalcons, peregrine falcons, laggar falcons and saker falcons can all be infected with the same strain of falconpox (*Avipox falconi*).

Transmission of the virus occurs primarily through biting insects or direct contact with open skin lesions and mucus membranes. The virus is thought to remain active in the salivary glands of mosquitoes (*Culex* spp.) for several weeks. Therefore the disease is seen most frequently in warm latitudes (Arab states along the Gulf) or during late summer in more temperate climates, when mosquitoes abound. Cooper (1969) suggests that poxviral infections in raptors are more common in Europe after Arab falcons have been imported.

Clinical disease
The course of disease is influenced by the virulence of the strain, the mode of infection and the resistance of the bird. Four basic forms of the disease are recognized, although combinations thereof can also occur.

Cutaneous form: This is the most common form seen in many raptors. The unfeathered areas of skin including the feet and eyelids, the commissures of the mouth and the cere will be affected. After an incubation period of 4 to 9 days, pinhead-sized papules develop, gradually enlarging and becoming crusty (Fig. 9.2). Some of the pox lesions may break open and exude thick serous fluid. Strong birds usually begin to recover after this point. Immunocompromised animals, on the other hand, may develop secondary infections with fungi or yeast, streptococcal or staphylococcal organisms. The papules then develop into deep lesions involving the dermis and underlying structures. The animal's feet and head develop generalized crusting and bleed easily. Pain and infection will result in depression and lethargy. Many birds are unable to stand on their infected feet and become recumbent. Septicemia may result in death.

Birds that survive the cutaneous form of poxvirus are often left with permanent scars. Abnormal talons lacking keratin sheaths can result from infections involving the base of the claw (Fig. 9.3). Scar tissue involving the palpebrae and periorbital skin can cause eyelid constrictions or closure of the palpebral fissure, impairing vision.

Diphtheroid form: Unlike with other groups of birds, the diphtheroid form of pox is only rarely seen in raptors. Some authors even suggest that it does not occur at all in birds of prey. Others describe the development of caseous yellow lesions in the oral cavity. These plaques may extend deep into the pharynx and the glottis. Attempts to remove them result in significant bleeding. Birds affected in this way are in danger of asphyxiation if these pseudomembranous deposits expand to obstruct the airways.

Tumorous form: Kuntze et al. (1968) described the development of cutaneous tumors in a broad-winged hawk (*Buteo platypterus*) that had previously been infected with poxvirus. These masses were described as wart-like and very prone to bleeding.

Neurological form: A group of falcons infected with falconpox in the Arab Gulf states was described as suffering from disturbances of the central nervous system, including inability to fly and vestibular problems. Because Newcastle disease virus is common in food animals from that area, it is possible that these falcons were suffering from both diseases.

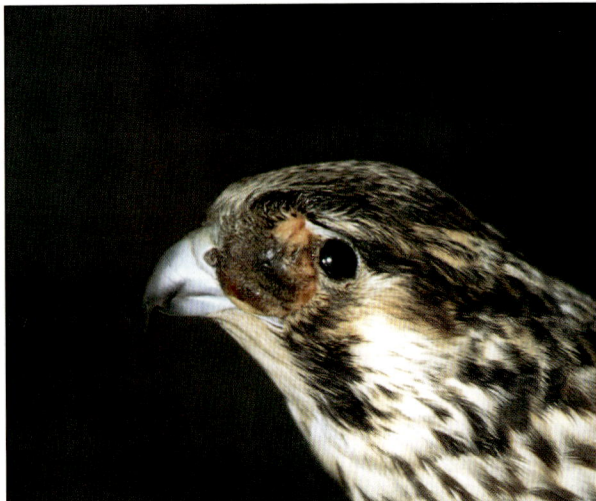

Fig. 9.2: A saker falcon (*F. cherrug*) with a severe case of cutaneous pox affecting the cere and the medial canthus of the eye. Early involvement of the lower eyelid is also noticeable.
(Photo: Lierz)

Prevention

A varied and nutritionally complete diet will do much to keep raptors healthy and immunologically strong, improving their ability to resist infection and disease. If a bird begins to show clinical signs of raptorpox, it should be immediately separated from uninfected birds. Secure insect netting for aviaries and breeding chambers is especially important during mosquito season.

Although effective vaccines have been developed for domestic poultry and canaries, none is yet available for raptors, especially falcons. Attempts to vaccinate falcons with pigeonpox vaccines have been carried out, but the long-term results are not yet known. Some authors have recommended vaccinating with fowlpox or turkeypox vaccines. Despite these supposedly effective vaccines, falconpox continues to be a problem, especially in Arab countries. Due to the narrow host spectrum of this virus, it is likely that a specific falconpox vaccine will be necessary to help control this disease in birds of prey.

Diagnosis

The cutaneous form of avian pox has a relatively characteristic presentation, making a preliminary diagnosis at the time of physical examination easy. The diphtheritic form can be more difficult to recognize if skin lesions are absent. Other diseases such as trichomoniasis, candidiasis, and oral capillariasis will show similar lesions. In either case, the diagnosis of pox should be confirmed and appropriate therapeutic measures instituted.

Confirmation of poxvirus disease can be accomplished in two ways. Direct confirmation requires culturing the virus from new, uninfected papules or lesions on the patient's skin. Older lesions or crusty material should not be used. The sample should be immediately transferred to a culture medium and sent to the lab, where the virus is cultured on chick embryo membranes.

Indirect confirmation involves histological examination of biopsy samples from affected skin. Special staining will reveal the characteristic viral inclusions known as Bollinger bodies.

Their presence constitutes a definitive diagnosis.

Treatment

The viral infection itself cannot be treated. Supportive care including broad spectrum antibacterial and antifungal therapy will help prevent or treat any secondary skin infections. Topical treatment of pox lesions with iodine-glycerin (1:4) and supplementation with vitamin A to promote epithelial regeneration may be helpful.

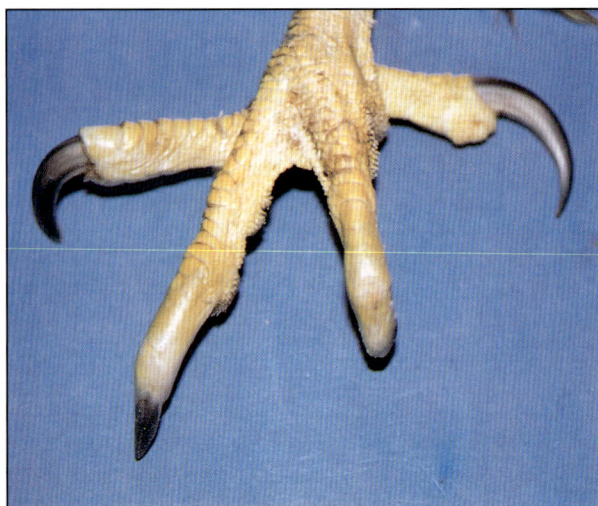

Fig. 9.3: The foot of a white gyrfalcon (*F. rusticolus*) which was infected with falconpox years ago.
The disease was transmitted by Arab falcons that were kept in the same facilities during the summer molting period.
(Photo: Heidenreich)

9.1.3   Herpesvirus infections

Herpesviruses are widespread among birds. In domestic fowl these include Marek's disease virus, turkey herpesvirus, infectious laryngotracheitis and duck plague. Herpesviruses have been isolated from wild birds as well, although they are not always associated with clinical disease. Table 9.1 summarizes the various strains of avian herpesviridae that have been isolated and described.

9.1.3.1 Falcon herpesvirus (Inclusion Body Disease of falcons)

Pigeon herpesvirus is often cited as the source for herpesvirus disease in falcons. Indeed, the pigeon and owl herpesviruses show a close antigenic relationship with the strain isolated from infected falcons (Aini et al., 1993). Because infection with and death from herpes in falcons are frequently associated with the feeding of pigeons, these food animals are suspected of transmitting the virus. This has not been definitively proven. Doubts as to this mode of transmission are strengthened by the fact that attempts to experimentally infect pigeons and doves with falcon herpesvirus succeeded only with African collared doves and failed in most other species including domestic pigeons.

Whether transmission of herpesvirus between falcons is possible remains unknown as well. Massive oral inoculation attempts involving the feeding of fresh liver and spleen from falcons that had died of the disease to other falcons were unable to induce clinical infections in the recipient birds.

Many herpesviruses are capable of producing latent infections in their host. These viruses will remain inactive until the host's immune system is compromised by stress or illness. This could occur in falcons as well, but is unlikely. Three siblings and both parents of a falcon that died of falcon herpesvirus infection remained

Table 9.1 : Avian herpesviruses

Herpesvirus	Host species	Disease
Infectious laryngotracheitis	Chickens, peafowl, pheasants	Upper respiratory system infection
Marek's disease virus	Gallinaceous species	Peripheral nerve disease, tumors
Colinus herpesvirus	Quail	Inflammation of liver and spleen
Turkey herpesvirus	Gallinaceous species	no disease
Duck plague	Ducks, geese, swans	Duck virus enteritis, hemorrhages
Pacheco's disease virus	Psittaciformes	Acute liver, spleen and kidney disease
Amazon tracheitis	Genus *Amazona*, chickens	Upper respiratory system infection
Pigeon inclusion body hepatitis	Pigeons, budgerigars	Conjunctivitis, rhinitis, ingluvitis
Pigeon herpes encephalomyelitis	Pigeons	Encephalomyelitis
Stork inclusion body hepatitis	White stork, black stork	Inflammation of liver and spleen
Crane inclusion body hepatitis	Various crane species	Inflammation of liver and spleen
Lake Victoria cormorant virus	Little pied cormorant	Unknown
Eagle herpesvirus	Bald eagle, booted eagle	Unknown
Owl herpesvirus	Eagle owl, great horned owl, striped owl, long-eared owl, snowy owl, little owl, Tengmalm's owl, forest eagle owl	Hepatosplenitis infectiosa strigum
Falcon herpesvirus	Peregrine falcon, prairie falcon, saker falcon, gyrfalcon, merlin, American kestrel, common kestrel, red-headed falcon	Inflammation of liver and spleen Inclusion body hepatitis of falcons

healthy and failed to develop antibodies to the virus despite being maintained under the same conditions as the affected bird and being exposed to the disease. Another observation made in the summer of 1994 also contradicts the theory of possible latent herpesvirus infections in falcons. That summer was unusually warm and a large falcon breeding facility experienced abnormally high mortality rates, especially among its young gyrfalcons. Approximately half the birds died of aspergillosis, the other half succumbed to herpesvirus infections. In no case were we able to diagnose a mixed infection involving both pathogens. It would seem that if latency and immunocompetence were factors in this disease, some of the birds suffering from aspergillosis should have developed herpes as well.

Although this virus can affect many different falcon species, gyrfalcons seem to be particularly susceptible.

Clinical disease
Because the route of infection is not fully understood, little is known about the incubation period or initial clinical signs of falcon herpes. Experiments with owl herpesvirus indicate that the period between infection and death in these birds ranges from 9 to 11 days.

Falcons that develop the disease appear suddenly depressed and unresponsive. They refuse to eat and produce lime green urates. Death usually occurs two or three days after signs of illness are first noted.

Pathology
This disease strikes so rapidly that the affected bird will still be in good body condition at the time of death. As in owls, herpesvirus infection in falcons produces easily-observed lesions involving the liver and spleen. Both organs will be enlarged and covered with pinhead-sized yellowish-white foci of necrosis (Figs. 9.4 and 9.5). Intranuclear inclusion bodies can be seen histopathologically.

Diagnosis
The rapid course and nonspecific signs of this disease in falcons make an antemortem diagnosis difficult unless other birds from the same facility have recently succumbed and been previously diagnosed. It would theoretically be possible to identify the characteristic necrotic foci on the liver and spleen laparoscopically. However, the risk of anesthesia is increased in affected birds, especially if injectable anesthetics that are metabolized or excreted by the liver and kidney are used.

In other bird species, particularly pigeons, gross necropsy findings similar to those described above may occur with generalized salmonellosis. It is therefore likely that necropsies of falcons performed prior to the isolation and description of falcon herpesvirus as a disease entity sometimes resulted in a misdiagnosis of salmonellosis, especially when the animal had a history of exposure to pigeons. In numerous microbial cultures performed by the author over the years in animals with suspicious liver lesions, *Salmonella* organisms were never isolated from any organ except the gastrointestinal tract of those animals that died. These isolates were presumably incidental, stemming from the consumption of pigeons.

A definitive diagnosis requires isolation of the virus or histological identification of intranuclear inclusion bodies in affected organs. It is always wise to rule out bacterial disease by requesting a microbial culture as well.

Treatment and prevention
Affected falcons have an almost 100% mortality rate. Effective treatment options are not known and vaccines are not available. Although pigeons have not been directly implicated in this disease, feeding pigeons to falcons should generally be avoided, especially in gyrfalcons. Some American breeders of gyrfalcons maintain their own, isolated pigeon colony and test the birds in it regularly for serologic evidence of exposure to herpesvirus (Berry, 1994). Only pigeons that test negative are fed to the falcons.

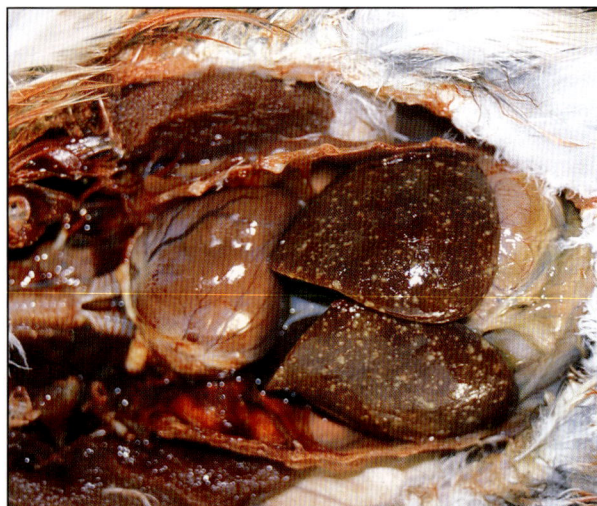

Fig. 9.4: The coelomic cavity of a white gyrfalcon (*F. rusticolus*) that died of falcon herpesvirus. The liver shows the typical yellowish-white foci of necrosis associated with this infection. Pigeons with salmonellosis have a similar postmortem appearance. It is possible that this resulted in misdiagnosis of this disease in falcons prior to the identification of falcon herpesvirus.
(Photo: Heidenreich)

9.1.3.2 Marek's disease

This disease is distributed worldwide and of special importance in the poultry industry. Also caused by a herpesvirus, it affects primarily young animals. Three different forms of Marek's disease have been described in gallinaceous species, the **nervous** form characterized by ataxia or lameness, the **ocular** form and a **tumorous** form in which lymphoid tumors may develop in various internal organs.

Marek's disease virus infection has been reported in a great horned owl and a European sparrowhawk (*Accipiter nisus*). The latter case involved three nestlings which developed "neurolymphomatosis (fowl paralysis)" (Woodford and Glasier, 1955).

Keymer (1972) described Marek's disease-like lesions involving the internal organs of a gray kestrel (*Falco ardosiaceus*) and an Ayre's hawk-eagle (*Hieraaetus dubius)* He described the lesions as "visceral lymphomatosis", but did not differentiate them from the very similar changes seen with leukosis virus infections.

9.1.3.3 Eagle herpesvirus

A herpesvirus was isolated from cloacal swabs taken from clinically healthy, wild bald eagle (*Haliaeetus leucocephalus*) nestlings (Docherty et al, 1983). It was also isolated from a South American eagle that developed lesions similar to those seen in falcons (Kaleta, 1990). The eagle strain is distinct from the one that

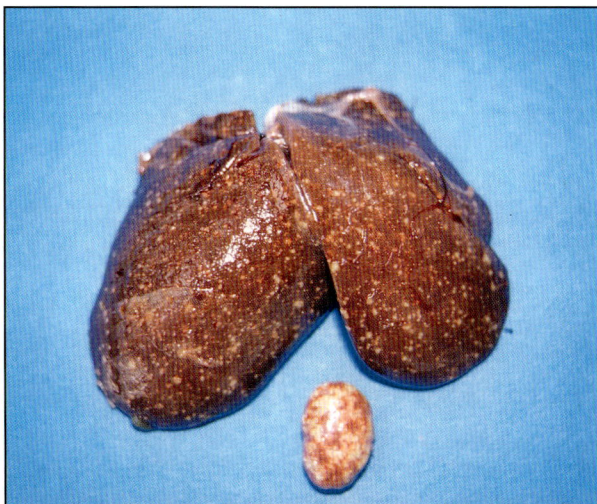

Fig. 9.5: Falcon herpesvirus affects not only the liver, but also the spleen. Hypertrophy of the white pulp of the spleen gives this organ a typical marbled appearance.
(Photo: Heidenreich)

causes falcon herpesvirus, making it likely that various groups of raptors harbor host-specific herpesvirus isolates.

9.1.4   Rabies

Rabies is a viral disease of great concern in mammals, which are infected by exposure of an open wound to the saliva or other tissues from infected animals. Birds of prey are thus at risk of exposure if they consume an animal infected with the rabies virus.

It is not known, however, whether raptors can actually become infected with the virus. Reports in the older literature (Paarmann, 1955; Roemmele, 1959; and CLAUSING, 1963) describe natural cases of rabies in goshawks (*Accipiter* sp.), buzzards (*Buteo* sp.) and kites (*Milvus* sp.) as well as in falcons and goshawks after experimental infection. Gough and Jorgenson (1976) were able to detect antibodies to the virus in birds of prey, but found no evidence of clinical disease. In other studies, immunosuppression using large doses of glucocorticoids was required to induce the production of antibodies in raptors after experimental infection with rabies virus. Again, the birds did not show clinical signs of infection.

In a case observed by the author himself, several golden eagles were bitten and seriously injured by a fox that was subsequently proven to be rabid. None of the birds developed the disease.

More recent research (Shannon et al., 1988; Artois, 1990) examining blood samples from a wide variety of American raptors indicated that these birds probably do not play a significant role in the spread and transmission of rabies to other animals.

There are several reports of supposedly rabid birds of prey attacking human beings. None of these birds was proven to carry the virus and it is more likely that these were human-imprinted animals or that they had escaped from captivity and were flying at people in search of food or mates.

Clinical disease
After experimental infection with the rabies virus in birds, three weeks to several months may pass before clinical signs are seen. This seems to depend on the site of inoculation. A brief excitable stage characterized by aggression and convulsions is followed by ataxia, lameness, paresis and then somnolence, culminating in death after a few days.

Diagnosis
A presumptive diagnosis can be reached on the basis of history and clinical signs. Histologic confirmation of Negri bodies or positive results of immunofluorescent

staining of nervous tissue are required to confirm the diagnosis.

Treatment and prevention

There is no known treatment for rabies in people or animals once clinical signs are evident. Some birds of prey have been reported to recover spontaneously after experimentally induced cases of rabies.

Despite the small likelihood that raptors can contract or transmit the rabies virus, exposure to potentially rabid animals such as foxes or raccoons should be avoided.

9.1.5   Adenovirus infection in american kestrels

A group of captive American kestrels with hemorrhagic enteritis showed evidence of being infected with a presumptive adenovirus (Sileo, 1983). Mortality was high. Necropsies revealed gastrointestinal petechiae and hepatocellular necrosis with intranuclear inclusions.

9.1.5.1 CELO-virus

This group of viruses belongs to the Adenoviridae family. CELO-viruses have been isolated from common buzzards (*Buteo buteo*) and the common kestrel (*Falco tinnunculus*). The clinical relevance of these findings is unknown, since the isolation occurred from birds that had been delivered already dead. A wild goshawk (*Accipiter gentilis*) was found alive but unable to fly and died shortly thereafter with convulsions. CELO-virus was isolated from this bird as well, but the clinical signs could not be definitely ascribed to it. It remains unclear whether this group of viruses is responsible for disease in birds of prey. Buteos, in particular, frequently have serologic evidence of antibodies to CELO-viruses without showing signs of illness.

9.1.6   Reovirus

A reovirus was isolated from a dead laggar falcon (*Falco jugger*). Antemortem clinical signs and the role of this virus in the bird's death remain unknown. In other birds, reoviruses cause diarrhea and swelling of the liver.

References and literature of further interest

AINI, I., SHIH, L.M., CASTRO, A.E. and Y.C. ZEE (1993):
Comparison of herpesvirus isolates from falcons, pigeons and psittacines by restriction endonuclease analysis.
J. Wildl. Dis. **29**, 196–202

AKRAE, M. (1980):
Die Identifizierung und Charakterisierung eines Falkenpocken- und eines Psittacidenpockenvirus aufgrund ihres Verhaltens in der Eikultur, sowie serologischer Reaktionen und ihres Wirtsspektrums im Tierversuch.
Vet. Med. Diss. München

ARTOIS, M., CHARLTON, K.M., TOLSON, N.D., CASEY, G.A., KNOWLES, M.K. and J.B. CAMPBELL (1990):
Vaccinia recombinant virus expressing the rabies virus glycoprotein: safety and efficacy trials in Canadian wildlife.
Can. J. Vet. Res. **54**, 504–507

BLANDFORD, T.B. and I.F. KEYMER (1987):
Inclusion body hepatitis in captive birds of prey (*Falco spp.*) in Great Britain.
Int. Symp. Erkrank. Zootiere **29**, 97–100

BORLAND, E.D. (1972):
Newcastle Disease in pheasants, partridges and wild birds in East Anglia.
Vet. Rec. **90**, 481–482

BURTSCHER, H. and M. SIBALIN (1975):
Herpesvirus strigis: Hostspectrum and distribution in infected owls.
J. Wildl. Dis. **11**, 164–169

CHU, H.P., TROW, E.W., GREENWOOD, A.G., JENNINGS, A.R. and I.F. KEYMER (1976):
Isolation of Newcastle disease virus from birds of prey.
Avian Path. **5**, 227–233

CLAUSING, D. (1963):
Zur Problematik der Tollwutbekämpfung.
Mhefte Vet. Med. **18**, 29–33

COOPER, J.E. (1969):
Two cases of pox in recently imported Peregrine Falcons (*Falco peregrinus*).
Vet. Rec. **85**, 683–684

COOPER, J.E. (1993):
Avian Pox in Birds of Prey (Order: *Falconiformes*)
Vet. Rec. **132**, 343–345

DOCHERTY, D.E., ROMAINE, R.I. and R.L. KNIGHT (1983):
Isolation of a Herpesvirus from a Bald Eagle nestling.
Avian Dis. **27**, 1162–1165

DRÜNER, K. (1978):
Die Hepatosplenitis infectiosa strigum und andere Todesursachen in Gefangenschaft gehaltener und freilebender Greifvögel und Eulen. Literaturstudie und epizootiologische Untersuchungen.
Vet. Med. Diss. Hannover

FITZNER, R.E., MILLER, R.A., PIERCE, C.A. and S.E. ROWE (1985):
Avian pox in a red-tailed hawk (*Buteo jamaicensis*).
J. Wildl. Dis. **21**, 298–301

GARNER, M.M. (1989):
Bumblefoot associated with poxvirus in a wild golden eagle (*Aquila chrysaetos*).
Companion-Animal-Practice **19**,17–20

GREENWOOD, A.G. and W.F. BLAKEMORE (1973):
Pox infection in falcons.
Vet. Rec. **93**, 468–470

GRIMM, F. (1978):
Newcastle-Krankheit beim Greifvogel.
Prakt. Tierarzt **59**, 641–642

GOUGH, P.M. and R.D. JORGENSON (1976):
Rabies antibodies in sera of wild birds.
J. Wildl. Dis. **12**, 392–395

GRAHAM, D.L. (1973):
Studies on inclusion body disease (herpesvirus infection) of falcons.
Diss. Abstracts-International **34** B, 2364

GRAHAM, D.L., MARE, C.J., WARD, F.P. and M.C. PECKHAM (1975):
Inclusion body disease (herpesvirus infection) of falcons (IBDF).
J. Wildl. Dis. **11**, 83–91

GREENWOOD, A.G. and J.E. COOPER (1982):
Herpesvirus infections in falcons.
Vet. Rec. **111**, 514

GUITTRE, C., ARTOIS, M. and A. FLAMAND (1992):
Utilisation d'un mutant avirulent du virus rabique pour la vaccination orale des especes sauvages: innocuite chez plusieurs especes non cibles.
Ann. Med. Vet. **136**, 329–332

HALLIWELL, W.H. (1972):
Avian pox in an immature red-tailed hawk.
J. Wildl. Dis. **8**, 104–105

HEIDENREICH, M. (1976):
Die Empfänglichkeit des Mäusebussards (*Buteo buteo*) für das Newcastle Disease Virus. Ein Beitrag zur Epizootologie der Newcastle Disease, sowie zur Immunprophylaxe bei Greifvögeln.
Vet. Med. Diss. Hannover

HEIDENREICH, M. (1977):
Newcastle Disease-Virusinfektion bei einem freilebenden Seeadler (Haliaeetus albicilla).
Int. Symp. Erkr. Zootiere **19**, 183–188

HEIDENREICH, M. (1978):
Newcastle disease in birds of prey (*Falconiformes, Strigiformes*). Prevalence, epidemiology, clinical features, diagnosis and immunoprophylaxis.
Prakt. Tierarzt **59**, 650–656

HEIDENREICH, M. and E.F. KALETA (1978):
Hepatosplenitis infectiosa strigum: Beitrag zum Wirtsspektrum
und zur Übertragbarkeit des Eulen-Herpesvirus.
Fortschr. Veterinärmedizin **28**, 198–203

HILL, J.R. and G. BOGUE (1977):
Epornitic of pox in a wild bird population.
J. Amer.Vet. Med. Ass. **171**, 993–994

JENNINGS, A.R. (1954):
Diseases in wild birds.
J. Comp. Path. **64**, 356–395

KALETA, E.F. (1983):
Herpesvirus-induzierte Infektionen und Krankheiten des
Vogels.
Tierärztl. Praxis **11**, 67–75

KALETA, E.F. (1990):
Herpesviruses of birds. A Review.
Avian Path. **19**, 193–211

KEYMER, I.F. (1972):
Diseases in birds of prey.
Vet. Rec. **90**, 579–594

KIEL, H. (1985):
Pockeninfektion bei Jagdfalken.
IV. Tagung der Fachgruppe »Geflügelkrankheiten«, München
202–206

KITZING, D. (1980):
Neuere Erkenntnisse über das Falkenpockenvirus.
Prakt. Tierarzt **61**, 952–954, 956

KOCAN, A.A., POTGIETER, L.N.D. and K.M. KOCAN (1977):
Inclusion body disease of falcons (herpesvirus infection) in an
American kestrel.
J. Wildl. Dis. **13**, 199–201

KÖSTERS, J. and J.R. JAKOBY (1987):
Aktuelle Probleme von Schutzimpfungen bei Vögeln.
Berl. Münch.Tierärztl. Wschrift. **100**, 297–300

KUNTZE, A., SCHRÖDER, H.D. and R. IPPEN (1968):
Geflügelpocken bei einem Breitschwingenbussard (*Buteo
platypterus*)
Int. Symp. Erkr. Zootiere **10**, 161–164

LOUPAL, G., SCHONBAUER, M. and J. JAHN (1985):
Pocken bei Zoo- und Wildvögeln. Licht- und elektronenmikro-
skopische Untersuchungen.
Zbl. Vet. Med. B **32**, 326–336

MARE, C.J. and D.L. GRAHAM (1972):
Isolation and characterization of herpesviruses of birds
of prey.
Proc. United States Animal Health Ass. **76**, 444–451

MARE, C.J. and D.L. GRAHAM (1973):
Falcon herpesvirus, the etiologic agent of inclusion body
disease in falcons.
Infection and Immunity **8**, 118–126

MARE, C.J. (1975):
Herpesviruses of birds of prey.
J. Zoo Animal Medicine **6**, 6-11

MOFFAT, R.E. (1972):
Natural pox infection in a golden eagle.
J. Wildl. Dis. **8**, 161–162

MOUSA, S. (1979):
Die Identifizierung und Charakterisierung eines Falkenpocken-
und eines Psittacidenpockenvirus unter Verwendung von Zell-
kulturmethoden.
Vet. Med. Diss. München

MOZOS, E., HERVAS, J., MOYANO, T., DIAZ, J., GOMEZ-VILLA-
MANDOS, J.C. (1994):
Inclusion body disease in a Peregrine falcon (*Falco pere-
grinus*): histological and ultrastructural study.
Avian Path. **23**, 175–181

OKOH, A.E.J. (1979):
Newcastle disease in falcons.
J. Wildl. Dis. **15**, 479–480

PAARMANN, E. (1955):
Das klinische Bild der Vogellyssa.
Mhefte Vet. Med. **10**, 346–350

PAARMANN, E. (1955a):
Ein Beitrag zur Lyssa der Vögel.
Zschr. Hyg. **141**, 103–109

PEARSON, G.L., PASS, D.A. and E.C. BEGGS (1975):
Fatal pox infection in a rough-legged hawk.
J. Wildl. Dis. **11**, 224–228

PECKHAM, M.C. (1975):
Herpesviruses of pigeons, owls, and falcons.
in: HITCHNER, S.B. et al.: Isolation and identification of avian
pathogens. 256–262
Amer. Ass. Avian Patholog. Ithaca, New York,

POTGIETER, L.N.D., KOCAN, A.A. and K.M. KOCAN (1979):
Isolation of a herpesvirus from an American kestrel with
inclusion body disease.
J. Wildl. Dis. **15**, 143–149

RAMIS, A., MAJO, N., PUMAROLA, M., FONDEVILA, D. and
L. FERRER (1994):
Herpesvirus hepatitis in two eagles in Spain.
Avian Dis. **38**, 197–200

RATCLIFFE, H.L. (1955):
Newcastle Disease in an osprey.
Rep. Penrose Res. Lab. Zool. Soc., Philadelphia

SAMOUR, J.H. and J.E. COOPER (1993):
Avian Pox in Birds of Prey (Order Falconiformes)
Vet. Rec. **132**, 343–345

SCHNEEGANSS, D. and R. KORBEL (1988):
Zum aktuellen Vorkommen aviärer Paramyxovirosen.
Tierärztl. Praxis **16**, 159–160

SCHNEEGANSS, D. (1990):
Nachweise von Paramyxovirus-1 bei Bartgeiern.
VII. Tagung über Vogelkrankheiten, München 262–269
D. V. G.

SCHOOP, G.R., SIEGERT, D., GALASSI, D. and G. KLÖPPEL (1955):
Newcastle-Infektion beim Steinkauz (*Athene noctua*), Horn-
raben (*Bucorvus sp.*), Seeadler (*Haliaeetus albicilla*) und
Rieseneisvogel (*Dacelo gigas*).
Mhefte. Tierhk. 7, 232-235

SEKIZAKI,T., IZAWA, H., ONUMA, M. and T. MIKAMI (1988):
Studies on a paramyxovirus isolated from Japanese sparrow-
hawks (*Accipiter virgatus gularis*).
IV. Hemagglutinating activity of two clones of the virus.
Jap. J. Vet. Sci. 44 275–282

SHANNON, L.M., POULTON, J.L., EMMONS, R.W., WOODIE,
J.D. and M.E. FOWLER (1988):
Serological survey for rabies antibodies in raptors from
California.
J. Wildl. Dis. 24, 264–267

SILEO,L., FRANSON, J.C., GRAHAM, D.L., DOMERMUTH, C.H.,
RATTNER, B.A. and O.H. PATTEE (1983):
Hemorrhagic enteritis in captive American kestrels (*Falco
sparverius*).
J. Wildl. Dis. 19, 244–247

TANTAWI, H.H., SHEIKHLYL-AL, S. and F.K. HASSAN (1981):
Avian pox in buzzard (*Accipiter nisus*) in Iraq.
J. Wildl. Dis. 17, 145–146

TANTAWI, H.H., IMAN, Z.I., MARE, C.J., EL-KARAMANY,
R., SHALABY, M.A. and F. TAYEB (1983):
Antigenic relatedness of pigeon herpes encephalomyelitis
virus to other avian herpesviruses.
Avian Dis. 27, 563–568

THIELE, J., KIEL, H. and H.D. ADOLPHS (1979):
Avian poxvirus – an ultrastructural study on a cherrug falcon.
Brief report.
Arch. Virol. 62, 77–82

TROMMER, G. (1969):
Ein Beitrag zu Greifvogelkrankheiten und deren
Behandlung.
Jahrb. Dtsch. Falkenorden 21–23

WARD, F.P. (1971):
Inclusion body hepatitis in a prairie falcon.
J. Wildl. Dis. 7, 120–124

WERNERY, U., REMPLE, J.D., NEUMANN, U., ALEXANDER, D.J.,
MANVELL, R.J. and O.R. KAADEN (1992):
Avian paramyxovirus serotype 1 (Newcastle disease virus)
infections in falcons.
J. Vet. Med. B 39, 153–158

WHEELDON, E.B., SEDGWICK, C.J. and T.A. SCHULZ (1993):
Epornitic of avian pox in a raptor rehabilitation
center.
J. Amer. Vet. Med. Ass. 187, 1202

WHELER, C.L. (1993):
Herpesvirus disease in raptors: A review of the literature.
in: COOPER, J.E., J.D. Remple and D.B. Hunter (1993):
Raptor Biomedicine. 103–107
Ciron Publ. Ltd., Keighley, West Yorkshire, England

WINTEROLL, G. (1976):
Newcastle-Disease bei Greifen und Eulen.
Prakt. Tierarzt 57, 76–78

WINTEROLL, G., MOUSA, S. and M. AKRAE (1979):
Pockenisolate aus Psittaciden und Falken – Nähere Charak-
terisierung.
Fachgruppe Geflügelkrankheiten München 117–129

WOODFORD, M.H. and P.E.B. GLASIER (1955):
Sub-committees report on diseases in hawks.
The Falconer 3, 63–65

ZUYDAM, D.M. (1952):
Isolation of Newcastle Disease Virus from osprey and the
parakeet.
J. Amer. Vet. Med. Ass. 120, 88

9.2   Bacterial, chlamydial and mycoplasmal diseases

Diagnostic procedures in birds of prey often reveal the presence of bacterial, chlamydial or mycoplasmal microorganisms. The exact role these potential pathogens play in an individual patient is not always clear. Tests on fecal samples, pharyngeal swabs or skin scrapes, in particular, often reveal microbes whose significance is questionable and which may merely be part of the animal's normal flora.

Frequently, only the isolation of large numbers of a single organism in conjunction with obvious disease in a certain organ make it reasonable to link an illness to the presence of the particular pathogen.

Many of these microorganisms are capable of producing disease on their own or as secondary invaders in cases where other diseases permit them to overwhelm the host's defenses. For practical purposes, the diseases listed below have been loosely organized based on the etiologic agent and include only those caused directly by a microbial infection.

9.2.1   *Erysipelothrix* infection

Erysipelothrix rhusiopathiae is a bacterium that can cause an acute, or occasionally chronic infection in turkeys. Infections with this pathogen are occasionally seen in other types of birds as well, including birds of prey. They have been reported in a golden eagle (*Aquila chryseatos*), a European sparrowhawk (*Accipiter nisus*), a northern goshawk (*Accipiter gentilis)* and a hen harrier (*Circus cyaneus*).

Domestic animals, rats, mice, and other birds are thought to act as reservoirs for *E. rhusiopathiae*. Insects may play a role as vectors. Any injury to the skin or mucus membranes will permit this bacterium to enter and infect the body.

Clinical disease
Unlike other birds and mammals, raptors are known only to acquire the acute form of *Erysipelothrix* infection. Several hours after initial exposure, pronounced swelling and red discoloration will be noted in the infected areas of skin (Fig. 9.6). Death will ensue within two or three days if treatment is not begun immediately. Occasionally the disease will progress more slowly and, in that case, be more amenable to treatment.

Treatment
Antibiotics such as tetracycline, doxycycline or penicillins are very effective in treating this infection. Im-

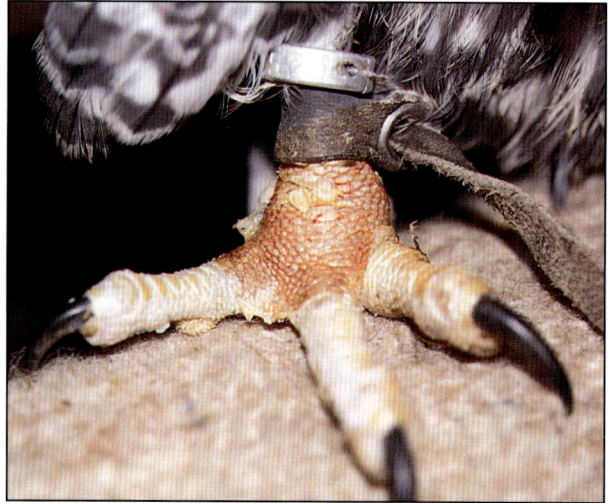

Fig. 9.6: A three year old gray gyrfalcon (*F. rusticolus*) acutely developed a pronounced swelling involving the base of the foot. Within a few hours the outer layer of skin peeled off and the underlying dermis was so hemorrhagic that serum oozed from between the scales. A pure culture of *Erysipelothrix rhusiopathiae* was obtained from a fine needle aspirate. Immediate treatment with doxycycline helped resolve these dramatic changes within two days. The source of infection was probably a bite wound from a wild rat.
(Photo: Heidenreich)

mediate therapy is required since this disease has a very rapid course.

Prevention
Vaccination with *E. rhusiopathiae* bacterins has proven effective in turkeys, although protection lasts only one or two months. This type of vaccination seems impractical in raptors, especially since the disease is encountered only rarely.

9.2.2   Clostridial infections

9.2.2.1   *Clostridium perfringens* enterotoxemia

Clostridium perfringens is a ubiquitous bacterium that will rapidly proliferate under conditions of low oxygen and warm temperature, especially in protein-rich substrates. Different types of this organism produce a group of highly potent exotoxins that can rapidly result in illness and death in a wide variety of animals (Koehler and Baumgart, 1972).

Large raptor facilities often freeze larger quantities of meat for later thawing and feeding as needed. If the freezing process is delayed, proliferation of clostridia and clostridial toxin production can begin to take place. Even more dangerous is the thawing process, during which a protein-rich puddle of water can form in the bottom of the container overnight and act as a culture medium for clostridial organisms. When this normal-appearing meat is offered as food, massive infection with the bacteria or ingestion of the toxin will rapidly result in deadly disease for the raptor.

Another risky practice is the "watering down" of meat practiced by some falconers to bring their hunting hawks into condition faster. The food is soaked in water overnight to leach out some of the nutritional content. If the meat was previously contaminated with clostridia and is not kept refrigerated, bacterial proliferation can occur just as described above.

Even meat that is only mildly contaminated with clostridia can pose a problem if enough of it is consumed, especially by debilitated birds. These raptors often have a delayed digestive transit time (see Ch. 4.4). This allows bacterial proliferation and toxin production to take place within the warm, anaerobic conditions of the animal's digestive tract, with often deadly results.

Clinical disease

The clinical picture associated with this disease will vary depending upon whether the problem is caused by the ingestion of bacteria or by uptake of previously formed clostridial toxins:

Peracute course: With the ingestion of sufficient amounts of clostridial exotoxin, severe generalized illness, depression and death are seen within only a few hours. No distinctive clinical signs are associated with this rapid course of disease.

Acute course: If infectious quantities of the clostridial bacteria themselves are consumed with the food, the infected bird will rapidly become depressed and reluctant to eat. Any food consumed will be regurgitated. The feces become initially soft and brown, then progress to reddish and bloody. As with other diseases involving the liver and/or kidneys (aspergillosis, Newcastle disease, herpesvirus), the urates will show a characteristic pastel green discoloration. Affected animals that are not treated usually die within one to three days.

Pathology

Gross necropsy findings will vary depending on the course of the disease. With the peracute form, there may only be swelling of the liver, kidney and spleen. More prolonged illness will result in hemorrhagic, inflammatory and necrotic changes involving the intestinal mucosa.

Diagnosis

Clostridium perfringens enterotoxemia can usually be suspected on the basis of the extremely rapid course of disease. Since the origin of the infection commonly lies in the food, more than one bird in a facility is usually affected or dies during the same time. For confirmation, an examination of the food or the intestinal contents of deceased birds will reveal the presence of clostridial bacteria or the associated toxin.

Treatment and prevention

The peracute form of clostridial enterotoxemia is not amenable to therapy. The less rapid course of disease seen with the acute form should be immediately treated with broad spectrum antibiotics. There is no time to wait for microbial culture and sensitivity results. Clostridia are sensitive to a variety of antibacterial drugs. Affected raptors can be treated with intramuscular oxytetracycline at a dose of 100 mg/kg body weight SID for five days or with the long-acting form of doxycycline at 100 mg/kg IM once (Vibravenös, available only in Europe and Canada) or intravenously at 50 mg/kg SID (Vibramycin hyclate – will cause severe muscle necrosis if given IM). If treated immediately, many birds can still be saved.

Prevention is key with a disease that is as lethal and rapid as clostridial enterotoxemia. Careful attention to feeding practices and avoidance of frozen food are most important in this regard.

If the freezing of food animals can not be avoided, every effort should be made to freeze and thaw the carcasses as rapidly as possible. Frozen meat can be placed on grates so that water and juices do not accumulate during the thawing process. This also prevents the creation of anaerobic conditions conducive to clostridial proliferation. Poultry processing plant byproducts like chicken heads and necks are often contaminated with blood, mucus and regurgitated stomach contents. They should be thoroughly rinsed with cold water both before and after freezing. If meat is to be soaked before feeding, this should be done only in flowing cold water.

9.2.2.2 Clostridial dermatomyositis

Clostridium perfringens, as well as other clostridia such as *Clostridium septicum* and *Clostridium novyi*, are implicated in this disease, also known as necrotic dermatitis or gas gangrene. The initiating cause is usually a traumatic injury to the skin that becomes infected. Although birds are generally very resistant to skin infections, clostridial infections seem to be an exception to the rule. Small, almost invisible, but relatively deep wounds such as those created by raptor talons during disagreements between birds in aviaries are more likely to become infected this way than are large open wounds. Talons are usually contaminated with food remnants and dirt that are deposited deep into the muscle tissue when the animals grasp at each other. Clostridial bacteria thus injected find themselves in an ideal, anaerobic environment for proliferation and the production of exotoxins.

Clinical disease

The skin covering an infected area will become bluish-red within hours, then jelly-like and soft (Fig. 9.7). Palpation often reveals crepitation in the subcutis and underlying musculature as bacterial gases accumulate (Fig 9.8). The bird will become rapidly depressed and unresponsive, often succumbing to the infection within 48 hours.

Treatment

Although small injuries in birds usually heal without special attention, any talon injury requires immediate treatment with broad spectrum antibiotics. Because clostridia require anaerobic conditions to multiply, deep cleaning of the wound with hydrogen peroxide (3%) is helpful in preventing infection. Topical antibacterial therapy as well as systemic antibiotics are recommended.

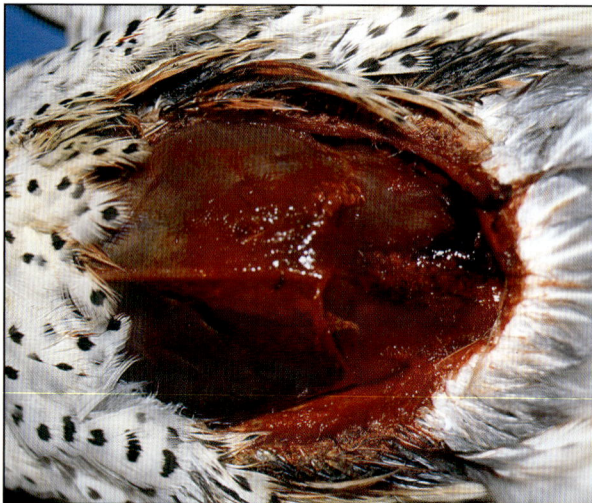

Fig. 9.8: A white gyrfalcon (*F. rusticolus*) tiercel presented with severe depression and lameness in one leg. He had been grabbed in that leg by another bird in the aviary the day before. On physical examination, black discoloration of the skin in the stifle area was noted. Removal of the necrotic tissue revealed underlying foamy fluid in which clostridia were present. Debridement of the affected area and flushing with antibiotic solutions in addition to parenteral treatment with tetracycline antibiotics eventually resulted in this bird's recovery. (Photo: Heidenreich)

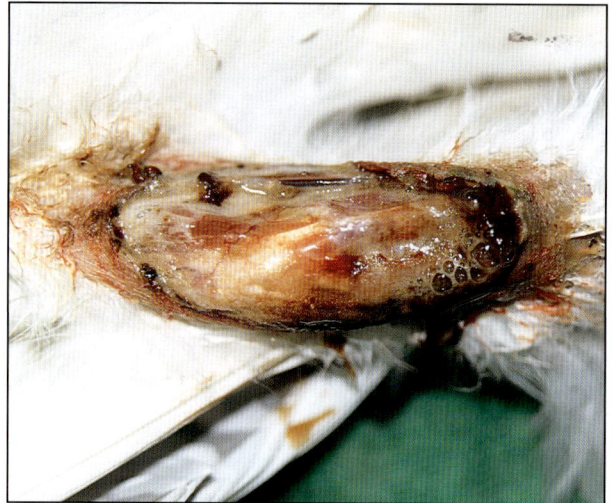

Fig. 9.7: A hybrid peregrine (*F. peregrinus*) X gyrfalcon (*F. rusticolus*) tiercel was injured in the caudal pectoral area by the talons of another raptor. An immediate examination by the falconer did not reveal any obvious wounds. Twenty-four hours later, the bird became depressed and the following day it died. Several puncture wounds are clearly visible near the keel. Also noticeable are the spongy, gelatinous changes involving the muscle tissue and a dark red exudate. Postmortem samples from this case came back with a pure culture of *Clostridium perfringens*. (Photo: Heidenreich)

9.2.2.3 Botulism

Botulism does not result directly from a bacterial infection, but is instead an intoxication due to the absorption of *Clostridium botulinum* toxin. *Cl. botulinum* multiplies in rotting cadavers and produces a potent neurotoxin that will result in paralysis after ingestion of the contaminated meat or of maggots that have fed from it.

Wild birds of prey are rarely affected by this disease. Most of them do not eat carrion and only occasionally consume animals found already dead. The exception occurs with vultures, but this group of birds is resistant to the botulinum toxin. In captivity, botulism can occur if extremely hungry hawks are forced to eat decaying meat contaminated with the toxin.

Clinical disease

The primary clinical sign is a characteristic flaccid paralysis involving the neck and limbs. This has given the disease its common name of "limberneck". The animal will become recumbent and make feeble, uncoordinated movements. Paralysis of the pharyngeal muscles renders the bird incapable of swallowing food or water. If enough of the toxin has been absorbed, respiratory paralysis can lead to death in anywhere from a few hours to several days. Less serious cases can recover within a few days, especially if given medical support.

Treatment

A presumptive diagnosis of botulism will be supported if there is evidence of consumption of rotting meat. Treatment with guanidine at 15 to 30 mg per day can be attempted. Cathartics and laxatives may help flush any unabsorbed toxin from the body.

Nutritional and respiratory support as well as fluid therapy will help keep the affected bird alive until the toxin is eliminated from the body and recovery occurs.

9.2.2.4 Tetanus

Tetanus is also caused by a clostridial neurotoxin. In humans and other mammals, this disease, caused by *Clostridium tetani*, is often fatal. Infection of a deep puncture wound with these ubiquitous bacteria allows them to proliferate under anaerobic conditions. The toxin then released enters the nerves and interferes with their normal function, resulting in strong contractions of the body's extensor muscles.

The occurrence of this disease in birds, including birds of prey, is debated. Gylstorff and Grimm (1987) mention tetanus in a turkey and three geese. Ritchie et al. (1994) consider birds generally resistant to this disease and suspect that earlier reports represent misdiagnosed cases. A recent report of possible tetanus in a falcon by Lierz (1995) is therefore of interest.

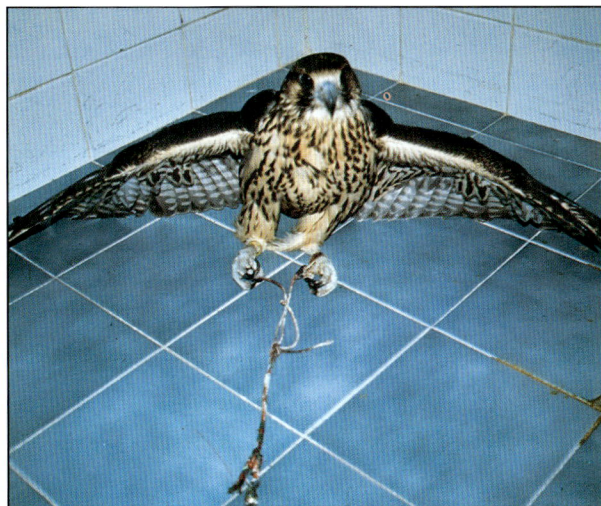

Fig. 9.9: A saker falcon (*F. cherrug)* with a suspected case of tetanus showing extensor rigidity.
(Photo: Lierz)

Case description: A saker falcon suffered talon puncture wounds during an altercation with another raptor. Several days later, the injured bird developed muscle spasms in both legs. This extensor rigidity quickly spread to involve the pelvic muscles and wings (Fig. 9.9).

Similar signs are associated with other diseases, and a definitive diagnosis can not be based on physical examination alone. In this case, however, administration of tetanus toxoid seemed to result in rapid improvement of the bird's condition.

That this falcon never fully recovered and had to be euthanatized after several weeks does not invalidate the presumptive diagnosis. Advanced cases of tetanus are often not curable.

9.2.3 Avian tuberculosis (Mycobacteriosis)

Avian tuberculosis is widespread among wild and, particularly, captive birds of prey. Most people who own raptors have lost a bird to this disease at some point or another.

Pathogen

Tuberculosis in birds is caused primarily by *Mycobacterium avium*, a microorganism that is particularly resistant to common disinfection agents and has an outstanding ability to persist in the environment. It remains infectious in soil for years and in surface waters for several months.

Common sources of infection in raptors include other infected birds consumed as prey or direct contact with fecal material from such animals. The usual route of infection is oral, with occasional transmission by the respiratory tract or through open skin lesions. Insects can act as mechanical vectors for mycobacteria if they come in contact with contaminated feces or soil.

Clinical disease

Avian mycobacteriosis is a chronic disease that presents with progressive weight loss despite a good appetite. Depending on the primary site of infection, different clinical courses may be observed.

Respiratory form: Only rarely are tuberculous lesions confined to the lungs. In the advanced stage, these patients may present with increased respiratory sounds or other signs similar to aspergillosis (Fig. 9.10).

Skin and Muscle form: Localized tuberculosis lesions involving the skin, subcutis or muscle are usually caused by talon injuries inflicted by another raptor. Aggression involving the establishment of dominance or territorial defense among conspecific birds of prey frequently results in talon injuries to the legs. Tuberculous skin lesions are therefore commonly seen on the upper thighs or in the shank region of affected birds.

The site of infection initially develops a small nodule which gradually enlarges over several months to form an easily palpated, walnut-sized granuloma. Although chronic wasting is seen in these birds as well, the animal will appear generally normal in behavior and appetite. If the lesion gets large enough, the affected limb may be carried at an odd angle or become lame.

Generalized form: This is the most common form of mycobacteriosis in birds and usually involves the visceral organs, particularly the liver and the intestinal tract. Clinical signs consist predominantly of a chronic wasting syndrome developing over months. Affected birds will appear ravenously hungry, attacking offered food items and beginning to consume them voraciously. After a brief time, they suddenly lose interest in eating and begin to pick listlessly at the meat. Small bits of food are flung away with the beak, resulting in an accumulation of food particles circumferentially around the feeding area. With fluffed plumage, the sick raptor remains standing over the uneaten remains, grasping them tightly for some time without making further attempts to eat. If force-fed, the animal will regurgitate.

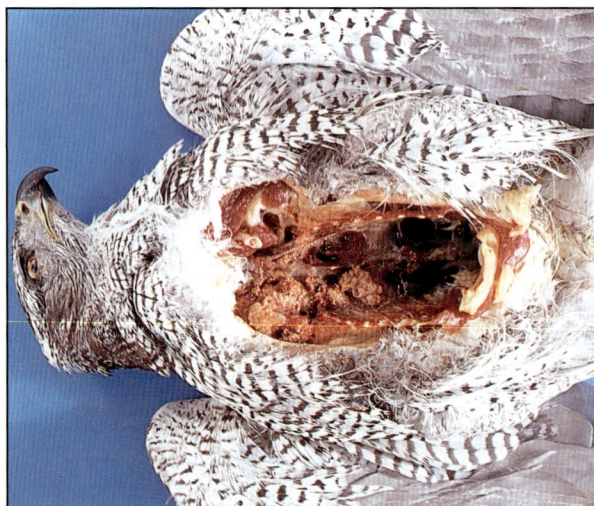

Fig. 9.10: A four year old female northern goshawk (*Accipiter gentilis*) suffered from chronic weight loss and became dyspneic a few days before death. Aspergillosis was initially suspected. At necropsy, caseous granulomas were present in the lungs. *M. avium* was identified in these lesions, confirming this as a rare case of pulmonary tuberculosis in a raptor.
(Photo: Heidenreich)

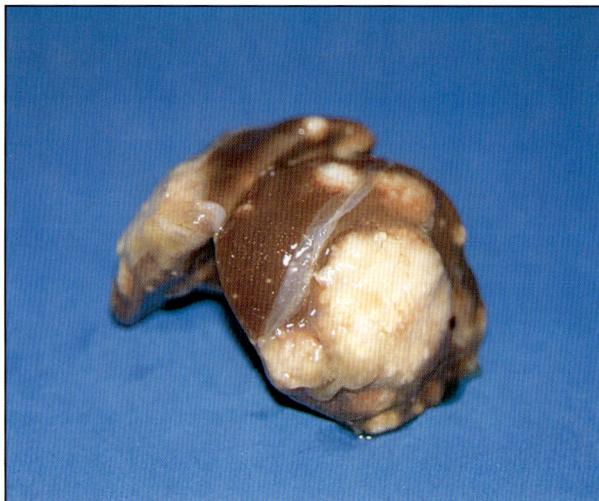

Fig. 9.11: Typical tuberculous granulomas in the liver of a raptor.
(Photo: Heidenreich)

These late stages of the disease are often accompanied by abdominal enlargement. Large granulomas can sometimes be palpated through the abdominal wall.

Pathology
Gross necropsy of affected animals usually reveals a body in emaciated condition, most noticeable in the pronounced atrophy of the pectoral muscles. Although lesions may be found in any organ system, the liver, spleen, intestine, kidneys and bone marrow are most commonly involved. Yellowish-white nodules filled with crumbly caseous exudate and ranging from pinhead to walnut-sized are typical for avian tuberculosis (Fig. 9.11). Herpesvirus infection should be on the list of differential diagnoses if the lesions appear small and are confined to liver and spleen. Chronic hypoproteinemia and liver involvement may result in ascites (Fig. 9.12) or pericardial effusion.

Diagnosis
In most cases the animal's history and a thorough physical examination will suffice for a presumptive diagnosis. Chronic weight loss, sometimes associated with diarrhea or lameness, especially in an older bird, are strong indications of possible mycobacterial infection. In the author's own experience, no bird with tuberculosis has ever been less than three years of age.

Radiography: Radiographs are often helpful in the diagnosis of this disease, especially in cases with respiratory involvement or when palpable abdominal masses or abdominal swelling are present. Tuberculous granulomas in birds do not mineralize and may

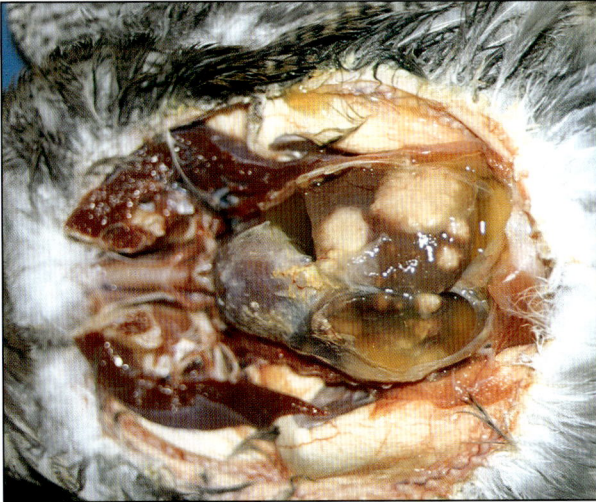

Fig. 9.12: The body cavity of a peregrine falcon (*F. peregrinus*) tiercel only three years old. The lesions are typical for tuberculosis in birds of prey. Several large, deep granulomas in the liver resulted in chronic weight loss and the development of ascites. The excess amber fluid is visible around the liver.
(Photo: Heidenreich)

be difficult to distinguish radiographically from similar soft tissue densities associated with aspergillosis or tumors (Fig. 9.13).

Biopsy: If skin lesions are present, these can easily be surgically removed and submitted for biopsy. Ziehl-Neelson staining of cytologic smears or fixed tissues will reveal the presence of acid-fast mycobacteria. Satterfield (1981) recommends an endoscopic liver biopsy for early diagnosis of the disease in birds affected with the generalized form of tuberculosis.

Endoscopy: Depending on the location of the lesions, endoscopic examination of the body cavity and, if possible, biopsy of suspicious lesions, can assist in the diagnosis of avian tuberculosis. One should take into account that the risk with both injectable or inhalant anesthetics is significantly greater in diseased animals.

Tuberculosis testing: Two different types of tests are mentioned in the literature:

Tuberculin test (allergenic test): 0.1 ml avian tuberculin is injected into the skin, preferably in the fold of skin near a raptor's ear. If there is a positive reaction, an obvious doughy swelling will be noticeable at the site 48 to 72 hours after injection.

Slide agglutination test (serologic test): Plasma or serum from the patient is mixed with a suspension of mycobacterial antigens. If clumping or agglutination is seen after 60 seconds, this test is considered positive for tuberculosis.

Both tests have the disadvantage that a definitive answer is possible only in the case of a positive result. False negative results are common. A negative result can therefore not be interpreted to mean that the patient does not carry the disease.

Fecal examinations: The most common form of tuberculosis in raptors involves the gastrointestinal tract. Intestinal granulomas are often in communication with the lumen of the gut (open infection), so that mycobacteria may be shed into the feces. Microscopic examination of fecal samples may thus aid in the diagnosis of this disease.

The procedure involves taking four grams of feces and mixing them with 12 ml of a human sputum solvent such as 15% Sputofluol® solution (Merck). This suspension is mixed well and then centrifuged. The resulting pellet is smeared on a slide and stained with Ziehl-Neelsen stain.

Not all acid-fast bacilli identified this way are necessarily pathogenic mycobacteria. Harmless mycobacteria may also stain positive and can be hard to differentiate. This test is therefore difficult to interpret.

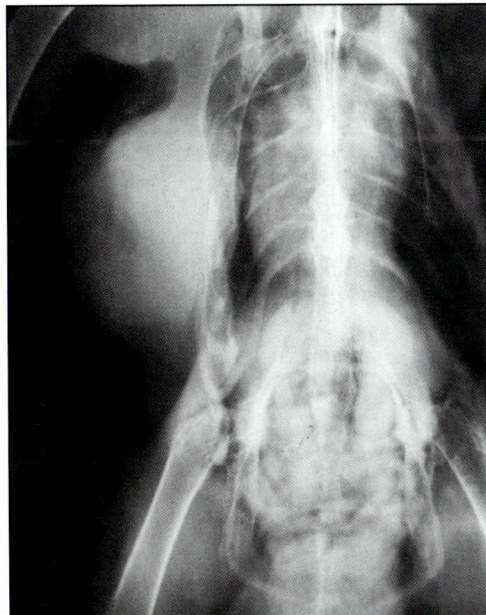

Fig. 9.13: This radiograph of a northern goshawk (*Accipiter gentilis*) shows two large subcutaneous masses in the right axillary region and along the body wall. These tuberculosis lesions were easily detectable on physical examination.
(Photo: Heidenreich)

Treatment

Before attempting to treat avian tuberculosis, one should take into account that this is a potentially zoonotic disease. *M. avium* is most likely to infect immuno-suppressed people and can result in serious disease that is refractory to treatment and sometimes fatal. It is therefore not wise to treat infected raptors that are in close contact with human beings or other birds. Humane euthanasia is the recommended alternative. Some people feel that birds known to have been in close contact with a diseased animal should also be separated and quarantined for two years with regular testing throughout that period.

In cases where good reason exists for attempting treatment, a combination of the following drugs can be tried:

Isoniazid 30 mg/kg PO SID plus ethambutol 30 mg/kg PO SID plus rifampin 45 mg/kg PO SID, all for at least 8 weeks.

Despite such intensive treatment, the prognosis for a complete cure is poor. Shedding of mycobacteria and progression of the disease may be stopped, but the infection usually remains and can be reactivated at any time.

Prevention

The primary method of prevention involves the reduction or elimination of exposure to *M. avium* in the environment. This requires strict hygienic measures for birds housed in captivity. Contact with excretions from other potentially infected animals should be avoided (see Ch. 3.2.6 – aviary hygiene).

Because tuberculosis can be spread by birds such as pigeons, quail and chickens that are commonly used as food animals, these should always be examined for signs of tuberculosis before being used. Even in the field, captured prey can be quickly examined for suspicious lesions in the abdominal cavity before letting the hawk eat. This process takes less than a minute and can be done while the hawk is still plucking feathers from the animal.

Once tuberculosis has been diagnosed in a bird, the soil or other substrate in the aviary or around the animal's perch must be removed as thoroughly as possible and completely replaced. All aviary furniture and equipment should be burned. Disinfection is not reliable.

9.2.4 Salmonellosis

The older literature mentions salmonellosis as an occasional cause of illness, even in birds of prey (Kirkpatrick and Trexler-Myren, 1970). The fear of salmonellosis is therefore widespread among falcon-

ers, especially those who feed their birds with pigeons, which are known carriers of *Salmonella* sp. bacteria.

Indeed, necropsies and bacterial cultures performed on raptors occasionally reveal the presence of salmonella organisms. The significance of such findings and their association with any disease present is usually unclear and remains speculative (SYKES et al., 1981).

Pigeons that succumb to salmonellosis show a miliary pattern of necrotic foci in the liver. It is likely that similar lesions seen in falcons were interpreted to be the same infection, although falcon herpes, unknown at the time, was more likely the cause (see Ch. 9.1.3.1).

It is certain, in any case, that various species of salmonellae can be isolated from the feces of perfectly healthy birds of prey. Many of these may simply be carried by prey animals and be only transiently present in the hawk's mutes (Khan, 1970).

Neither the published literature nor the author's own experiences have been able to assign a clear clinical disease to the presence of salmonellae in raptors. It is therefore likely that these bacteria play a minor role in the disease processes affecting birds of prey (Lüthgen, 1978).

Nothelfer and Wernery (1995) recently isolated *Salmonella typhimurium* and *Salmonella münster* from a group of imported saker and gyrfalcons in Dubai that died with distinct clinical and postmortem findings. The animals were depressed, dehydrated, and had greenish urates. Bloodwork showed elevated liver enzymes. At necropsy, enlarged livers and spleens with subcapsular hemorrhages and necrosis predominated. The source of infection was traced to the feeding of pigeons and quail that were proven to carry the same salmonellae. Other causes of death, such as falcon herpesvirus and Newcastle disease, were ruled out by the investigators. It seems, therefore, that some *Salmonella* species can cause clinical disease in falcons under certain circumstances.

9.2.5 Pasteurellosis

Pasteurellosis is the name for a number of diseases caused by members of the bacterial genus *Pasteurella* in mammals and birds. Avian cholera, caused by *Pasteurella multocida*, is an infection of importance in the commercial poultry industry, especially among turkey and duck producers. It can cause outbreaks of disease with high rates of death. Large groups of migrating or wintering wild waterfowl are also subject to epornitics of this disease. Klukas and Locke (1970) and Rosen (1972) describe one such massive infection that killed approximately 37,000 birds in California during the winter of 1970/1971. Raptors are subject to infection by *P. multocida* as well. Bald and golden eagles that had consumed dead or dying ducks during the outbreak in California were found dead in the same area (Locke et al., 1972; Rosen and D'Amico, 1973).

Transmission of *P. multocida* to raptors is direct via the consumption of infected prey. The bacteria, present primarily in the upper respiratory tract of infected birds, rodents and rabbits, are easily transferred to the mucus membranes of the oral cavity or eyes in birds of prey (Williams et al., 1987). The feeding of turkey and duck heads obtained from meat processing plants should therefore always be avoided!

Clinical disease
There are two main forms of the disease, depending on the virulence of the strain, level of exposure and resistance of the bird:

Acute form: In these cases, septicemia occurs only a few hours after infection. The bird will become depressed and die without any further signs. An endotoxin produced by the more virulent strains of *P. multocida* is responsible for the shock, rapid course of disease and death seen in these animals.

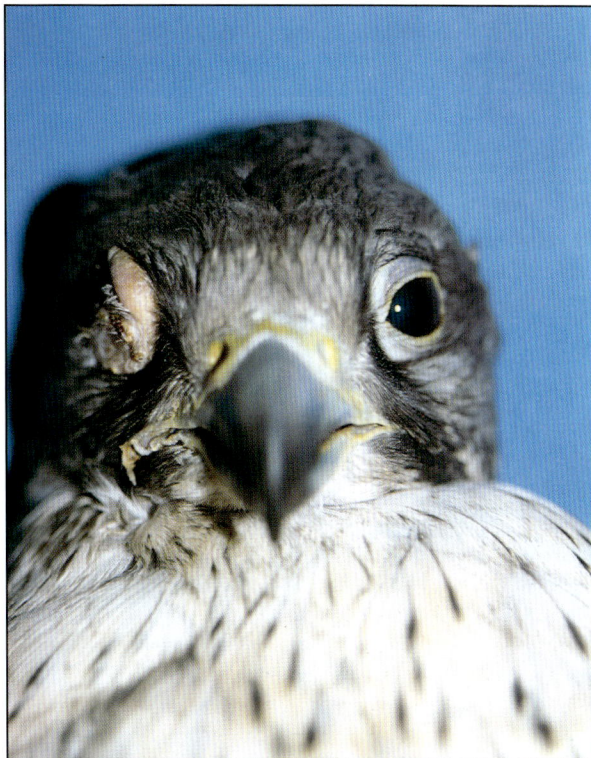

Fig. 9.15: In the early stages, localized pasteurellosis can result in swelling of the eyelids and conjunctivitis so severe that the bird is unable to open the eye, as in this gray gyrfalcon tiercel (*F. rusticolus*). (Photo: Heidenreich)

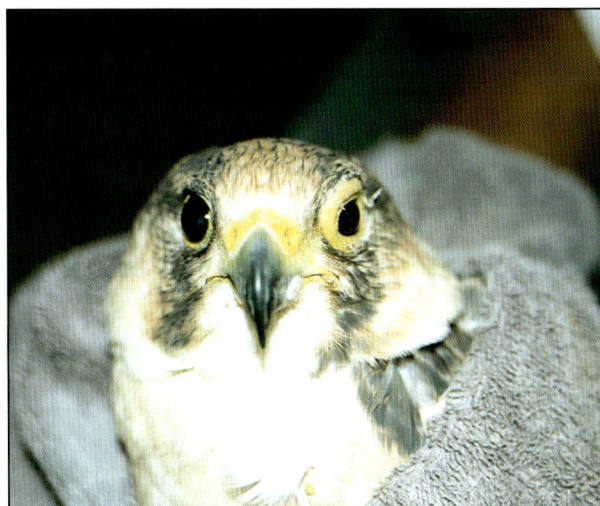

Fig. 9.14: Unilateral inflammation and swelling of the eyelids, as seen in this female red-naped shaheen (*F. pelegrinoides babylonicus)*, are more common with pasteurellosis than is bilateral involvement. (Photo: Heidenreich)

Chronic form: Initial signs with this less virulent form of pasteurellosis include watery nasal discharge and swelling of the infraorbital sinuses as well as inflammation and swelling of the eyelids and conjunctival membranes (Figs. 9.14 and 9.15). This is similar to the clinical picture seen in turkeys with this disease.

Inflammation of the trachea, bronchi and syrinx in infected birds may lead to hoarse vocalizations or loss of voice altogether. Infections involving the joints and tendon sheaths are also common. Painful, doughy swelling of the hock joint may be noted clinically.

Death is rare with this chronic form of infection. Clinical signs may persist for months, however, and permanent damage to joints or eyes may result if the disease remains untreated.

Pathology
Postmortem findings with the acute septicemic form of pasteurellosis are absent or limited to enlargement of liver and kidneys with ecchymotic hemorrhages on the serosal surfaces of abdominal organs. More chronic disease may result in pneumonia and inflammatory

changes involving the air sacs. Hydropericardium and infections of the oviduct are sometimes also seen.

Birds with joint involvement will have flocculent yellowish-white material suspended in cloudy joint fluid.

Diagnosis

Microbial culturing is required to prove that a bird is infected with *P. multocida*. A history of exposure to potentially infected ducks or turkeys and the typical clinical signs can aid in making a presumptive diagnosis while culture results are pending.

Birds with the acute septicemic form will have positive blood culture results. A serologic test is available to detect the presence of antibodies to *P. multocida* in chronically infected birds.

Treatment

Birds suffering from the acute disease can occasionally be saved by the immediate, preferably intravenous, administration of antibiotics. Even these efforts often come too late to prevent death.

More chronic cases are treated with long-term administration of broad spectrum penicillins, tetracyclines or sulfonamides. Even better is antibiotic treatment based on the results of culture and sensitivity testing. The goal is to eliminate the chronic carrier state that can pose a risk to other birds. A rapid response to therapy is usually seen.

Prevention

Various vaccines are available commercially for poultry. These have not been tested in raptors and are unlikely to be very effective. Pasteurellosis is a frequent problem in large raptor breeding facilities, and the emphasis there should focus on preventing introduction of the pathogen by way of food animals such as ducks and turkeys. Every effort should be made to avoid exposure to wild rodents as well.

9.2.6 Chlamydiosis

This infection, also known as psittacosis (in parrots) or ornithosis (in other species), is caused by *Chlamydia psittaci*. It is a disease with worldwide distribution that is of particular importance in parrots and other birds. Chlamydia can also be transmitted to mammals including humans, where they may result in serious illness. For this reason, avian chlamydiosis is a reportable disease in many countries. The strains seen in ducks and turkeys are particularly virulent for other avian species.

Chlamydia psittaci infection has been reported in various raptors, including the common buzzard (*Buteo buteo)*, the red-tailed hawk (*Buteo jamaicensis*), kites

(*Milvus* sp.), goshawks (*Accipiter* sp.) and harriers (*Circus* sp.) (Fowler, 1990; Gerbermann and Korbel, 1992).

Chlamydia organisms are transmitted primarily by aerosol, although insects may act as vectors. Direct transmission is suspected in some cases such as with buzzards or hawks. Their primary prey animals are rodents, a group of animals frequently known to be latent carriers of the disease. Latent infections also occur in birds. This can result in long-term carrier states and in sudden outbreaks of chlamydiosis with fecal shedding of the organism when a bird is stressed or otherwise immunosuppressed.

Clinical disease

Various forms of chlamydiosis are seen, depending on the virulence of the particular strain and the resistance of the host. The acute form with rapid death described in other avian species is not seen in birds of prey. Raptors seem to suffer more commonly from chronic infections that may last for months. A discharge from eyes and nose, accompanied sometimes by diarrhea and weight loss, may be the only clinical signs.

Pathology

The main postmortem finding is pronounced splenomegaly, sometimes up to several times normal size. Enlargement of the liver and kidneys may also be present. Cloudy or gelatinous air sac changes are observed only in the more chronic cases.

Diagnosis

Clinical signs are usually nonspecific, making diagnostic testing important in presumptive cases of chlamydiosis.

Postmortem samples can be relatively rapidly tested by special staining of impression smears from affected organs (STAMP). Diagnosis in the living patient is somewhat more difficult. Conjunctival smears can sometimes be examined using the stains mentioned above.

Chlamydia psittaci is intermittently shed in the feces. The organism is very sensitive and dies quickly at room temperature. Samples to be submitted for culture should be frozen immediately for submission to the laboratory or placed in special culture media. Even so, false negatives are common with this diagnostic method.

Relatively sensitive and rapid ELISA tests for detecting chlamydial antibodies or antigens are now available in many laboratories. These, also, are occasionally subject to false negative and false positive results.

Because latent infections are common, serologic tests that measure antibody levels are not reliable indicators of active infection. Paired samples indicating a rapid rise in titer can be more useful in such cases.

Treatment

In psittacines, treatment with chlortetracycline or doxycycline is usually dictated by the chlamydiosis regulations established by individual countries (1991 [BGB1. I, S. 2111]).

Doxycycline is effective also for treatment of raptors. The long-acting preparation available in Europe is well-tolerated and should be administered at 100 mg/kg IM once every 5 days for a total of six doses.

Intravenous preparations available in the United States cannot be given intramuscularly. Recommendations in that case are oral doxycycline at 40 to 50 mg/kg PO SID or BID for at least 30 days.

Enrofloxacin has shown great promise as an effective antichlamydial agent in preliminary trials with various species of psittacines. Normal antibacterial dosages of this drug administered for at least 14 days are recommended. It should be kept in mind that enrofloxacin is not yet approved for treatment of chlamydiosis in birds.

Prevention

The avoidance of ducks, turkeys and pigeons as food animals is the only way to minimize the risk of infection in raptors. Nevertheless, latent infections in raptors are most common and the danger of this disease should not be overstated.

9.2.7 *Mycoplasma* infection

Mycoplasma sp. frequently cause infections in commercial chicken and poultry facilities and usually result in a chronic inflammatory disease involving the upper respiratory tract. Recently, an epornitic of mycoplasma conjunctivitis has also been seen among wild passerines in the eastern United States.

In raptors, *Mycoplasma* sp. infections have been reported by Furr et al. (1977) in large falcons (*F. peregrinus, F. mexicanus* and *F. cherrug)*, as well as in common kestrels (*F. tinnunculus*), in buzzards (*Buteo* sp.) (Bolske and Morner, 1982) and in griffon vultures (*Gyps fulvus)* (POVEDA et al., 1990).

These reports describe dyspnea with crackles and wheezes indicating air sac involvement. *Mycoplasma* organisms were demonstrated in tracheal swabs taken from affected birds. One falcon responded well to treatment with tylosin initially but redeveloped the infection one year later.

Because the demonstration of *Mycoplasma* sp. by culture from potentially infected birds is difficult, few cases of this disease have been described in birds of prey. The significance of *Mycoplasma* infection in raptors thus remains unclear. Pigeons are known carriers of several *Mycoplasma* species. Initial results indicate that enrofloxacin may be an effective drug for the treatment of mycoplasma infections in birds.

9.2.8 *Aegyptianella* infection

Aegyptianella sp. are rickettsial parasites of red blood cells in birds. They can cause anemia and icterus. Ticks of the genus *Argas*, found only in warmer climates, act as the agents of transmission. This disease is therefore encountered only in raptors from tropical or Mediterranean areas.

Young animals or adult birds whose resistance has been somehow compromised can develop acute infections with sudden death. More chronic cases will show signs of anemia due to red blood cell destruction and icterus with liver involvement.

The causative agent is easily identified by the small inclusion bodies seen within erythrocytes on a routine blood smear. Tetracycline antibiotics are recommended for treatment. Prevention involves avoiding exposure to ticks in endemic areas.

References and literature of further interest

BANGERT, R.L., WARD, A.C.S., STAUBER, E.H., CHO, B.R. and P.R. WIDDERS (1988):
A survey of the aerobic bacteria in the feces of captive raptors.
Avian Dis. **32**, 53–62

BOLSKE, G. and T. MORNER (1982):
Isolation of a Mycoplasma sp. from three buzzards (*Buteo spp.*).
Avian. Dis. **26**, 406–411

CLARK, F.D. (1986):
Mycobacteriosis in a red-tailed hawk (*Buteo jamaicensis*).
Southwest. Vet. **37**, 200–201

COOPER, J.E. (1968):
Tuberculosis in birds of prey.
Vet. Rec. **100**, 61

ENDERSON, J.H. and M.D. BERTHRONG (1984):
Pseudomembraneous gastritis compatible with Clostridium sp. in a captive peregrine falcon.
Raptor Research **18**, 72–74

FOWLER, M.E., SCHULZ,T., ARDANS, A., REYNOLDS, B. and D. BEHYMER (1990):
Chlamydiosis in captive raptors.
Avian Dis. **34**, 657–662

FURR, P.M., COOPER, J.E. and D. TAYLOR-ROBINSON (1977):
Isolation of mycoplasmas from three falcons (*Falco spp*).
Vet. Rec. **100**, 72–73

GERBERMANN, H. and R. KORBEL (1992):
Chlamydienbefunde bei Greifvögeln aus freier Wildbahn.
VIII. Tagung der Fachgruppe Geflügelkrankheiten 105–123
D. V. G.

GERBERMANN, H., JAKOBY, J.R. and J. KÖSTERS (1990):
Chlamydienbefunde aus einer größeren Greifvogelhaltung.
J. Vet. Med. B. **37**, 739–749

GERBERMANN, H. and P. JANECZEK (1991):
Chlamydiose bei Vögeln: Gegenwärtige Situation und Alternativen der Diagnose und Bekämpfung.
Prakt. Tierarzt. **72**, 521–524, 526–528

GYLSTORFF, I. and F. GRIMM (1987):
Vogelkrankheiten.
Verlag Eugen Ulmer, Stuttgart

HINZ, K.H. (1993):
Botulismus in: SIEGMANN, O. (1993):
Kompendium der Geflügelkrankheiten.
Verlag Paul Parey, Berlin und Hamburg

KALINER, G. and J.E. COOPER (1973):
Dual infection of an African fish eagle with acid-fast bacilli and *Aspergillus* sp.
J. Wildl. Dis. **9**, 51–55

KHAN, A.Q. (1970):
Salmonella infections in birds in the Sudan.
Bull. epizoot. Dis. Afr. **18**, 207–212

KIRKPATRICK, C.E. and V.P. TREXLER-MYREN (1986):
A survey of free-living falconiform birds for Salmonella.
J. Amer. Vet. Med. Ass. **189**, 997–998

KLUKAS, R.W. and L.N. LOCKE (1970):
An outbreak of fowl cholera in Everglades National Park.
J. Wildl. Dis. **6**, 77–79

KÖHLER, B. and W. BAUMGART (1972):
Toxi-Infektionen durch Clostridium perfringens Typ A bei Greifvögeln
Mhfte. Vet. Med. **25**, 348–352

KOSHIMIZU, K., KOTANI, H., ITO, M., TASHIRO, K., MASUI, M., TANABE, K., KAWASAKI, I., SAITO, K., and H. HIRAMATSU (1984): Further isolation of mycoplasmas from zoo-animals.
Japan. J. Vet. Sci. **46**, 129–132

KRAUTWALD-JUNGHANNS, M.E., KOSTKA, V. and K. PIEPER (1991): Pathologische Röntgenzeichen bei der Tuberkulose von Zier- und Greifvögeln.
Tierärztl. Praxis **19**, 156–162

KRONBERGER, H., SCHÜPPEL, K.F. and G. KUNZ (1976):
Tuberkulose bei Turmfalken (*Falco tinnunculus*).
Int. Symp. Erkrank. Zootiere **18**, 167–169

LAIRMORE, M., SPRAKER, T. and R. JONES (1985):
Two cases of tuberculosis in raptors in Colorado.
J. Wildl. Dis. **21**, 54–57

LIERZ, M. (1995):
personal communication

LOCKE, L.N., NEWMAN, J.A. and B.M. MULHERN (1972):
Avian Cholera in a Bald Eagle from Ohio.
Ohio J. Sci. **72**, 294

LÜTHGEN, W. (1978):
Salmonelleninfektion oder Salmonellose bei Greifvögeln.
Prakt. Tierarzt **59**, 663–666

LUMEIJ, J.T., DORRESTEIN, G.M. and J.W.E. STAM (1981):
Observations on tuberculosis in raptors.
in: Recent advances in the study of raptor diseases.
Proceedings of the International Symposium on Diseases of Birds of Prey, 137–139
Publ. Ltd. Keighley, West Yorkshire, England

LUMEIJ, J.T., STAM, J.W.E. and W.T.C. WOLVEKAMP (1980):
Tuberculose bij een havik.
Tijdschrift Diergeneesk. **105**, 729–730

LUMEIJ, J.T. and G.J. VAN-NIE (1982):
Tuberculose bij roofvogels. II. Literatuuroverzicht en suggesties voor klinische diagnostiek en vaccinatie.
Tijdschrift Diergeneesk. **107**, 573–579

MIRANDE, L.A., HOWERTH, E.W. and R.P. POSTON (1992):
Chlamydiosis in a red-tailed hawk (*Buteo jamaicensis*).
J. Wildl. Dis. **28**, 284–287

MONTALI, R.J., BUSH, M., THOEN, C.O. and E. SMITH (1976):
Tuberculosis in captive exotic birds.
J. Amer.Vet. Med. Ass. **169**, 920–927

NEEDHAM, J.R., KIRKWOOD, J.K. and J.E. COOPER (1979):
A survey of the aerobic bacteria in the droppings of captive birds of prey.
Res. Vet. Sci. **27**, 125–126

NEEDHAM, J.R., COOPER, J.E. and R.E. KENWARD (1979):
A survey of the bacterial flora of the feet of free-living goshawks (*Accipiter gentilis*).
Avian Path. **8**, 285–288

NIE, G.J.-VAN (1981):
Tuberculose bij een buizerd met bumblefoot.
Tijdschrift Diergeneesk. **106**, 1033–1036

NOTHELFER, H.B. and U. WERNERY:
Salmonella septicemia as cause of death in falcons in the United Arab Emirates.
In print

PIECHOCKI, R. (1981):
Tuberkulose bei wildlebenden Greifvögeln (*Falconiformes*) und Eulen (*Strigiformes*).
Int. Symp. Erkrank. Zootiere **23**, 55–66

POVEDA, J.B., CARRANZA, J., MIRANDA, A., GARRIDO, A., HERMOSO, M., FERNANDEZ, A. and J. DOMENECH (1990):
An epizootiological study of avian mycoplasmas in southern Spain.
Avian Path. **19**, 627–633

POVEDA, J.B., GIEBEL, J., KIRCHHOFF, H. and A. FERNANDEZ (1990):
Isolation of mycoplasmas from a buzzard, falcons and vultures.
Avian Path. **19**, 779–783

POVEDA, J.B., GIEBEL, J., FLOSSDORF, J., MEIER, J. and H. KIRCHHOFF (1994):
Mycoplasma buteonis sp. nov., *Mycoplasma falconis* sp. nov., and *Mycoplasma gypis* sp. nov., three species from birds of prey.
Int. J. System. Bacteriol. **44**, 94–98

RITCHIE, B.W., HARRISON, G.J. and L.R. HARRISON (1994):
Avian medicine: Principles and application.
Wingers Publishing, Inc. Lake Worth, Florida

ROSEN, M.N. (1972):
The 1970–71 avian Cholera epornitic impact on certain species.
J. Wildl. Dis. **8**, 75–78

ROSEN, M.N. and K. D'AMICO (1973):
First record of a golden eagle death due to avian cholera.
California Fish Game **59**, 209–210

SABISCH, G. (1977):
Ornithose bei einem Mäusebussard (*Buteo buteo*).
Berl. Münch. Tierärztl. Wschrift. **90**, 441–442

SATTERFIELD, W.C. (1981):
Early diagnosis of avian tuberculosis by laparoscopy and liver biopsy.
in: Recent advances in the study of raptor diseases.105–106
Chiron Publ. Ltd. Keighley, West Yorkshire, England

STIKA, V., CERMAK, S. and V. RACHAC (1989):
Tuberkuloza dennich dravcu.
Veterinarstvi. **39**, 86–88

SMIT, T., EGER, A., HAAGSMA, J. and T. BAKHUIZEN (1987):
Avian tuberculosis in wild birds in the Netherlands.
J. Wildl. Dis. **23**, 485–487

SYKES, G.P., MURPHY, C. and V. HARDASWICK (1981):
Salmonella infection in a captive peregrine falcon.
J. Am. Vet. Med. Ass. **179**, 1269–1271

SYKES, G.P. (1982):
Tuberculosis in a red-tailed hawk (*Buteo jamaicensis*).
J. Wildl. Dis. **18**, 495–499

WERNERY, U. (1995):
personal communication

WILLIAMS, E.S., RUNDE, D.E., MILLS, K. and L.D. HOLLER (1987):
Avian Cholera in a Gyrfalcon (*Falco rusticolus*).
Avian Dis. **31**, 380–382

9.3 Fungal infections

Fungi are always present in the environment and around birds without necessarily causing disease. On the contrary, some fungi are part of the normal flora of the skin and mucus membranes. Only when the animal's immune system is compromised in some way can an imbalance between fungus and host lead to disease.

Understanding this relationship is important in the treatment of such infections. Any therapy aimed at controlling avian fungal diseases must include the recognition and elimination of any predisposing factors that allowed the infection to occur in the first place.

9.3.1 Aspergillosis

Aspergillosis is a common and usually lethal fungal infection of captive birds of prey (Forbes, 1991). Loupal (1983) reports that this disease is responsible for between 15 and 30 % of the deaths of raptors exhibited in zoos. It is much less of a problem in wild raptors (Redig et al., 1980).

Pathogen

The fungus *Aspergillus fumigatus* is isolated from 95% of raptors with aspergillosis. *Aspergillus flavus* and *Aspergillus niger* are occasionally found as well. These fungi are ubiquitous and proliferate rapidly in moist, warm conditions on suitable organic substrates such as bark mulch or wet straw.

Poor aviary conditions such as those that foster excess humidity or extreme dryness combined with poor ventilation are most likely to result in high concentrations of airborne aspergillus spores that can invade and infect a bird's respiratory system.

Improper feeding practices, especially those resulting in excessive weight loss for hunting hawks, reduce the animal's resistance to infection and can promote the development of this disease. Any other source of stress that reduces a bird's immunocompetence will act similarly. Wild birds, especially falcons and goshawks, that are ill or injured and find themselves suddenly in captivity are especially vulnerable to aspergillosis.

Aspergillosis is thus an opportunistic infection, influenced by environmental hygienic factors and the animal's resistance to infection, and not truly an infectious disease that can be spread from one bird to another.

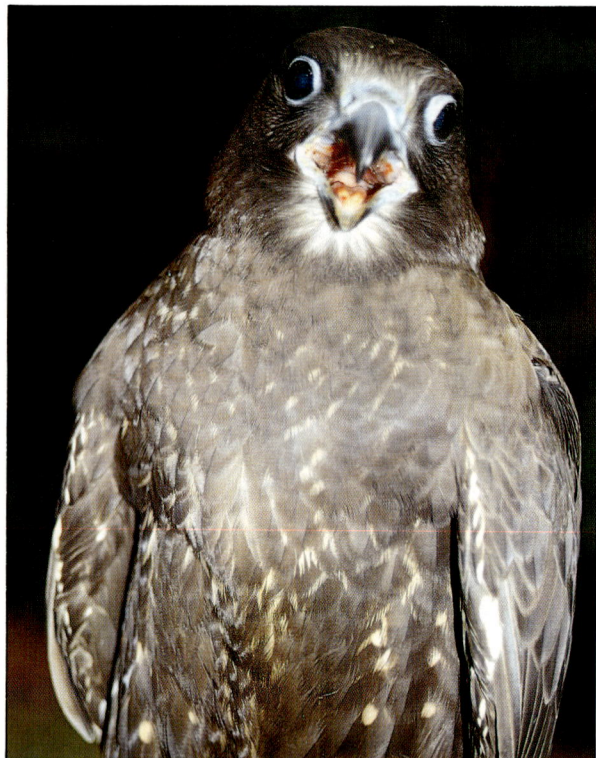

Fig. 9.16: A male hybrid falcon [gyrfalcon X (gyrfalcon X saker falcon)] developed aspergillosis while still a young bird. Initial signs included decreased appetite and generalized depression progressing to unresponsiveness. Only two days before death did respiratory signs, including open-mouth and abdominal breathing, become evident.
(Photo: Heidenreich)

Younger animals are particularly susceptible, but older birds that have been in captivity for years can develop aspergillosis as well. Birds that have been in captivity for up to four generations are as vulnerable to aspergillosis as wild-caught ones. This period of time is obviously too short for selective pressures to have affected their susceptibility.

Clinical disease

Aspergillosis is a disease that primarily affects the avian respiratory apparatus, including lungs, air sacs and occasionally the trachea. Surprisingly, respiratory signs do not dominate the clinical picture. Noticeable weakness, exercise intolerance and dyspnea with open-mouth and abdominal breathing are seen only towards the very end of the disease process (Fig. 9.16). Earlier signs tend to be nonspecific and mild. Within this general pattern, several forms of aspergillosis in birds have been recognized:

Acute course: After an incubation period that can range from a few days to several weeks, the infected bird will suddenly become depressed, dyspneic and then die within a few days. Occasionally the animal dies suddenly without any signs of respiratory involvement.

Chronic course: This more common form of aspergillosis involves a gradual loss of body condition and a decrease in appetite with respiratory signs noticeable only shortly before death. The duration varies greatly and can be up to several weeks, depending on the resistance of the host. Changes in voice quality or loss of

Northern raptor species such as gyrfalcons (*Falco rusticolus*) and merlins (*Falco columbarius)* as well as eagles (genus *Aquila*) and goshawks (genus *Accipiter*) are particularly prone to developing respiratory fungal infections. Aspergillosis was described in gyrfalcons as early as the Middle Ages, giving this species the nickname "the falcons that are short of breath". Almost all the falcons imported from Greenland and Iceland in those days died of aspergillosis within a few weeks of reaching their new home.

The unusual susceptibility to fungal infections seen in birds native to cold climates is evident also among penguins from the Antarctic. Aspergillosis is the primary cause of death of penguins held in captivity (Heidenreich, 1978). The reasons for this may lie in the inability of cold adapted birds to adjust to changes in climate, which in turn can lead to stress and immunosuppression. There may also be genetic or evolutionary factors involved, related to the fact that these species evolved in an environment relatively free of fungal spores.

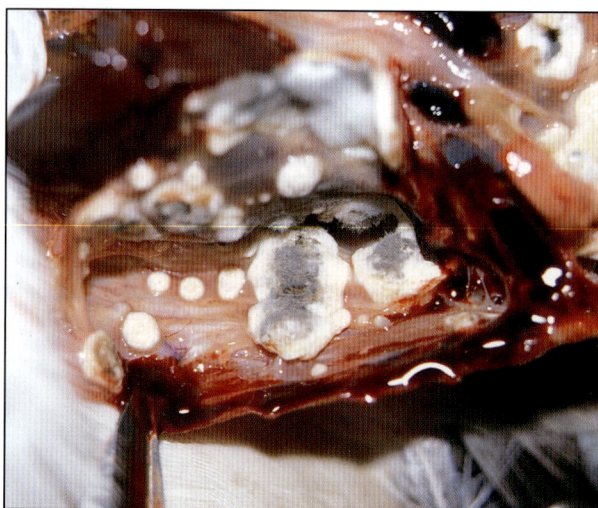

Fig. 9.17: This bird with aspergillosis has fungal colonies of various sizes showing the characteristic *Aspergillus fumigatus* coloration in the abdominal air sac.
(Photo: Heidenreich)

voice may be among the earliest signs. As with other diseases that involve the kidney, pastel green urates can be seen in the later stages of disease.

Affected birds do not die of respiratory insufficiency, but rather from the effects of aflatoxins produced by the fungus. This explains why birds may die with only a few fungal granulomas present in the lungs or just one or two colonies of mold in the air sacs.

Localized form: In rare cases, well-encapsulated aspergillus granulomas (aspergillomas) can be found in the trachea, esophagus or under the skin. These probably represent an effective walling-off of early fungal infections on the part of the bird. Such lesions can become a source of reinfection in situations that lower host resistance, or they may cause problems as space-occupying masses, especially in the upper airways.

Pathology

Postmortem findings will vary, depending on the course and duration of disease. With the acute form of aspergillosis, pinpoint foci of infection will be distributed throughout the lung parenchyma. In birds that succumb to the chronic form, extensive fungal colonies with a characteristic pigmentation may cover the air sac regions. *Aspergillus fumigatus* colonies form fuzzy, grayish-green plaques (Fig. 9.17) that can spread out to cover the entire air sac surface in severe cases (Fig. 9.18). All other parts of the respiratory tract will be infected as well (Fig. 9.19). Additionally, the lung, and occasionally the liver, will be distorted by yellowish-white fungal granulomas of varying size.

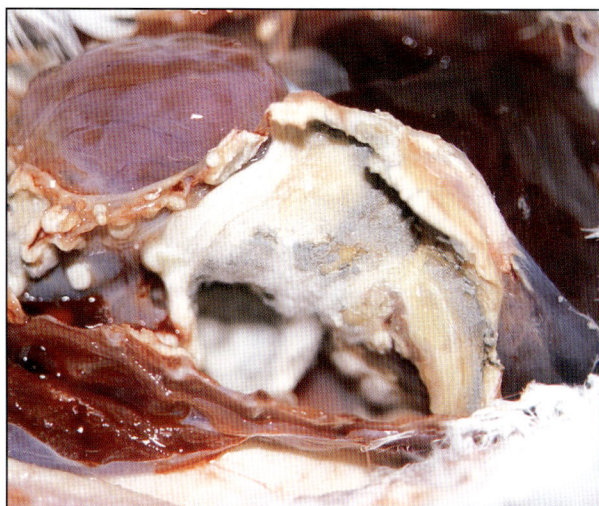

Fig. 9.18: In advanced cases, the air sacs can be completely covered with a thick, cottony growth of fungal mycelia.
(Photo: Heidenreich)

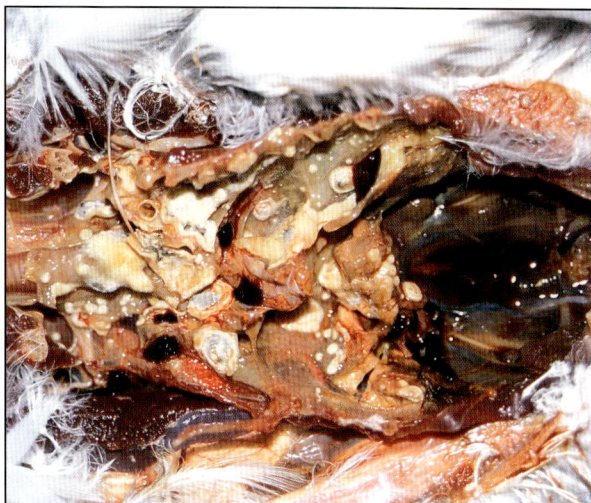

Fig. 9.19: In the final stages of disease, the entire respiratory system can be affected by fungal growth and aspergillus granulomas. It is easy to see why such advanced cases of aspergillosis are rarely amenable to treatment.
(Photo: Heidenreich)

Diagnosis

In view of the various possible forms of this disease and the vague initial clinical signs, early diagnosis of aspergillosis is relatively difficult. A thorough history and physical exam combined with a variety of diagnostic procedures can help confirm a presumptive diagnosis. Diagnostic procedures that may be of assistance are listed below.

Radiography

This modality is useful primarily in the later stages of disease, when granulomas and air sac changes are advanced enough to be visible. High-detail film-screen combinations will make interpretation easier. Soft tissue masses in the lung parenchyma, thickening of air sac membranes or opacities within the air sac lumen are suggestive of aspergillosis. By the time such changes are visible, the prognosis for successful treatment of the disease is poor.

Endoscopy

An endoscopic examination of the trachea or air sacs can reveal the presence of fungal colonies or granulomas. The lesions can be biopsied and submitted for culture or histopathology, and impression smears can be examined cytologically for evidence of fungal hyphae and spores. An air sac wash with 0.5 ml of physiologic saline can sometimes be similarly useful.

These procedures require injectable or inhalant anesthesia, a risky undertaking in debilitated birds often suffering from some degree of respiratory compromise. The stress of such procedures is also a factor, acting to reduce the animal's resistance even further and potentially allowing the disease processes to accelerate.

Bloodwork

As with any infectious disease, elevations in white blood cell count (heterophilia) are usually present. The hematocrit is often low and liver enzymes may be elevated, especially AST (SGOT), probably as a result of the hepatotoxic effects of aflatoxins.

Pat Redig (1993) has developed an ELISA that tests specifically for antibodies to *Aspergillus* sp. in raptors and other birds. Experimentally, antibodies to the fungus are detectable only one week after infection, much earlier than clinical signs of the disease become evident. This test may be prove to be useful both for diagnostic purposes and in monitoring the progress or response to therapy in infected birds.

Tracheal culture

This procedure involves taking a sterile moistened cotton swab and inserting it deeply into the bird's trachea. Gently grasping the tongue and pulling it forward will make access to the glottis easier. Care must be taken not to come into contact with the oral mucus membranes and contaminating the swab during the procedure. The material thus obtained is streaked out on appropriate media and incubated at 37 °C. Fungal colonies will become visible after only 18 to 24 hours if the animal is infected.

Treatment

Treatment of aspergillosis is always difficult and success is possible only if therapy is instituted early in the disease process. Advanced cases presenting with emaciation and dyspnea are no longer likely to respond to treatment.

Recommended drugs and dosages can be obtained from the Table 8.3 in Chapter 8.2.2. Redig (1993) claims that the only effective treatment involves oral flucytosine in combination with amphotericin B.

Almost all antifungal drugs can cause vomiting if giving at high enough dosages. In such cases, the daily dose should be divided and given on a full stomach if possible.

Also important during treatment are supportive measures designed to strengthen the animal and boost its immune system. Any underlying stress factors that may have contributed to the development of aspergillosis should be addressed. In gyrfalcons, psychological well-being seems to play an important role. A sudden change of owner or environment can easily lead to depression and decreased disease resistance in these sensitive birds. It is easy to see that any benefits derived from diagnostic and therapeutic efforts in these falcons could be negated by the stress accompanying the long period of treatment necessary with this disease.

Prevention

In recent years, some breeders have tried to counteract the susceptibility of gyrfalcons to aspergillosis by crossing them with the relatively resistant saker falcons. Indeed, gyrfalcon X saker falcon hybrids appear to be less vulnerable to fungal infections. As these hybrids are back-crossed to gyrfalcons, their susceptibility seems to rise proportionally to the degree of gyrfalcon genes.

Optimal nutrition, good management and maintenance of adequate body condition, even during hunting season, will go far towards minimizing the risk of aspergillosis in raptors. Prophylactic treatment with 50–60 mg/kg flucytosine BID for ten days (see Table 8.3) has proven helpful in preventing the disease in young gyrfalcons that have just been moved to a new location or that are beginning to be manned or trained. This type of prophylaxis is of value for any endangered raptor species during stressful periods such as transport or after injuries and during medical treatment.

Experiments with vaccines against aspergillosis have been underway since the 1980's. These heat-inactivated fungal preparations have not yet proven effective.

9.3.2　Candidiasis

The yeast *Candida albicans* is an opportunistic pathogen affecting primarily the oropharyngeal mucus membranes and esophagus. Like many other opportunistic organisms, trichomonads for instance (see Ch. 10.1.2), candida yeast can be considered a frequent commensal in the oral cavity of raptors. Disease occurs only in situations which reduce the host's resistance to infection, upsetting the normal balance be-

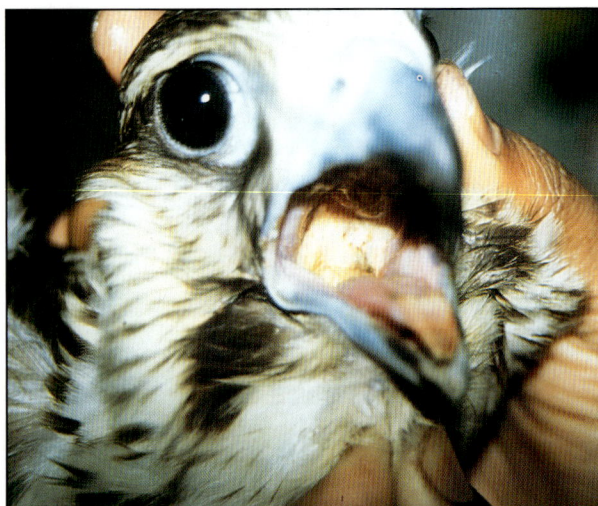

Fig. 9.20: Yellowish plaques are visible in the oropharynx of this saker falcon (*F. cherrug*) with candidiasis. (Photo: Lierz)

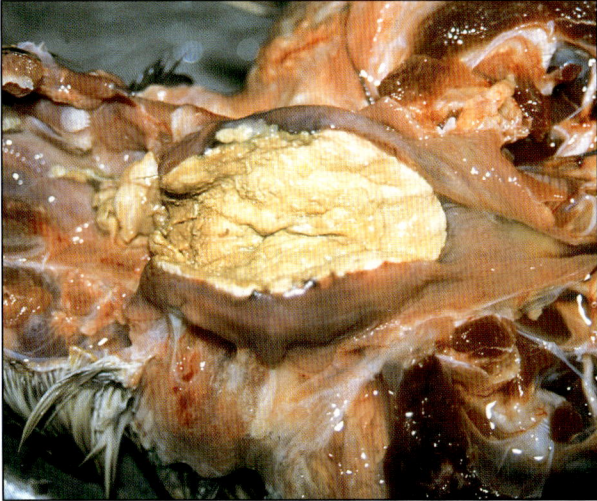

Fig. 9.21: Candidiasis is frequently characterized by membranous lesions of the esophagus that are difficult to identify on a routine physical exam. (Photo: Lierz)

tween it and the potential pathogen. Careless or excessive use of antibiotics or the presence of other primary diseases can permit the development of candidiasis. Young birds in their first few weeks of life are particularly vulnerable.

Clinical disease

Raptors suffering from infection with *C. albicans* initially show very few signs of disease. After a while, reduced food intake may alert the owner or veterinarian to examine the oral cavity. Yellowish-white plaques will be visible on the oral mucosa (Fig. 9.20). The typical mouth odor of a healthy raptor will disappear. Infections of the esophagus and crop are more common (Fig. 9.21), but also more difficult to diagnose. Palpation of the neck may reveal thickening of the esophageal mucosa. The lesions can often be visualized endoscopically.

Diagnosis

Clinical signs of candidiasis are similar to those seen with a number of other diseases. Identification of the pathogen is therefore very important. Both trichomoniasis and capillariasis can produce similar lesions in the oral cavity of birds of prey. In contrast to these two parasitic infections, early candida plaques can be rubbed off with a cotton-tipped swab without resulting in excessive bleeding from the underlying tissues.

The diagnosis is easily confirmed by microscopic examination of a smear from the mucus membranes. Dark blue, oval, occasionally budding yeast are seen with a Gram's stain. Typical round white colonies will develop in culture. A diagnosis of candidiasis is only justified, however, if the clinical picture corresponds to the diagnostic findings.

Pathology

In severe cases, the esophagus will be greatly thickened and covered with whitish plaques or membranes. The mucus membranes may peel off easily.

Treatment and prevention

Candidiasis is relatively easily treated with broad spectrum antifungal drugs. Nystatin is safe and effective for mild cases, while ketoconazole and itraconazole have proven effective for severe or refractory infections with this yeast (see Table 8.3, Ch. 8.2.2).

Since candidiasis is an opportunistic infection, all predisposing factors should be addressed. This includes underlying diseases, faulty management or feeding practices and excessive or unnecessary use of antibiotics.

9.3.3 Rhodotoruliasis

Rhodotorula mucilaginosa is a yeast that infects the skin. It has been occasionally diagnosed in raptors by the author, especially in falcons, where it seems to cause dermatologic lesions in the axillary area of the wing or between the thigh and body wall.

Clinical disease

Infections with this yeast are not usually irritating or pruritic. The problem is therefore often only recognized by the falconer after it has advanced to the point where significant lesions are present. Greasy yellowish-brown crusts overlying cracked and discolored areas of skin are seen initially (Fig. 9.22). Long-standing lesions become hyperkeratotic along their edges as

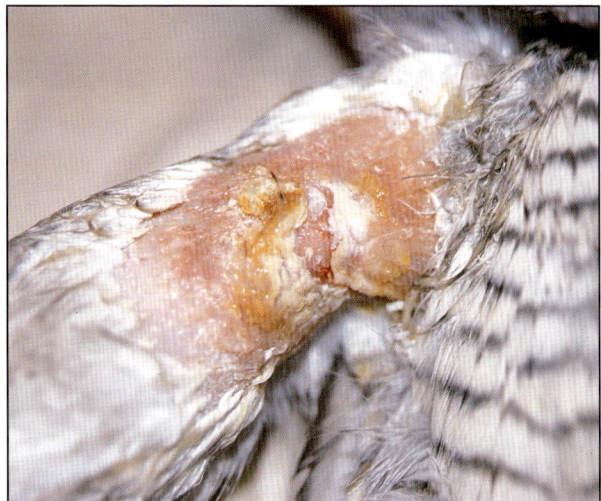

Fig. 9.22: An early infection with *Rhodotorula mucilaginosa* on the inner thigh of a peregrine falcon (*F. peregrinus*). These small skin lesions are easy to overlook.   (Photo: Heidenreich)

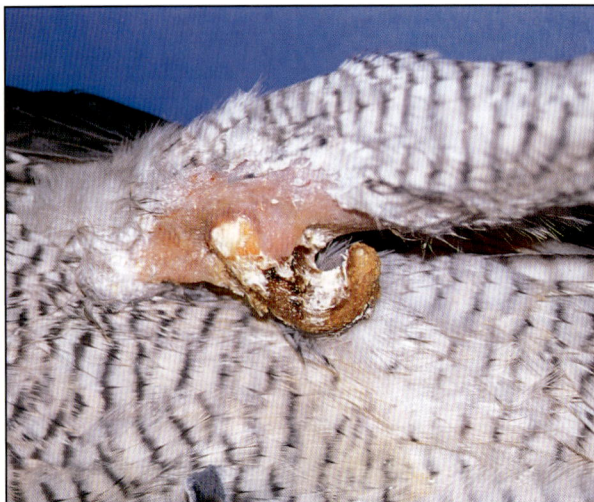

Fig. 9.23: Several weeks or months after initial infection, proliferative growths can be seen growing in areas affected with rhodotoruliasis.
(Photo: Heidenreich)

the body attempts to respond to the infection. Proliferative, horny growths may develop on infected skin over time (Fig. 9.23).

Treatment

Physical removal of any horny growths and several weeks of topical treatment with an antifungal cream are required to treat this infection. Because the lesions are often secondarily infected with bacteria, alternating applications of broad spectrum topical antibiotic ointment may be necessary. As with any treatment involving topical creams or ointments, care should be taken that the bird can not ingest the medication after it has been applied.

Treatment efforts may be complicated by repeated tearing of the healing areas of skin. Exercise restriction during this time is often unavoidable.

The few cases of rhodotoruliasis treated by the author have not given any indication as to the underlying causes for the infection. One can probably assume that this yeast is also an opportunist, and that earlier dermatologic changes of some sort permit the infection to become established.

References and literature of further interest

Cooper, J.E. (1969):
Some diseases of birds of prey.
Vet. Rec. **84**, 454–457

Cutsem, J.-van and J. Fransen (1987):
Fungal infections in birds in captivity - six case reports.
Mykosen **30**, 166–171

Donnelly, C.C., Picket, C. and M. Bush (1983):
Prophylactic antimycotic treatment and vaccination trials in American eider ducks for the prevention of aspergillosis.
Int. Symp. Erkr. Zootiere, 1983, 117–122

Fatunmbi, O.O. and A. Bankole (1984):
Severe disseminated aspergillosis in a captive Abyssinian tawny eagle (*Aquila rapax*).
J. Wildl. Dis. **20**, 52–54

Forbes, N.A. (1991):
Aspergillosis in raptors.
Vet. Rec. **128**, 263

Grimm, F.H. (1979):
Der indirekte Haemagglutinationstest zur Diagnose der Aspergillose.
DVG-Tagung, München 135–149

Heidenreich, M. (1978):
Abgangsursachen von Pinguinen in Gefangenschaft.
Tierärztl. Praxis **6**, 395–401

Keymer, I. F. (1972):
Diseases of birds of prey.
Vet. Rec. **90**, 579–594

Lawrence, K. (1983):
Treatment of aspergillosis in raptors.
Vet. Rec. **112**, 88

Loupal, G. (1983):
Pathomorphologischer Beitrag zum Vorkommen von Mykosen bei Zoo- und Wildvögeln.
Int. Symp. Erkrank. Zootiere **25**, 123–133

Parrott, T. (1991):
Clinical treatment regimes with fluconazole.
Proc. Ann. Meeting Assoc. Avian Vet., Chicago 15–17

Redig, P.T. (1981):
Aspergillosis in raptors.
in: Cooper, J.E. and A.G. Greenwood (1981):
Recent advances in the study of raptor diseases.
Chiron Public. Ltd. Keighley, West Yorkshire, UK

Redig, P.T. (1993):
Medical management of birds of prey.
A collection of notes on selected topics. 115–124
Raptor Center, Minnesota

Redig, P.T., Fuller, M.R. and D.L. Evans (1980):
Prevalence of *Aspergillus fumigatus* in free-living goshawks (*Accipiter gentilis atricapillus*).
J. Wildl. Dis. **16**, 169–174

Wagner, C., Hochleithner, M. and W.D. Rausch (1991):
Ketoconazole plasma levels in buzzards.
Proc. Conf. Europ. Comm. Ass. Avian Vet. 333–340

10　Parasitic diseases

A parasitic relationship implies that one organism (the parasite) is dependent on another (the host) for fulfillment of its needs during part or all of its life cycle. The host generally derives no benefit from this relationship, and may even be impaired by it. As with infectious microorganisms, parasites often achieve a fine balance with the host animals they depend on in nature. Serious illness or death of the host animal would interfere with the parasite's ability to survive, multiply and distribute itself.

Parasitic organisms can live **on** their host as "ectoparasites", or **inside** the animal as "endoparasites". These broad categories are not sufficient to describe the complexity of parasitic lifestyles, however. Some parasites require a host only for certain stages of their life cycle, while others may be found both externally and internally on a host at different times. For these reasons, the structure of the following chapter is based on the taxonomic classification, rather than on the location of the parasite inside or on the bird.

10.1　Protozoa

10.1.1　Trypanosomiasis

Trypanosomes are unicellular organisms that live in the blood of birds. Unlike other avian blood parasites, they remain free-swimming and do not invade blood cells. Transmission occurs primarily via biting insects or ticks. The distribution of these parasites therefore correlates closely with climatic conditions. Studies examining the incidence of trypanosomal infection in North American wild raptors found the protozoan in 1.2% of the birds examined. Similar investigations in Egypt and East Africa found trypanosomes in up to 7% of the animals tested.

Trypanosoma avium is the most common trypanosome found in birds. A different species (*Trypanosoma benetti*) has been described in American kestrels (*Falco sparverius*).

Trypanosomal infections in birds are sometimes incidentally discovered on examination of stained blood smears, but they have not been linked to clinical disease in birds. Treatment for this parasite in birds of prey has not been described, nor is it likely to be necessary.

10.1.2　Trichomoniasis (Frounce)

Trichomonas gallinae is a flagellated organism that preferentially colonizes the mucosae of the avian oropharynx, esophagus and crop. It is particularly common in pigeons and doves. Almost all wild and domestic columbiformes are latently infected with this parasite and should be considered carriers of the infection. Transmission of *T. gallinae* to birds of prey is therefore relatively easy, especially since trichomonads are not particularly host specific, being capable of infecting and causing disease in a number of avian species.

For these reasons, some authors recommend never feeding fresh pigeons to raptors, or at least freezing the birds for a short time before offering them as food. The freezing process will kill any trichomonads present in the carcass. These precautions are probably unnecessary. *Trichomonas gallinae* is usually a facultatively pathogenic mucosal organism, present in many healthy birds of prey without causing disease. In situations where an injury to the upper digestive tract or immunosuppression in the bird create an opportunity for pathogenesis, the parasite may proliferate and cause clinical disease (frounce). In 1992, Pepler and Oettle described a very serious outbreak of trichomoniasis in various raptor species in South Africa. This situation may have involved an unusually pathogenic strain of *T. gallinae*.

Goshawks, sparrowhawks and falcons seem to be more vulnerable to trichomoniasis than other raptor species. The disease is more common in young animals, although it is also seen in adults that are weakened by other diseases, injuries or stress.

Clinical Disease
Various forms of trichomoniasis are seen, depending on the pathogenicity of the parasite and the resistance of the host:

Oropharyngeal Form: Yellowish caseous lesions develop in the oral cavity, primarily at the base of the tongue (Fig. 10.1). A foul, necrotic odor is usually associated with this infection. The bird's appetite is unaffected and it will continue to eat until the lesions get big enough to obstruct the esophageal opening. Ob-

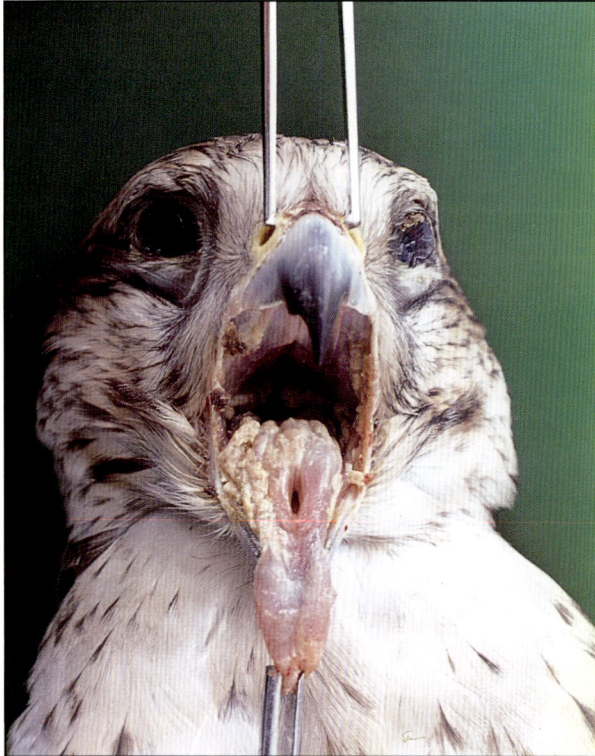

Fig. 10.1: This adult male saker falcon (*F. cherrug*) escaped while hunting and was later found by a lay person who fed him fish parts from a mink farm. The falcon became ill and died within a few days. Weight loss and an inappropriate diet had led to a severe case of trichomoniasis.
(Photo: Heidenreich)

struction of the glottis may also occur, and will result in signs of dyspnea. If the caseous plaques are manually removed, the underlying mucosa is injured. This can lead to severe bleeding.

Occasionally, esophageal lesions will develop into thick walnut-sized granulomas that interfere with swallowing. Birds affected in this way quickly lose weight.

Generalized form: In particularly serious cases, the infection can spread to internal organs and cause disseminated disease (Fig. 10.2). This occurs most often in young birds.

Diagnosis
Although the lesions of trichomoniasis are usually easily identified, they are so similar to those of candidiasis and oral capillariasis that further tests are required to confirm the diagnosis. This usually involves identification of the motile trophozoite in a sample from a lesion. A cotton-tipped swab is moistened with physiologic saline and used to swab the oropharynx. Trichomonads are very sensitive to environmental conditions, especially changes in temperature. The sample needs to be immediately examined for the motile uni-

cellular organisms on a warmed direct mount. Sending the samples to a lab or evaluating swabs from deceased birds is not possible.

Treatment
Very effective medications are available to treat this infection. Carnidazole (Spartrix®) has proven particularly successful at a one-time dose of one tablet per 500 g of body weight. Within a few days, clinical resolution of the lesions will be evident. In very serious cases, the treatment may need to be repeated.

This class of drugs is so effective that they can be used to confirm the diagnosis. If the lesions do not respond to carnidazole or metronidazole, a different etiology should be suspected.

Prevention
Preventive measures should focus primarily on maintaining healthy, disease resistant birds and less on avoiding high quality, fresh food such as pigeons. A monotonous, vitamin-deficient or otherwise inappropriate diet will quickly lead to disease, especially in sparrowhawk nestlings. Sudden weight loss can also predispose to the development of trichomoniasis.

Frequent monitoring of the oral cavity for lesions or an abnormal odor is a good practice. Carnidazole is so well-tolerated and safe that it can be used prophylactically in young or immunosuppressed birds at risk for the disease.

10.1.3 Coccidioses

Several different coccidial species from four different genera have been identified in birds of prey (see Table

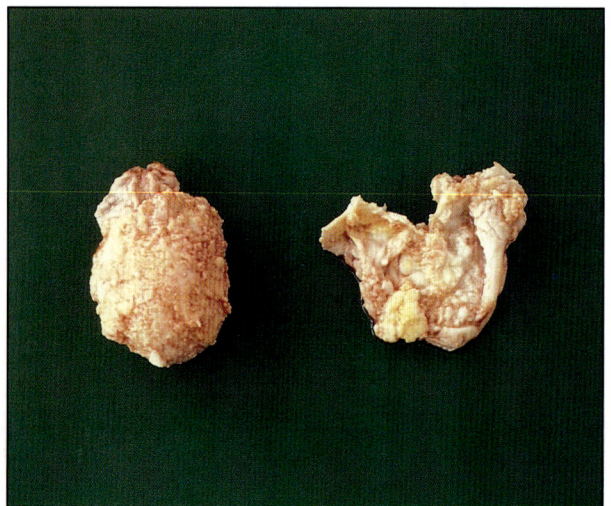

Fig. 10.2: The generalized form of trichomoniasis affects the internal organs as well as the upper GI tract. In this case, extensive lesions are seen involving the pericardium and heart of a falcon.   (Photo: Heidenreich)

10.1). They have been well studied in falcons (Boeer, 1982; Klueh, 1994) because this group of raptors is particularly vulnerable to coccidial infections, especially under captive conditions.

The four coccidial genera, *Eimeria, Caryospora, Sarcocystis* and *Frenkelia,* have different life cycles. *Eimeria* species have a direct life cycle. Their oocysts are excreted in the feces of infected birds and then directly taken up by another avian host. *Caryospora* rely primarily on the direct route of infection, but are also capable of passing through an intermediate host. An intermediate host is always necessary for infection with *Sarcocystis* species.

Because the life cycle, clinical signs, treatment and prevention of *Eimeria* coccidiosis are almost identical to those of *Caryospora,* only the latter will be discussed in detail.

10.1.3.1 *Caryospora*

Clinical disease linked to infection with various species of *Caryospora* is recognized primarily in captive falcons and can be a significant problem in large falcon breeding facilities.

Infected birds pass *Caryospora* oocysts in their feces. Two to four days are required for the oocysts to become infectious (sporulate), depending on temperature and humidity levels. They then remain viable in the environment for several months. Water, food, perches and even gauntlets contaminated with feces from an infected bird can thus become sources of infection for other falcons. Earthworms can also serve as intermediate hosts. Falcons kept on block or bow perches have easy access to the ground and to worms, and can be infected that way.

Eight to thirteen days after inoculation, an infected bird will begin passing *Caryospora* oocysts, sometimes up to 500,000 oocysts per gram of fecal material (Klueh, 1994). It is obvious that the animal's environment can become heavily contaminated in very little time.

Caryospora coccidiosis is primarily a problem in young falcons being manned or trained, while adult birds are thought to develop some degree of immunity. Adult falcons can develop clinical infections under conditions of improper feeding and management.

Clinical disease
Affected birds usually have a history of significant weight loss and other stresses associated with manning or training. This makes them vulnerable to infection and disease.

Initial clinical signs often involve changes in fecal consistency. The feces will initially be just soft, then progress to runny brown, eventually turning foul-smelling reddish or bloody. In advanced cases, red-

Table 10.1:
Coccidial species found in various birds of prey

Coccidial species	Raptor hosts
Caryospora falconis	Peregrine falcon (*Falco peregrinus*) European hobby (*F. subbuteo*) Common kestrel (*F. tinnunculus*)
Caryospora kutzeri	Gyrfalcon (*Falco rusticolus*) Saker falcon (*F. cherrug*) Peregrine falcon (*F. peregrinus*) Prairie falcon (*F. mexicanus*) Lanner falcon (*F. biarmicus*) Laggar falcon (*F. jugger*) European hobby (*F. subbuteo*) Common kestrel (*F. tinnunculus*)
Caryospora neofalconis	Peregrine falcon (*Falco peregrinus*) Prairie falcon (*F. mexicanus*) Lanner falcon (*F. biarmicus*) European hobby (*F. subbuteo*) Common kestrel (*F. tinnunculus*)
Caryospora boeri	Common kestrel (*F. tinnunculus*)
Caryospora megafalconis	Gyrfalcon (*Falco rusticolus*) Saker falcon (*F. cherrug*) Gyrfalcon X saker falcon hybrid (*F. rust. X F. cherrug*) Common kestrel (*F. tinnunculus*)
Caryospora henryae	Black kite (*Milvus migrans*) European hobby (*F. subbuteo*) Common kestrel (*F. tinnunculus*) Turkey vulture (*Cathartes aura*)
Caryospora uptoni	Red-tailed hawk (*Buteo j. borealis*)
Eimeria accipitris	European sparrowhawk (*Accipiter nisus*) Booted eagle (*Hieraaetus pennatus*)
Eimeria asturi	Northern goshawk (*Accipiter gentilis*)
Sarcocystis cernae	Common kestrel (*Falco tinnunculus*)
Sarcocystis sp.	Brown hawk (*Falco berigora*) Red kite (*Milvus milvus*) Northern goshawk (*Accipiter gentilis*) European sparrowhawk (*Accipiter nisus*) Common buzzard (*Buteo buteo*) Marsh harrier (*Circus aeruginosus*)
Frenkelia glareoli	Common buzzard (*Buteo buteo*)
Frenkelia microti	Red-tailed hawk (*Buteo jamaicensis*)

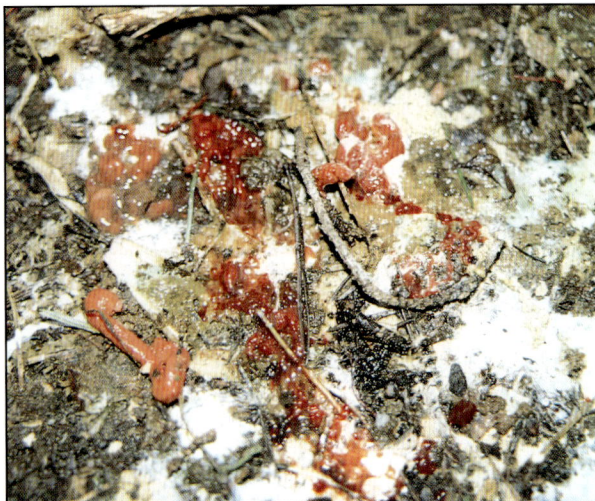

Fig. 10.3: Changes in fecal consistency this severe are seen only with overwhelming coccidial infections. Bloody fibrinous casts or pseudomembranes are produced and excreted by the inflamed intestinal tract.
(Photo: Heidenreich)

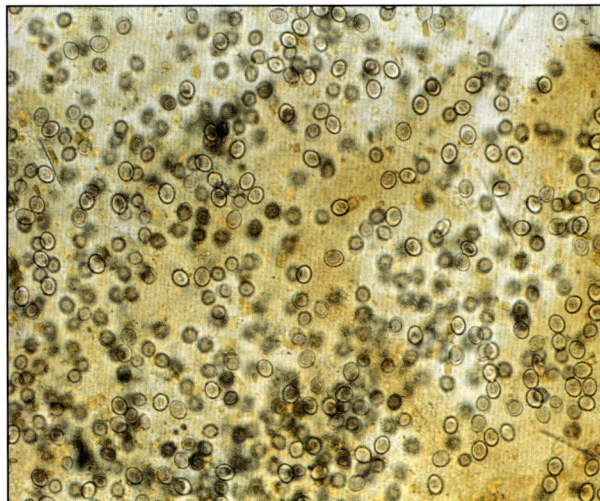

Fig. 10.4: Microscopic appearance of a fecal sample from a falcon with severe coccidiosis.
(Photo: Lierz, with kind help from B. Nothelfer, Central Veterinary Research Laboratory, U.A.E.)

dish-brown sausage-like casts of blood, intestinal mucosa and undigested particles of food may be excreted (Fig. 10.3).

Affected animals are typically lethargic and depressed, perching with fluffed plumage. Their appetite is poor and the rate of digestive passage slow. As the disease progresses, they may begin to vomit and regurgitate if force-fed. Death occurs due to dehydration caused by anorexia and diarrhea.

If the infected bird is being flown, a slow, ponderous style of flight will be noted. The falcon will be less aggressive in its pursuit of prey, preferring to simply follow the animal. It may appear that he would like to fly better and faster, but is unable to do so. Vitamin B deficiencies result in similar changes in flight style. Indeed, coccidia utilize B vitamins for their own metabolism and thus deprive their host of them. In addition, the inflammation associated with infections of this kind impairs the intestinal synthesis of B vitamins, further depriving the bird of these vital nutrients. Coccidiosis is often associated with clinical hypovitaminosis B.

Pathology

The degree of weight loss will depend on the severity and duration of coccidial enteritis. Inflammation of the intestinal mucosa is common and the contents of the digestive tract may appear hemorrhagic.

Diagnosis

A diagnosis of coccidiosis is quickly established by fecal examination. *Caryospora* oocysts are larger than those of other coccidia found in avian species and can be easily demonstrated with routine flotation techniques (Figs. 10.5 and 10.6). Their large size also makes them easy to differentiate from other coccidial oocysts ingested with prey and passed incidentally in the feces. Identification is aided by the fact that *Caryospora* develop only a single sporocyst containing eight sporozoites (Fig. 10.6), while *Eimeria* have four sporocysts with two sporozoites each and *Isospora* have two sporocysts with four sporozoites each.

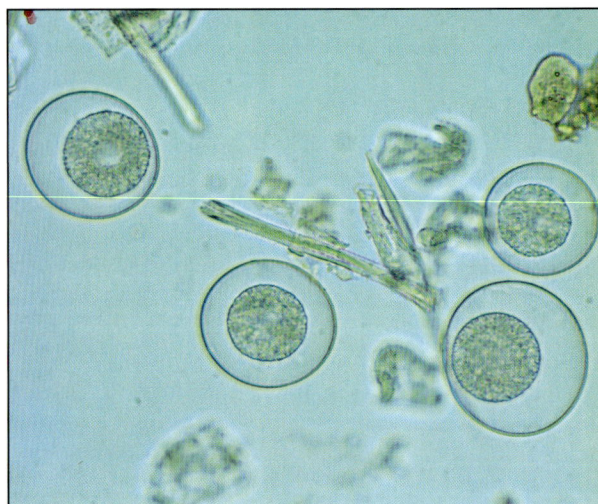

Fig. 10.5: The size difference between *C. megafalconis* and *C. falconis* is easily seen on this microscopic view (160X).
(Photo: Klueh)

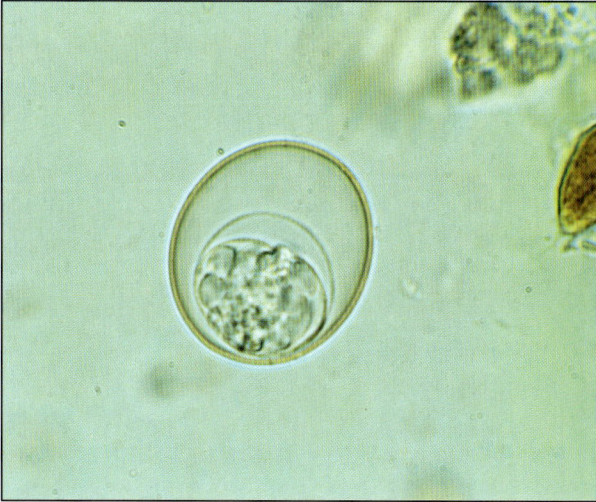

Fig 10.6: A sporulated *Caryospora* oocyst contains only a single sporocyst with 8 sporozoites. This differentiates *Caryospora* from other coccidial genera. (Photo: Klueh)

Prevention

It is practically impossible for captive raptors to avoid all exposure to coccidia. The goal is to minimize exposure as much as possible and to avoid situations which could reduce host resistance. If reinfection is strictly prevented, oocysts will disappear from the feces within 2 or 3 weeks, even without medical therapy. This proves that hygienic measures, especially the maintenance of a clean, dry environment, are particularly important (Fig. 10.7).

In aviaries, a substrate consisting of a thick layer of 2 or 3 cm diameter pea gravel over a layer of lime is effective. It allows the mutes to drop below the surface, away from the bird, and prevents exposure to earthworms.

Hawks can be fed on the fist or on feeding platforms, but never on the ground. All perches, blocks and water baths should be cleaned daily.

Treatment

In large-scale poultry operations, coccidiosis is commonly treated by medicating the feed or water. In contrast, raptors are treated individually, and this makes many of the preparations available for large-scale use impractical.

Sulfonamides are quite effective in treating coccidial infections. They should be used with caution, however. In several cases, illness and death due to kidney failure and gout have been noted in falcons several months after treatment with sulfonamide antibiotics.

There are other drugs that are equally effective and better tolerated by birds of prey. Amprolium at a dose of 30 mg/kg PO SID for 5 days, alone or in combination with ethopabate (Amprolvet Super®) at a dose of 0.5 mg/kg SID for 5 days is effective. These medications come in a bitter liquid form that requires repeated handling for oral administration. This is a drawback, as the birds become increasingly resistant to their administration.

Toltrazuril (Baycox®) is a liquid that requires only two doses of 25 mg/kg 24 hours apart. The bird will cease shedding oocysts one day after the second treatment (Klueh, 1994). Drawbacks are the same as with amprolium.

The drug of choice for the treatment of coccidiosis in falcons is clazuril (Appertex®), a product in tablet form that was developed for the individual treatment of pigeons. It has proven safe and effective in raptors as well. At a dose of 5 to 10 mg/kg once daily for two days, clazuril will eliminate fecal shedding of coccidia within 24 hours of initiation of therapy.

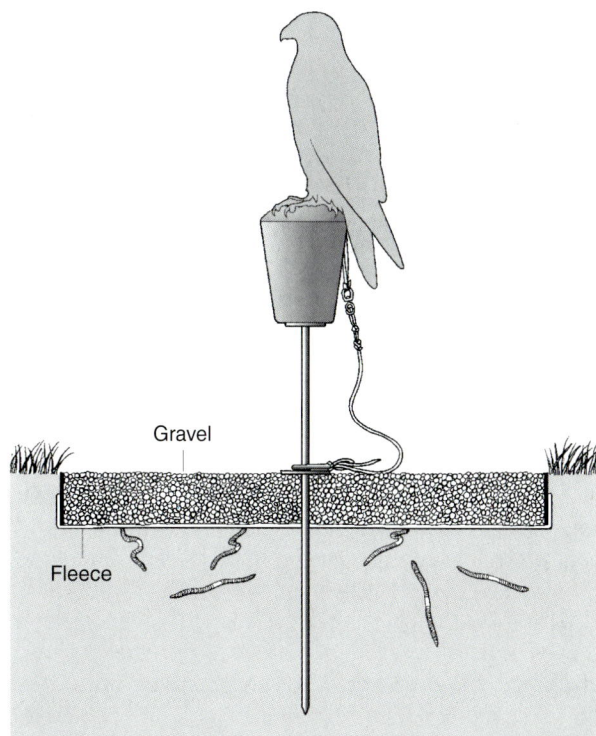

Gravel

Fleece

Fig. 10.7: Parasitic infections transmitted by the ingestion of earthworms can be avoided by providing a clean, dry substrate around the perch. (Illustration: R. Gattung-Petith and A. Gattung)

10.1.3.2 *Sarcocystis*

Raptors are the definitive host for the *Sarcocystis* species they harbor. The sporulated oocysts or individual sporocysts are passed in their feces and are ingested by an intermediate host, usually a common prey animal. Whitish, tubular sarcocysts containing bradyzoites form in the intermediate host's muscle tissue. The animal is probably weakened by this infection, and therefore more vulnerable to predation. Capture and ingestion by another bird of prey then completes the cycle of infection.

Clinical signs in raptors vary, but are usually no worse than a mild diarrhea. Aguilar et al. (1991) and Dubey et al. (1991) describe *Sarcocystis* infections in a northern goshawk *(Accipiter gentilis)* and a golden eagle *(Aquila chryseatos)* that involved CNS disturbances including vestibular problems and lameness.

There are more than 100 known species of *Sarcocystis*. Both hosts in the parasite's life cycle are known only for slightly over half of them. Two coccidian life cycles have been worked out in birds of prey – one in common kestrels *(Falco tinnunculus)* and one in the common buzzard *(Buteo buteo)*. In the kestrel, the intermediate host for *Sarcocystis cernae* is the earth mouse *(Microtus arvalis)*, while *Frenkelia glareoli*, found in the buzzard, utilizes the red mouse *(Clethrionomys glareolus)* (Rommel, 1978, 1978a).

10.1.4 Toxoplasmosis

Only cats can serve as the definitive host for the coccidian parasite *Toxoplasma gondii*. Sexual reproduction occurs in the intestine and the oocysts are subsequently shed in the feces. As with coccidia, several days are required before the oocysts sporulate and become infectious. They are then ingested by other animals, most commonly small rodents. These serve as intermediate hosts, developing intramuscular cysts that are infectious to many other animals. If a cat consumes the infected rodent, the cycle is completed.

Raptors also frequently ingest rodents carrying *Toxoplasma* cysts. Extensive studies in eastern Europe have shown that approximately 34% of all wild birds of prey from that region carry antibodies to the parasite. Similar levels of infection were found by LINDSAY et al. (1993) in the United States. They obtained positive results in 20 to 64% of the various raptor species examined for antibody levels to *T. gondii* and intramuscular cysts.

Raptors are not the definitive host for *Toxoplasma* organisms. They can become infected, but do not shed oocysts in their feces as do cats. Instead, the parasites reproduce asexually in the bird's internal organs, musculature and central nervous system.

In contrast to some other avian species such as finches, in which infections of this type lead to serious disease and death, toxoplasmosis in raptors is typically asymptomatic and results merely in latent infection.

T. gondii can be spread from cat feces by vectors such as flies, cockroaches, worms and snails. This is one of the reasons why cats should not be permitted in areas where raptors are kept.

10.1.5 Babesiosis

Babesia is a tick borne protozoan organism that invades the erythrocytes of its definitive host. It reproduces inside the erythrocyte, destroying it when the offspring exit into the plasma to invade new cells.

Babesia species have been reported in bearded vultures *(Gypaetus barbatus)*, common kestrels *(Falco tinnunculus)* and prairie falcons *(Falco mexicanus)* (Croft and Kingston, 1975). In the case involving the prairie falcons, *Babesia moshkovskii* was present in 6 out of 30 nestlings and absent in all the adults.

This hemoparasite is most common in areas with a warm climate and can cause serious illness in other animal species. Raptors seem to be asymptomatic carriers and *Babesia* organisms are usually an incidental finding on a stained blood smear.

10.1.6 Hemoparasites

The family Plasmodiidae includes the genera *Plasmodium*, *Haemoproteus* and *Leukocytozoon*. All three of them are hemoparasites in raptors and are transmitted by biting insects. This mode of transmission means that infection rates are greatest in tropical climates or during the summer months in temperate zones.

10.1.6.1 *Plasmodium*

Avian malaria in raptors is caused by two species of *Plasmodium*, *P. circumflexum* in sharp-shinned hawks *(Accipiter striatus)* and *P. relictum* in large falcons. Mosquitoes serve as vectors.

Like penguins, which come from cold climates and suffer frequently from avian malaria in captivity, gyrfalcons hail from arctic regions and are also particularly vulnerable to avian malaria. Infection with *Plasmodium* in one gyrfalcon resulted in signs of weakness, dyspnea, vomiting and convulsions. Sixteen percent of this bird's erythrocytes were infected. Peregrine falcons housed in the same facilities had subclinical infections that affected only 0.01 to 0.4% of their red blood cells. If not treated, infected gyrfalcons can die within a few days of showing initial clinical signs (Remple, 1981). Redig (1993) reported that two out of four gyrfalcons infected in the US succumbed to plasmodial infections despite medical therapy.

Other birds of prey generally harbor the parasite without signs of illness.

A diagnosis is quickly made by examining a stained blood smear. The parasite can be identified by the characteristic intraerythrocytic gametocytes, although various stages of the parasite can also be found in other blood cells.

The same drugs used for malaria in humans are effective in birds. Chloroquine at an initial dose of 25 mg/kg PO followed by 15 mg/kg at 12, 24 and 48 hours has been recommended. The addition of primaquine at 0.75 mg/kg PO improves the effectiveness of the therapeutic regimen. Intramuscular administration of these drugs reduces the required dose of chloroquine to 1 mg/kg SID for 5 days. Quinacrine can also be used IM at a dose of 1.6 mg/kg for 5 days.

10.1.6.2 *Haemoproteus*

Haemoproteus is a normally apathogenic protozoan that infects the tissues and red blood cells of many different birds. Five different species have been identified in birds of prey (Kucera, 1981; Apanius and Kirkpatrick, 1988; Mikaelian and Bayol, 1991):

Family: Falconidae
Haemoproteus nisi
Haemoproteus elani
Haemoproteus janovyi

Family: Accipitridae
Haemoproteus tinnunculi
Haemoproteus brachiatus

Haemoproteus seems to be common in buzzards (buteos). In one study, more than 50% of these birds were found to be carriers of the parasite. Younger animals had higher rates of infection.

Hippoboscid flies are thought to transmit *Haemoproteus* from one bird to another. Clinical disease is rare with this infection. Immunosuppressed or otherwise injured and weakened birds may have large numbers of erythrocytes infected with the curved or "halter-shaped" gametocytes.

10.1.6.3 *Leucocytozoon*

This parasite of avian blood cells is also common in birds of prey (Sacchi and Prigioni, 1984; Peirce et al., 1990; Simpson, 1991). As with other hemoparasites, *Leucocytozoon* is transmitted by biting insects.

Birds in the family Accipitridae serve as hosts for *Leucocytozoon toddi*, while members of the Falconidae are infected by *L. lanilewsky*. Unlike leukocytozoonosis in ducks and geese, which is a serious clinical disease, raptors infected with this parasite rarely show clinical signs. As with *Haemoproteus*, disease is seen only with severe infections, usually in young or weakened birds of prey. These animals will be anemic, showing pale mucous membranes and weakness. Respiratory signs may occasionally be seen.

A diagnosis is easily made by examining a stained blood smear. The large, nucleated parasites severely distort the cells they infect.

Treatment can be attempted with sulfonamides or pyrimethamine. There are no reports of specific therapeutic trials in infected raptors.

References and literature of further interest

AGUILAR, R.F., SHAW, D.P., DUBEY, J.P. and P. REDIG (1991):
Sarcocystis-associated encephalitis in an immature northern goshawk (*Accipiter gentilis atricapillus*).
J. Zoo Wild. Med. **22**, 466–469

ALVAREZ-CALVO, J.A. and J.A.A. CALVO (1977):
Nuevo hospedador para *Haemoproteus multiparasitans* (Ortega & Gallego 1950) (*Haemosporidiida: Haemoproteidas*).
Rev. Iberica Parasitol. **37**, 387-391

APANIUS, V. and C.E. KIRKPATRICK (1988):
Preliminary report of *Haemoproteus tinnunculi* infection in a breeding population of American kestrels (*Falco sparverius*).
J. Wildl. Dis. **24**, 150–153

BENNETT, G.F., EARLE, R.A. and M.A. PEIRCE (1992):
New species of avian *Hepatozoon* (Apicomplexa: Haemogregarinidae) and a re-description of *Hepatozoon neophrontis* (Todd & Wohlbach, 1912) Wenyon, 1926.
System. Parasitol. **23**, 183–193

BÖER, B. (1982):
Untersuchungen über das Vorkommen von Kokzidien bei Greifvögeln und über die Entwicklung von zwei *Caryospora*-Arten der Falken (*Caryospora neofalconis* n. sp. und *Caryospora kutzeri* n. sp.).
Vet. Med. Diss. Hannover

CAWTHORN, R.J. (1993):
Cyst-forming coccidia of raptors: significant pathogens or not?
in: REDIG, T.P. et al. (1993):
Raptor Biomedicine, Chiron Pub. Ltd. Keighley, West Yorkshire, England

CERNA, Z., KOLAROVA, I. and P. SULC (1978):
Sarcocystis cernae (Levine, 1977), excystation, life-cycle and
comparison with other heteroxenous coccidians from rodents
and birds.
Fol. Parasitol. **25**, 201–207

CERNA, Z., KOLAROVA, I. and L. KOLAROVA (1982):
What we know about the Sarcosporidia of carnivorous birds.
J. Protozool. **29**, 505

CERNA, Z. (1984):
The role of birds as definitive hosts and intermediate hosts of
heteroxenous coccidians.
J. Protozool. **31**, 579–581

CERNA, Z. and Z. KVASNOVSKA (1986):
Life cycle involving bird-bird relation in *Sarcocystis coccidia*
with the description of *Sarcocystis accipitris* sp.n.
Fol. Parasitol. **33**, 305–309

CROFT, R.E. and N. KINGSTON (1975):
Babesia moshkovskii (Schurenkova, 1938) Laird and Lari,
1957; from the prairie falcon, *Falco mexicanus,* in Wyoming;
with comments on other parasites found in this host.
J. Wildl. Dis. **11**, 229–233

DUBEY, J.P., PORTER, S.L., HATTEL, A.L., KRADEL, D.C.,
TOPPER, M.J. and L. JOHNSON (1991):
Sarcocystosis-associated clinical encephalitis in a golden eagle
(*Aquila chrysaetos*).
J. Zoo Wildl. Med. **22**, 233–236

GEISEL, O., KAISER, E., KRAMPITZ, H.E. and M. ROMMEL
(1978):
Beiträge zum Lebenszyklus der Frenkelien. IV. Pathomor-
phologische Befunde an den Organen experimentell infizierter
Rötelmause.
Vet. Pathol. **15**, 621–360

GHORBANI, M. (1983):
Animal toxoplasmosis in Iran.
J. Trop. Med. Hyg. **86**, 73-76

GREINER, E.C. and A.A. KOCAN (1977):
Leucocytozoon (*Haemosporida: Leucocytozoidae*) of the
Falconiformes.
Can. J. Zool. **55**, 761–770

HOOGENBOOM, I. and C. DIJKSTRA (1987):
Sarcocystis cernae: a parasite increasing the risk of predation
of its intermediate host, *Microtus arvalis.*
Oecologia **74**, 86–92

KINGSTON, N., REMPLE, J.D. and W. BURNHAM (1976):
Malaria in a captively-produced F1 gyrfalcon and in two F1
peregrine falcons.
J. Wildl. Dis. **12**, 562–565

KIRKPATRICK, C.E. and D.M. LAUER (1985):
Hematozoa of raptors from southern New Jersey and adjacent
areas.
J. Wildl. Dis. **21**, 1–6

KIRKPATRICK, C.E. and C.A. TERWAY-THOMPSON (1986):
Biochemical characterization of some raptor trypanosomes. I.
In vitro cultivation and lectin-binding studies.
Can. J. Zool. **64**, 189–194

KIRKPATRICK, C.E., TERWAY-THOMPSON, C.A. and
M.R. IYENGAR (1986):
Biochemical characterization of some raptor trypanosomes.
II. Enzyme studies, with a description of *Trypanosoma
bennetti* n.sp.
Can. J. Zool. **64**, 195–203

KLÜH, P.N. (1994):
Untersuchungen zur Therapie und Prophylaxe der *Caryospora*-
Infektion der Falken (*Falconiformes: Falconidae*) mit
Toltrazuril sowie die Beschreibung von zwei neuen *Caryo-
spora*-Arten (*C. megafalconis* n. sp. und *C. boeri* n. sp.).
Vet. Med. Diss. Hannover

KOLAROVA, L. (1986):
Mouse (*Mus musculus*) as intermediate host of *Sarcocystis* sp.
from the goshawk (*Accipiter gentilis*).
Fol. Parasitol. **33**, 15–19

KUCERA, J. (1981):
Blood parasites of birds in Central Europe. 3. *Plasmodium* and
Haemoproteus.
Fol. Parasitol. **28**, 303–312

LINDSAY, D.S. and B.L. BLAGBURN (1989):
Caryospora uptoni and *Frenkelia* sp.-like coccidial infections
in red-tailed hawks (*Buteo borealis*).
J. Wildl. Dis. **25**, 407–409

LINDSAY, D.S., UPTON, S.J., TOIVIO-KINNUCAN, M.,
MCKOWN, R.D. and B.L. BLAGBURN (1992):
Ultrastructure of *Frenkelia microti* in prairie voles inoculated
with sporocysts from red-tailed hawks.
J. Helminthol. Soc. Wash. **59**, 170–176

LINDSAY, D.S., SMITH, P.C., HOERR, F.J. and B.L. BLAGBURN
(1993):
Prevalence of encysted *Toxoplasma gondii* in raptors from
Alabama.
J. Parasitol.**79**, 870–873

MATHEY, W.J. (1966):
Isospora buteonis Henry 1932 in an American kestrel (*Falco
sparverius*) and a golden eagle (*Aquila chrysaetos*).
Bull. Wildl. Dis. Ass. **2**, 20

MIKAELIAN, I. and P. BAYOL (1991):
Hemoprotozoaires chez les rapaces en rehabilitation.
Point Veterinaire **22**, 857–860

OLSEN, G.H. and S.D. GAUNT (1985):
Effect of hemoprotozoal infections on rehabilitation of wild
raptors.
J. Am. Vet. Med. Ass. **187**, 1204–1205

PAK, S.M. (1975):
Toksoplazmoz dikikh ptits.
Akadem. Nauk **7**, 64–78

PEIRCE, M.A. and J.E. COOPER (1977):
Haematozoa of birds of prey in Great Britain.
Vet. Rec. **100**, 493

PEIRCE, M.A. and J.E. COOPER (1977):
Haematozoa of East African birds. V. Blood parasites of birds
of prey.
East Afric. Wildl. J. **15**, 213–216

PEIRCE, M.A. (1981):
Current knowledge of the haematozoa of raptors.
in: COOPER et al. (1981):
Recent advances in the study of raptor diseases, 15–19
Chiron Publ. Ltd.Keighley, W. Yorkshire, England

PEIRCE, M.A. and M. MARQUISS (1983):
Haematozoa of British birds. VII. Haematozoa of raptors in
Scotland with a description of *Haemoproteus nisi sp. nov.* from
the sparrowhawk (*Accipiter nisus*).
J. Nat. Hist. **17**, 813–821

PEIRCE, M.A., GREENWOOD, A.G. and J.E. COOPER (1983):
Haematozoa of raptors and other birds from Britain, Spain and
the United Arab Emirates.
Avian Pathol. **12**, 443–446

PEIRCE, M.A., BENNETT, G.F. and M. BISHOP (1990):
The haemoproteids of the avian order Falconiformes.
J. Nat. Hist. **24**, 1091–1100

PEPLER, D. and E.E. OETTLÉ (1992):
Trichomonas gallinae in wild raptors on the Cape Peninsula.
South African J. Wildl. Res. **22**, 87–88

REDIG, P.T. (1993):
Avian malaria.
Medical management of birds of prey.
A collection of notes on selected topics. 127–138
Raptor Center, Minnesota

REMPLE, J.D. (1981):
Avian malaria with comments on other haemosporidia in large
falcons.
in: COOPER et al. (1981):
Recent advances in the study of raptor diseases. 107–110
Chiron Pub. Ltd., Keighley, W. Yorkshire, England

ROMMEL, M. and H.E. KRAMPITZ (1978):
Weitere Untersuchungen über das Zwischenwirtsspektrum und
den Entwicklungszyklus von *Frenkelia microti* aus der Erd-
maus.
Zbl. Vet. Med. B **25**, 273–281

ROMMEL, M. (1978):
Vergleichende Darstellung der Entwicklungsbiologie der
Gattungen *Sarcocystis, Frenkelia, Isospora, Cystoisospora,
Hammondia, Toxoplasma* und *Besnoitia.*
Z. Parasitenk. **57**, 269–283

ROMMEL, M. (1981):
Toxoplasma, Sarcocystis- und Frenkeliainfektionen der Klein-
und Heimtiere sowie der Greifvögel.
Prakt. Tierarzt **62**, 52–56

SACCHI, L. and C. PRIGIONI (1984):
Occurrence of *Leucocytozoon* and *Haemoproteus* (Apicom-
plexa, Haemosporina) in Falconiformes and Strigiformes of
Italy.
Ann. Parasitol. Hum. Comp. **59**, 219–226

SCHAFFRATH-BÖER, A. (1983):
Untersuchungen über den endogenen Entwicklungszyklus von
Caryospora kutzeri (Böer, 1982).
Vet. Med. Diss. Hannover

SHARMA, R.K. and H.L. SHAH (1990):
Pariah kite (*Milvus migrans*) as a definitive host of an
unknown *Sarcocystis* species.
Indian J. Anim. Sci. **60**, 804–805

SIMPSON, V.R. (1991):
Leucocytozoon-like infection in parakeets, budgerigars and a
common buzzard.
Vet. Rec. **129**, 30–32

TADROS, W. (1981):
Studies on Sarcosporidia of rodents with birds of prey as
definitive hosts.
in: CANNING, E.U. (1981):
Parasitological topics, 248–259
Soc. Protozool. Inc. Lawrence, Kansas, USA

TAFT, S.J., ROSENFIELD, R.N. and J. BIELEFELDT (1994):
Avian hematozoa of adult and nestling Cooper's hawks
(*Accipiter cooperii*) in Wisconsin.
J. Helminth. Soc. Washington **61**, 146–148

UPTON, S.J. and R.D. MCKOWN (1992):
The red-tailed hawk (*Buteo jamaicensis*), a native definitive
host of *Frenkelia microti* (Apicomplexa) in North America.
J. Wildl. Dis **28**, 85–90

VAL'KYUNAS, G.A. and T.A. EZHOVA (1990):
Infection of sparrow-hawks with haemosporidia (*Sporozoa,
Haemosporidia*) in the West-European and Indo-Asiatic
migration routes.
Parazit. **24**, 113–120

10.2 Helminths

10.2.1 Trematodes (Flukes)

Trematodes, commonly called flukes, are small (0.5–5 mm) elongated parasites that require one or more intermediate hosts to complete their life cycle. Several types of flukes found in birds of prey are listed in Table 10.2.

Table 10.2: Trematodes found in birds of prey

Trematode	Identified hosts
Strigea falconis	Northern goshawk (*Accipiter gentilis*) Common buzzard (*Buteo buteo*) Saker falcon (*Falco cherrug*) Peregrine falcon (*Falco peregrinus*)
Clinostomum complanatum	Bald eagle (*H. leucocephalus*)
Neodisplostomum attenuatum	Common buzzard (*Buteo buteo*)
Opistorchis sp.	Marsh harrier (*Circus aeruginosus*) Hen harrier (*Circus cyaneus*)
Pseudostrigea buteonis	Common buzzard (*Buteo buteo*) Kite (*Milvus korshun*) Osprey (*Pandion haliaetus*)
Cryptocotyle lingua	Bald eagle (*H. leucocephalus*)
Echinostomum goldi	Marsh harrier (*Circus aeruginosus*)
Diplostomum spathaceum	Osprey (*Pandion haliaetus*)

The eggs are excreted in the feces and then develop into miracidia, which in turn infect an intermediate host (usually a snail). There they develop into cercariae and are excreted again, sometimes to develop into metacercariae in another intermediate host (arthropod). The cercariae or metacercariae are ingested by the definitive host, where they develop into flukes, thus completing the life cycle.

The typical thin-walled, operculated eggs are frequently found in fecal samples from birds of prey. One study found that 71% of the saker falcons and 46% of the peregrine falcons in the United Arab Emirates carry this parasite (Greenwood et al., 1984).

In raptors, flukes reside primarily in the small intestine. With severe infections, diarrhea and weakness may be seen. Samedov (1979) described a trematode found in the bile ducts of kites. A bile duct fluke was also reported in American kestrels (*Falco sparverius*) (Shell, 1957). Severe liver pathology led to death in some infected birds.

Fluke eggs are shed intermittently, sometimes requiring several direct smears or fecal flotations for diagnosis. Treatment involves administration of praziquantel (Droncit®) at 10 mg/kg once, with a follow-up dose one week later. Fenbendazole has also been recommended for flukes in birds.

Trematodes are probably rare under normal captive conditions. Certainly reinfection is unlikely, since the intermediate hosts are usually not present in the environment.

10.2.2 Cestodes (Tapeworms)

Tapeworms are very well-adapted to their hosts and only rarely cause clinical disease. Raptors imported from warmer climates are sometimes heavily infected and require treatment for cestodes.

Tapeworm segments may be found in the feces. The eggs will be seen in fecal sediment smears.

Praziquantel (Droncit®) at a one-time dose of 10 mg/kg is effective in eliminating the parasite. Since the required intermediate hosts are absent, reinfection is unlikely in captivity.

Table 10.3 lists some tapeworm species found in birds of prey. Most of these were incidentally identified during postmortem examinations.

10.2.3 Nematodes (Roundworms)

10.2.3.1 Ascarids

Ascarids are among the most common nematode parasites found in wild and, especially, captive birds of prey. Their prevalence in captive hawks can be traced to their direct life cycle, which permits immediate

Table 10.3: Tapeworms identified in selected birds of prey

Tapeworm	Identified hosts
Hymenolepis exilis	Gyrfalcon (*Falco rusticolus*) Laggar falcon (*Falco jugger*)
Plagiorchis elegans	Gyrfalcon (*Falco rusticolus*)
Claotaenia sp.	Many falcon species (*Falconidae*)
Dileptididae	Northern goshawk (*Accipiter gentilis*) Bonelli's eagle (*Hieraetus fasciatus spilogaster*)

reinfection by ingestion of eggs shed in an infected animal's feces or present in the aviary substrate. Ascarid eggs are very resistant to environmental conditions and will persist in the ground for months.

Once inside the host, a larva hatches from the egg and invades the intestinal mucosa. After a period of development, it reenters the intestinal lumen as a small worm, eventually reaching a length of several centimeters as an adult. It takes the ascarid worm about 5 or 6 weeks to achieve sexual maturity and begin putting out eggs of its own. Although the bird is infected, negative fecal samples will be obtained during the prepatent period between infection and the first appearance of eggs.

Clinical disease

Clinical infections with ascarids are primarily a problem in young birds. Heavy infections can result in significant clinical disease. Weight loss and depression are seen, but diarrhea is rare. There are occasional reports of lameness associated with ascarid infections in raptors, purportedly resulting from toxic metabolites produced by the parasite. Very heavy infections can lead to intestinal obstruction by masses of adult worms (Fig. 10.8).

Diagnosis

The round eggs with their thick, rough coat are easily identified in the feces. Goshawks have been known to excrete eggs in their castings as well.

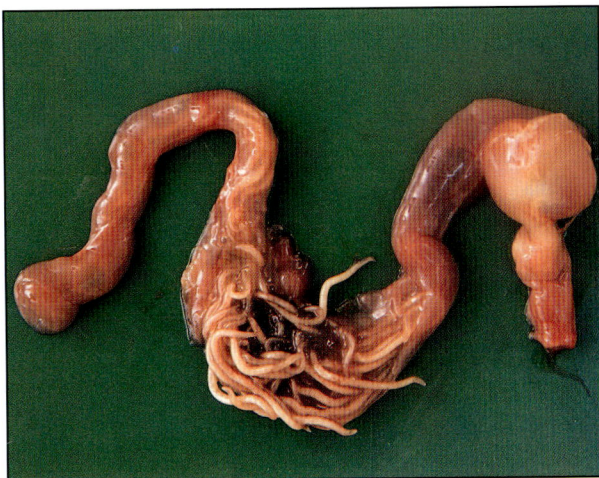

Fig. 10.8: Heavy ascarid infections can lead to complete intestinal obstruction.
(Photo: Heidenreich)

Treatment

Fenbendazole (Panacur®) is safe and effective for the treatment of avian ascarid infections. Table 8.4 (Ch. 8.2.3) gives a range of recommended dosages. Personal experience has shown a dose of 20 mg/kg SID for 7 days to be effective against both ascarids and *Capillaria* (see below), which are known to be more resistant. Very high doses of fenbendazole may lead to impairment of peripheral circulation, causing developing blood feathers to die of ischemia and fall out.

Caution! Vultures do not seem to tolerate fenbendazole well.

Prevention

Reducing the risk of infection is difficult in aviary situations. Ascarid eggs are quite resistant to disinfectants and remain viable in the environment for long periods of time. It takes 14 days for the eggs to become infectious after being excreted. Therefore, concurrent deworming of all birds in an aviary and immediate replacement of the substrate thereafter can be helpful in reducing exposure levels. Hygienic practices discussed for coccidia are valid for these infections as well.

10.2.3.2 *Capillaria*

Capillaria spp. nematodes are also common in birds of prey. Various species of the threadlike, 1 to 5 cm long worms live in the avian host's intestine, esophagus or oropharynx. *Capillaria* can have a direct life cycle, or they may require an intermediate host (see Table 10.4).

After the infectious eggs or the intermediate hosts carrying the *Capillaria* larvae are ingested by a bird, the parasites burrow into the intestinal mucosa. The worms mature into reproductive adults after a prepatent period of 3 to 4 weeks. The eggs can be detected in fecal samples or scrapings and washes from the oral cavity and esophagus.

Table 10. 4: A Selection of common capillarids in birds of prey

Capillarid species	Intermediate host	Organ infected
Eucoleus annulatus	Earthworm	Oropharynx and esophagus
Eucoleus contortus	None (direct life cycle)	Oropharynx and esophagus
Eucoleus dispar	Earthworm	Esophagus
Capillaria falconis	Earthworm	Small intestine

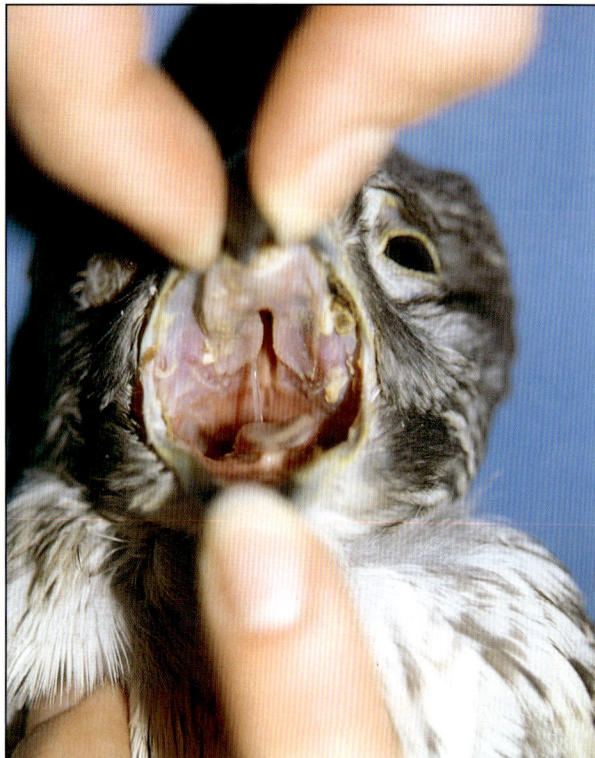

Fig. 10.9: The early stages of a *Capillaria* infection show up as small yellowish plaques on the oral mucosa of this gray gyrfalcon (*F. rusticolus*) and are easily overlooked. (Photo: Heidenreich)

Clinical disease

Three different forms of the disease are recognized. They are based on the location of the infection.

Oropharyngeal Form: Mild infections of this type will produce stringy yellow deposits on the mucosa of the pharynx, around the base of the tongue or at the inner corners of the mouth. These lesions can be wiped away to reveal the mildly inflamed tissues underneath (Fig. 10.9).

In more advanced cases, yellowish-brown, bean-sized granulomas will occur in the affected area (Figs. 10.10 – 10.12). Removal of these lesions is more difficult and results in heavy bleeding. Secondary infections of the damaged mucosal tissue can lead to localized abscesses. Occasionally, such infections spread to the mandibular bones as well.

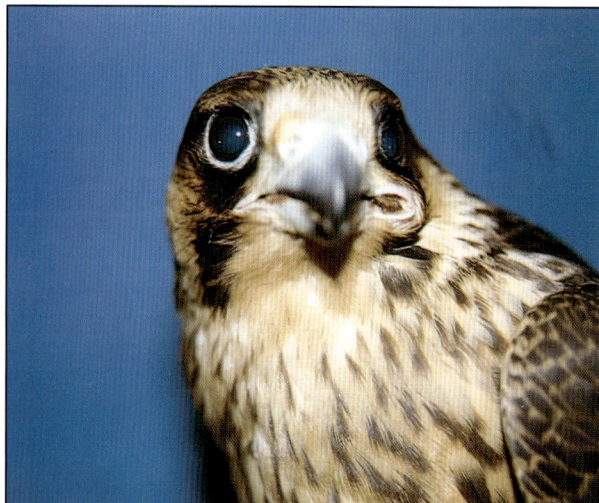

10.10

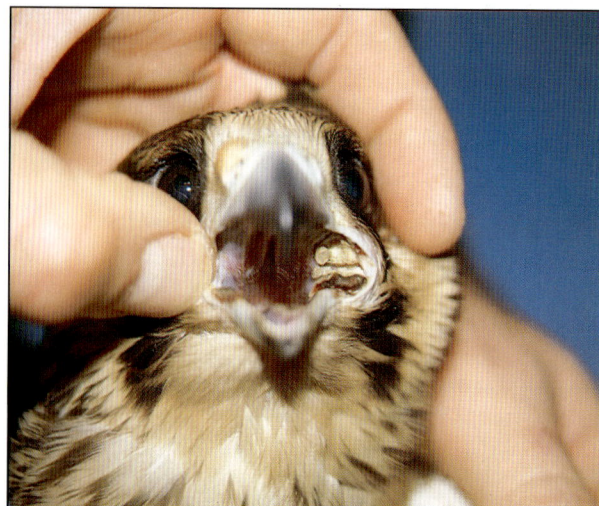

10.11

Figs. 10.10, 10.11 and 10.12: A young male peregrine falcon (*F. peregrinus*) presented with a peanut-sized lesion in the left commissure of the mouth (10.10). The affected mucosa was covered with thick yellowish-brown plaques (10.11). Large quantities of Capillaria eggs were seen in samples obtained from the lesion. Five days of treatment with fenbendazole resulted in resolution of the infection. Within three weeks, the falcon had regained a normal appearance (10.12). (Photo: Heidenreich)

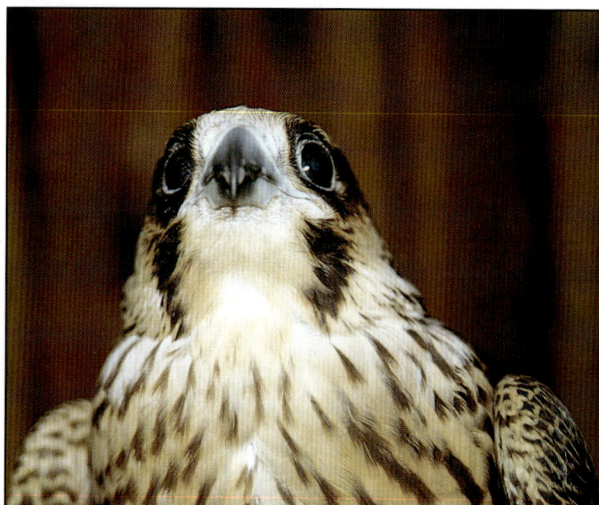

10.12

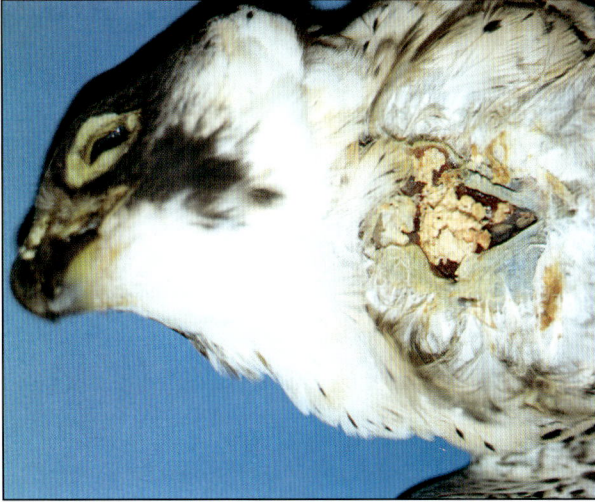

Fig. 10.13: This female peregrine falcon (*F. peregrinus*) died from the effects of esophageal rupture caused by a *Capillaria*-related abscess. If such cases are identified early enough, death can be prevented by appropriate medical therapy and, if necessary, surgical intervention to treat the abscess.
(Photo: Heidenreich)

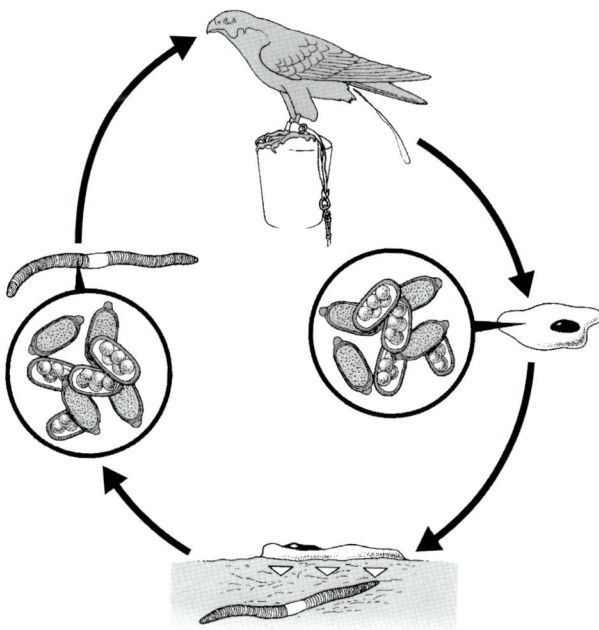

Fig. 10.14: A representative parasitic life cycle involving earthworms as transport hosts. Further development of the parasite does not occur in the earthworm.
(Illustration: R. Gattung-Petith and A. Gattung)

Esophageal Form: Infections of the esophagus are more difficult to detect, especially when they occur in the absence of visible oral lesions. A thickening of the esophagus may be palpable in some cases. Nevertheless, esophageal *Capillaria* infections are often detected late in the course of disease, usually after the lesions have progressed to the point where they rupture through the skin of the neck, revealing accumulations of malodorous caseous exudate (Fig. 10.13).

Intestinal Form: Some species of *Capillaria* can infect the small intestine of raptors, resulting in inflammatory changes and destruction of the mucosa. Initial clinical signs may be mild and limited to diarrhea. Hunting falcons may perform poorly when flown. They will appear to fly unevenly and have difficulty balancing during landing or while flying to the lure. In extreme cases, the bird will be unable to fly. It is likely that these signs stem from CNS disturbances secondary to vitamin B deficiency.

Diagnosis

The presence of *Capillaria* is easily identified by microscopic examination of fecal samples, mucosal scrapings from suspect lesions or esophageal flushes. Capillaria eggs are oval and have characteristic bipolar plugs, making them easy to identify.

Treatment

The reader is referred to Chapter 8.2.3 for a list of anthelmintic drugs. Abscessed or perforated esophageal lesions will also require surgical debridement and antibacterial therapy (see Ch. 13.8.2).

Prevention

Earthworms can play a major role in the transmission of *Capillaria* to birds of prey (Fig. 10.14). Measures to prevent exposure to soil and uptake of worms should be instituted as described for *Caryospora* coccidiosis (Fig. 10.7).

Hunting hawks appear to be capable of becoming infected with *Capillaria* by ingestion of infected prey, particularly gulls and crows. The bird will begin passing parasite eggs approximately four weeks after consuming the infected prey. These are definitely not eggs ingested with the animal and then incidentally passed in the feces. Most hunting hawks do not consume the intestinal tract of their prey, and any eggs taken up in this way are not yet infectious anyway. The mode of transmission in these cases remains uncertain. Maybe some embryonated eggs are present on the cloacal feathers of the infected bird and are then ingested by the hawk during plucking. Another possibility is that infectious eggs present in the mucosa of the upper digestive tract are ingested with the head of the animal. Clausen and Gudmundson (1981) made observations

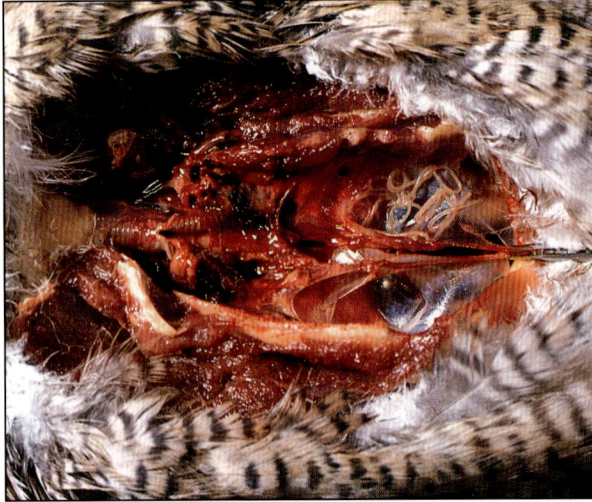

Fig. 10.15: This female peregrine falcon (*F. peregrinus*) was imported from the Middle East and succumbed to avian tuberculosis. A tangled mass of filariid worms (*Serratospiculum* sp.) was found incidentally in the right abdominal air sac during postmortem examination. (Photo: Heidenreich)

to this effect in Icelandic gyrfalcons, which apparently became infected by ingesting wild ptarmigan.

Regular fecal examinations in hunting hawks will permit timely identification of *Capillaria* infections so that treatment can be instituted before clinical signs occur.

10.2.3.3 Filariid nematodes

Various species of worms belonging to the family Filariidae can occur in falcons from tropical climates and in Accipiters. Many of the wild-caught birds used for falconry in Arab countries carry these parasites. *Diplotriaena falconis* and *Serratospiculum* spp., both parasites of the respiratory system, are most commonly identified.

Filarial worms are long, threadlike organisms that can be found bunched up like spaghetti inside the falcon's air sacs (Fig. 10.15), often partially attached to the serosal membranes. The thin-shelled, embryonated ova are coughed out of the trachea, then swallowed and excreted in the feces. Insects, particularly beetles or grasshoppers, may consume the eggs with the fecal material and then act as vectors or intermediate hosts for the filarial parasites (Fig. 10.16).

Clinical disease

These worms appear to be relatively apathogenic. Respiratory signs or vomiting are only rarely seen. The parasites are most often discovered by chance during necropsies of birds that succumbed to other diseases.

The ova can also be found in feces and saliva. Death may occur from this infection in situations of extreme stress or in very heavily infected animals (Kocan and Gordon, 1976).

Treatment

Filariid nematodes are difficult to treat successfully. Their location within the poorly-perfused air sac membranes makes them relatively immune to medical therapy. Another consideration is that the dead worms will remain in the respiratory system and could cause problems as they decay.

For these reasons, it is recommended that these parasites be endoscopically removed. Postoperative treatment with 10 mg fenbendazole into the air sac and 25 mg/kg fenbendazole PO SID for three days should result in a complete cure.

Prevention

Most wild-caught falcons acquired in the fall in Arab countries already carry filarial parasites. Reinfection is unlikely to occur under local conditions. In temperate zones, only birds imported from warmer climates are

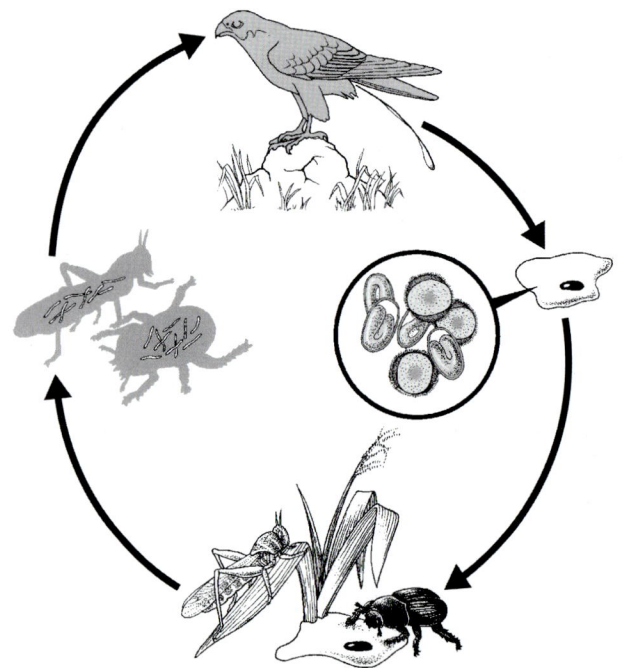

Fig. 10.16: A representative parasitic life cycle requiring intermediate hosts for development of certain life stages. In the case of *Serratospiculum*, beetles and grasshoppers are presumed to act as intermediate hosts for the development of microfilariae.
(Illustration: R. Gattung-Petith and A. Gattung)

likely to be infected. In these cases also, reinfection or transmission of the parasite to other birds is highly unlikely since the intermediate hosts are not available.

10.2.3.4 *Syngamus*

Many wild birds, including pheasants, grouse, thrushes, crows and magpies, as well as birds of prey, can be infected with the bright red nematode *Syngamus trachea*. The adult worms live in the host bird's trachea, interfering with respiration if they become numerous enough. The typical gasping for air seen in affected birds has given *Syngamus* the popular name "gapeworm".

There is a marked sexual dimorphism in this species. The female can be up to 20 mm long, while the male is typically only 6 mm in length. The pair is permanently joined in copulation, giving them a Y-shaped appearance together.

Although this parasite has a direct life cycle and does not require an intermediate host, they are often transmitted by ingestion of transport hosts such as earthworms and snails. These invertebrates do not support further development of the parasite, but they can concentrate relatively large numbers of infectious larvae within themselves. These larvae sometimes encapsulate and remain infectious for long periods of time inside the earthworm or snail.

When a bird ingests these transport hosts or the embryonated ova directly, the larvae hatch and migrate to the liver and then to the lung. The large females attach themselves to the tracheal mucosa, often producing a strong inflammatory response accompanied by significant mucus production. The eggs are coughed up with the mucus and swallowed, to be excreted with the feces.

Clinical disease
Affected birds present with raspy sounds of upper airway obstruction even in cases of mild or recent infection. Unlike with aspergillosis, there is no abdominal breathing. Frequent sneezing and head shaking may be observed as the hawk tries to rid itself of the irritating parasites. Heavier infections result in open-mouthed breathing and dyspnea. These bloodsucking worms can also cause anemia, further weakening the bird. Death can occur due to asphyxiation.

Diagnosis
Syngamus trachea can frequently be seen in the upper airways with the naked eye. The glottis is usually wide open as the bird gasps for air, allowing easy visual access to the tracheal lumen. Endoscopic examination may also be helpful in visualizing the parasites. After a prepatent period of about 3 weeks, the thick-walled oval eggs with the small bipolar plugs are easily identified in the feces.

Treatment
This worm consumes the blood of its host, making systemic antiparasitic therapy easy and effective. A variety of anthelmintics can be used (see Table 8.4 in Ch. 8.2.3).

Prevention
Uptake of the transport hosts should be prevented. If an aviary is being converted for use with raptors, care should be taken that it was not previously inhabited by poultry or other commonly infected birds that could have contaminated the substrate with *Syngamus* ova.

10.2.3.5 *Trichinella*

Trichinella spp. are parasites of some importance in pigs and certain wild animals. They are of concern for their zoonotic potential as well. The older literature suggests that trichinosis does not occur in birds of prey thanks to their rapid gastrointestinal transit time. These studies examined only *Trichinella spiralis*, found most commonly in pigs.

Trichinella pseudospiralis is a species first described in 1972. Research has shown this nematode to be a parasite of some significance in raptors, both through natural infection and experimentally (see Table 10.5).

Raptors acquire the infection by ingesting prey animals carrying encysted *T. pseudospiralis* larvae in their muscle tissue. The larvae are released from the cyst during digestion and quickly penetrate the small intestinal mucosa. Within a few days, they develop into sexually mature adults and spend approximately three weeks producing new larval offspring before dying. These new young larvae enter the portal circulation

Table 10.5: Reports of *Trichinella pseudospiralis* in birds of prey

Identified host	Author
Marsh harrier (*Circus aeruginosus*)	OBENDORF and CLARKE (1992)
American kestrel (*Falco sparverius*)	SAUMIER et al. (1988) MEEROVITCH and CHADEE (1982)
Common buzzard (*Buteo buteo*)	CALERO et al. (1978)
Cooper's hawk (*Accipiter cooperi*)	WHEELDON (1984) TITCHIE (1985)

and lymphatic system, traveling to striated muscle tissues, where they become encysted and remain viable for years.

Clinical disease

Experimental infections in American kestrels (*Falco sparverius*) resulted in a noticeable reduction in flight activity between days 5 and 35 after infection. This corresponds to the period in which the larvae migrate and become encapsulated within the muscle tissue. Oral infection with 1000 larvae per bird resulted in death for all affected falcons. Up to 89 larvae per gram of muscle were found in these animals on the 40th day after infection.

Trichinosis also had a negative effect on reproduction in these kestrels. Infected females laid fewer eggs, while the eggs themselves had higher rates of breakage (29%) and embryo mortality (40%) when compared with uninfected controls. Overall reproductive success rate was 1/3 less than in uninfected falcons (SAUMIER et al., 1986, 1988).

A wild Cooper's hawk (*Accipiter cooperi*) was found unable to walk or fly. It survived for five months before being euthanatized. Large numbers of *Trichinella* larvae were found in the pectoral and leg muscles.

Diagnosis

Since the female worm produces live larvae that immediately invade the host and are rarely excreted, a fecal examination is not diagnostic for trichinosis. Encapsulated larvae may be found in the muscle tissue during postmortem examination. The cysts do not mineralize in birds, making radiographic diagnosis also not feasible.

Treatment and prevention

Freezing of food animals may kill the larvae encysted in muscle tissue. The administration of corticosteroids can help reduce inflammation during the period of larval migration and encystment. Once the larvae have encysted, there is no known treatment.

10.2.3.6 *Cyathostoma*

Simpson and Harris (1992) found nematode parasites identified as *Cyathostoma lari* in the lower eyelid and around the eye of wild common kestrels (*Falco tinnunculus*), a common buzzard (*Buteo buteo*) and a European sparrowhawk (*Accipiter nisus*). They appeared to produce no tissue reaction or pathologic changes in their conjunctival location. One worm in the eyelid itself caused some local tissue necrosis. Surgical removal probably suffices for the treatment of this nematode in raptors.

10.3 Acanthocephalans

These "thorny-headed" worms are several centimeters long and have a proboscis armed with a hook for attaching to the intestinal mucosa. Several different species have been described in birds of prey (see Table 10.6). Disease has only rarely been reported in association with this infection.

Kasimov and Samedov (1975) found an infection rate of almost 20% among Eastern European raptors.

All acanthocephalans require an insect intermediate host to complete their life cycle. Heavy infections can lead to diarrhea and weight loss. The parasite's eggs contain a small larva complete with hooked proboscis and can be identified in a fecal sediment sample. A specific therapeutic regimen for infected raptors has not been established. Other avian species have been treated with fenbendazole at a dose of 20 mg/kg SID for 5 days or 40 mg/kg TID for 3 days.

Table 10.6: Acanthocephalans identified in various birds of prey

Identified host	Acanthocephalan
Lesser kestrel (*Falco naumanni*)	*Centrorhynchus buteonis* *Centrorhynchus spinosus* *Mediorhynchus papillosus* *Mediorhynchus micracanthus*
Common kestrel (*Falco tinnunculus*)	*Centrorhynchus cylindraceus*
European sparrowhawk (*Accipiter nisus*)	*Centrorhynchus cylindraceus*
Peregrine falcon (*Falco peregrinus*)	*Centrorhynchus globocaudatus*
Osprey (*Pandion haliaetus*)	*Centrorhynchus milvus*
Tawny (Stepe) eagle (*Aquila rapax*)	*Centrorhynchus itatsinis*
Milan (*Milvus korshun*)	*Mediorhynchus micracanthus* *Centrorhynchus erraticus*
Marsh harrier (*Circus aeruginosus*) Hen harrier (*Circus cyaneus*)	*Centrorhynchus teres* *Centrorhynchus amphibius*

References and literature of further interest

BRGLEZ, J. (1982):
Nematodes of suborder Filariata Skrjabin, 1915, in falconiform and passeriform birds in Yugoslavia – incidence and
pathogenicity.
Int. Symp. Erkr. Zootiere **24**, 341–345

CALERO, R., BECERRA, C., MARTINEZ, F. and S. HERNANDEZ
(1978):
Epidemiologia de la triquinelosis en la provincia de Cordoba.
Rev. Iberica Parasitol. **38**, 239–248

CLAUSEN, B. and F. GUDMUNDSSON (1981):
Causes of mortality among free-ranging gyrfalcons in Iceland.
J. Wildl. Dis. **17**, 105–109

DEDRICK, M.L. (1965):
Notes on a strigeid trematode – an intestinal parasite of a
prairie falcon.
J. North. Am. Falcon. Ass. **4**, 12–14

FREY, H. and E. KUTZER (1982):
Zur Diagnostik heimischer Greifvogel- und Eulenparasiten.
Prakt. Tierarzt **3**, 894–902

GREENWOOD, A.G., FURLEY, C.W. and J.E. COOPER (1984):
Intestinal trematodiasis in falcons (order Falconiformes).
Vet. Rec. **114**, 477–478

HALLIWELL, W.H. (1979):
Diseases of birds of prey.
Small Anim. Pract. **9**, 541–568

HOPPE, R. (1975):
Haarwürmer bedrohen isländische Gerfalken.
Falke **22**, 209, 212

IMAI, S., IKEDA, S.I., ISHII, T. and K. UEMATSU (1989):
Diplotriaena falconis (Connal, 1912) (Filariidae, Nematoda)
from a red-legged falconet, *Microhierax caerulescens*.
Japan. J. Vet. Sci. **51**, 209–212

KASIMOV, G.S. and G.A. SAMEDOV (1975):
The acanthocephalan fauna of diurnal birds of prey in
Azerbaidzhan.
Akad. Nauk Gel'mintol. 56–59

KOCAN, A.A. and L.R. GORDON (1976):
Fatal air sac infection with *Serratospiculum amaculata* in a
prairie falcon.
J. Am. Vet. Med. Ass. **169**, 908

KOCAN, A.A., SNELLING, J. and E.C. GREINER (1977):
Some infectious and parasitic diseases in Oklahoma
raptors.
J. Wildl. Dis. **13**, 304–306

KOTREMBA, J. (1978):
Beitrag zur Helminthen- und Acanthocephalenfauna
heimischer Greifvögel.
Vet. Med. Diss. Wien

KUTZER, E., FREY, H. and J. KOTREMBA (1980):
Zur Parasitenfauna österreichischer Greifvogel
(Falconiformes).
Angew. Parasitol. **21**, 183–205

LAWRENCE, K. (1983):
Efficacy of fenbendazole against nematodes of captive birds.
Vet. Rec. **112**, 433–434

MEEROVITCH, E. and K. CHADEE (1982):
Experimental infection of American kestrels, *Falco sparverius*,
with *Trichinella pseudospiralis* (Garkavi, 1972) and *T. spiralis*.
Can. J. Zool. **60**, 3150–3152

NIE, G.J.-VAN (1974):
Capillaria in keel en krop van wilde buizerden.
Tijdschr. Diergeneesk. **99**, 494

OBENDORF, D.L. and K.P. CLARKE (1992):
Trichinella pseudospiralis infections in free-living Tasmanian
birds.
J. Helminth. Soc. Wash. **59**, 144–147

OKULEWICZ, A. (1988):
Fauna nicieni ptakow drapieznych i sow (Falconiformes i
Strigiformes) Dolnego Slaska.
Wiadom. Parazyt. **34**, 137–149

RAMISZ, A. and J. SKOTNICKI (1981):
Behandlung des Capillaria-Befalles bei Zoovögeln mit
Fenbendazol.
Int. Symp. Erkr. Zootiere **23**, 237–241

RATHORE, G.S. and H.S. NAMA (1985):
Helminth parasites of birds of the arid zone.
Sci. Rev. Arid Zone Res. **3**, 129–148

SAMEDOV, G.A. (1967):
Acanthocephalans and nematodes in birds of prey in the
Lenkoran region of Azerbaidzhan.
Biol. Nauki **2**, 44–50

SAMEDOV, G.A. (1979):
Trematodes and acanthocephalans of birds of prey in
Azerbaidzhan.
Biol. Nauki **1**, 60–63

SANTIAGO, C., MILLS, P.A. and C.E. KIRKPATRICK (1985):
Oral capillariasis in a red-tailed hawk: treatment with
fenbendazole.
J. Am. Vet. Med. Ass. **187**, 1205–1206

SAUMIER, M.D., RAU, M.E. and D.M. BIRD (1986):
The effect of *Trichinella pseudospiralis* infection on the
reproductive success of captive American kestrels
(*Falco sparverius*).
Can. J. Zool. **64**, 2123–2125

SAUMIER, M.D., RAU M.E. and D.M. BIRD (1988):
The influence of *Trichinella pseudospiralis* infection on the
behaviour of captive, nonbreeding American kestrels
(*Falco sparverius*).
Can. J. Zool. **66**, 1685–1692

SCHELL, S. C. (1957):
Dicrocoeliidae from birds in the Pacific Northwest.
Trans Am. Microsc. Soc. **76**, 184

SCHELLNER, H.P. and S. RODLER (1971):
Ein Trematoden- und Kokzidienbefall bei einem Luggerfalken (*Falco jugger*).
Jb. Dtsch. Falkenorden 90–93

SCHÜTZE, H.R. and D. ZASTROW (1974):
Zur Diagnose der Filarien bei Großfalken.
Dtsch. Tierärztl. Wschr. **81**, 313

SHAIKENOV, B. (1980):
Spontaneous infection of birds with *Trichinella pseudospiralis* (Garkavi, 1972).
Fol. Parasitol. **27**, 227–230

SIMPSON, V.R. and E.A. HARRIS (1992):
Cyathostoma lari (Nematoda) infection in birds of prey.
J. Zool. **227**, 655–659

SMITH, S.A. (1993)
Diagnosis and treatment of helminths in birds of prey.
in: REDIG P.T. et al. (1993):
Raptor Biomedicine, Chiron Pub. Ltd. Keighley, West Yorkshire, England

STEHLE, S. (1977):
Behandlung von Helminthosen bei Greifvögeln (Falconiformes) mit Fenbendazol (Panacur).
Kleintierpraxis **22**, 261–266

STERNER, M.C. and R.H. ESPINOSA (1988):
Serratospiculoides amaculata in a Cooper's hawk (*Accipiter cooperii*).
J. Wildl. Dis. **24**, 378–379

TITCHE, A.R. (1985):
Host responses to experimental trichinellosis in raptors and quail.
Diss. Abstracts Int. B, **46**, 432

WARD, F.P. and D.G. FAIRCHILD (1972):
Air sac parasites of the genus *Serratospiculum* in falcons.
J. Wildl. Dis. **8**, 165–168

WHEELDON, E.B., DICK, T.A. and T.A. SCHULZ (1983):
First report of *Trichinella spiralis* var. *pseudospiralis* in North America.
J. Parasitol. **69**, 781–782

WHEELDON, E.B. (1984):
Trichinellosis in a Cooper's hawk.
J. Am. Vet. Med. Ass. **181**, 1385–1386

10.4   Arthropods

The phylum Arthropoda is incredibly diverse, encompassing more than $^2/_3$ of all living animal species. Representatives from this group can be found in all possible environments, filling many different niches. It is therefore not surprising that a large variety of arthropods are associated with birds of prey, primarily as parasites. Describing them all is beyond the scope of this book. The following discussion limits itself to clinically important arthropod parasites of raptors.

Ticks and mites (subclass Acarina) are the most important members of the class Arachnida to be discussed, while lice, hippoboscid flies, blow flies and feather flies are the representatives of the class Insecta.

10.4.1   Arachnids

10.4.1.1 Ticks (*Argas* sp., *Ixodes* sp.)

Two families, the soft ticks (Argasidae) and the hard ticks (Ixodidae) are widespread among raptors. The Argasidae are more common in warmer climates. Both will periodically attach themselves to the unfeathered portions of the skin, eyelids and cere of raptors to suck blood. Ticks are particularly significant as vectors of bloodborne pathogens (for example *Aegyptianella* and *Babesia*). Their presence causes problems only in cases of very heavy infestation. Nestlings are sometimes so heavily parasitized that they succumb to blood loss. Mechanical removal of ticks usually suffices as treatment of affected birds. If large numbers of the very small nymphs are present, topical application of oil to the ticks will cause them to die and fall off.

10.4.1.2 Fowl mites and red mites (*Ornithonyssus* spp., *Dermanyssus* spp.)

The northern fowl mite (*Ornithonyssus sylvarium*) is a common parasite of many avian species, especially wild birds and poultry. The mite spends its brief life on the host, sucking blood and reproducing among the feathers and skin. It is rare in young birds. In adults, the mites can often be found along the edges of small contour feathers.

The red mite (*Dermanyssus gallinae*) differs from the northern fowl mite in being a temporary parasite on the bird, leaving its hiding places among the small cracks and crevices in the environment to feed on the bird's blood only at night. This makes it difficult to recognize an infestation by this parasite. Anemic nestlings are often the first sign of a *D. gallinae* problem.

Mite infestations are controlled by spraying or dusting with pyrethrin products (Permethrin, Flumethrin). Northern fowl mites are treated directly on the bird, while *Dermanyssus* requires thorough treatment of the aviary environment as well.

10.4.1.3 Quill mites (*Harpyrhynchus* spp.)

Quill mites can be a significant parasite in some species of birds. These tiny animals live within the shaft of a mature or developing feather. The damage they do to the pulp of a blood feather can result in its death midway in development. An hourglass-like constriction will appear in the shaft and the feather will break at that point. Once the remaining portion of the feather dries up, the mites leave and find a new blood feather to feed on.

This type of feather damage can result in the loss of all flight and tail feathers. It has been observed in buteos, golden eagles and sea eagle, both in captivity and in the wild.

There is currently no known treatment for quill mites. The parasites are well-protected from topical insecticides by their location inside the feather shaft. Those feeding on blood feathers may be vulnerable to systemically administered ivermectin (Ivomec®). Cau-

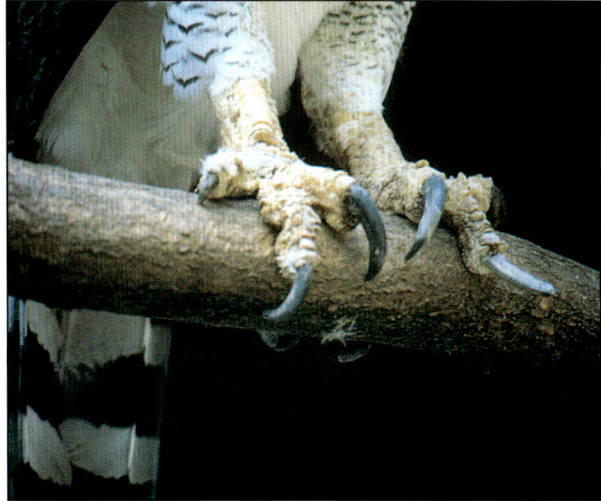

Fig. 10.18: The legs and feet of this harpy eagle (*Harpia harpyja*) resemble those of chickens affected by *Knemidocoptes* mange mites. Although a mite was not identified in this case, the lesions resolved after several washings and topical treatment with mineral oil, making epidermoptid mites the likely cause.
(Photo: Heidenreich)

tion should be exercised with the use of this drug, as its safety and efficacy have not been established in many raptor species.

10.4.1.4 Epidermoptid mites (*Knemidocoptes* spp.)

Epidermoptid mites inhabit the external layers of the skin, usually limiting themselves to the unfeathered areas of the body. *Knemidocoptes mutans* affects poultry and *Knemidocoptes pilae* is well-known in budgerigars as the scaly leg and face mite.

The lesions these parasites produce are typically quite visible and include grayish crusty, hyperkeratotic or spongy proliferations of the eyelids, cere and legs. Closer inspection will reveal the tiny tunnels dug by the mites that give these lesions their porous appearance.

Epidermoptid mites have only rarely been reported in birds of prey. The cases described below (Figs. 10.17 and 10.18) represent, to the author's knowledge, only the second report of these mites in raptors. Bougerol described this disease first in 1967.

Knemidocoptes mites are often found in the cere and around the base of the beak. This can adversely affect growth and development of the beak, leading to deformities. Ivermectin (Ivomec®) has been used successfully in budgerigars at a dose of 0.2 mg/kg once, with a follow-up treatment 14 days later. Alternatives in-

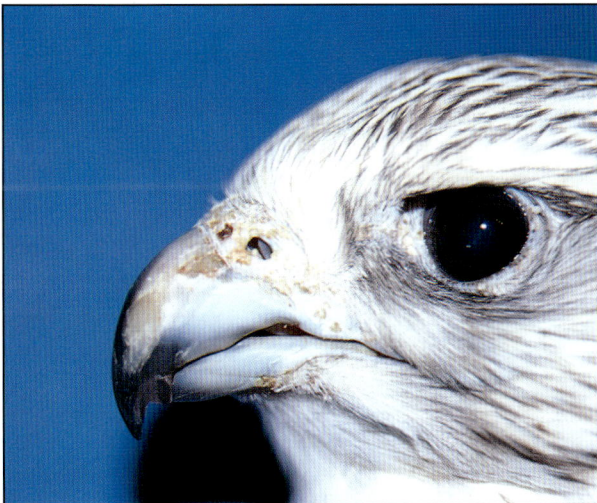

Fig. 10.17: This falcon hybrid (saker falcon X gyrfalcon) developed crusty lesions involving the base of the beak, the upper beak and the cere over a period of several weeks. A skin scraping revealed a knemidocoptic mite. Since this was the only area affected, the bird was treated topically with mineral oil applied once a week for three weeks to the affected area. Although the cere returned to normal within a few weeks, the pitted defects of the upper beak took several months to grow out.
(Photo: Heidenreich)

clude topical treatment of affected areas with mineral oil or several applications of Odylen® (Bayer) diluted 1:10.

10.4.2   Insects

10.4.2.1 Feather lice (*Mallophaga*)

The order Mallophaga includes two families of importance to birds, the Ischnocera, which subsist exclusively on dead feather material and flakes of skin, and the Amblycera, which also consume the blood of their host.

Feather lice are highly specialized parasites that irritate birds and make them restless without seriously affecting their health. They live on the feather surface (Fig 10.19), sometimes consuming large portions thereof. Very heavy infestations may cause enough damage to impair a bird's ability to fly (Fig. 10.20).

Feather lice are easily found by examining the undersides of feathers. Hooded falcons standing quietly in a warm room may have these parasites crawling around on their hood. Drops in body temperature associated with anesthesia or death will force feather lice to flock to the surface in large numbers (Fig. 10.21).

Treatment is easily accomplished with topical application of pyrethroid sprays or powders twice at an interval of 10 days.

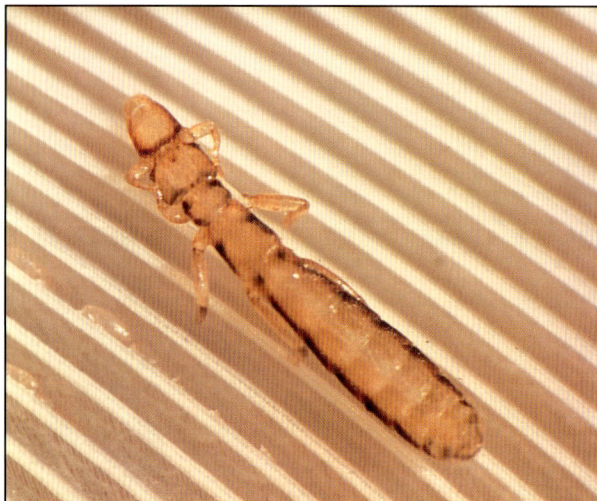

10.19

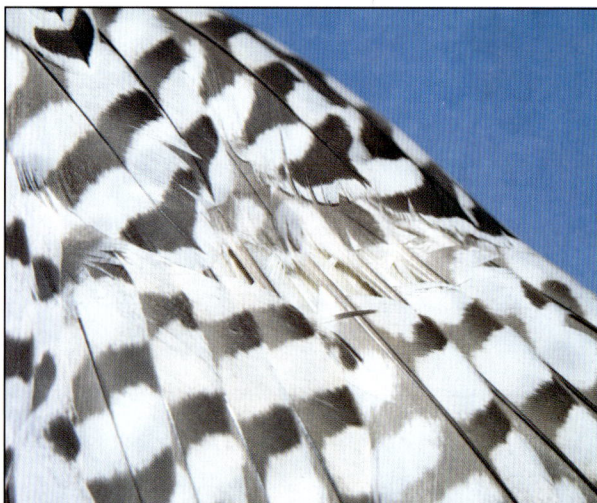

10.20

Fig. 10.19: Avian lice can vary considerably in shape and size. This enlargement shows a louse from a common kestrel (*F. tinnunculus*).
(Photo: Heidenreich)

Fig. 10.20: Since feather lice prefer to hide underneath the feathers of their avian host, they commonly restrict their feeding to the base of the large flight feathers, as seen in the damage done to the remiges of this gyrfalcon (*F. rusticolus*).
(Photo: Heidenreich)

Fig. 10.21: If the host's body temperature drops [in this case, a saker falcon (*F. cherrug*)], or the bird is placed in a warm, dark place, previously unnoticed feather lice will suddenly come to the surface in large numbers.
(Photo: Heidenreich)

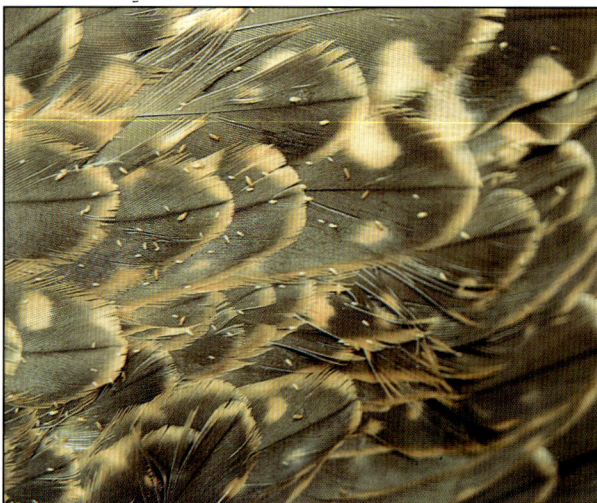

10.21

10.4.2.2 Louse flies (*Hippoboscidae*)

Hippoboscid or louse flies are found on all birds of prey, although infestations as heavy as those seen in swallows and swifts are rare. Swallow nestlings sometimes die of the blood loss incurred with this type of parasitism. Louse flies are similar in size to houseflies, often green in color, and have an oval, flattened abdomen. They are able to move with great agility and speed both in the air and among the feathers in which they normally hide.

Hippoboscid flies are so good at hiding among the bird's plumage that they are easily overlooked. Their shiny dark brown pupae are the size of a pinhead and can occasionally be found under a hawk's perch. They act as vectors for a variety of pathogens and should be eliminated with pyrethroid dusts or sprays.

10.4.2.3 Feather flies (*Carnus* spp.)

Carnus hemapterus is a parasitic fly that has been a problem in raptor nestlings, primarily among falcon chicks, since the earliest days of captive breeding. Feather flies are not host-specific, having been reported in various other avian species (Walter and Hudde, 1987). They are very common in starling nestlings, for example. The author has seen these flies leave the nest area and fly away to seek new hosts once the young starlings lose their down feathers and acquire adult plumage. On their new nestling host, they lose their wings and, in the case of falcons, aggregate on folds of skin underneath the wings and inside the thigh. This parasite is found only on downy chicks and occurs primarily in the months between May and July.

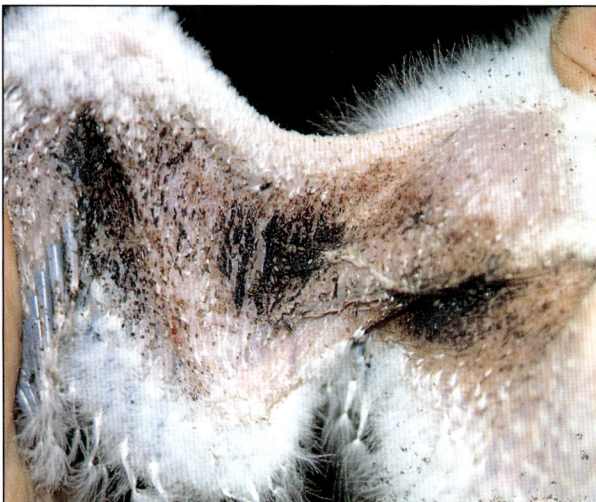

Fig. 10.22: Feather flies affect only downy nestlings.
(Photo: Heidenreich)

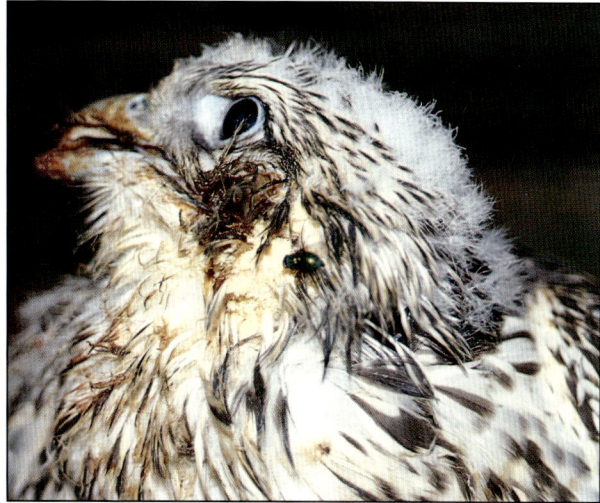

Fig. 10.23: This white gyrfalcon (*F. rusticolus*) nestling suffered from metabolic bone disease (rickets). It developed a beak deformity that made it difficult for the bird to eat or preen. Blow flies were able to lay great masses of eggs among the contaminated feathers underneath the falcon's eye. This bird was euthanatized.
(Photo: Heidenreich)

There are various opinions regarding the pathogenicity of *C. hemapterus*. On the one hand, the flies may be bloodsucking, a suspicion based on the brownish-red excretions found on affected areas of skin (Fig. 10.22). Affected nestlings occasionally even die. On the other hand, Liebisch (1995) suggests that these flies are incapable of feeding this way, possessing a feeding apparatus that appears to resemble the sucking mouth parts of a housefly more than the biting or piercing ones of bloodsucking insects.

In any case, it is advisable to check the skin of downy nestlings regularly so that treatment can take place early in cases of *C. hemapterus* infestation. Topical pyrethroid sprays or powders are immediately effective. Treatment may need to be repeated at later times if indicated.

10.4.2.4 Blow flies (*Calliphoridae*)

Blow flies are not generally parasitic, normally laying their eggs or larvae on carrion. They can also do so on open, contaminated wounds of animals, causing damage as their larvae proceed to invade and consume the surrounding tissue (myiasis) (Fig. 10.23).

Myiasis is a problem in nestlings or in injured adults unable to clean themselves. Young birds with diarrhea often contaminate the vent feathers with fecal material. Blow flies are attracted by the odor of decay and lay their eggs in the area. The larvae that hatch proceed to invade the pericloacal tissues, sometimes progressing from there into the abdomen and literally eating the poor bird from the inside out.

Open wounds contaminated with blow fly eggs or larvae should be immediately cleaned by manual re-moval of the maggots and rinsing with a surgical dis-infectant. In many cases, the tissue damage is so severe that euthanasia is the only humane option. The presence of flies or their larvae on a bird often indicate the animal's impending death.

References and literature of further interest

BOUGEROL, C. (1967)
in: COOPER, J.E. (1978):
Veterinary aspects of captive birds of prey.
Standfast Press, Saul, Gloustershire, England

BÜTTIKER, W. (1975):
Die Gefiederfliege (*Carnus hemapterus* Nitzsch) in der Schweiz.
Schw. Entomol. Ges. **48**, 3–4

COOPER, J.E. and N.A. FORBES (1986):
Studies on morbidity and mortality in the merlin (*Falco columbarius*).
Vet. Rec. **118**, 232–235

JUREK, V. (1988):
Über Erfahrungen mit Ivomec bei Zoovögeln.
Int. Symp. Erkrank. Zootiere **30**, 343–347

LIEBISCH (1995):
personal communication

MARTIN-MATEO, M.P. and G. MANILLA (1988):
Nuevos malofagos de aves en Italia.
Rivista Parasitol. **5**, 141–150

PEREZ-JIMENEZ, J.M. (1988):
Mallophaga of *Buteo b. buteo* in southern Spain.
Angew. Parasitol. **29**, 189–200

RÖDDER, A. (1985):
Stoßmauser bei einem Bussard-Nestling?
Jb. Dtsch. Falkenorden 47

SCHULZ, T.A. (1990):
New and unusual ectoparasites on raptors.
in: LUDWIG, D. R. (1990):
Wildlife rehabilitation. **8**. Sartell, Minnesota, USA 205–213

SMITH, S.A. and B.J. SMITH (1988):
Lice in birds of prey.
Comp. Anim. Prac. **2**, 35–37

TENDEIRO, J. (1988):
Etudes sur les Colpocephalum (Mallophaga, Menoponidae) parasites des Falconiformes. III – Invalidation du Colpoce-phalum mutabile Tendeiro et al., 1979.
Garcia-de-Orta.-Serie-de-Zoologia. **15**, 153–162

TENDEIRO, J. (1988):
Observations sur deux Kurodaia (Mallophaga, Menoponidae), parasites des Falconiformes, avec description d'une nouvelle espece, au Bresil.
Garcia-de-Orta.-Serie-de-Zoologia. **15**, 163–169

TENDEIRO, J. (1988):
Presence du Falcoliperus quadripustulatus (Burmeister) (Mallophaga, Ischnocera) a l'Afghanistan.
Garcia-de-Orta.-Serie-de-Zoologia. **15**, 171–174

TROMMER, G. (1994):
Die eigenartigen Falkenlausfliegen gehören in Wirklichkeit zu den Gefiederfliegen.
Greifvögel u. Falknerei 1993
Verlag Neumann-Neudamm 60–61

WALTER, G. and H. HUDDE (1987):
Die Gefiederfliege, *Carnus hemapterus* (Milichiidae, Diptera), ein Ektoparasit der Nestlinge.
J. Ornithol. **128**, 251–255

WARD, F.P. (1975):
A clinical evaluation of parasites of birds of prey.
J. Zoo Anim. Med. **6**, 3–8

WILKINSON, P.R., FYFE, R. and J.E.H. MARTIN (1980):
Further records of Ornithodoros ticks on prairie falcons and in bat-inhabited buildings in Canada.
Can. Field Nat. **94**, 191–193

ZIEGLER, H. (1969):
Systematische und morphologische Bearbeitung der Federling-sammlung des parasitologischen Instituts der Tierärztlichen Hochschule in Wien.
Vet. Med. Diss. Wien

11 Nutritional deficiencies and metabolic disorders

The incidence of nutritional deficiencies and metabolic disorders in captive birds of prey is directly related to the quality of the nutrition and environment with which they are provided. When a diverse diet appropriate to the species and adequate opportunities for exercise are available, these types of problems are rare, occurring only occasionally in the presence of other underlying disease.

This discussion is limited to disorders that are relevant to raptors.

11.1 Vitamin deficiencies

Inadequate levels of certain critical vitamins in the diet can result in a variety of metabolic disturbances.

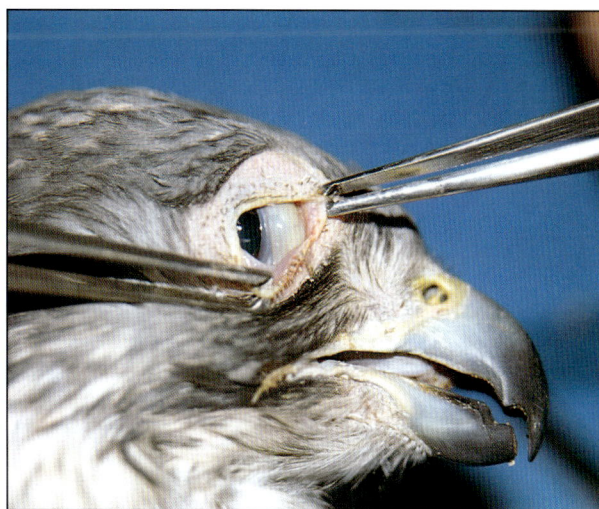

Fig. 11.1: The nictitating membrane of raptors is normally transparent. In this gyrfalcon (*F. rusticolus*) with vitamin A deficiency it has become opaque white and the underlying Harderian gland is swollen. The bird had been fed only rabbit muscle meat for a long period of time.
(Photo: Heidenreich)

11.1.1 Vitamin A deficiency

Raptors have a higher requirement for vitamin A than do mammals. Deficiencies can develop with long-term feeding of a diet consisting exclusively of muscle meat.

Signs of vitamin A deficiency develop gradually. Initial changes include opacification of the nictitans and enlargement of the associated lacrimal glands. The eyelids become hyperkeratotic and the conjunctival epithelium undergoes squamous metaplasia. Lacrimal secretions are reduced. As the cornea dries out and the eye's normal bacterial defense mechanisms are impaired, keratoconjunctivitis sicca develops. Corneal and conjunctival inflammation and infection will be accompanied by swelling of the eyelids and ocular discharge. (Konstaninov and Ippen, 1979).

Poor hatching rates and reduced hatchling viability have also been linked to hypovitaminosis A.

In cases where this deficiency is suspected, immediate diversification of the diet to include liver, as well as kidneys and blood, should be instituted. Until clinical signs resolve, vitamin A supplementation at a dose of 1500 to 2000 IU/kg is recommended.

It is possible to supplement with excess amounts of vitamin A, resulting in toxicity. Signs of hypervitaminosis A are similar to those of the deficiency.

11.1.2 Vitamin B deficiency

As with vitamin A, a diet limited to muscle meat is capable of resulting in deficiencies of some B vitamins, particularly B_1, B_2 and B_6. Intestinal inflammatory disorders and coccidiosis can also reduce the uptake of B vitamins (Ward, 1971; Stauber, 1973). Fish-eating raptors (osprey and sea eagles) can develop a thiamine deficiency on an unsupplemented diet of ocean fish. Most of these fish contain the enzyme thiaminase, which inactivates this B vitamin. A diet consisting exclusively of day-old chicks can result in similar problems.

Clinical signs of hypovitaminosis B in adult birds will develop gradually, while they may appear suddenly in juveniles. Mild ataxia will progress to pronounced incoordination, convulsions and opisthotonus (ex-

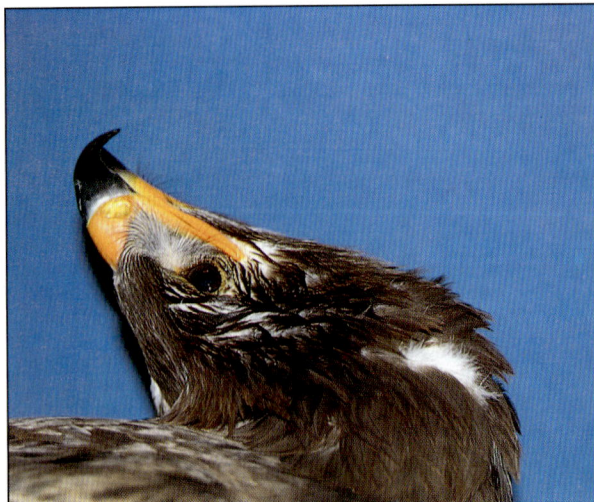

Fig. 11.2: This tawny eagle (*Aquila rapax*) suffered from chronic diarrhea of unknown etiology. Pronounced opisthotonus was the primary sign of a vitamin B deficiency that developed as a result of the diarrhea and its negative effect on intestinal vitamin synthesis and absorption.
(Photo: Heidenreich)

tension of head and neck backward) (Fig. 11.2). Any type of stimulation or excitement will exacerbate these neurological signs.

Besides addressing the underlying causes of the problem, treatment should be instituted with vitamin B complex preparations (10–30 mg/kg thiamine) administered daily until signs resolve. Toxicity is not a problem with administration of this water-soluble group of vitamins. Excess vitamins are eliminated by the kidneys. The urates of birds receiving vitamin B supplements usually develop a yellow color and a characteristic, sweet odor.

Response to therapy depends a great deal on the duration of the deficiency. If clinical signs have been present for only a few days, the prognosis is quite good and recovery should occur within one or two days. Permanent damage to the central nervous system occurs when hypovitaminosis B is not recognized and treated quickly. The prognosis for full recovery is poor in such cases and permanent neurological deficits such as head tilt may remain (Fig. 11.3).

11.1.3 Vitamin D deficiency

Vitamin D_3 is important in maintaining the physiologic balance between calcium and phosphorus in the body. Ingested vitamin D precursors are activated in the skin by ultraviolet radiation from sunlight. Only 45 minutes of daily exposure to sunlight suffice to prevent signs of hypovitaminosis D.

Deficiencies of this vitamin are responsible for rickets (see Ch. 11.2.1.1), a condition in which an imbalance of calcium and phosphorus in the body of a young, growing animal results in bone deformities. In older birds, similar imbalances will result in demineralization of existing bones and a predisposition to pathologic fractures (osteomalacia). Egg-laying females that are unable to obtain enough calcium may lay eggs with thin or defective shells.

A nutritionally complete diet of whole animals is all that is required to avoid these problems. Liver is especially rich in vitamin D. Like vitamin A, vitamin D is a fat-soluble vitamin and oversupplementation can lead to toxicity.

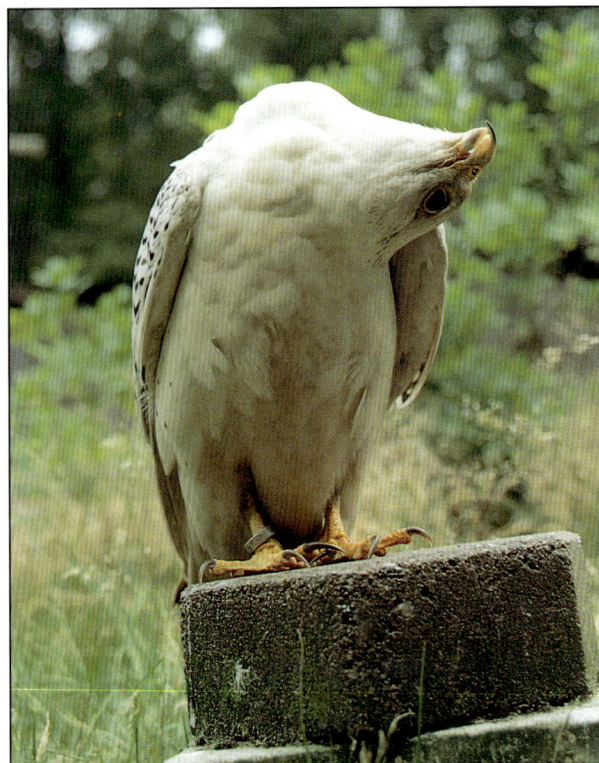

Fig. 11.3: A noticeable head tilt was present for many years in this white gyrfalcon (*F. rusticolus*). When calm and relaxed, he was able to eat and fly almost normally. The slightest excitement, however, elicited strong signs of CNS disturbance such that he would almost topple over backward. Since there was no indication of past trauma or other disease, it was assumed that these clinical signs were the result of permanent damage resulting from a past episode of hypovitaminosis B. Treatment at this point was ineffective and the falcon was euthanatized for humane reasons.
(Photo: Heidenreich)

11.2 Metabolic disorders

11.2.1 Disorders of mineral metabolism

The effect of mineral levels in the diet on the health and development of poultry is well known. Since a raptor's meat-based diet is fundamentally different from that of granivorous birds, this information can not always be directly applied to the nutrition of birds of prey. This discussion is therefore limited to disorders of calcium and phosphorus metabolism, which are relatively common and well-understood in birds of prey.

Adequate levels of both calcium and phosphorus are present in the natural diet of raptors. The bones and tissues of prey animals contain the correct Ca:P ratio of 1.5:1. Deficiencies occur only when the birds are not offered a complete or balanced diet.

All-meat diets deficient in bone are most often responsible for calcium deficiencies. Clean meat is relatively high in phosphorus and low in calcium. Beef, for instance, has a Ca:P ratio of 1:17, while liver is even worse, with a ratio of 1:44.

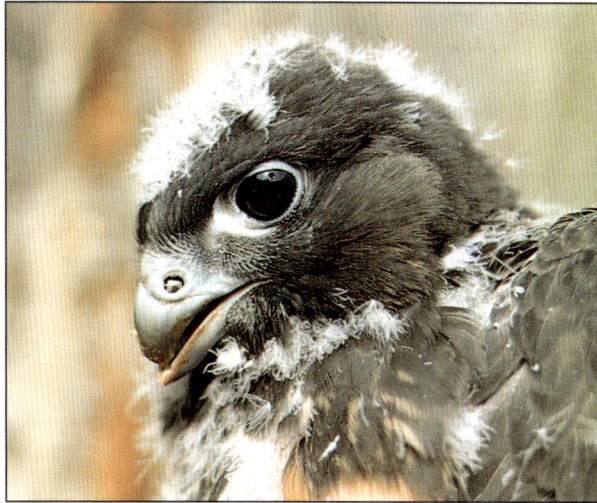

Fig. 11.5: This six week old peregrine falcon X gyrfalcon hybrid presented with a beak deformity attributed to rickets. Repeated efforts to realign the beak were unsuccessful. Despite the permanent defect, this bird was able to feed independently and undergo falconry training. (Photo: Heidenreich)

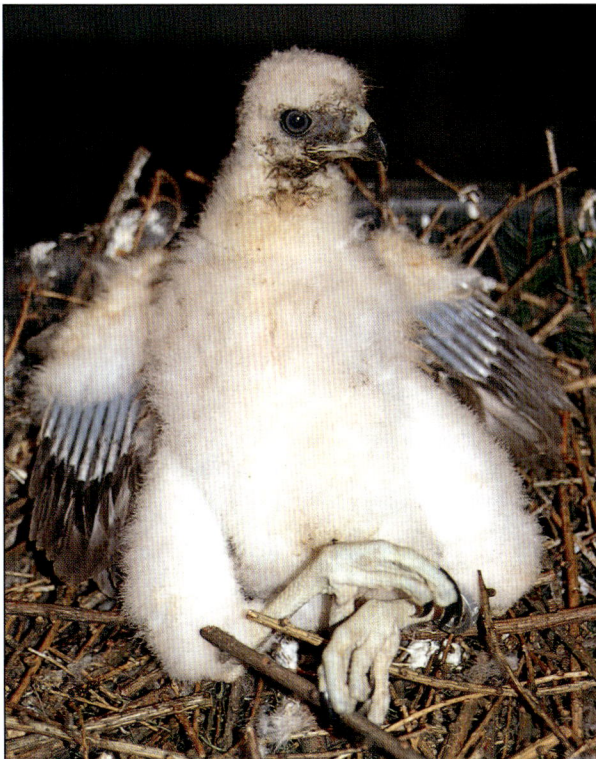

Fig. 11.4: A northern goshawk (*Accipiter gentilis*) was removed from the nest at 18 days of age and hand-raised. A calcium and vitamin deficient diet consisting of cleaned pigeon meat resulted in severe deformities of the long bones within days. The young bird was unable to stand and had episodic seizures.
(Photo: Heidenreich)

Adult birds are capable of tolerating this type of mineral imbalance for relatively long periods of time without obvious ill effects. Young, growing animals, however, have a relatively active bone metabolism and will develop problems very rapidly. Recently hatched chicks can show signs of rickets within days.

Deficiencies or imbalances in dietary calcium and phosphorus are most easily avoided by feeding a natural, whole animal diet. Vitamin and mineral supplements are difficult to administer at appropriate levels, especially since many of them are not formulated for meat-eating animals.

11.2.1.1 Rickets

A deficiency in available calcium for normal body function will show up in the bones first and causes syndromes known as rickets in growing birds or osteomalacia in adults. Either excessive phosphorus or insufficient calcium levels in the food can cause these diseases by producing an inappropriate dietary Ca:P ratio.

In the early days of captive raptor breeding, rickets was a common problem. It was always caused by the feeding of cleaned meat without the inclusion of bones or calcium supplements. Breeders were attempting to give the chicks what they thought was the best food, imitating the type of feeding practiced by adult birds in the wild. They were unaware that the saliva of raptors is naturally high in calcium and thus balances the soft diet of parent-raised chicks.

Clinical disease

Bending and distortion of the long bones can be seen in chicks with rickets by two to three weeks of age. The birds are unable to stand up to defecate, resulting in pasting of the vent and underbelly with urates and feces. This is sometimes misdiagnosed as diarrhea. As the birds grow and gain weight, the long bones of the legs become increasingly deformed (Fig. 11.4). In advanced cases, even the wings will be affected and spontaneous fractures can occur in any weight bearing bone. Malformations can develop in any part of the skeletal system. The keel can become bent and beak deformities may develop (Fig. 11.5).

Juvenile birds suffer greatly with this painful condition and will begin to complain vocally soon after the initial signs are noted. Many become depressed and refuse to eat, dying before they reach adulthood.

Diagnosis

A diagnosis is easily established based on the dietary history and careful palpation of the long bones. These bones will be obviously deformed and of a rubbery flexibility. Familiarity with normal avian anatomy is helpful to avoid mistaking bending fractures for limb joints (Fig. 11.6). A radiograph will confirm the presence of bony deformations, pathologic fractures and reduced bone density (Fig. 11.7).

Treatment

Treatment of metabolic bone disease in young birds is effective and worthwhile only in the early stages of rickets. Oral and injectable (calcium borogluconate 500 mg/kg/day) calcium supplements are employed

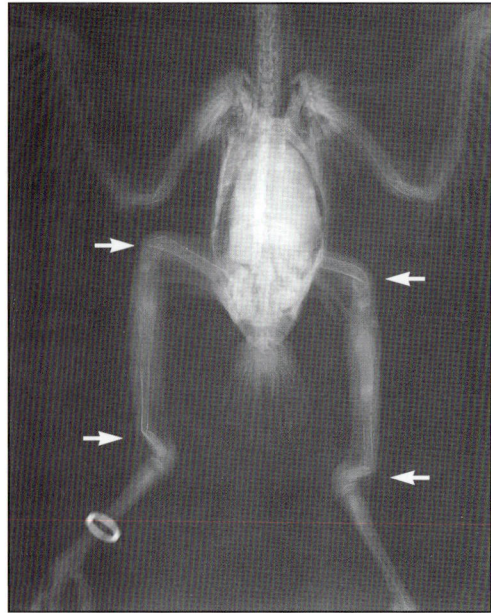

Fig. 11.7: Radiographs are often necessary for a definitive diagnosis of metabolic bone disease or rickets. Bilaterally symmetrical spontaneous fractures (arrows) and a lack of bone density are clearly visible in this ventrodorsal view of a young goshawk (*Accipiter gentilis*). (Photo: Heidenreich)

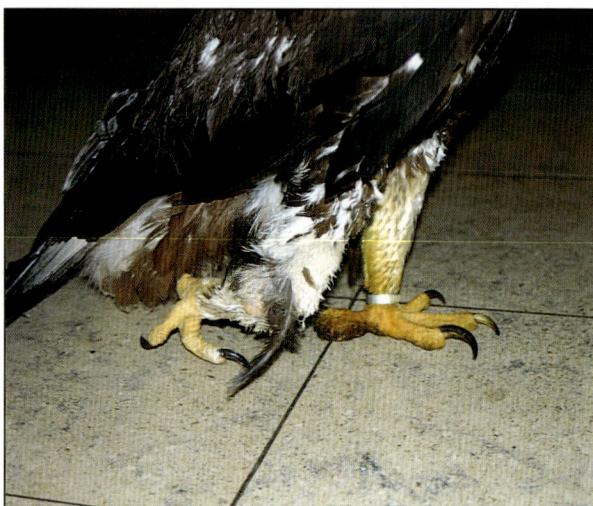

Fig. 11.6: A two year old male golden eagle (*Aquila chrysaetos*) suffered from a mild case of rickets as a nestling. This later led to a pronounced bend of the right tibiotarsus. (Photo: Heidenreich)

until adequate uptake of calcium in the diet is assured. Calcium carbonate can be sprinkled on the food. Young chicks will recover very rapidly. If bone deformities are already present, treatment generally comes too late. Calcium supplementation will result in mineralization and fixation of the bony fractures and bends, resulting in permanently crippled birds. Young birds with advanced cases of rickets should therefore be humanely euthanatized.

Prevention

Prevention of rickets in young birds is easy if correct feeding practices are employed. Chicks being fed cleaned meat in the first few days of life should receive a calcium supplement (such as Vitakalk®). The addition of ground bones from food animals or chopped mouse tails is even better. The small, rounded vertebrae present in mouse tails are not damaging to the intestinal tract and provide a good source of calcium. Human saliva (nonsmokers only!) can make the food morsels easier to swallow and contains valuable minerals and enzymes that further aid digestion in young chicks.

When the birds are a few days old, small pieces of bone from young food animals can easily be incorporated into the diet. Chopped rat or mouse pinkies have proven very successful for early feeding of young raptors.

11.2.2   Gout

Avian gout is a disorder in which uric acid, a nitrogenous waste product normally secreted by the kidneys, is improperly deposited in various parts of the body. Any condition that impairs renal function can contribute to the development of this disease. Infections that affect the kidneys, vitamin A deficiency with squamous metaplasia of the ureters, exposure to mycotoxins, the feeding of horsemeat and dehydration are all considered possible contributing factors to gout in raptors.

In birds of prey dehydration may play the most important role in the development of gout. Although many falcons, especially desert falcons and saker falcons, almost never drink water and obtain most of their fluids from the food they consume, dehydration can develop if food consumption is reduced. This often occurs during conditioning for the hunting season, when the birds are partially deprived of food to reduce their weight and stimulate their desire to pursue game. The accompanying reduction in fluid intake can result in elevated blood levels of urea and uric acid. If these are not excreted from the body, azotemia and hyperuricemia develop and may lead to death.

Clinical disease

In falcons, gout is always a chronic disease that takes weeks or months from the time that initial signs are noted until the bird dies. Affected hunting hawks that can be observed during flight will appear reluctant to expend energy, flying slowly and resting frequently or refusing to return when called from a longer distance.

There are two forms of avian gout, depending on the location of uric acid crystal deposition:

Articular gout: Birds in whom uric acid is deposited in limb joints show signs of joint pain, flying only reluctantly or acting lame when at rest. They may shift their weight from one leg to the other frequently or even lie down when they can. On palpation, doughy swelling and tenderness are evident in the joints and along tendons. Occasionally, even the feet become swollen, giving the appearance of bumblefoot. In combination with uneven weight bearing resulting from articular pain, avian gout does occasionally lead to true pododermatitis (see Ch. 13.10.4.1).

Visceral gout: The deposition of uric acid crystals on visceral organs, especially the pericardium and the serosa of the liver, is more difficult to detect. These birds show no initial clinical signs. As the disease progresses, increased water intake becomes noticeable. This polydipsia may progress to the point where the bird remains standing in his water bath most of the time, drinking almost continuously. Later, they become lethargic and anorectic and die.

Pathology

Visceral gout is easy to recognize on gross necropsy. The internal organs look as if they were covered in white powder and the kidneys appear whitish pink from the accumulations of uric acid within the renal tubules (Fig. 11.8).

Diagnosis

A presumptive diagnosis of avian gout can often be based on clinical signs alone. Radiographs help confirm the presence of uric acid on visceral organs and especially in the kidneys. The latter will appear abnormally dense (mineralized) on the x-ray film.

Endoscopic examination can also be used to confirm a diagnosis of visceral gout. Injectable anesthetics should never be used in these animals, since renal function is severely compromised and excretion of drugs by that route is impaired.

There have been many attempts to detect avian gout early by determining serum uric acid levels. Very high values, far above theoretical solubility limits for uric acid, were found in normal raptors, especially after consumption of meat. This diagnostic test is therefore of limited value. If performed, the bird should have fasted for at least 24 hours.

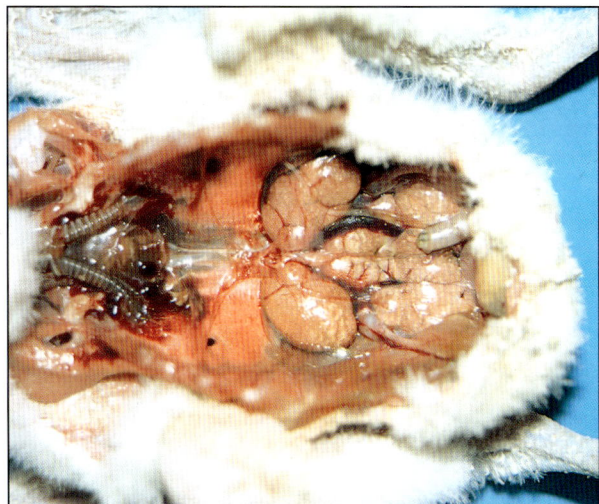

Fig. 11.8: Gout is not a disease restricted to adult birds. This three week old shaheen falcon chick shows the typical pale discoloration and enlargement of the kidneys that results from the accumulation of uric acid crystals in the renal tubules.
(Photo: Heidenreich)

Treatment and Prevention

There is currently no reliable treatment for this disease in birds. Supplementation with vitamin A and oral administration of 1% sodium bicarbonate solution for 10 days have been suggested. Gylstorff and Grimm (1987) recommend treatment with allopurinol, while Lumeij and Redig (1992) suggest avoiding its use, having been able to induce gout in three out of six healthy red-tailed hawks (*Buteo jamaicensis*) that were treated with allopurinol experimentally.

When bringing hunting hawks down in weight, special attention should be paid to providing adequate amounts of fluid. This can be accomplished by keeping the water bath filled or, for falcons that do not drink, offering soaked meat, which is depleted of nutrients but provides adequate amounts of water. Soaked meat should always be prepared in cold, running water to guard against clostridial diseases (see Ch. 9.2.2).

11.2.3   Diabetes mellitus

In diabetic birds, hyperglycemia is caused by any of a number of possible conditions that interfere with glucose metabolism, especially fatty livers or pathologic changes involving the pancreatic islet cells. Diabetes mellitus has been described in a variety of avian species, including parrots, geese, pigeons and, particularly, toucans (Worell, 1988; Altman and Kirmayer, 1976). Wallner-Pendleton et al. (1993) were the first to report on a case of diabetes mellitus in a raptor, a red-tailed hawk (*Buteo jamaicensis*).

Clinical disease

As in mammals, the most noticeable abnormality in affected birds is a great increase in water consumption. This polydipsia is associated with the production of copious quantities of watery urates. Depending on the severity of the disease, the bird's general demeanor may be affected as well. A case of diabetes mellitus in a young gyrfalcon (*Falco rusticolus*) from the author's own experience presented as follows:

The captive-bred falcon was removed from the breeding chamber at ten weeks of age. At that time, it appeared clinically normal. It was kept hooded for 24 hours and then placed on a block perch on the lawn. The bird's appetite was poor initially, but this is to be expected at the beginning of manning. He was, however, unusually calm and tame, never jumping from the perch the way other young falcons do. Since the falcon's appetite remained poor, he was offered a water bath and watched for signs of dehydration in the warm summer weather. He immediately jumped into the water and remained there for many hours, drinking frequently and greedily. Large amounts of very watery urates were produced, and when these were tested for

glucose with a test strip, the results were strongly positive. A blood sample submitted to the lab came back with a serum glucose value of 1848 mmol/l, almost ten times the normal value for birds.

The falcon's attitude improved somewhat with ad libitum water consumption, but he was not very interested in the lure. When supplied with a telemetry device and released from the creance, he only jumped off his perch and hopped over to the feeding area. Larger distances were also always covered on foot. When thrown up into the air, he glided clumsily back to the ground, unable to fly. Treatment with insulin was not attempted and the bird was eventually euthanatized.

The inability to fly seems to be common in diabetic raptors. The wild hawk described by Wallner-Pendleton was also found unable to fly.

11.2.4   Fatty liver syndrome

Common in poultry, especially laying hens, fatty liver syndrome or hepatic lipidosis is a multifactorial disease (Siegmann, 1993). High carbohydrate diets, a lack of exercise and high levels of estrogen are involved in stimulating hepatic lipogenesis and deposition of fat in the liver. This fatty degeneration greatly impairs the liver's normal metabolic functioning. Similar syndromes have been described in a variety of captive exotic bird species, especially parrots on high-fat all seed diets.

Cooper and Forbes (1983) and Forbes and Cooper (1993) describe a fatty liver and kidney syndrome seen only in captive merlins (*Falco columbarius*). All 12 merlins they examined were breeding birds that had been kept confined in aviaries for prolonged periods of time. None of the birds were used for hunting or exercised in any way. Clinical signs are unknown, since the birds all died suddenly, presumably of a fat embolus. The diagnosis of fatty liver syndrome was made at necropsy.

Pathology

Affected birds are approximately 5% overweight. Pronounced hepatomegaly (approximately 30% heavier than normal) as well as enlargement of spleen and kidneys are evident. These organs have a yellowish color due to fatty infiltration of the parenchyma (Fig. 11.9).

Presumptive etiology

Cooper and Forbes speculate that fatty liver syndrome in merlins may be related to a variety of vitamin and mineral deficiencies. A diet high in fat may contribute as well. This disease has never been seen in birds used for hunting, which are generally kept lean and in good physical condition. It may therefore simply result from inappropriate feeding and maintenance practices.

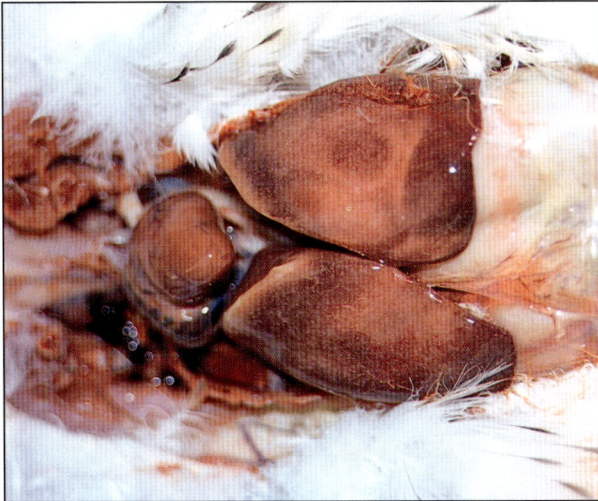

Fig. 11.9: Fatty infiltration of the liver is evident in the pale color of the liver parenchyma in this white gyrfalcon (*F. rusticolus*).The well-nourished (possibly overweight) bird died suddenly and without prior signs of illness. (Photo: Heidenreich)

References and literature of further interest

ALTMAN, R.B. and B.A. KIRMAYER (1976):
Diabetes mellitus in the avian species.
J. Amer. Animal Hosp. Assoc. **12**, 531–537

BAUMANN, C.R. (1980):
Harnsäurebestimmungen im Blutplasma bei verschiedenen Vogelarten.
Vet. Med. Diss. München

CALLE, P.P., DIERENFELD, E.S. and M.E. ROBERT (1989):
Serum alpha-tocopherol in raptors fed vitamin E-supplemented diets.
J. Zoo Wildl. Med. **20**, 62–67

COOPER, J.E. (1975):
Osteodystrophy in birds of prey.
Vet. Rec. **97**, 307

COOPER, J.E. and N.A. FORBES (1983):
A fatty liver kidney syndrome of merlins.
Vet. Rec. **112**, 182–183

DÖTTLINGER, H.:
Influence of diet on haematological parameters in captive peregrine falcons (*Falco peregrinus*).
In print

FERNANDEZ-REPOLLET, E., J. ROWLEY and A. SCHWARTZ (1982):
Renal damage in gentamicin-treated Lanner falcons (*Falco biarmicus*).
J. Am. Vet., Med. Ass. **181**, 1392

FORBES, N.A. and J.E. COOPER (1993):
Fatty liver-kidney syndrome of merlins.
in: REDIG, P.T. et al. (1993): Raptor Biomedicine, 45–48
Chiron Pub. Ltd. Keighley, West Yorkshire, England

GYLSTORFF, I. and F. GRIMM (1987):
Vogelkrankheiten.
Verlag Eugen Ulmer, Stuttgart

HALLIWELL, W.H. and D.L. GRAHAM (1973):
Nutritional diseases in birds of prey.
J. Zoo Anim. Med. **4**, 18–20

KIEL, H. (1986):
Nierengicht beim Uhu und Falken.
DVG V. Tagung über Vogelkrankheiten, 208–212

KONSTANTINOV, A and R. IPPEN (1979):
Vitamin-A-Mangel bei Zoo- und Wildvögeln.
Int. Symp. Erkrank. Zootiere **21**, 41–46

LUMEIJ, J.T. and J.D. REMPLE (1991):
Plasma urea, creatinine and uric acid concentrations in relation to feeding in peregrine falcons (*Falco peregrinus*).
Avian Path. **20**, 79–83

LUMEIJ, J.T. and P.T. REDIG (1992):
Hyperuricaemia and visceral gout induced by allopurinol in red-tailed hawks (*Buteo jamaicensis*).
DVG, VIII. Tagung der Fachgruppe »Geflügelkrankheiten« 265–269

RITCHIE, B.W. and HARRISON, G.J. (1994):
in: RITCHIE, B.W., HARRISON, G.J. and L.R. HARRISON (1995):
Avian medicine: principles and application.
Wingers Publishing, Lake Worth, Florida

SCHWEIGERT, F.J., UEHLEIN-HARRELL, S., HEGEL, G.V. and
H. WIESNER (1991):
Vitamin A (retinol and retinyl esters), alpha-tocopherol and
lipid levels in plasma of captive wild mammals and birds.
J. Vet. Med. A. **38**, 35–42

SIEGMANN, O. (1993):
Kompendium der Geflügelkrankheiten.
Verlag Paul Parey, Berlin u. Hamburg

SLINDEE, C. (1975):
Exotic case history (nephritis in a hawk).
Iowa State Univ. Vet. **37**, 76–77

STAUBER, E. (1973):
Suspected riboflavin deficiency in a golden eagle.
J. Am. Vet. Med. Ass. **163**, 645–646

WALLACH, J.D. (1970):
Nutritional diseases of exotic animals.
J. Am. Vet. Med. Ass. **157**, 583–599

WALLACH, J.D. and G.M. FLIEG (1970):
Cramps and fits in carnivorous birds.
Int. Zoo Yearbook **10**, 3–4

WALLNER-PENDLETON, E.A., ROGERS, D. and A. EPPLE
(1993):
Diabetes mellitus in a red-tailed hawk (*Buteo jamaicensis*).
Avian Path. **22**, 631–635

WARD, F.P. (1971):
Thiamine deficiency in a peregrine falcon.
J. Am. Vet. Med. Ass. **159**, 599–601

WORELL, A. (1988):
Management and medicine of toucans.
Proc. Ass. Avian Vet. 1988, 253–261

12 Toxicoses

In the second half of this century, birds of prey have become well known for their tragic vulnerability to environmental contaminants, especially pesticides. As predators at the top of the food chain, they are most likely to ingest and accumulate high levels of toxins present in their surroundings and in the animals they eat. A dramatic drop in the populations of some raptor species during the decades of the 60's and 70's alerted the world to this problem. Since then, many of the substances responsible, especially DDT, have been banned from use or are no longer produced in Western countries.

12.1 Lead intoxication

Intoxication with the heavy metal lead is relatively common in both wild and captive birds of prey. Lead is usually ingested in the form of shotgun pellets present in the tissues of an animal that was shot or that had ingested the pellets (common in waterfowl). If the raptor is fed only clean meat from the contaminated animal, the problem will be exacerbated because he will be unable to cast a pellet incorporating the lead shot, thus expelling it quickly. Lead particles that remain in the digestive tract are exposed to corrosive stomach acids and dissolve over a period of several weeks. The lead thus released is absorbed into the systemic circulation and deposited throughout the body, free to exert its toxic effects on almost every system. Experiments with bald eagles (Pattee et al., 1981) showed that lead poisoning led to death within 10 to 125 days after oral ingestion of between 10 and 156 four millimeter lead pellets.

Lead particles not exposed to acids, such as those lodged in muscle or bone, remain intact and pose almost no threat to the animal.

Lead competes with calcium in the body, interfering with many of that mineral's vitally important functions. It also produces anemia in affected animals by interfering with the action of some important enzymes, especially those involved in hemoglobin synthesis.

Clinical disease
Raptor species vary greatly in their sensitivity to lead intoxication. The amount ingested and its rate of passage through the digestive tract also influence the range and severity of clinical signs in affected birds.

Mild (sublethal) intoxication: Wild birds of prey are often exposed to infrequent, low levels of lead. They will eat animals containing lead shot only occasionally and usually regurgitate the pellets in their castings after only brief exposure to the toxin. Mildly elevated blood or organ lead levels (0.6–1 ppm) are often discovered in these animals coincidentally during treatment for other disorders or on necropsy. Repeated exposure to small amounts of lead can, over time, lead to clinically significant accumulation of the heavy metal in the body.

Lethal toxicity: Initial clinical signs of serious lead intoxication include green diarrhea, inappetance, weight loss and visual disturbances. After a few days or weeks, convulsions and paresis may set in (Fig. 12.1). Blood or organ lead levels are above 1 ppm.

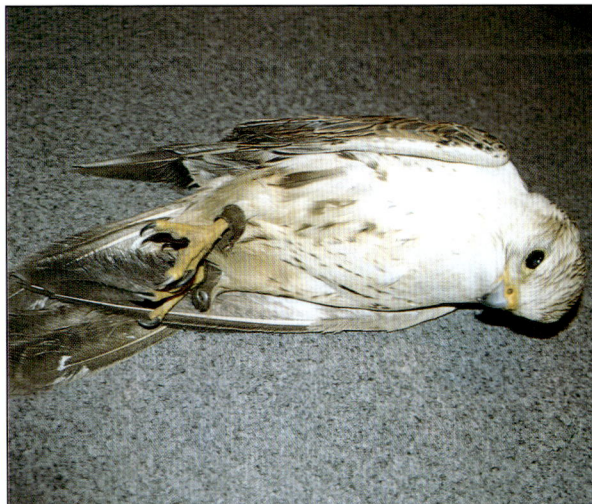

Fig. 12.1: An adult saker falcon (*F. cherrug*) presented with tonic-clonic convulsions that were exacerbated by any kind of stimulation. The bird's plumage had been severely damaged by the its uncoordinated activity on the ground. Samples of liver tissue obtained at necropsy contained 55 ppm of lead. The source of this intoxication was a lure weighted with lead shot. The falcon had been feeding from it for weeks.   (Photo: Heidenreich)

Diagnosis

Because this problem is often chronic in nature, a diagnosis is not easily made. A variety of ancillary tests are available to help confirm the presence of lead in the animal's tissues.

Radiographs: Lead pellets are extremely radiodense and thus easily visualized radiographically. An absence of metallic densities within the digestive tract of the affected bird does not rule out lead poisoning.

Blood lead levels: Blood lead levels above 60 μg/dl will support a diagnosis of lead toxicity.

ALAD activity: Delta-aminolevulenic acid dehydratase (ALAD) is an enzyme that is rapidly inhibited by the presence of lead. It is therefore considered a reliable and sensitive indicator of exposure to this toxin. Table 12.1 lists normal values of ALAD in some representative birds of prey. Units of measurement may vary in the US.

In common buzzards, ALAD levels drop from a normal of 3.52 U/l to 1.11 U/l only four days after oral ingestion of lead and remain at or below 40% of normal for weeks. In contrast, hemoglobin levels take 10 to 14 weeks to fall below normal after an animal's exposure to lead. Hemoglobin levels are therefore not useful as an early indicator of lead toxicity (Meister, 1981).

Treatment

If ingestion of lead occurred recently and pellets are still present in the digestive tract, every effort should be made to remove them. If the feeding of fibrous casting material such as animal skins and fur does not result in regurgitation of the lead shot, surgical intervention may be necessary.

Several chelating agents are available for the removal of heavy metals from the systemic circulation. They are generally very effective, although complete removal of lead may take a relatively long time.

Table 12.1: ALAD activity levels (U/l) in normal raptors (from MEISTER, 1981)

Peregrine falcon (*Falco peregrinus*)	1.28 ± 0.08
Common kestrel (*Falco tinnunculus*)	3.77 ± 0.15
Common buzzard (*Buteo buteo*)	3.58 ± 0.44
Red kite (*Milvus milvus*)	3.26 ± 0.68
Black kite (*Milvus migrans*)	3.21 ± 0.40

Ca EDTA is given at a dose of 10 to 40 mg/kg BID intramuscularly for five days. After 5 days, blood lead levels can be remeasured and treatment repeated if necessary.

D-penicillamine (PA) at a dose of 55 mg/kg SID to BID can be given orally for several days to weeks until clinical signs resolve and blood lead levels return to normal. Lethargy, anemia and weight loss may develop secondary to copper deficiency with excessive use of this drug.

Dimercaprol (BAL - British Anti-Lewisite) is considered the most effective drug for eliminating lead from the central nervous system. The dose is 2.5 mg/kg IM every four hours for two days, then BID for another 10 days.

Prevention

The main source of lead for raptors is lead shot used in hunting. Wild animals killed this way should never be fed to raptors. In some countries, efforts to ban lead shot may help reduce the incidence of this problem.

12.2 Chloralose intoxication

Alpha-chloralose is an anesthetic sometimes placed in bait for the capture or control of gulls, pigeons, crows and rodents. Depending on the dose, animals that have ingested this drug may die or, with lower doses, recover after several hours of anesthesia. The induction period varies greatly, but always takes at least 10 or 20 minutes. Intoxicated birds can therefore fly relatively far before succumbing to the effects of chloralose. Then they become vulnerable to birds of prey looking for an easy meal.

Raptors that capture and eat such animals show the same signs as the poisoned gull or pigeon that they consumed. Their flight becomes uncoordinated, causing them to collide with obstacles or fall to the ground, where they will lie with twitching wings. When stimulated by handling, they may respond with strong excitement. Affected birds can also salivate profusely or vomit, putting themselves at risk of aspiration pneumonia. Mild intoxication usually resolves within a day. With higher levels of exposure, death may ensue as a result of hypothermia or respiratory paralysis.

Diagnosis

It is difficult to confirm a presumptive diagnosis of chloralose intoxication. Often several birds in the area are found showing similar clinical signs or dead. Special toxicological laboratories may be able to test gastrointestinal contents from affected birds for the presence of chloralose.

Treatment

Birds suspected to have ingested chloralose should have all remaining stomach contents flushed out as soon as possible. This involves pumping large quantities of water or physiologic saline solution into the crop and proventriculus while the bird is suspended with its head down to prevent aspiration of food or fluids as they are removed. Sleeping birds should be kept warm and doxapram can be given to help stimulate respiration. In the field, the oral administration of strong coffee seems to help speed up recovery. Sodium sulfate (Glauber's salts) 5 g in 100 ml of water or two to three pieces of candy sugar crystals given by mouth act as cathartics and help speed the elimination of chloralose from the lower GI tract.

12.3   Barbiturate intoxication

Very high doses of barbiturates are frequently used for the euthanasia of animals. In most countries, the use of these drugs is limited by law to veterinarians or people with special licenses for this purpose. However, barbiturates are sometimes used illegally by lay people, for instance in the euthanasia of farm-raised fur animals. In Europe, mink are often killed by gassing with car exhaust or by injection with embutramide and mebenzonium iodide (T 61®). Pentobarbital solutions are used for similar purposes in the US. If the bodies are sold as a cheap source of meat and fed to birds of prey, they will induce a deep, anesthesia-like state of sleep which can last hours or days and might even lead to death if not treated.

Initial therapy involves the removal of all stomach contents to minimize further absorption of the drug. If the respiratory rate is low, doxapram (Dopram V®) can be administered at a dose of 5–10 mg/kg IM. This may have to be repeated several times, depending on the animal's response.

Body temperature should be monitored regularly. Hypothermia can be treated with warm water bottles placed under the wings. Animals suffering from longer anesthetic episodes will also benefit from intravenous fluid supplementation.

The recovery period may be accompanied by strong excitatory behavior. The awakening bird may beat its wings or struggle in an uncoordinated fashion. Loosely wrapping the animal in a towel during this phase will help prevent injuries.

12.4   Coumarin intoxication

Products containing the potent anticoagulant coumarin or its derivatives (Brumolin®, Warfarin®, etc.) are available commercially as rodenticides, usually in the form of treated grains. The anticoagulant action of this class of drugs is based on the inhibition of vitamin K and causes death by slow internal hemorrhaging in affected animals. Raptors can become exposed to coumarin in the course of rodenticide use in and around their perches or aviaries.

Ingestion of coumarin-intoxicated rodents is generally not harmful, since the poison is rapidly degraded and rendered inactive inside the body. Direct ingestion of coumarin is necessary for clinical signs to occur. The rodenticide can be spread to the raptor's food or water by rodents, or undigested portions may remain in the stomach of a rat eaten by the bird. MARTIN et al. (1994) reported that a dose of only 0.25 mg/kg was sufficient to cause clinical signs in an eagle. In this case, the product used was "Pindon®", a potent coumarin derivative used to control rabbit populations in Australia.

Clinical disease

The inhibition of blood clotting functions results in internal hemorrhaging and the excretion of reddish-brown, bloody urates and feces. Affected birds will be weak, depressed and anemic, with pale mucous membranes.

Treatment

In animals suspected of having been exposed to coumarin compounds, immediate administration of large doses of vitamin K (Konakion®) will act as an antidote. Blood transfusions or iron supplementation may be indicated, depending on the severity of the anemia. Every effort should be made to avoid physical trauma that could induce further hemorrhage.

12.5   Pesticide intoxications

12.5.1   Organophosphates

Organophosphates are present in a variety of commercially available fungicides, herbicides and insecticides (Malathion, Parathion, Dichlorvos and others). Some topical insecticides for use on pets also contain these toxic compounds. The indiscriminate use of products intended for use in dogs or cats on a bird of prey can quickly lead to death. Wild raptors can also be exposed to organophosphates, especially in agricultural areas where the environment or their prey may be contaminated.

Clinical disease

Organophosphates act as inhibitors of acetylcholinesterase, an enzyme involved in neuromuscular transmission and the parasympathetic nervous system. Signs of intoxication include muscle tremors, convulsions, diarrhea, vomiting and pupillary constriction. The latter is a strong indicator for organophosphate or carbamate poisoning.

Treatment

With acute intoxication and very high doses, the bird will die within minutes. Treatment is not possible. Mild or chronic exposure to organophosphates is treatable with atropine (0.2–0.5 mg/kg IM). Treatment can be repeated if necessary.

Pralidoxime hydrochloride (2-PAM) at a dosage of 10 mg/kg IM has proven effective for the treatment of organophosphate poisoning in other types of birds. Information on its use in raptors is still lacking.

Prevention

The use of topical insecticides for the treatment of ectoparasites in birds of prey should be considered carefully. Powdered preparations permit oral uptake of the toxins during preening. Liquid sprays are often capable of penetrating through the of bird's thin skin and being absorbed into the systemic circulation. The safest products for topical use are based on pyrethrins, an insecticide derived from chrysanthemums. Pyrethrins are often mixed with synergistic compounds or synthetic derivatives (pyrethroids). The latter should also be avoided or used with great care. It is wise to always carefully read the labels on these types of products before applying them to a bird. Labels indicating that the ingredients are not toxic to man or animals should be interpreted with skepticism regarding birds.

To avoid the inadvertent use of pesticide-contaminated animals or meat as food, ill animals or those found dead should never be fed to birds of prey.

12.5.2   Carbamates

Carbamate insecticides are similar to organophosphates in their mechanism of action, although they are not as potent. They are often broadly applied in poultry facilities or to crops in agricultural areas. Although carbamates were long considered to be relatively safe, more recent evaluations have concluded that as many as 2 million birds a year may succumb to the effects of carbofuran (a carbamate insecticide) in the United States alone.

Clinical signs are similar but generally less severe than with organophosphate poisoning. Atropine is the antidote of choice in these cases as well. Pralidoxime should not be used, however, as it may actually exacerbate the toxicity of carbamate compounds.

12.5.3   Chlorinated Hydrocarbons

This class of insecticides includes various groups, among them those containing DDT and benzene hexachloride (lindane). DDT is particularly notorious for its negative impact on the environment, especially on wild birds, including birds of prey. Chlorinated hydrocarbons tend to accumulate in the fatty tissues of the body over time. They reach particularly high levels in predatory animals at the top of the food chain, such as raptors. Their effect in birds is to interfere with egg shell production, resulting in abnormally thin-shelled, fragile eggs. The long term result is frequent breaking of the eggs before hatching and a marked reduction in nesting success, with potentially disastrous effects on population levels.

The use of DDT is now forbidden in many countries. However, many of our migratory species are still exposed to this pesticide in their wintering grounds to the south.

Chlorinated cyclodiene insecticides (heptachlor, octachlor, dieldrin, endrin, etc.) are also used as insecticides in agriculture and forestry. Their use has been drastically reduced in the countries of the European Union, but they are still applied frequently outside this area.

Raptors are very sensitive to this class of compounds and die with only low levels of exposure. Barely 5 ppm in the brain of a falcon are sufficient to cause death. Clinical signs of exposure include abnormal posture, excitability, convulsions, vomiting and hypersalivation.

Because chlorinated hydrocarbons are stored in the fat, any situation involving weight loss, such as preparing a hawk for the hunting season, can result in release of these toxins into the systemic circulation. No specific treatment is available.

12.5.4   Polychlorinated Biphenyls (PCB's)

These chemicals are found in coolants, lubricants, wood protectants and as softeners in plastics. From there they can contaminate the environment and enter the food chain for man and animals. As with chlorinated hydrocarbons, these compounds bioaccumulate, so that the animals at the top of the food chain are most seriously affected. Fish-eating birds of prey show the highest levels in their tissues. PCB's are stored in adipose tissue for years and can be deposited in the yolk during egg production. They result in increased rates of embryo mortality, but there is no evidence that they affect egg shell thickness. No treatment has proven effective against these toxins.

References and literature of further interest

ADLAM, R.P. (1972):
Pollution and birds of prey.
Hawk Trust annual report. 1972, 21–42
Hawk Trust, Newent, Gloucestershire. England

BEAN, J.R. and R.H. HUDSON (1976):
Acute oral toxicity and tissue residues of thallium sulfate in golden eagles, *Aquila chrysaetos.*
Bull. Environment. Contam. Toxicol. **15**, 118–121

BENSON, W.W., PHARAOH, B. and P. MILLER (1974):
Lead poisoning in a bird of prey.
Bull. Environment. Contam. Toxicol. **11**, 105–108

BOSCHOFF, A.F., KOCK, A.C. and A.C. DE-KOCK (1988):
Further evidence of organo-chlorine contamination in Cape Vultures.
Ostrich **59**, 40–41

BOWES, V., PULS, R. and M. PETERS (1992):
Fenthion toxicity in bald eagles.
Canad. Vet. J. **33**, 678

CLAUSEN, B. and O. KARLOG (1977):
Thalliumgehalt bei Eulen und anderen Raubvögeln in Dänemark.
Nord. Vet. Med. **29**, 227–231

COOKE, A.S. (1979):
Changes in the egg shell characteristics of the sparrowhawk (*Accipiter nisus*) and peregrine (*Falco peregrinus*) associated with exposure to environmental pollutants during recent decades.
J. Zool. **187**, 245–263

CRICK, H. (1990):
Poisoned prey in the heart of Africa.
New Scientist **128**, 1744

DECKER, R.A., MCDERMID, A.M. and J.W. PRIDEAUX (1979):
Lead poisoning in two captive king vultures.
J. Am. Vet. Med. Ass. **175**, 1009

DELBEKE, K., JOIRIS, C. and G. DECADT (1984):
Mercury contamination of the Belgian avifauna 1970–1981.
Environment. Pollution, B **7**, 205-221

DEMENT, S.H., CHISOLM, J.J., BARBER, J.C. and J.D. STRANDBERG (1986):
Lead exposure in an »urban« peregrine falcon and its avian prey.
J. Wildl. Dis. **22**, 238–244

ENDERSON, J.H., CRAIG, G.R., BURNHAM, W.A. and D.D. BERGER (1982):
Eggshell thinning and organochlorine residues in Rocky Mountain peregrines, *Falco peregrinus*, and their prey.
Canad. Field Natur. **96**, 255–264

FOX, N.C. and J.W. LOCK (1978):
Organochlorine residues in New Zealand birds of prey.
New Zealand J. Ecol. **1**, 118-125

FRANSON, J.C., SILEO, L., PATTEE, O.H. and J.F. MOORE (1983):
Effects of chronic dietary lead in American kestrels (*Falco sparverius*).
J. Wildl. Dis. **19**, 110–113

FROSLIE, A., HOLT, G. and G. NORHEIM (1986):
Mercury and persistent chlorinated hydrocarbons in owls (Strigiformes) and birds of prey (Falconiformes) collected in Norway during the period 1965–1983.
Environment. Pollution B. **11**, 91–108

FYFE, R.W. and W. WALKER (1976):
Pollutant effects on the reproduction of the Prairie Falcons and Merlins of the Canadian prairies.
Canad. Field Natur. **90**, 346–355

GARNER, M. (1991):
Suspected lead toxicosis in a captive goshawk.
J. Am. Vet. Med. Ass. **199**, 1069–1070

GERRIETS, D. and C. SAAR (1985):
Einfluß der Pestizide auf die Wildpopulationen und auf in Gefangenschaft gehaltene Wanderfalken (*Falco peregrinus*).
Int. Symp. Erkrank. Zootiere **27**, 227–236

GILSLEIDER, E. and F.W. OEHME (1982):
Some common toxicoses in raptors [organic chlorine compounds, lead, mercury, nicotine].
Vet. Human Toxicol. **24**, 169–170

HAHN, E., HAHN, K. and G. KLEINSTÄUBER (1992):
Quecksilbergehalt in Wanderfalken aus Ostdeutschland.
Greifvögel und Falknerei, 87–93
Verlag Neumann-Neudamm, Morschen-Heina

HAVERA, S.P. and R.E. DUZAN (1986):
Organochlorine and PCB residues in tissues of raptors from Illinois, 1966-1981.
Bull. Environment. Contam. Toxicol. **36**, 23–32

HENNY, C.J., PRESCOTT-WARD, F., RIDDLE, K.E. and R.M. PROUTY (1982):
Migratory peregrine falcons, *Falco peregrinus*, accumulate pesticides in Latin America during winter.
Canad. Field Natur. **96**, 333–338

HENNY, C.J., KOLBE, E.J., HILL, E.F. and L.J. BLUS (1987):
Case histories of bald eagles and other raptors killed by organophosphorus insecticides topically applied to livestock.
J. Wildl. Dis. **23**, 292–295

Hernandez, L.M., Gonzalez, M.J. and M.A. Fernandez (1988):
Organochlorines and metals in Spanish Imperial eagle eggs, 1986–87.
Environment. Conserv. **15**, 363-364

HOFFMAN, D.J., PATTEE, O.H., WIEMEYER, S.N. and B. MULHERN (1981):
Effects of lead shot ingestion on delta-aminolevulinic acid dehydratase activity, hemoglobin concentration, and serum chemistry in bald eagles (*Haliaeetus leucocephalus*).
J. Wildl. Dis. **17**, 423–431

Holt, G., Froeslie, A. and G. Norheim (1979):
Mercury, DDE, and PCB in the avian fauna in Norway
1965–1976.
Acta Vet. Scand. **70**, 28

Hunt, K.A., Bird, D.M., Mineau, P. and L. Shutt
(1992):
Selective predation of organophosphate-exposed prey by
American kestrels.
Animal Behaviour. **43**, 971–976

Janssen, D.L., Oosterhuis, J.E., Allen, J.L., Anderson, M.P.,
Kelts, D.G. and S.N. Wiemeyer (1986):
Lead poisoning in free-ranging California condors (*Gymnogyps californianus*).
J. Am. Vet. Med. Ass. **189**, 1115–1117

Johnston, D.W. (1978):
Organochlorine pesticide residues in Florida birds of prey,
1969-76.
Pestic. Monito. J. **12**, 8–15

Keck, G., Paubel, P. and R.J. Monneret (1982):
Organochlorine and mercury residues in peregrine falcon eggs
in France.
Bull. Environment. Contam. Toxicol. **28**, 705–709

Knapp, M. and H.A. Rüssel (1973):
Gefahren für Greifvögel bei der Möwenbekämpfung durch
Chloralose. Nachweis einer Chloralosevergiftung bei zwei
Bussarden.
Dtsch.Tierärztl. Wschrift. **80**, 573–574

Kösters, J., Busche, R. and B. Baumbach (1979):
Zur Frage der Verfütterung von mit Bleischrot erlegten Tierkadavern an Greifvögel.
Prakt. Tierarzt **60**, 988, 991–992

Langelier, K.M., Andress, C.E., Grey, T.K., Wooldridge,
C., Lewis, R.J. and R. Marchetti (1991):
Lead poisoning in bald eagles in British Columbia.
Canad. Vet. J. **32**, 108–109

Langelier, K.M. (1993):
Barbiturate poisoning in twenty-nine bald eagles.
in: Redig, P.T. et al. (1993): Raptor biomedicine 231–232
Chiron Pub. Ltd. Keighley, West Yorkshire, England

Lingle, G.R. and G.L. Krapu (1988):
Ingestion of lead shot and aluminum bands by bald eagles
during winter in Nebraska.
Wilson Bull. **100**, 326–327

Macdonald, J.W., Randall, C.J., Ross, H.M., Moon, G.M.
and A.D. Ruthven (1983):
Lead poisoning in captive birds of prey.
Vet. Rec. **113**, 65–66

Martin, G.R., Kirkpatrick, W.E., King, D.R., Robertson,
I.D., Hood, P.J. and J.R. Sutherland (1994):
Assessment of the potential toxicity of an anticoagulant, pindone (2-pivalyl-1,3-indandione) to some Australian birds.
Wildl. Res. **21**, 85–93

Meister, B. (1981):
Untersuchungen zur alimentären Bleivergiftung bei Greifvögeln.
Vet. Med. Diss. Gießen

Meister, B. and J. Kösters (1981):
Weitere Untersuchungen zur Bleivergiftung bei Greifvögeln.
Prakt. Tierarzt **62**, 870, 875–878

Mendelsohn, H. and U. Paz (1977):
Mass mortality of birds of prey caused by azodrin, an organophosphorus insecticide.
Biol. Conserv. **11**, 163–170

Nelson, T.A., Mitchell, C. and C. Abbott (1989):
Lead-shot ingestion by bald eagles in Western Arkansas.
Southwest. Naturalist **34**, 245–249

Newton, I., Bogan, J., Meek, E. and B. Little (1982):
Organochlorine compounds and shell-thinning in British
merlins *Falco columbarius*.
Ibis **124**, 328–335

Newton, I., Bogan, J.A. and P. Rothery (1986):
Trends and effects of organochlorine compounds in
sparrowhawk eggs.
J. App. Ecol. **23**, 461–478

Nie, G.J.-van (1975):
Mogelijke chloralose vergiftiging bij buizerds.
Tijdschr. Diergeneesk. 100, 1052–1053

Pattee, O.H., Wiemeyer, S.N., Mulhern, B.M., Sileo, L. and
J.W. Carpenter (1981):
Experimental lead-shot poisoning in bald eagles.
J. Wildl. Managem. **45**, 806–810

Peakall, D.B. (1976):
The Peregrine falcon (*Falco peregrinus*) and pesticides.
Canad. Field Natur. **90**, 301–307

Peakall, D.B. and L.F. Kiff (1979):
Eggshell thinning and DDE residue levels among peregrine
falcons (*Falco peregrinus*): a global perspective.
Ibis **121**, 200–204

Porter, S.L. and S.E. Snead (1990):
Pesticide poisoning in birds of prey.
J. Ass. Avian Vet. **4**, 84–85

Porter, S.L. (1993):
Pesticide poisoning in birds of Prey.
in: Redig, P.T. et al. (1993): Raptor biomedicine 239–245
Chiron Pub. Ltd. Keighley, West Yorkshire, England

Prouty, R.M., Pattee, O.H. and S.K. Schmeling (1982):
DDT poisoning in a Cooper's hawk collected in 1980.
Bull. Environment. Contam. Toxicol. **28**, 319–321

Radvanyi, A., Weaver, P., Massari, C., Bird, D. and
E. Broughton (1988):
Effects of chlorophacinone on captive kestrels.
Bull. Environment. Contam. Toxicol. **41**, 441–448

REDIG, P.T., STOWE, C.M., BARNES, D.M. and T.D. ARENT (1980):
Lead toxicosis in raptors.
J. Am. Vet. Med. Ass. **177**, 941–943

SHLOSBERG, A., LUBLIN, A., BAHAT, O., HEYMANN, G.D., HANJI, V., BELLAICHE, M., MECHANI, S. and A. NYSKA (1994):
Percutaneous exposure to ethyl parathion in a feral Griffon vulture (*Gyps fulvus*).
Vet. Human Toxicol. **36**, 224–226

SCHWARZBACH, S.E., FRY, D.M., ROSSON, B.E. and D.M. BIRD (1991):
Metabolism and storage of p,p' dicofol in American kestrels (*Falco sparverius*) with comparisons to ring neck doves (*Streptopelia risoria*).
Arch. Environ. Contam. Toxicol. **20**, 206–210

SHRUBB, M. (1985):
Breeding sparrowhawks (*Accipiter nisus*) and organo-chlorine pesticides in Sussex and Kent.
Bird Study **32**, 155–163

SPRONK, N. and G.C. HARTOG (1971):
Mercury in birds of prey.
Ardea **59**, 34–37

STEHLE, S. (1980):
Orale Bleivergiftung bei Greifvögeln (*Falconiformes*) – Vorläufige Mitteilung.
Kleintierpraxis **25**, 309–310

STENDELL, R.C. (1980):
Dietary exposure of kestrels to lead.
J. Wildl. Managem. **44**, 527–530

STENDELL, R.C., BEYER, W.N. and R.A. STEHN (1989):
Accumulation of lead and organochlorine residues in captive American kestrels fed pine voles from apple orchards.
J. Wildl. Dis. **25**, 388–391

STONE, W.B., OVERMANN, S.R. and J.C. OKONIEWSKI (1984):
Intentional poisoning of birds with parathion.
Condor **86**, 333–336

SUNDLOF, S.F., FORRESTER, D.J., THOMPSON, N.P. and M.W. COLLOPY (1986):
Residues of chlorinated hydrocarbons in tissues of raptors in Florida.
J. Wildl. Dis. **22**, 71–82

TERNES, W., PETERAT, B. and H.A. RÜSSEL-SINN (1986):
Belastung der Greifvögel in Norddeutschland mit den Schwermetallen Blei, Cadmium und Quecksilber.
DVG, V. Tagung über Vogelkrankheiten, München, 187–194

WHEELDON, E.B., BOGAN, J.A. and D.J. TAYLOR (1975):
Dieldrin poisoning in a captive bird of prey.
Vet. Rec. **97**, 412

WHITE, D.H., HAYES, L.E. and P.B. BUSH (1989):
Case histories of wild birds killed intentionally with famphur in Georgia and West Virginia.
J. Wildl. Dis. **25**, 184–188

13 Diseases of specific organ systems

13.1 Feathers and skin

Avian feathers function primarily to provide protection from the elements and to permit flight. Almost all raptor chicks are covered with down when they hatch, initially with the whitish early down (neoptil), which quickly changes into the denser gray mesoptil. The permanent feathers emerge from their follicles with a pulp-filled shaft and a covering sheath of keratin which gradually peels away to release the mature feather. When a young bird has completed the growth of its first real plumage and no pin feathers remain, it is said to be "full-summed."

Most of a bird's body surface is covered with contour feathers. In addition, the tail has 12 rectrices or tail feathers, and each wing has 10 primary and 12 secondary feathers, known together as flight feathers.

Gyr- or saker falcons occasionally grow feathers on their toes (Fig. 13.1). Whether this is an atavistic phenomenon indicating that their evolutionary ancestors once had feathered feet remains unknown.

All raptors regularly undergo a loss of all old, worn or damaged feathers and replace them with new ones. This moulting process occurs annually in small and medium-sized birds of prey and takes several months to be completed. Larger birds such as vultures and eagles may take several years to replace their entire set of feathers.

The moulting season corresponds to the period of nesting and raising young and is controlled by photoperiod and by hormonal mechanisms (see Ch. 13.9). Females generally lose their first feathers shortly after egg-laying, while males start moulting somewhat later. Under normal circumstances one can assume that no further eggs will be laid after a hawk begins to moult. This rule does not apply to second and third clutches, which can be laid quite a bit later.

The moult occurs in a definite pattern which ensures that the bird remains capable of hunting and flight during this period. No large gaps occur in the flight feathers or tail. The next feather is not lost until the previous one has regrown at least halfway.

Falconers and ornithologists do not agree on the numbering of primary feathers on the wing. This has led to repeated misunderstandings in the literature. While falconers begin counting with the outermost (most distal) feather and move proximally, ornithologists go the other way, beginning at the carpus and moving distally. The ornithological system used in science is applied from here on in this book.

Raptor groups differ in their moulting pattern, a fact that has been used in the systematic classification of birds of prey. Streseman and Streseman (1960) identified three different patterns of feather loss for primary feathers among birds of prey:

Descending molt: Accipiters, harriers, Harris' hawks, New World vultures and kites show this pattern. It begins with the first primary and proceeds consecutively until the tenth, or outermost feather is reached (see Fig. 13.2, goshawk).

Beginning with the fourth primary: All falcons have almost the same pattern of moulting regarding the primary wing feathers. It starts with the fourth feather and proceeds in both directions from there. There is a minor distinction between the hierofalcon group and peregrine falcons. Hierofalcons (saker, gyr-, lanner and laggar falcons) follow the pattern: 4, 5, 6, 3, 7, 2, 8, 9, 1, 10 (see Fig. 13.2, gyrfalcon).

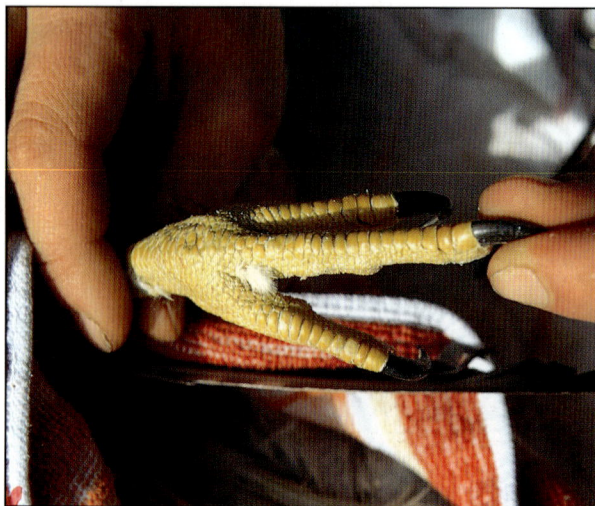

Fig. 13.1: "Atavistic" feather growth between the toes of a gyrfalcon (*Falco rusticolus*). (Photo: Heidenreich)

Peregrines, on the other hand, begin also with feather number four, but then proceed as follows: 4, 5, 3, 6, 7, 2, 8, 1, 9, 10 (see Fig. 13.2, peregrine falcon).

Mebs (1960) pursued this even further and determined that subtle differences in moulting patterns can be detected within the peregrine falcon species. Seventy percent of them lose the third feather before the sixth, while the remaining 30% of peregrines lose the sixth feather before the third.

Irregular moult: This pattern is seen in larger raptors, especially vultures and eagles. It begins in various locations along the wing and progresses in no predetermined order. Some species may moult in a "normal" descending pattern when young and then develop irre-

gular moults as they mature. Bearded vultures and golden eagles both fall into this category. A theory proposed by Streseman and Streseman suggests that this pattern reflects the phylogenetic connection between the original descending pattern and the newer irregular pattern, a form of ontogeny recapitulating phylogeny.

Very thin powder down feathers can be found close to the skin. They are constantly growing and disintegrating, releasing a fine keratin powder that helps condition feathers and reduce friction between them. The plumage is also conditioned by the secretions of the uropygial gland, a small structure located dorsally at the base of the tail. The oily substance produced there is collected with the beak and spread through the feathers during preening.

13.1.1 Moulting disorders

Feather loss of any kind occurring outside the moulting period is unusual. It may be associated with some types of drug therapy. Administration of chloramphenicol in growing young hawks, for instance, can lead to the development of damaged feathers or even permanent abnormalities of the plumage.

Similar circumstances were behind the "permanent" moult of the falcon depicted in Fig. 13.3. This patient

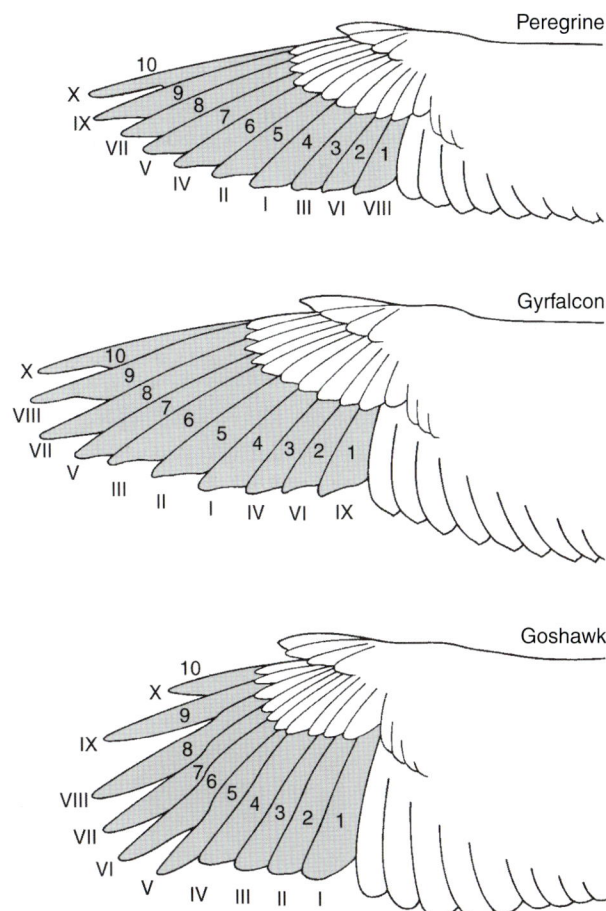

Fig. 13.2: Comparison of moulting patterns in a peregrine falcon, a hierofalcon (gyrfalcon), and a goshawk. (1–10, feather numbers; I–X, the order of feather growth). (Illustration: R. Gattung-Petith and A. Gattung)

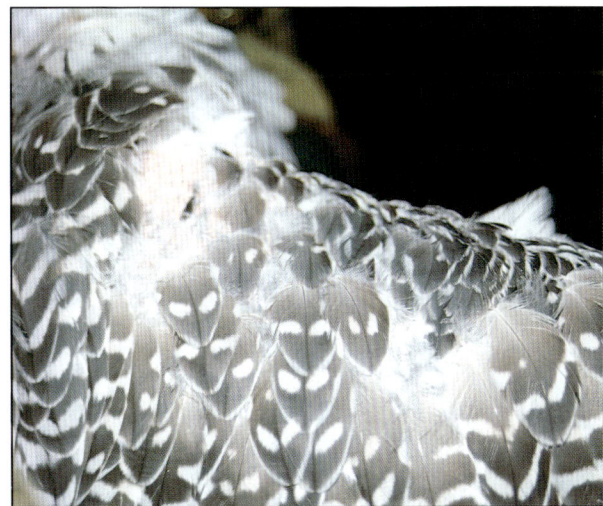

Fig. 13.3: A hybrid falcon (gyrfalcon X lanner falcon) was treated for inflammatory lesions of the feet with high-dose intramuscular injections of enrofloxacin for 8 days. Several days after that he began losing large tracts of feathers on the breast and on the dorsal aspects of the wings. Later, the flight feathers fell out as well, although it was not moulting season. Feathers that tried to regrow continued to fall out before reaching maturity.

was treated with enrofloxacin (Baytril®) for over a week. Shortly thereafter, the bird lost large numbers of feathers all over his body. He was unable to replace them for years afterward.

In 1976, a young white-tailed sea eagle (*Haliaeetus albicilla*) from a wild eyrie was found on the forest floor unable to fly. It had lost all flight feathers. This bird is still alive today, 20 years later, and has never developed a normal feather again. A similar syndrome with a viral etiology is known in cockatoos and parrots (Gylstorff and Grimm, 1987).

The distal-most primaries from both wings in an imperial eagle (*Aquila heliaca)* were so tightly grown together that they were moulted in bunches (Fig. 13.4). The cause of this problem was never discovered.

Falconers would often like to accelerate the moulting process, which normally takes several months, so that they can begin working their hawks earlier in the fall. This desire has ancient roots. Arab veterinarians as early as the 8th Century A.D. discussed methods by which this might be accomplished (Al Gitrif, 744). They recommended the feeding of a special type of "meat" obtained from sheep: "Use the meat that is found on either side of the airway at the site where the butcher slits the throat." Doubtless they were talking about the sheep's thyroid glands.

The influence that thyroid hormones have on moulting has apparently long been recognized. Indeed, supplementing with thyroxin will speed the moulting process. Such treatment involves significant risks for the bird, however.

Baronetzky-Mercer and Seidel (1995) recommend giving 1 mg/kg thyroxin PO SID to initiate moulting. This dose can be gradually increased if no response is seen.

In the author's own experience, the administration of thyroxin tablets at physiologic doses has never been successful. The feeding of approximately 25 grams of beef thyroid per kg of body weight, however, does induce moulting. About seven days after consuming this glandular material, the bird will begin massively losing feathers both large and small. A second treatment three weeks later generally results in the loss of all remaining feathers. The moulting sequence will not conform to the normal pattern and appears to be random. This type of treatment can not induce moulting, but only accelerates the process once it has begun.

Birds treated with beef thyroid will become markedly ravenous. The metabolic acceleration they undergo forces them to eat almost constantly. This phase lasts several days. Adequate amounts of top quality meat containing no casting materials such as fur or feathers must be offered during this period. Otherwise, the animal could literally starve to death on quantities of food that would normally be sufficient to sustain it!

As long as the bird's nutritional needs are fully met, the quality of the feathers that regrow after such treatment is as good as that of feathers produced during a normal moult.

A product called "Voliton" is available in Arab countries. According to the label, it is produced in Germany. The active ingredients are not listed, but presumably consist of thyroid hormones in some form. According to the instructions, the tablets should be given to falcons orally for 11 days to initiate and/or accelerate moulting. Since the manufacturer is not identified and the ingredients are unknown, such experimentation is not advised.

Thyroid supplementation strongly interferes with a bird's normal metabolic and endocrine processes and should not be undertaken simply to satisfy impatient falconers. There are, however, some situations in which acceleration of the moult may be justified – to permit the earlier release of a rehabilitated raptor with poor plumage, for instance.

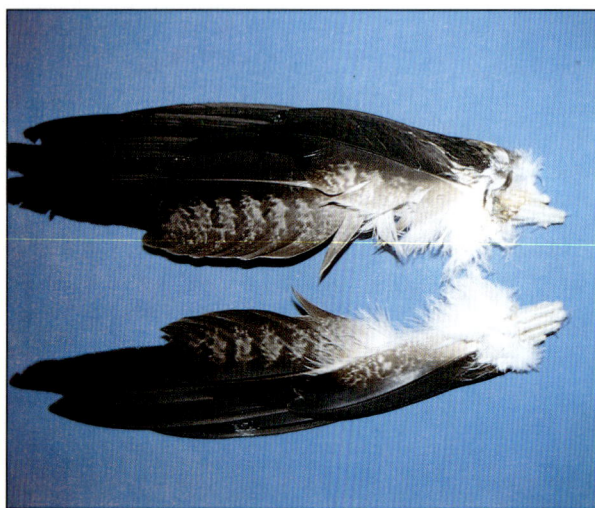

Fig. 13.4: An imperial eagle (*Aquila heliaca*) lost entire bundles of distal primary feathers during an otherwise normal moult. The feather follicles involved may have grown together as a result of bilateral injuries to the wing tips.
(Photo: Heidenreich)

13.1.2   Feather problems

13.1.2.1 Stress marks

Occasionally one can observe transparent lines that run straight across a feather (Fig. 13.5). These so-called stress marks are seen most commonly in young birds. Falconers call them "fret marks". They are often seen in nestlings taken from the wild who undergo a period of stress and refuse to eat when first brought into captivity.

Stress marks are rarely seen in wild birds although such birds are also subject to periods of insufficient food intake. It is therefore likely that stress, not malnutrition, is the primary factor in causing these disruptions in feather development. Episodes of stress or shock result in the shunting of blood to vital organs, leaving peripheral tissues like skin and growing feathers poorly perfused. The result is a temporary disruption in nourishment to the growing feather and a corresponding area of weakness in the emerging vane. The term "stress marks", as used by Cooper and Harrison (1994), is therefore appropriate.

If this type of feather damage is minimal and limited to only a few feathers, it will not affect a bird's ability to fly. Larger stress marks, on the other hand, can affect the strength of the shaft and make the feather vulnerable to breakage.

Wild-caught eyasses will often develop a band of stress marks across their entire tail. Until these feathers are molted the following year, they serve as a record indicating approximately how old the bird was when it was removed from the nest.

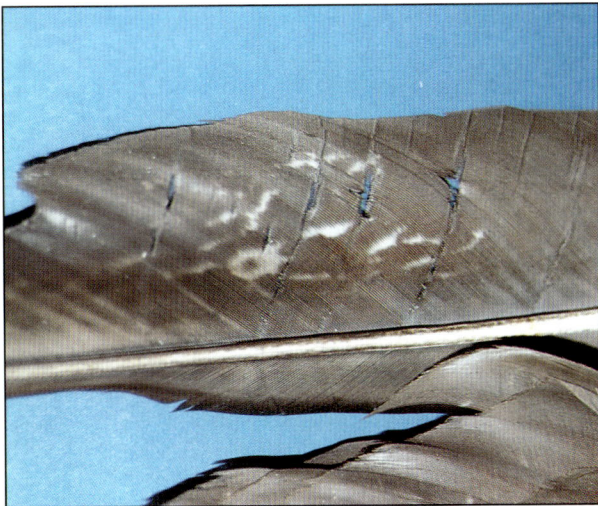

Fig. 13.5: A wing feather from a golden eagle (*Aquila chryseatos*) showing numerous stress marks. (Photo: Heidenreich)

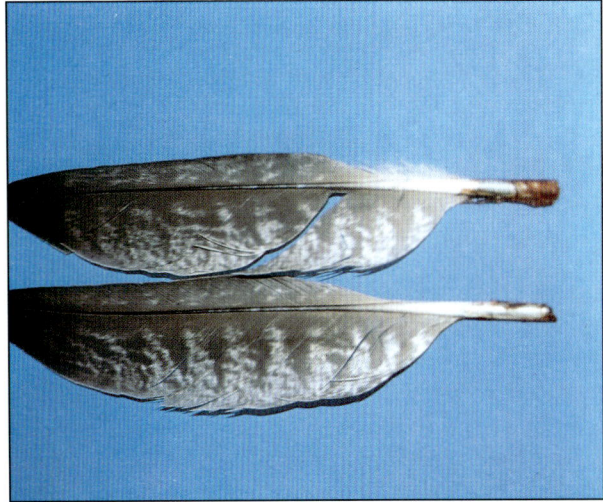

Fig. 13.6: The fourth and fifth primary feathers from the wing of a gyrfalcon (*Falco rusticolus*). They were injured while still in the pin feather stage and broke off. (Photo: Heidenreich)

13.1.2.2 Injuries to pin feathers

Injuries to the pulpy shaft of growing feathers always have a serious impact on feather development. Frequently all growth ceases, the pulp dries up and an hourglass-shaped constriction appears at the site of injury. The feather easily breaks off at the constriction (Fig. 13.6). The remaining proximal portion of the shaft is lost soon thereafter. Normally, a new feather will develop from that follicle. If several adjacent feathers have been damaged and lost at once, there is a great risk that these redeveloping feathers will be injured again. They will lack the protection normally provided for a fragile pin feather by the mature feathers surrounding it.

A bird's ability to fly, and therefore to hunt, is of critical importance to the falconer. Those who work with birds of prey pay close attention to each growing feather and take great care to avoid damage to them.

13.1.2.3 Pulled feathers

The loss of fully developed feathers outside the moulting period can occur in many different ways. Aggressive quarry can sometimes pull feathers from a hawk, or a transmitter attached to the tail feathers can pull them out if it gets caught on a wire or a branch. Raptors hit by cars frequently lose wing or tail feathers that get caught under the rolling wheel of the automobile.

While smaller contour feathers normally grow back without any trouble, the regrowth of a forcibly removed flight or tail feather is problematic. There has usually been some damage to the feather follicle or the surrounding skin. If the follicle grows shut during the healing process, the regrowing feather will be unable to emerge, curling subcutaneously within the follicle instead, and forming a cyst that can get as big as a walnut. When such cysts are cut open, they are filled with dark, dry feather material.

To prevent the development of feather cysts, it has long been a practice to insert a kernel of rice or wheat into the follicular opening to keep it patent during the healing process. Richter (1990) modified this technique, taking the shaft from the pulled feather, cutting it to a length of two centimeters, and suturing it back in place for three weeks.

In some cases, pulled flight feathers simply do not regrow at all, or there is disruption of the critical attachment to the periosteum of the wing bone that gives the feather its stability. These types of injuries have very serious consequences for the bird's ability to fly.

If, for some reason, a flight feather or a broken feather shaft needs to be pulled, this can be done without damage to the follicle by applying a few drops of hyaluronidase (Hylase®) to the lumen of the shaft at the base. This enzyme will soften the keratin structure of the feather and diffuse into the surrounding connective tissues to loosen them. In a matter of minutes, the feather can be firmly grasped with a pair of pliers and pulled out with a gentle tug. There will be no injury to the feather follicle or the surrounding tissues.

13.1.2.4 Broken feathers

Inappropriate housing and perches, or accidents during the hunt can result in damage and breaking of the large flight and tail feathers. If a gap is thus created, the surrounding feathers become vulnerable to damage themselves and a vicious cycle of feather damage begins. To avoid such a situation, and especially to keep the bird able to fly and hunt, broken feathers should be repaired or "imped".

Imping is an ancient practice. Traditionally, the old and new portions of the feather were connected with an edged steel needle that was treated with lemon juice or salt water to promote oxidation (rusting) and help glue it in place.

Nowadays, elastic fiberglass rods, thin bamboo sticks or the shaft of a discarded feather are used instead. Rapid-setting glue is used to help join the feather parts together with the rod inside the hollow shaft. This type of work demands a fair amount of experience and care, since the replacement feather needs to be matched closely to the original. As a replacement piece the broken-off portion, a previously molted feather from the same bird or feathers from a differ-

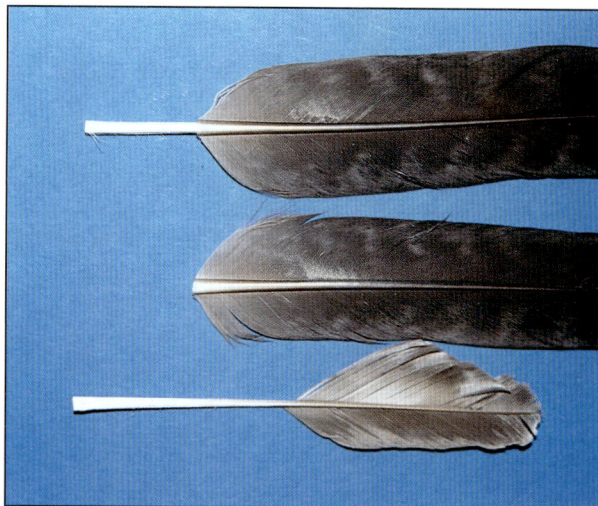

13.7

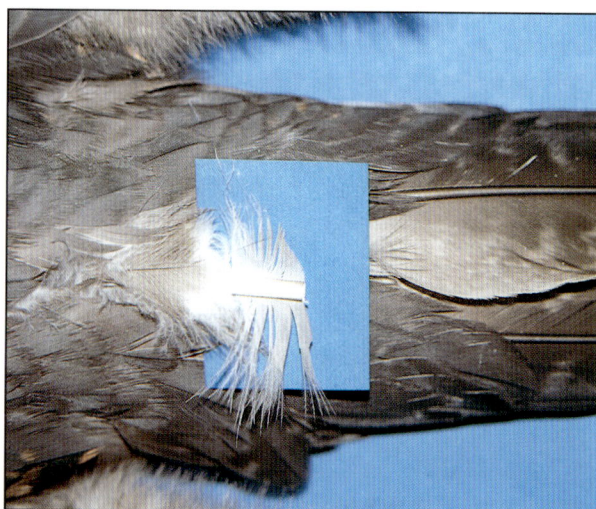

13.8

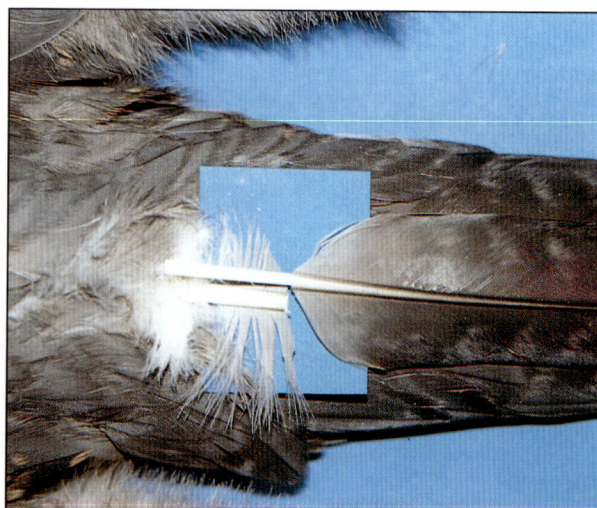

13.9

ent bird, preferably of the same species, can be used. Person (1990) gives a good description of imping using a feather shaft as shown in Figs. 13.7–13.10.

Since the bird must remain very still for these manipulations, and nearby feathers have to be pushed aside to prevent them from getting stuck with glue, it is usually best to anesthetize the hawk for this procedure (see Ch. 15).

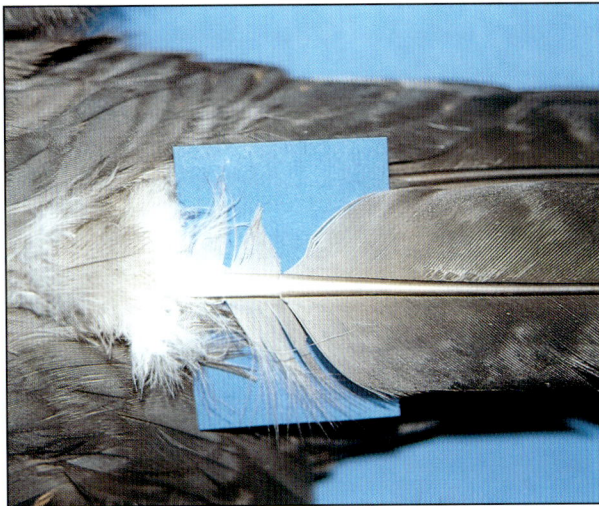

13.10

Figs. 13.7, 13.8, 13.9 and 13.10:
Among falconers, the practice of repairing broken feathers by imping is centuries old. The keratin shaft of another feather makes the best material for repair. It incorporates the necessary qualities of strength and flexibility better than do fiberglass, metal or bamboo needles.

First, a feather whose shaft has approximately the same size and shape as the one to be repaired is chosen. The vane is removed on both sides and the remaining shaft is trimmed to a length of a few centimeters. The pin thus created is inserted halfway into the new replacement feather (preferably the identical feather from a previous moult) and fixed in place with epoxy glue (13.7).

The broken feather on the bird is cut off a few centimeters above the skin and exposed by placing a small piece of paper between it and the other feathers (13.8). The replacement feather is fitted in place and any necessary corrections (13.9) are made before the whole thing is joined with epoxy (13.10). Care must be taken not to get glue on any of the other feathers. The length and position of the repaired feather can be checked and corrected before the epoxy has hardened.
(Photos: Heidenreich)

13.1.2.5 Bent feathers

Flight feathers that have been merely bent or kinked without actually disrupting the shaft can be straightened using steam or hot water. Heat and moisture cause the keratin to swell and straighten in a matter of seconds. Repeated exposure to hot water, however, can leach the oils from the feather, leaving it dry and brittle. It is helpful, therefore, to treat the straightened feather afterwards with uropygial gland secretions from a pigeon or duck.

A feather straightener is a small tweezer-like tool used for repairing bent feathers. Its flattened ends are heated with a match and then quickly applied to the kinked portion of the shaft. The natural moisture inside the feather works just as the steam described above, and the defect is straightened.

13.1.2.6 Deformed feathers

"Curly" feathers have occasionally been observed in hawks. Only a few wing coverts were thus affected in the bird depicted in Fig. 13.11. What role genetic or

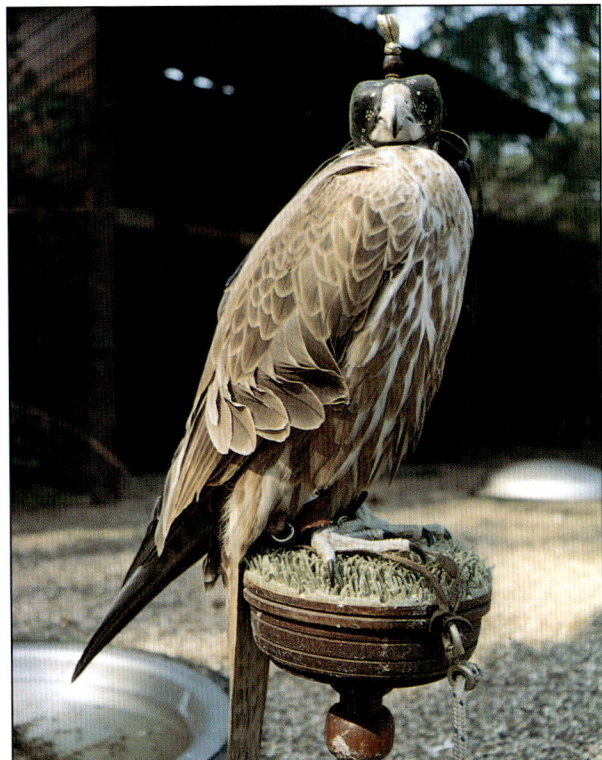

Fig. 13.11: This young saker falcon (*Falco cherrug*) developed curly feathers bilaterally among the wing coverts of his immature plumage.
(Photo: Heidenreich)

developmental factors play in such things is un-known. The siblings and parents of this bird were unaffected.

13.1.2.7 Disorders of feather development

As feathers grow, they are initially surrounded by a keratin sheath. This sheath splits at the tip and peels away to release the feather vane. Sometimes the sheath fails to come off, leaving the bird with long spiny shafts in place of the normal feather (Fig. 13.12).

The possible reasons for this type of disruption in feather development are many. Normally, the keratin sheath is removed by the bird in the daily process of preening. A hawk unaccustomed to its surroundings and under stress may not find the time to do this, and the feather will be left inside its sheath.

Excess humidity, insufficient exposure to sunlight or inadequate opportunities to bathe can also interfere with normal removal of the keratin covering. Wet keratin is soft and rubbery, making it difficult to peel off with the beak. If the sheath isn't allowed to dry well enough, it will not split open. A growing feather requires alternate periods of wetness and drying, as well as attention during preening, to develop and unfold normally.

If this type of problem occurs, it is almost impossible to obtain a completely normal feather, even if the keratin sheath is manually removed.

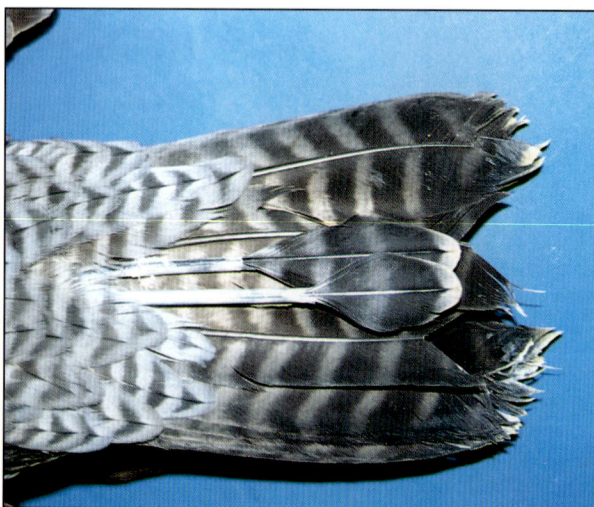

Fig. 13.12: Pin feather sheaths that fail to open, as in the tail of this peregrine falcon (*Falco peregrinus*), prevent the normal unfolding of the feather vanes.
(Photo: Heidenreich)

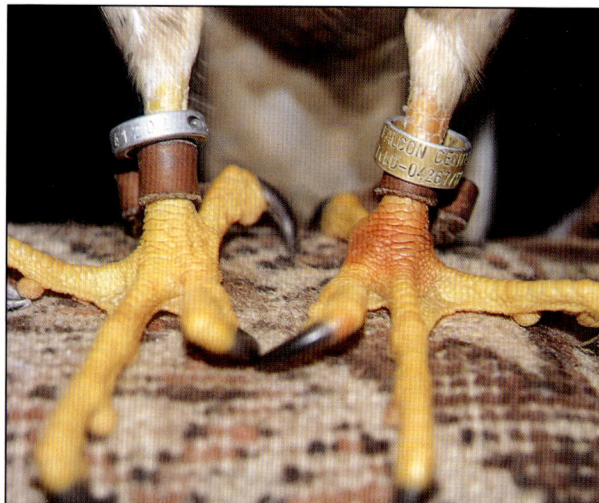

Fig. 13.13: Falcons sometimes strike their quarry at very high speeds. This can lead to foot injuries like the bruise seen on this bird. Some of the smaller, more aggressive falcons are prone to injuries of this type when they go after game that is too large for them.
(Photo: Heidenreich)

13.1.3 Subcutaneous emphysema

Injuries to the air sacs, after an impact with an obstacle for instance, can allow air to escape into the subcutaneous connective tissues. The emphysema that results may be limited to a small area around the site of the injury, or it may spread over large portions of the body. Affected birds may appear lumpy or inflated.

Palpation of the emphysematous areas will reveal a distinctive crackling. The thin avian skin may be tightly stretched over the air pockets and the feathers will stand on end. Otherwise, the hawk will seem unaffected.

Treating this condition is relatively simple. Small incisions are made in the skin at several locations. The air can be heard to escape with a small hissing sound. Any remaining air pockets can be gently massaged towards the skin openings and allowed to escape. The skin incisions generally close more quickly than the air sac rupture, and a second treatment is often required.

13.1.4 Hematomas

Subcutaneous hemorrhages or bruising are generally only recognized on the unfeathered portions of the avian integument. In hunting hawks they occur on the feet (Fig. 13.13) after altercations with large or aggressive quarry. If no external injuries posing a risk of infection are found, no further treatment is necessary. Resorption of the hematoma will occur within a few days. Larger bruises can be treated with topical gels (Hirudoid) that accelerate their resorption.

13.1.5   Abscesses

Injuries to the skin that become infected can quickly turn into abscesses. These will usually require surgical intervention to resolve. Unlike in mammals, avian pus is not liquid, but rather firm and cheesy in consistency (Fig. 13.14). A simple incision will therefore not suffice to drain the abscess. After exposing the purulent material, it is generally necessary to curette out the necrotic material and pus, then flush the wound thoroughly with some type of antiseptic to make sure that no residual infectious material remains.

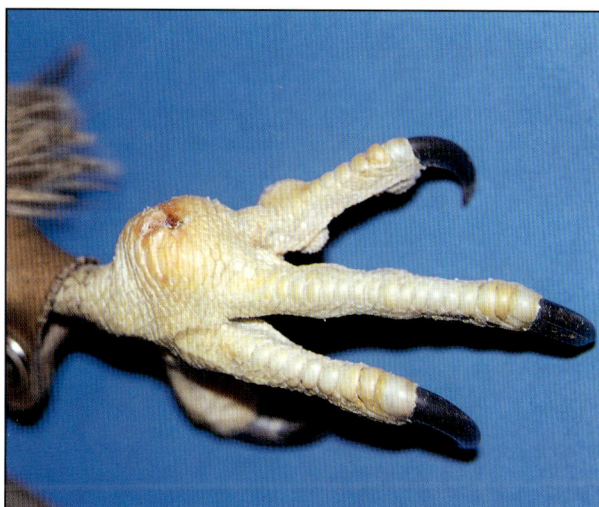

Fig. 13.14: This abscess on the dorsal aspect of the foot of a saker falcon (*Falco cherrug*) still shows the puncture site through which the bacterial pathogens gained entrance weeks ago.   (Photo: Heidenreich)

13.1.6   Wounds

Skin lacerations are common in hunting hawks, although their natural prey are rarely the cause. Barbed wire and other sharp objects in the environment are more commonly at fault. The mews or aviaries should therefore always be carefully checked for sharp wires, nails or other objects which could result in injury to the bird.

Avian skin is extremely thin and tears easily. The edges of the wound dry out quickly, making repair more difficult. Treatment of skin lacerations, even if performed promptly, will usually require surgical debridement and freshening of the skin edges before closure. Although this procedure will enlarge the wound, areas like the neck or abdomen generally have enough loose skin to compensate.

The breast area and back are covered relatively tightly with skin. Wound closure here can be difficult. Fortunately, healing by second intention, even for relatively large wounds, usually carries a good prognosis. Birds generally have a better healing capacity than mammals.

Small puncture wounds, especially those that penetrate into the muscle, are of much greater concern. Wounds of this type, often caused by the talons of another hawk, are prone to developing clostridial dermatomyositis (see Ch. 9.2.2.2). They should be immediately flushed with hydrogen peroxide.

References and literature of further interest

AL GITRIF (744):
Die Beizvögel. Übersetzung Georg Olms Verlag, Hildesheim, Zürich, New York

BARONETZKY-MERCIER, A. and B. SEIDEL (1995):
in: Göltenboth, R. and H.G. Klös: Krankheiten der Zoo- und Wildtiere. 443–465
Blackwell Wissenschafts-Verlag, Berlin

BRÜLL, H. (1981):
Über Verhalten und Mauser brutpflegender Seeadler (*Haliaeetus albicilla*) in offenen Zuchtvolieren im »Wildpark Eekholt«.
Jb. Dtsch. Falkenorden, 17–23

BRÜLL, H. (1986):
Stoßmauser eines jungen Seeadlers (*Haliaeetus albicilla*) bis zur Geschlechtsreife.
Jb. Dtsch. Falkenorden, 46–48

COOPER, J.E. and G.J. HARRISON (1994):
in: RITCHIE, B.W., HARRISON, G.J. and L.R. HARRISON (1994):
Avian medicine, 608–639
Wingers Publishing, Lake Worth, Florida, USA

DORSCHNER, K. (1975):
Ein Vergleich von vier Mauserperioden eines Beizsperbers.
Jb. Dtsch. Falkenorden, 43–46

GRÜNHAGEN, H. (1985):
Vorschlag zur Verbesserung des Schiftens.
Jb. Dtsch. Falkenorden, 65–66

GRÜNHAGEN, H. (1988):
Federanomalien bei Greifvögeln.
Greifvögel und Falknerei, 73–76
Verlag Neumann-Neudamm, Morschen-Heina

GYLSTORFF, I. and F. GRIMM (1987):
Vogelkrankheiten.
Verlag Euen Ulmer, Stuttgart

KÖSTERS, J. (1979):
Die physiologische Mauser bei Greifvögeln und Möglichkeiten
ihrer Beeinflussung.
Prakt. Tierarzt **60**, 226–233

LAWNICZAK, W. (1980):
Das Schiften gebrochener Pennen mit Glasfiber.
Jb. Dtsch. Falkenorden, 75

MEBS, T. (1960):
Untersuchungen über den Rhythmus der Schwingen- und
Schwanzmauser bei großen Falken.
J. Orn. **101**, 175–194

PERSON, M. (1990):
Dr. Mike's foolproof imping method.
Hawk Chalk **29**, 59–61

RICHTER, T. (1990):
Ausgerissene Schwanzfeder bei einem Beizfalken
Greifvögel und Falknerei, 107
Verlag Neumann-Neudamm, Morschen Heina

RÖDDER, A. (1985):
Stoßmauser bei einem Bussard-Nestling?
Jb. Dtsch. Falkenorden, 47

STRESEMANN, V. and E. STRESEMANN (1960):
Die Handschwingenmauser der Tagraubvögel.
J. Orn. **101**, 373–403

13.2 Beak and talons

13.2.1 Beak disorders

Raptors possess variously shaped and specialized beaks, depending on their manner of killing and/or consuming prey. With the exception of a few highly specialized species, beaks among raptors can be roughly separated into two categories (Figs. 13.15 and 13.16).

13.2.1.1 Traumatic injuries to the beak

The normal beak is a strong horny structure with a shiny smooth surface. It grows continuously outward from the base and the underlying bone. Even minor injuries to this area can result in abnormal ridges or gaps in the beak as it grows out (Fig. 13.17). If loose fragments are present, they should be removed to prevent further tearing of the beak material.

Continuous injury and irritation to the zone of beak growth, as occurs with shy birds that habitually fly into their aviary wires nose first, can lead to permanent and non-correctable malformations of the upper beak (Fig. 13.18).

Incorrect feeding practices can prevent a hawk from experiencing normal beak wear and lead to overgrowth of the upper beak. An exclusive diet of soft day-old chicks is often at fault. The overgrown horny tip sometimes breaks off. If it does not, the long horny structure may interfere with normal closure of the beak (Fig. 13.19).

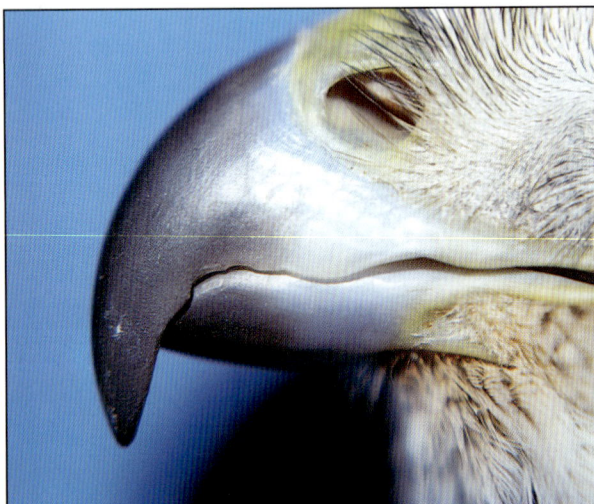

Fig. 13.15: The hooked cutting beak of accipiters and buteos is designed only for tearing and ingesting food. Birds with this type of beak kill their prey by footing and have well-developed talons.
(Photo: Heidenreich)

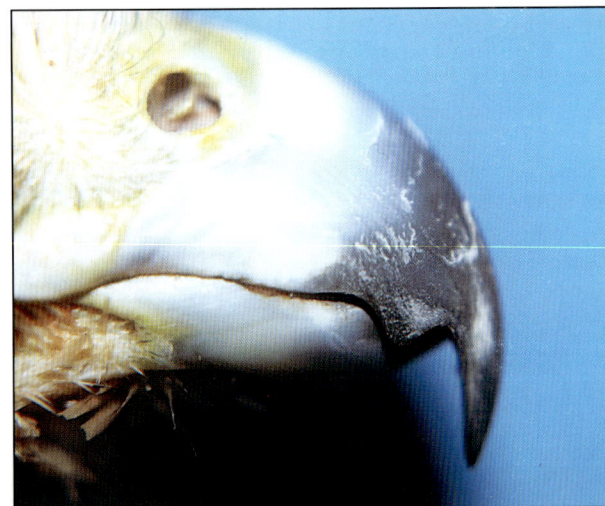

Fig. 13.16: The hooked biting beak of falcons functions both in tearing or ingesting meat, and in the killing of prey by biting the nape of the neck. The distinctive "tooth" found on falcon beaks probably aids in the killing function. These birds of prey merely grasp with their feet and have relatively short talons. (Photo: Heidenreich).

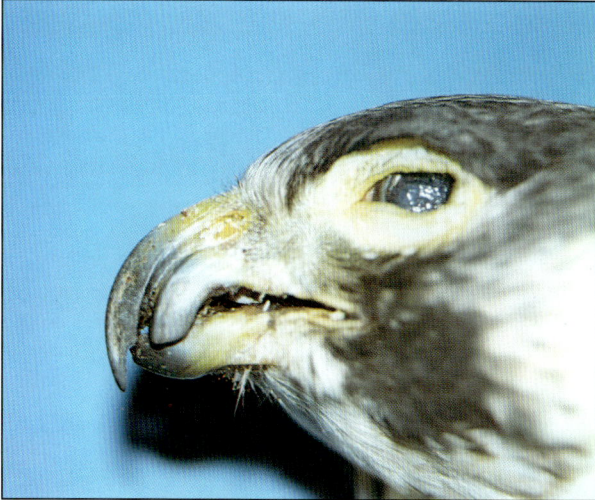

13.17

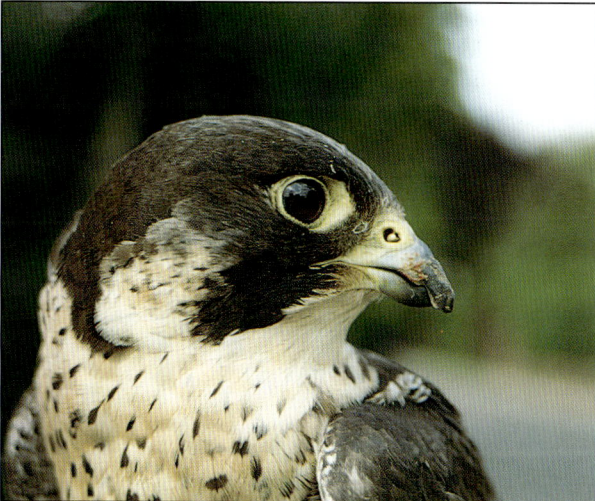

△ 13.18

▽ 13.19

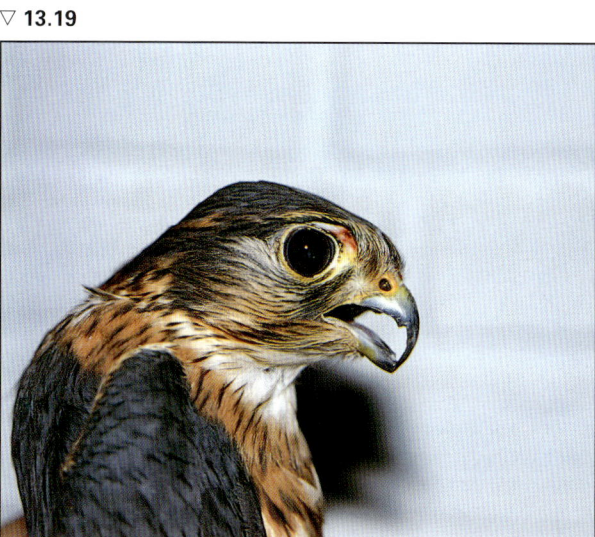

Since growth and development of the upper and lower beaks are interdependent and influenced by mutual wear, injuries to one of them often result in abnormal growth of the other (Fig. 13.20).

Falcons occasionally develop an overgrown tooth on the upper beak. This can tear and lead to injury (Fig. 13.21) or even break off completely. Such damage to the beak heals very slowly, repair being dependent on the characteristically slow rate of beak regeneration.

Overgrown beaks, in contrast, are easily corrected. Careful cutting with nail clippers or filing with a fine electric sander (Dremel tool) will quickly restore the beak to its original shape.

Uni- or bilateral brown crusty lesions occurring at the base of the beak are usually caused by a poorly fitting hood (Fig. 13.22). Prolonged periods of continuous pressure will result in barely noticeable oozing lesions within hours. Later these areas develop varying degrees of necrosis. The affected bird should immediately be fitted with a suitable hood that will permit the pressure sores to heal.

13.2.1.2 Beak damage due to disease

In birds of prey, severe cases of rickets (see Ch. 11.2.1.1) affect not only the long bones of the wings and legs, but also cause beak deformities. This is due to softening of the bony maxilla and mandibles that lie underneath the horny coverings.

Vitamin or mineral deficiencies can also affect the growth of the keratin covering of the beak. Hypovitaminosis A, for example, can result in dry, hyperkeratotic lesions strongly resembling the pathologic changes caused by epidermoptid mites (see Ch. 10.4.1.4).

Figs. 13.17, 13.18 and 13.19: Even minor injuries to the zone of growth at the base of the bill can result in permanent damage to the horny tissue, manifested as grooves in the growing beak (13.17). More extensive damage to the cere area may produce permanent abnormalities in the development of the upper beak (13.18). Inappropriate feeding practices, including the excessive feeding of soft foods (day-old chicks) can result in insufficient wear on the upper beak and beak overgrowth (13.19), such as seen in this merlin tiercel (*Falco columbarius*).
(Photos: Heidenreich)

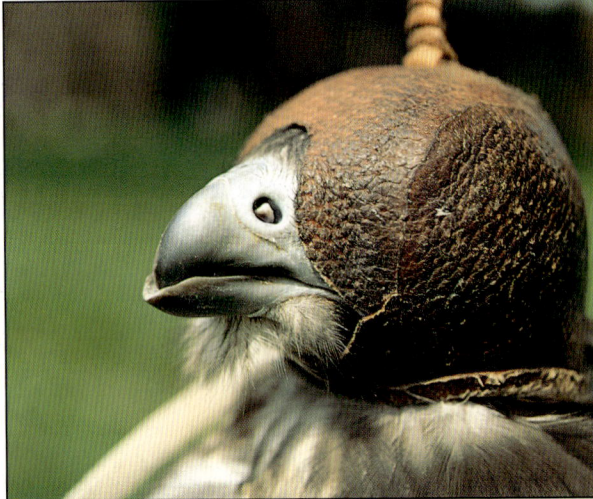

13.20

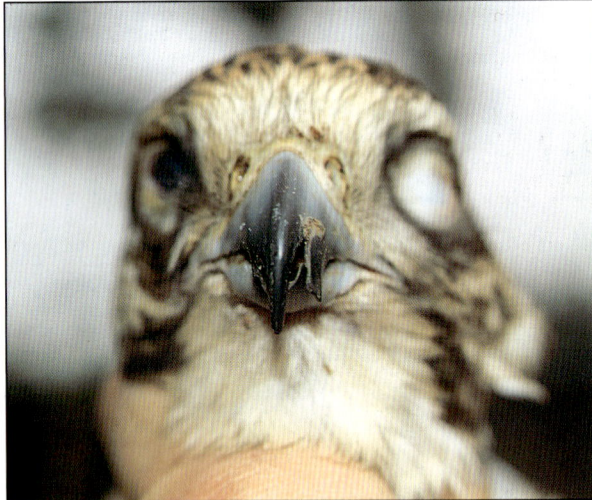

△ 13.21

▽ 13.22

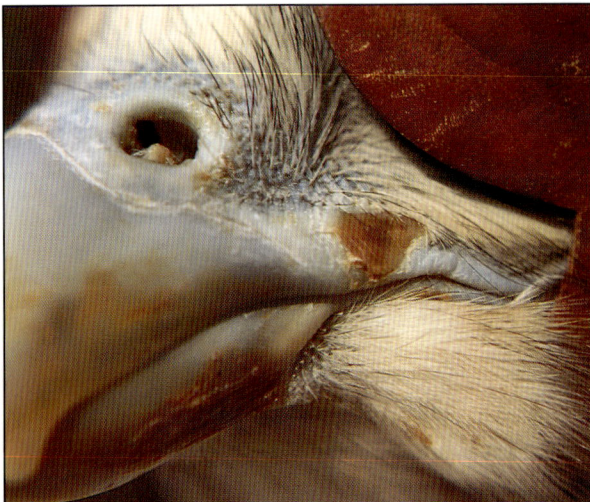

13.2.2   Talon disorders

As with beaks, the structure of a raptor's feet and talons reflects the way in which that particular species captures and kills prey. Two primary forms are recognized among those that grasp their quarry (Fig. 13.23).

Ospreys (*Pandion haliaetus*) are unique in having an outer toe that can be brought backward to grasp fish better. Also for that purpose, they are endowed with a very rough-textured epidermis on the grasping surfaces of their feet. The secretary bird (*Sagittarius serpentarius*), has short toes and dull claws suited for rapid movement on the ground and for stomping snakes to death. Other groups, such as the vultures, who do not hunt, have only minimally modified claws.

Like the beak, the talons grow continuously from their base. Injuries to this zone of proliferation can interfere with development of the horny tissue of the claws. Trauma or disease can result in a complete loss of the hard, keratinous covering of the talon. If the nail bed is injured as well, the talon will be unable to regrow (Fig. 13.25), or it will regrow abnormally.

Loss of the talon's horny covering leaves the underlying phalangeal bone exposed. It should be immediately covered with an ointment such as cod liver oil salve to keep the periosteum from desiccating. This will improve the chances that a normal talon will be able to grow back. The process of regrowth can take many weeks. The bandage should be changed regularly and left off only after the bone is completely protected by a healthy black covering of horny tissue.

Figs. 13.20, 13.21 and 13.22: If the hooked portion of the upper beak is missing, normal wear of the lower beak is disrupted and the lower beak overgrows, as in the hybrid falcon (*Falco peregrinus X Falco rusticolus)* depicted here (13.20). The toothed portion of a falcon's beak can overgrow as well. It is then at risk of breaking off or cracking, and injuring the upper beak, as in this saker falcon (*Falco cherrug).* Loose pieces should be removed immediately to prevent further damage.
Improperly fitted hoods that cover and put pressure on the corners of the mouth can lead to pressure necrosis of the affected areas in a matter of hours. A well-designed and properly fitted hood leaves these areas exposed (13.22).
(Photos: Heidenreich)

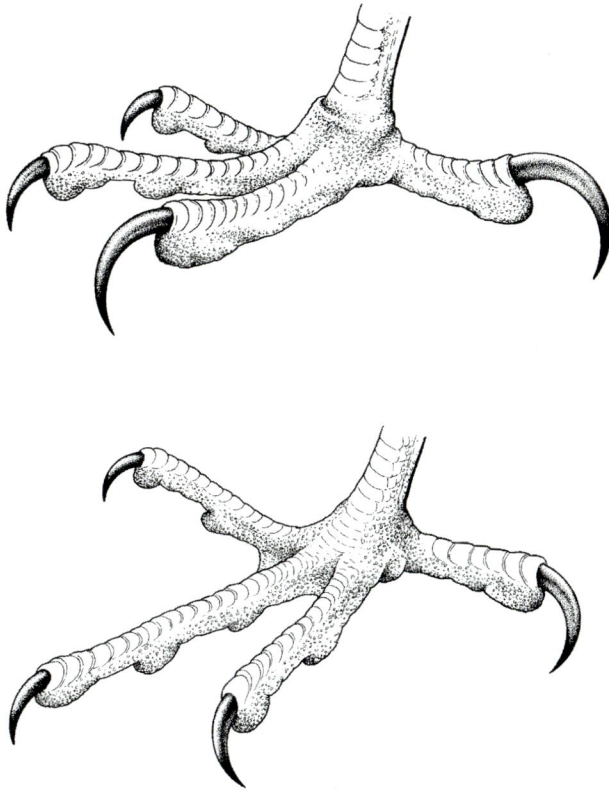

Fig. 13.23: A bird of prey that kills with its feet (top) has longer talons than one who uses the feet only for grasping (bottom).
(Illustration: R. Gattung-Petith and A. Gattung)

Insufficient wear of the talons occurs when birds are kept on unsuitable perches. As the talon continues to grow, it will curl in a corkscrew fashion (Fig. 13.24). Trimming or "coping" is necessary to return the claws to normal.

Young birds just removed from the aviary, or any raptor that is still shy and unpredictable, should have the sharp tips of the talons coped before beginning training. This will prevent the bird from injuring itself or others, especially if it decides to lash out while hooded. This practice will also reduce the risk that the hawk will tear off its own hood during the early stages of manning. By the time the bird has been manned and trained for the hunt, the talons will have regained their original sharpness.

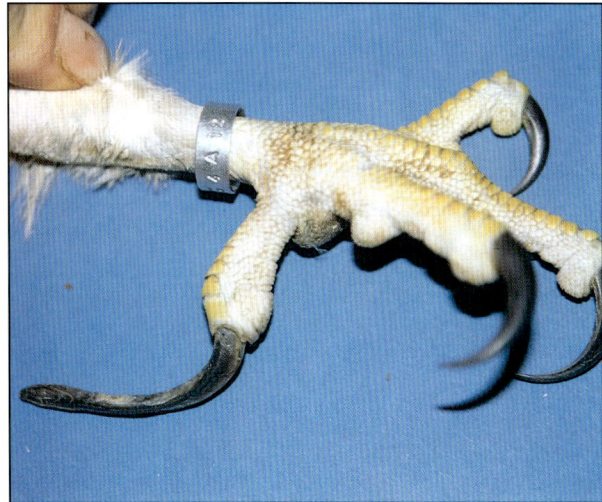

Fig. 13.24: Insufficient wear results in overgrowth of the continuously growing talons. Such overgrown talons put the bird at risk of injuring itself.
(Photo: Heidenreich)

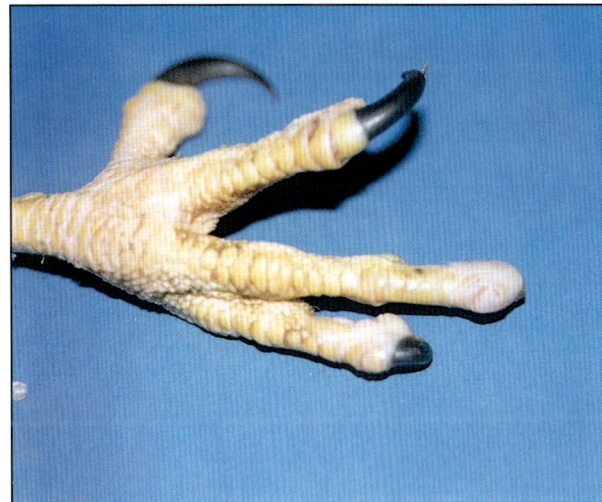

Fig. 13.25:
Severe injuries that result in loss of the distal phalanx and the base of the claw cause permanent loss of the corresponding talon. This picture shows the foot of a gyrfalcon (*Falco rusticolus*) that suffered permanent damage to the talons after a bout of pox. Pox lesions involving the feet did irreversible damage to the bird's nail beds.
(Foto: Heidenreich)

References and literature of further interest

KRUSE, D. (1988):
Überschnabel bei Lannerfalken und die Folgen.
Greifvögel und Falknerei 77–79
Verlag Neumann-Neudamm, Morschen-Heina

13.3   Eyes

Raptors are visually oriented animals. It is therefore not surprising that they have very well-developed eyes. The globe is surprisingly large in relation to the size of the skull. The visual acuity of raptors is eight times better than that of humans and is said to be one of the best in the animal kingdom. Fischer (1969) was able to prove that vultures have eyes sharp enough to accurately identify an object only eight centimeters in size from a height of 1000 meters.

In contrast to humans, birds of prey have two foveae, or areas of sharp focusing ability, in their retinas. One fovea is positioned to receive images from the side of the bird's head, the other focuses in front. The four foveae of both eyes combined permit raptors to judge distances with much greater accuracy than simple binocular vision would allow.

Because the globe is so large, its mobility within the orbit is limited. Birds compensate for this by having a very flexible and mobile head that can turn to provide visual images from all directions.

The supraorbital bone of many species extends over the dorsal aspect of the orbit, providing some protection for the large eye. This same feature gives accipiters and eagles their "stern" expression (Fig. 13.26). Raptors also have a well-developed third eyelid, or nictitans, which is capable of moving across the cornea to protect and lubricate it (Fig. 13.27).

13.3.1   Traumatic injuries to eyes

Murphy et al. reported a 15% incidence of eye disease in raptors. Ninety percent of that is a result of traumatic injury, primarily from automobile and train collisions (33%), or gunshot wounds (13%). Injuries of this type are usually unilateral.

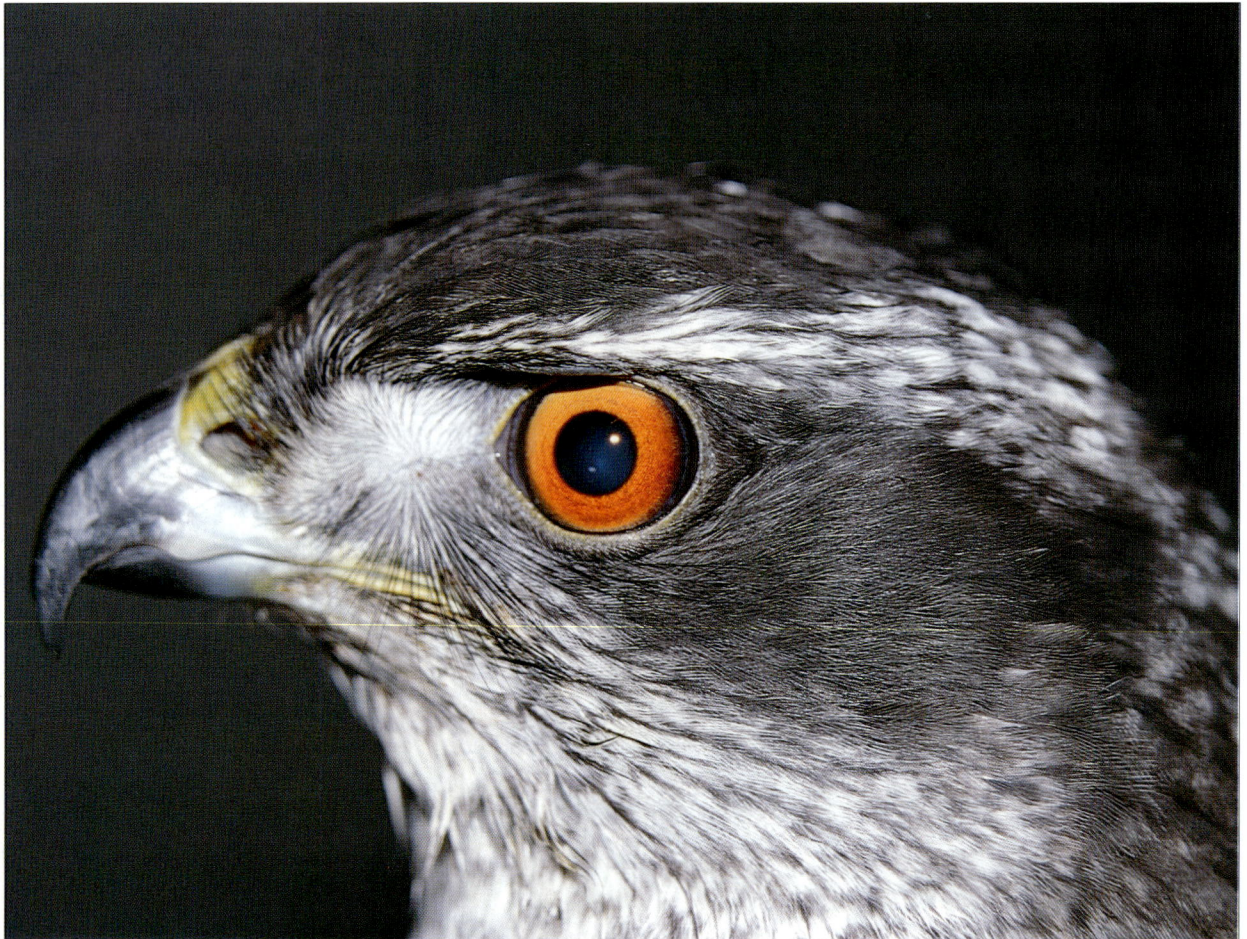

Fig. 13.26: The supraorbital bone jutting out above this goshawk (*Accipiter gentilis*) tiercel's eye serves not only to protect the eye, but also to provide shade for the exposed part of the globe. That is why the iris is less deeply pigmented dorsally where it is shaded best (see also Ch. 17.1).
(Photo: Heidenreich)

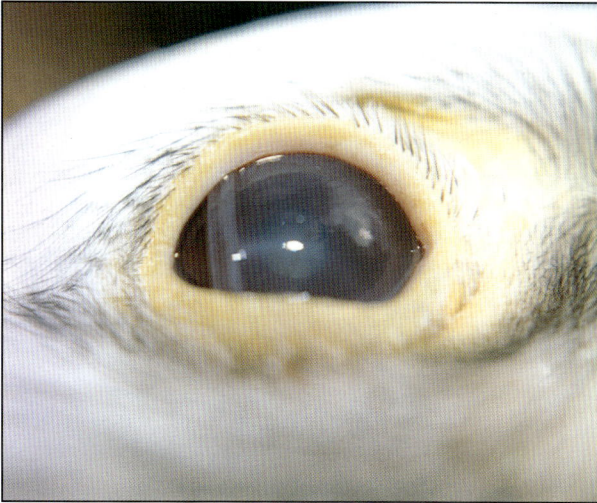

Fig. 13.27: The third eyelid (membrana nictitans) functions in the protection of the cornea and distribution of the precorneal tear film. It is often transparent, as seen in this white gyrfalcon (*Falco rusticolus*).
(Photo: Heidenreich)

eyelids up and over the eye, temporarily blinding the bird. Although such measures may seem cruel at first glance, Remple and Gross (1993) claim that this is not painful for the bird. Indeed, it immediately calms newly captured falcons and reduces the stress they experience.

The hawk's attempts to open its eyes produce permanent tension on the sutures. As the thin tissue of the eyelids stretches, the eyes gradually open and the bird is able to see a little more each day (Fig. 13.31). The passage hawk thus gradually becomes accustomed to its environment. It loses its initial fear and is ready for training sooner than is a bird manned using only a hood.

Blunt trauma to the eye can result in hemorrhages within the anterior chamber, easily visualized as a dark red discoloration in front of the iris. Hyphema like this is usually resorbed within a few days. Fundic exams sometimes reveal retinal detachments or blood in the posterior chamber.

More severe trauma can cause tearing of the iris or lens luxation. Adhesions of the iris to other structures in the eye, called synechiae, may develop as the eye heals. They often result in serious visual impairment for the bird.

Penetrating injuries of the cornea allow escape of the aqueous humor and collapse of the eye.

Any injury resulting in loss of sight may manifest as a loss of pupillary light reflexes. The pupil will appear dilated and the animal will try to compensate by turning its head so that the normal eye is focused on objects of interest in the environment.

Trauma to the eyelids in the form of lacerations is common in birds of prey. If such damage is not immediately surgically repaired, permanent disfigurement and visual impairment can result (Figs. 13.28 and 13.29).

Wild-caught falcons in the Middle East often have small notches located centrally on the edge of each lower eyelid. These stem from the practice of "seeling", a procedure applied to almost every wild-caught bird in those regions.

In this procedure, the eyes are sutured closed (Fig. 13.30). A fine thread is placed through each lower eyelid and then the threads from both sides are tied together at the top of the head. This pulls the

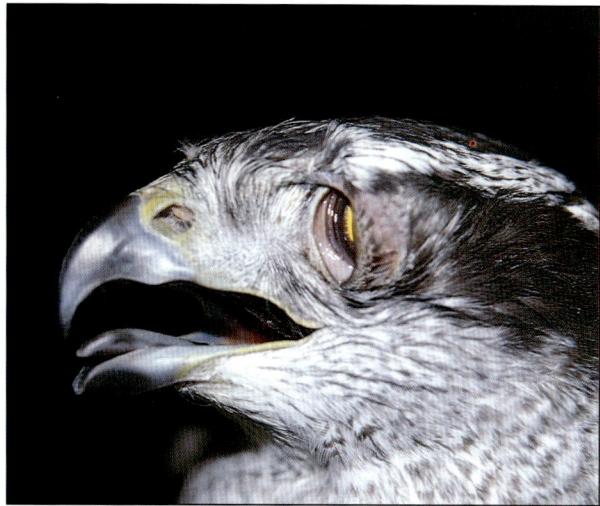

13.28

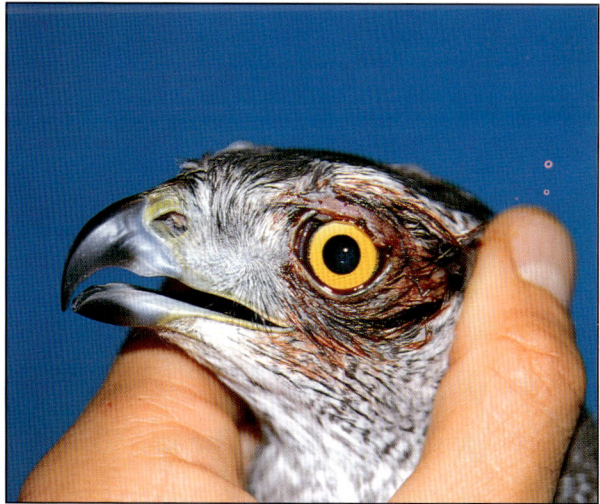

13.29

Figs. 13.28 and 13.29: An injury involving the left eyelids of this goshawk (*Accipiter gentilis*) resulted in almost complete fusion of the lids as they healed (13.28). Surgical intervention was required to separate them and allow the eye to function normally again (13.29). (Fotos: Heidenreich)

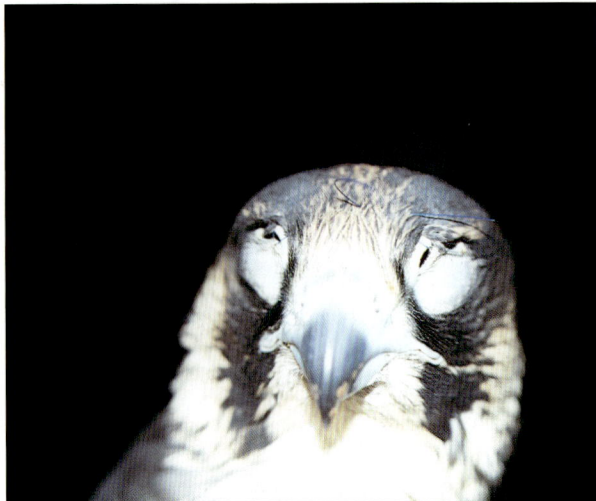

△ 13.30   13.31 ▽

notches like this is generally assumed to be a wild-caught bird imported from the Middle East.

13.3.2   Cataracts

Cataracts are whitish opacities involving the lens, most commonly seen in older birds of prey (Fig. 13.32). Changes in lens fiber composition interfere with the penetration of light into the eye and result in some degree of visual impairment. Kern et al. (1984) and Koch (1992) describe a surgical technique for lens extraction in birds of prey suffering from cataracts. This type of surgery may improve the cosmetic appearance of a bird and allow some improvement in vision. However, aphakic vision is unlikely to be good enough to allow a bird to hunt or to be released to the wild.

Medical treatment of cataracts is not possible.

13.3.3   Disorders of the eyelids and conjunctiva

Various infectious diseases of raptors (see Ch. 9) can involve the eyelids (palpebrae) or conjunctiva. Signs will range from mild swelling to complete closure of the lids (Fig. 13.33).

There is usually an increase in tear production resulting in wetness of the periocular feathers (Fig. 13.34) and causing the hawk to rub its face on the ipsilateral wing.

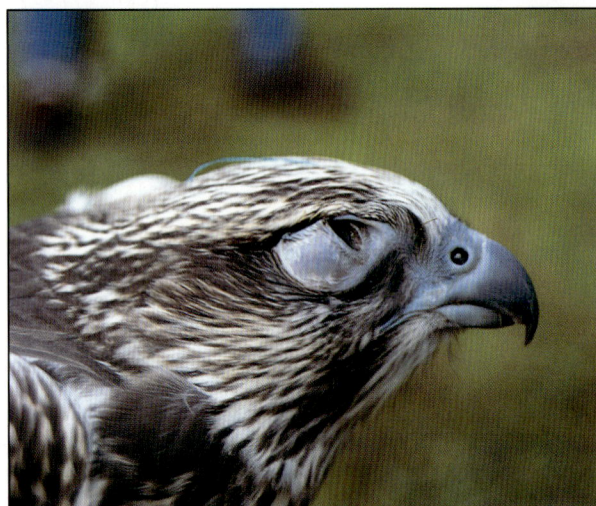

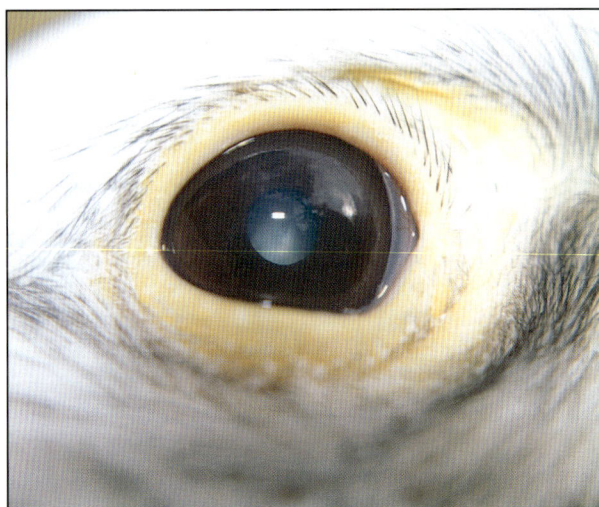

Fig. 13.30 and 13.31: The practice of suturing a bird's eyes closed, here shown in a peregrine falcon (*Falco peregrinus*), is a pain-free method of reducing stress and shortening the manning period for a falcon. The lids are held closed in a normal position (birds cover the eye primarily with the lower lid) by means of fine threads tied together at the top of the head (13.30).

Only one day later, the lids are starting to stretch open (13.31) so that the bird can begin to observe its surroundings. Vision is still sufficiently impaired, however, to keep it calm.
(Photos: Heidenreich)

After approximately five days, the eyes have opened enough that the bird can see almost normally. The sutures are then removed. The tension they produced usually results in some necrosis and scarring of the palpebral edge, visible from then on in the form of a tiny notch. The lid's function in protecting the eye and retaining tears is in no way impaired by this tiny scar.

Since this practice is not common among European or American falconers, a bird showing bilateral eyelid

Fig. 13.32: This 20-year old white gyrfalcon (*Falco rusticolus*) is suffering from a cataract. Such lens opacities are most common in older birds of prey and result in significant loss of visual capacity.
(Photo: Heidenreich)

13.3.5 Sinusitis

The infraorbital sinus is a complex air-filled bony cavity below the avian eye. Infectious diseases involving this area (see Ch. 9.2.5) produce inflammation and swelling. In severe cases the affected bird is said to have an "owl's head" appearance as a result of the pronounced periocular swelling.

Mild sinusitis can sometimes be treated with local and/or systemic antibiotics. A fine needle aspirate with cytologic evaluation and culture and sensitivity will increase the chances of success. Advanced cases in which pus and necrotic debris occlude the normally air-filled cavities require surgical curettage if there is to be any chance of resolving the infection. Avian pus is too caseous to drain from the sinuses by natural means. After removal of the inspissated material, thorough flushing with antibiotics prior to wound closure will help prevent recurrence of the infection. If necessary, the wound can be left open to heal by second intention. Avian sinusitis can sometimes lead to scarring and obstruction of the sinus openings into the nasal cavity, which frequently results in repeated infections.

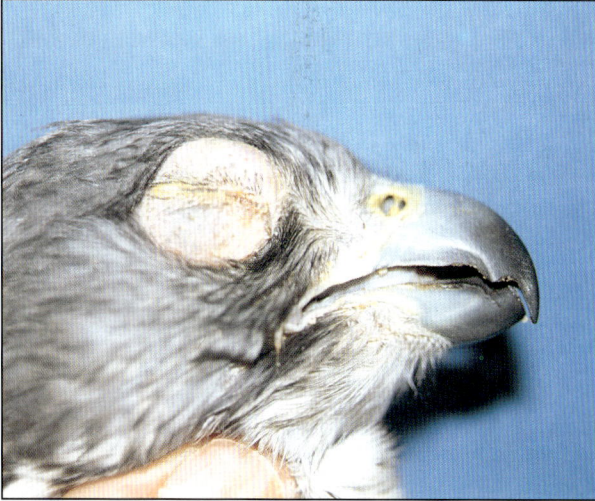

Fig. 13.33: Systemic diseases (pasteurellosis, for example), as well as localized inflammatory disorders, can involve the eyelids and conjunctival membranes. This gray gyrfalcon (*Falco rusticolus*) tiercel's eyes are so severely affected that the lids have swollen shut. (Photo: Heidenreich)

The course of treatment depends on the underlying disease. Topical therapy with ophthalmic medications can help speed resolution of ocular signs and prevent further injury from rubbing. Topical solutions or ointments containing corticosteroids should never be used in the presence of bacterial infections or corneal ulcers. A fluorescein dye test can help rule out the latter. Corticosteroids can delay healing or even promote corneal erosion and perforation.

13.3.4 Disorders involving the lacrimal duct

The lacrimal duct leads from the medial canthus of the eye to the nasal cavity and functions in the drainage of tears to the nose. Infections and swelling can easily obstruct this very fine canal (see also Ch. 13.5.1). Signs of such obstruction include the accumulation of foamy bubbles in the corner of the eye and the spilling of tears over the lower lid and down the face. In larger animals the duct can be flushed to help restore patency, but the lacrimal puncta in raptors are too small to permit such procedures. Therapy is limited to systemic and topical treatment of the underlying disease.

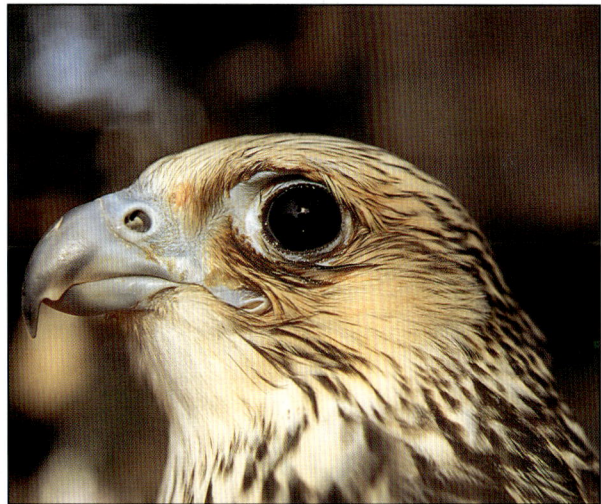

Fig. 13.34: Tearing (epiphora) in raptors can be associated with conjunctivitis or obstruction of the nasolacrimal duct. The bird, in this case a red-naped shaheen X gyrfalcon hybrid, will rub its face along the wing, further irritating the affected eye with wet feathers and dust. (Foto: Heidenreich)

References and literature of further interest

BRAEKEVELT, C.R. (1991):
Fine structure of the pecten oculi of the red-tailed hawk
(*Buteo jamaicensis*).
Anat. Hist. Embryol. **20**, 354–362

BUYUKMIHCI, N.C. (1985):
Lesions in the ocular posterior segment of raptors.
J. Amer. Vet. Med. Ass. **187**, 1121–1124

BUYUKMIHCI, N.C., MURPHY, C.J. and T. SCHULZ (1988):
Developmental ocular disease of raptors.
J. Wildl. Dis. **24**, 207–213

DUKES, T.W. and G.A. FOX (1983):
Blindness associated with retinal dysplasia in a prairie falcon
(*Falco mexicanus*).
J. Wildlife-Diseases. **19**, 66–69

FISCHER, A.B. (1969):
Laboruntersuchungen und Freilandbeobachtungen zum
Sehvermögen und Verhalten von Altweltgeiern.
Zool. Jb. Syst. **96**, 81–132

GRANITZ, U. (1989):
Das physiologische Elektroretinogramm des Greifvogels –
klinische und theoretische Aspekte.
Archiv Experiment. Veterinärmedizin **43**, 185–190

GRANITZ, U., REICHENBACH, A. and B. SEIDEL (1987):
Zur Retinaatrophie bei einem juvenilen Rotmilan – Fallbericht.
Zoolog. Garten **57**, 6–10

GREENWOOD, A.G. and K.C. BARNETT (1980):
The investigation of visual defects in raptors.
Proc. Int. Symp. Dis. Birds of Prey, 131–135
Chiron Pub. Ltd. Keighley, West Yorkshire, England

MARTIN-ROLDAN, R. and M.J. BLANQUEZ-LAYUNTA (1979):
Estudio anatomico y estructural del bulbo ocular del ratonero
comun (*Buteo buteo*).
Anat. Histol. Embryol. **8**, 205–219

KERN, T.J., MURPHY, C.J. and R.C. RIIS (1984):
Lens extraction by phacoemulsification in two raptors
(*Otus asio, Falco peregrinus pealei*).
J. Amer. Vet. Med. Ass. **185**, 1402–1406

KERN, T.J. (1990):
Ocular disorders of raptors.
in: Ludwig, D.R.: Wildlife rehabilitation 215–221
Sartell, USA; National Wildlife Rehabilitation Association.

KERN, T.J., PAUL-MURPHY, J., MURPHY, C.J., BUGUKMIHCI, N.C.,
BURLIN, K., MILLER, P.E., OPPENHEIM, Y. and R.C. RIIS (1996):
Disorders of the third eyelid in birds: 17 cases.
J. Avian Med. Surg. **10**, 12–18

KOCH, H. (1992):
Fallbericht: Kataraktchirurgie bei einem Falken.
Kleintierpraxis **37**, 479

LINDLEY, D.M., HATHCOCK, J.T., MILLER, W.W. and
M.N. DiPINTO (1988):
Fractured scleral ossicles in a Red Tail Hawk.
Vet. Radiol **29**, 209–212

MOORE, C.P., PICKETT, J.P. and B. BEEHLER (1985):
Extracapsular extraction of senile cataract in an Andean condor
(*Vultur gryphus*).
J. Amer. Vet. Med. Ass. **187**, 1211–1213

MURPHY, C.J., KERN, T.J. and R.C. RIIS (1982):
Intraocular trauma in a red-tailed hawk (*Buteo jamaiconsis*).
J. Amer. Vet. Med. Ass. **181**, 1390–1391

MURPHY, C.J., KERN, T.J., McKEEVER, K., McKEEVER, L. and
D. MacCOY (1982):
Ocular lesions in free-living raptors.
J. Amer. Vet. Med. Ass. **182**, 1207–1211

MURPHY, C.J., BROOKS, D.E., KERN, T.J., QUESENBERRY, K.E.
and R.C. RIIS (1983):
Enucleation in birds of prey.
J. Amer. Vet. Med. Ass. **183**, 1234–1237

MURPHY, C.J., KERN, T.J., LOEW, E., BUYUKMIHCI, N.C.,
BELLHORN, R.W., LAHUNTA, A., HECK, W. and D.L. GRAHAM
(1985):
Retinal dysplasia in a hybrid falcon.
J. Amer. Vet. Med. Ass.**187**, 1208–1209

MURPHY, C.J. (1987):
Raptor ophthalmology.
Comp. Educ. Pract. Vet. **9**, 241–257, 260–263

NIEKERK, W.H.-van and S.W. PETRICK (1990):
Unilaterale lentektomie in 'n blouvalkie.
J. South Afric. Vet. Ass. **61**, 124–125

REMPLE, D. and C. GROSS (1993):
Falconry and birds of prey in the gulf.
Motivate Publishing, Dubai

STILES, J., BUYUKMIHCI, N.C. and T.B. FARVER (1994):
Tonometry of normal eyes in raptors.
Amer. J. Vet. Res. **55**, 477–479

13.4 The cardiovascular system

Cooper and Pomerance reported finding pathologic changes involving the heart in 17 out of 66 raptors (26%) they examined at necropsy. In addition, there were 3 cases of atherosclerosis in obviously overweight and obese birds.

Lesions involving the heart are associated with systemic diseases such as trichomoniasis or tuberculosis (see Chapters 9 and 10), but can also be seen independently. The diagnosis of heart disease in birds is difficult and often based merely on clinical suspicion. Radiographs depicting the cardiac silhouette and pulmonary vessels may aid in confirming the diagnosis. Non-selective angiocardiography has also been performed in birds. Endoscopy is generally too risky for cardiac patients. The avian electrocardiogram (ECG) has been studied for decades and may provide useful information. Echocardiography is less well established, but promises to be a non-invasive and potentially useful tool for examining the avian heart.

Despite all these diagnostic possibilities, therapy for avian cardiovascular disease is still in the early stages and relatively limited, especially in wild birds of prey.

Most of the time, a diagnosis of disease involving the heart or vascular system is made incidentally at necropsy. Ischemic heart disease, pericardial effusions,

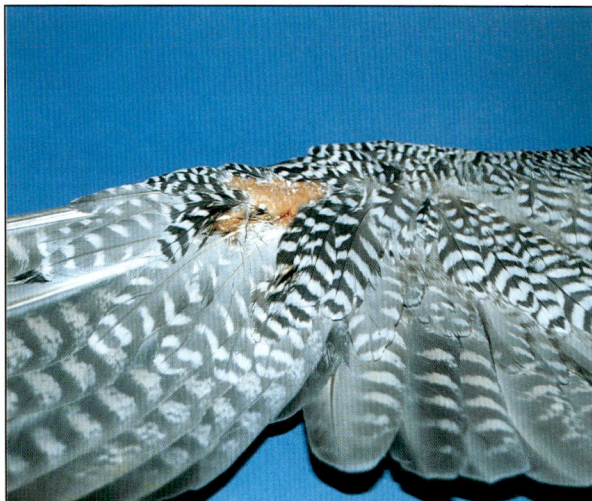

Fig. 13.36: All cases of wing tip edema treated by the author were limited to aspects of the wing distal to the alula. In the early stages, the skin covering the wing tip is edematous and swollen. Soon thereafter, a protein-rich fluid oozes from the affected area.
(Photo: Heidenreich)

vegetative endocarditis and aortic ruptures have been identified this way in raptors.

Atherosclerosis is common in a variety of avian species. Various authors (Lumeij and Ritchie, 1994; Nichols and Montali, 1985) describe this condition in birds of prey. It usually affects primarily the aorta (Fig. 13.35) and is characterized by degenerative changes and the deposition of collagen, cholesterol and calcium in the arterial wall. Overfeeding and lack of exercise are associated with atherosclerosis in birds. All affected raptors have been over five years of age. Risk factors such as elevated blood cholesterol and high serum lipids probably play a role in this disease in most animals, including man. Raptors easily become overweight under captive conditions, and those that do are at higher risk of developing atherosclerosis. One or two fasting days per week are recommended to prevent obesity in birds of prey that are not being exercised regularly.

Another disease of raptors, whose etiology has not yet been fully determined, is **wing tip edema** and necrosis. Because this condition may be related to deficiencies in venous drainage from the wing, it will be discussed here under vascular disorders. Forbes and Harcourt-Brown (1991) as well as Dallimore (1991) have described wing tip edema in various birds of prey.

Although generally reported to occur independently of the season, the author's personal experience suggests that wing tip edema is more common during

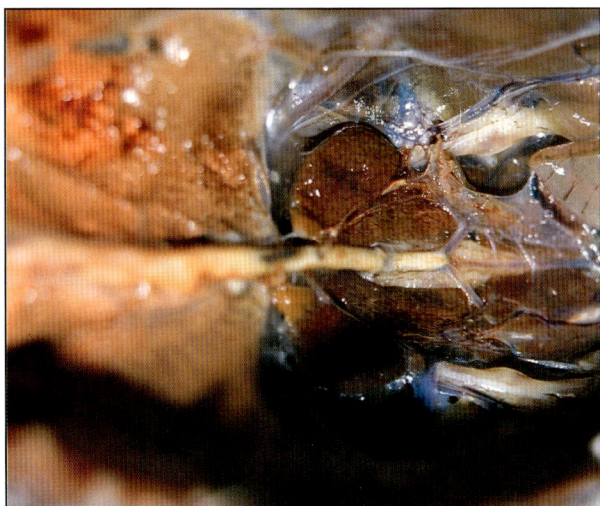

Fig. 13.35: A six-year old peregrine falcon (*Falco peregrinus*) appeared unusually lethargic and depressed inside its aviary. It died in the process of being caught up for examination. A markedly enlarged yellowish-white caudal aorta was noted at necropsy. The normally elastic artery was firmly calcified and crunched audibly when cut.
(Photo: Heidenreich)

summer and early fall. Initial signs include moist, sticky feathers at the distal aspects of the wings and slightly abnormal wing posture. Closer examination reveals gelatinous thickening of the skin in the carpal regions (Fig. 13.36). A sticky serous fluid often leaks from the affected areas.

Baronetzky-Mercier and Seidel (1995) suggest that this condition may also occur in the legs. In either case, the affected body parts generally become necrotic, dry (dry gangrene) and eventually slough off. In severe cases, the entire metacarpal and digital aspects of the wing are lost.

Although similar signs are seen with frostbite and high voltage injuries, these etiologies were ruled out in all patients diagnosed with wing tip edema.

Since the cause is unknown, no effective forms of treatment have been developed for this disease. Baronetzky-Mercier and Seidel recommend flushing with 0.3% hydrogen peroxide in the early stages. Forbes and Harcourt-Brown (1991) tried using antibiotics without success. The birds they treated developed necrotic wing tips after approximately six weeks and then lost the affected body parts.

Three cases presented to the author, one in a laggar falcon (*Falco jugger)* and two in steppe eagles (*Aquila rapax*) were treated successfully with corticosteroids (prednisolone 5 mg/kg every 72 hours) and antibiotics. The edema resolved completely within two days and the birds were fully capable of normal flight after cleaning their sticky wing feathers. A peregrine falcon (*Falco peregrinus*) which presented in a more advanced stage of the disease suffered necrosis and sloughing of the wing tip despite treatment with steroids.

13.5   The respiratory system

The avian respiratory system differs considerably from that of mammals. Birds have a single coelomic cavity not separated by a diaphragm. A small septum is present, but it does not function in respiration. The lung parenchyma is firmly fixed to the ribs and thoracic vertebrae and is rigid, rather than expandable. In addition, birds have an extensive system of air sacs that connect with the bronchi or lungs and play an important part in the breathing process (Fig. 13.37).

The air sacs can be divided into a single clavicular and paired cervical, cranial thoracic, caudal thoracic and abdominal air sacs. Extensions of these air-filled cavities are found throughout the body cavity, around the viscera, under the skin and, in mature birds, even in the femur and humerus, creating "pneumatic" bones.

Only half the inspired air is directed to the lungs. The other half enters the caudal thoracic and

References and literature of further interest

BARONETZKY-MERCIER, A. and B. SEIDEL (1995): in: GÖLTENBOTH, R. and H.G. KLÖS (1995): Krankheiten der Zoo- und Wildtiere, 455 Blackwell Wissenschafts-Verlag, Berlin

COOPER, J.E. and A. POMERANCE (1982): Cardiac lesions in birds of prey. J. Comp. Pathol. **92**, 161–168

DALLIMORE, M.J. (1991): Wing tip oedema in raptors. Vet. Rec. **129**, 19

FORBES, N.A. and N.H. HARCOURT-BROWN (1991): Wing tip oedema and dry gangrene of raptors. Vet. Rec. **128**, 575–576

LUMEIJ, J.T. and B.W. RITCHIE (1994): Cardiology in: RITCHIE et al.: Avian medicine, 695–722 Wingers Pub., Florida

NICHOLS, D. and R.J. MONTALI (1985): Atherosclerosis in zoo birds. Lab. Investigation **52**, 48–49

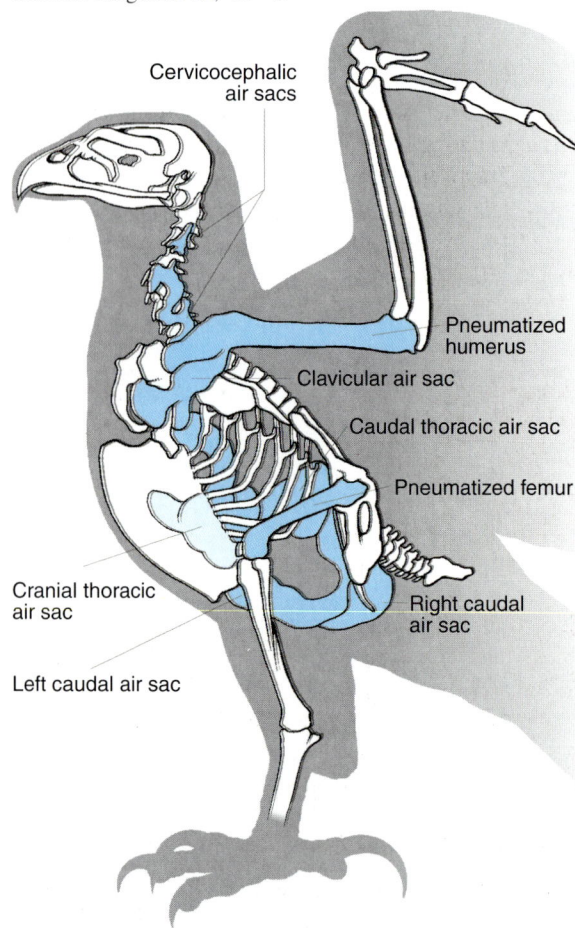

Fig. 13.37: Lateral view of a raptor depicting the system of air sacs (blue).
(Illustration: R. Gattung-Petith and A. Gattung)

abdominal air sacs. At the same time, the spent air sitting in the lungs from the previous breath is pushed out into the cranial air sacs.

During expiration, the unused air from the caudal air sacs is pumped into the lungs and the used air stored in cranial air sacs is exhaled. The avian lung is thus supplied with fresh air for gas exchange both during inspiration and expiration.

The unique avian respiratory anatomy and physiology have serious consequences for potential air sac disease. The caudal thoracic and abdominal air sacs receive inspired air directly without benefiting from the lung's filtering and immunologic defense functions. In addition, the air sac membranes are often poorly supplied with blood vessels, being thin enough to fulfill their oxygen needs by diffusion. The body of a bird thus contains a number of relatively large, warm and moist cavities that can provide optimal, incubator-like conditions for the proliferation of pathogens. Serious respiratory diseases, especially those of fungal etiology, are therefore relatively common in birds of prey.

13.5.1   Nares

The nares are the portals of entry for inspired air. They vary considerably in size and shape among different families of raptors. Vultures, for example, often find themselves reaching deep into a cadaver for food and have developed very narrow, slit-like nares (Fig. 13.38). Falcons, on the other hand, are rapid fliers and have large, round nares with a central

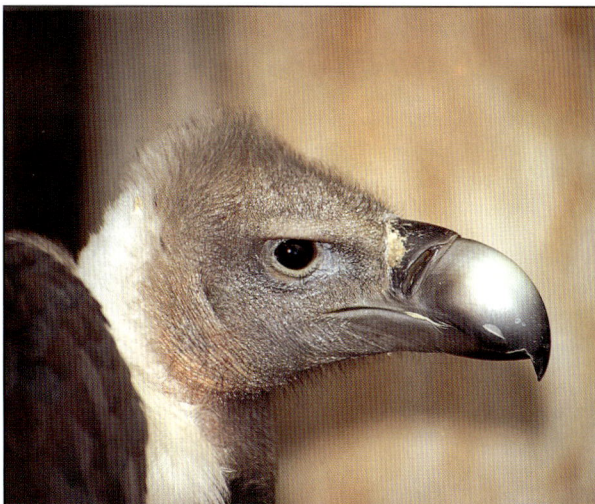

Fig. 13.39: The gyrfalcon (*Falco rusticolus*) is a rapid-flying bird that needs large nares to supply it with sufficient air. Since falcons can reach extreme speeds during the plunging descent upon their quarry, a small operculum inside the nasal cavity serves to redirect the incoming air and prevent it from entering the nasal cavities with too much pressure.
(Photo: Heidenreich)

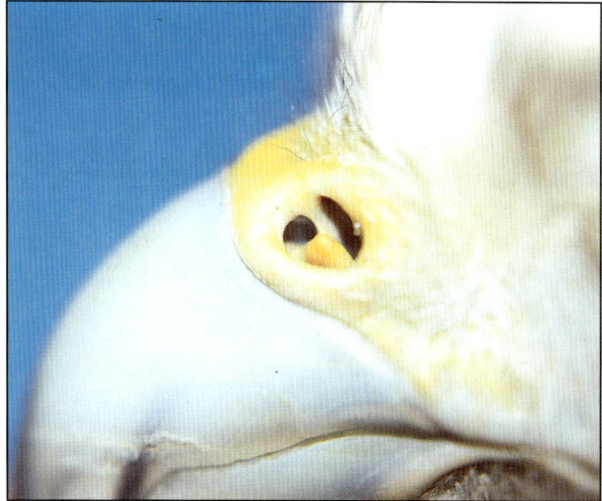

Fig. 13.38: The size and shape of the nares differ among families of raptors, depending on their way of life. The soaring and scavenging Indian white-backed vulture (*Pseudogyps bengalensis)* has slit-shaped openings that help prevent food from entering the nose.
(Photo: Heidenreich)

operculum (Fig. 13.39) that probably serves to reduce the pressure of incoming air during a hurtling descent that can reach speeds of more than 300 km/hr. The nasal cavities of all raptors are separated by a bony septum. The New World vultures, in contrast, lack such a division (see Ch. 2).

The nares and nasal cavities are subject to inflammatory disorders (rhinitis), generally accompanied by some kind of discharge which can result in obstruction of one or both sides as it accumulates and dries. Affected birds often present with open-mouthed breathing.

The patency of the nasal passages can be tested by placing a few drops of physiologic saline on the nasal aperture. If the fluid is sucked into the nose with inspiration, then that side is still patent. This procedure also helps soften dry crusts that may obstructing air flow inside the nose. After a few minutes, gentle pressure from the outside with a saline-filled syringe can help flush the dried secretions through.

Inflammation and swelling of the nasal mucosa occasionally results in obstruction of the nasolacrimal duct, preventing tears from draining normally into the nasal cavity. This duct also serves as a connection between the nose and eye through which pathogens can travel in either direction to cause secondary infections. In such cases, both nasal and ocular secretions will be present (Fig. 13.40).

Rhinitis in raptors is usually of bacterial origin. Sampling the secretions to perform cytologic evaluations as well as for culture and sensitivity (see

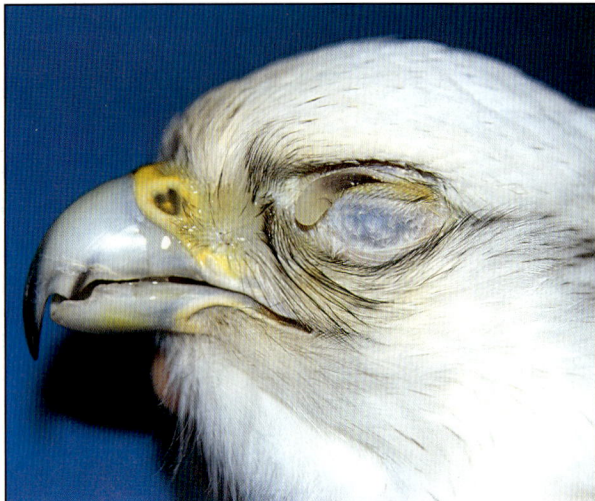

Fig. 13.40: Rhinitis that is associated with a serous discharge can sometimes lead to infection and discharge in the ipsilateral eye, as seen in this gyrfalcon (*Falco rusticolus*).
(Photo: Heidenreich)

Ch. 8.2.1.1) will help in the selection of suitable antibiotics. Since the eyes are often also involved, topical medications suitable for ophthalmic use should be selected. Liquid solutions are preferable to ointments although they have a shorter duration of action. Ointments can sometimes obstruct the fine network of sinuses in the avian skull.

See Ch. 13.3.5 for diseases involving the sinuses.

13.5.2 Trachea and lungs

Infection with the parasite *Syngamus trachea* (see Ch. 10.2.3.4) is the only primary tracheal disease of raptors. The airways and lungs are subject to involvement in other generalized infectious diseases of fungal or bacterial etiology that affect birds of prey (see Ch. 9).

Occasionally, raptors suffer from tracheal foreign bodies. These are usually feathers from the quarry that are accidentally inhaled during plucking or eating. This occurs most commonly during very warm weather when the hawk flies hard and lands breathing heavily with a wide-open glottis.

It is sometimes possible to reach such foreign bodies endoscopically and grasp them. If this is not an option, a tracheal wash using sterile saline with the bird positioned upside down may help flush the object out of the airway. A surgical tracheotomy is the last resort. The incision should be made as close to the location of the foreign body as possible. Cutting between tracheal rings, only part way around, will permit gentle angulation of the proximal and distal segments and make the foreign body accessible. Fine (5–0) absorbable suture material is used to close the tracheotomy site. Care should be taken to include a tracheal ring on either side during closure to prevent the sutures from tearing out.

13.5.3 Air sacs

Bacterial and fungal infections involving the air sacs present a challenge for the avian clinician. The aspects of avian respiratory anatomy that predispose to such infections and complicate treatment have been previously discussed. Aspergillosis is the most common air sac disease in birds of prey (see Ch. 9.3.1). Treatment of this fungal infection is difficult and carries a guarded to poor prognosis despite many recent therapeutic advances.

References and literature of further interest

DUNCKER, H.R. (1979):
Die funktionelle Anatomie des Lungen-Luftsack-Systems der Vögel – mit besonderer Berücksichtigung der Greifvögel.
Prakt. Tierarzt. **60**, 203–226

PETERSEN, A. (1992):
Vergleichende Anatomie der Nasenhöhle und Nasennebenhöhlen bei Greifvögeln (*Falconiformes*) und Eulen (*Strigiformes*).
Vet. Med. Diss., Hannover

TULLY, T.N. and G.J. HARRISON (1994):
in: Ritchie, B.W., Harrison, G.J. and L.R. Harrison:
Avian medicine: Principles and application, 556–581
Wingers Pub., Lake Worth, Florida

13.6   The digestive system

With a few specialized exceptions, most birds of prey are entirely carnivorous. The food is torn into manageable pieces using talons and beak, then swallowed and temporarily stored in the crop before undergoing digestion in the stomach. This form of food intake has forced raptors to develop a very powerful digestive system. The proventriculus and ventriculus, which together make up the avian stomach, can reach a pH between 1.2 and 2.5, a level so acidic that large pieces of meat and even bones are digested within a short time.

Birds of prey do not have a true crop, but make do with a dilatation of the caudal esophagus that serves to store food. The mucosa of that area is not supplied with secretory glands and no digestive processes take place there. Nevertheless, the term "crop" is still commonly used by falconers and will be applied in this book as well.

Like many other birds, raptors are capable of producing pellets or "castings" consisting of the indigestible fur, feather and bone portions of an ingested animal. These compact conglomerations of fiber and bone are produced in the proventriculus and regurgitated prior to the next meal. Because birds of prey consume such a nutrient-rich diet, their intestinal tract is relatively short and the ceca, so well developed in granivorous birds, are purely vestigial.

Diseases involving the gastrointestinal tract are relatively common in birds of prey.

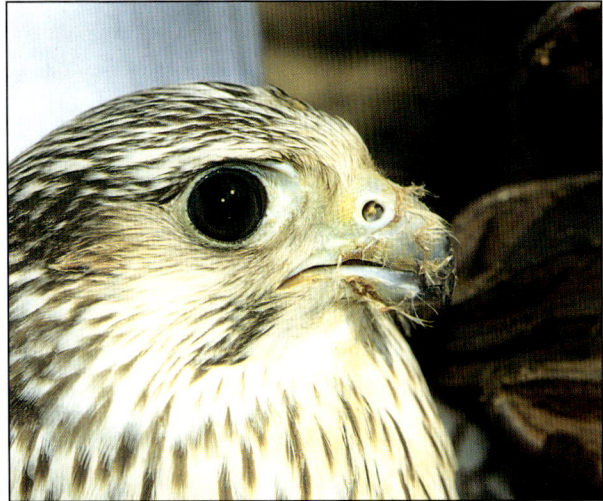

Fig. 13.42: A food-encrusted beak can be a sign of a fractured basihyoid bone. It can also occur in any situation involving generalized depression and unresponsiveness, indicating merely that the bird (in this case, a saker falcon, *F. cherrug*) is unable or uninterested in cleaning its beak after feeding. (Photo: Heidenreich)

13.6.1   Oral cavity

Infectious diseases that involve the oral cavity, including trichomoniasis, capillariasis and candidiasis, have been discussed in Chapters 9 and 10.

Injuries caused by sharp bones or feathers to the roof of the mouth, and secondary abscessation, are an occasional problem in hawks (Fig. 13.41). Food remains that adhere to the beak or remain in the oral cavity, especially under the tongue, and are not removed by the bird indicate a possible fracture of the basihyoid bones, beak damage (rickets), or general depression and unresponsiveness due to other causes.

Fractures of the delicate bones at the base of the tongue can occur after high speed collisions with chain link fences or similar structures that allow the bird's head to pass through and cause trauma to the throat area behind the mandibles. Birds injured in this manner are unable to use the tongue to help swallow morsels of food present in the oral cavity. Decaying meat will accumulate in pockets of the oropharynx. The location and delicate bony structure at the base of the avian tongue make treatment impossible. Many hawks remain unable to feed themselves. Hand-feeding or euthanasia are frequently the only options left.

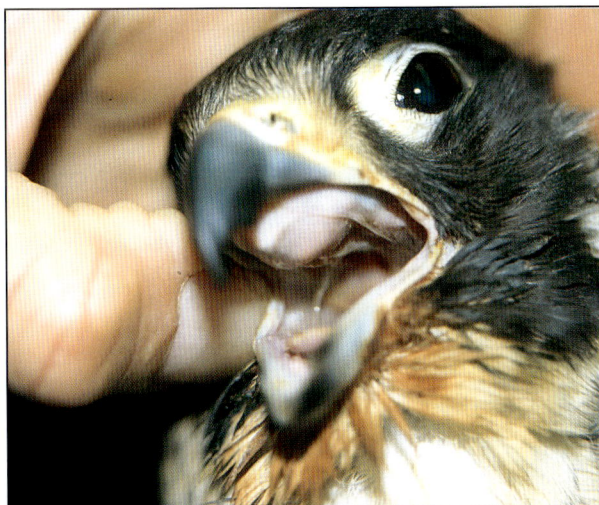

Fig. 13.41: Oral abscesses, like the one involving the roof of the mouth in this peregrine falcon (*Falco peregrinus*), can occur after mucosal injuries caused by sharp bone splinters or feather shafts. (Photo: Heidenreich)

13.6.2 Esophagus ("Crop")

The distensibility and storage function of the distal esophagus make this area vulnerable to injury when full. Wild raptors rarely stuff their crop to its limit, but hunting hawks in good condition will gorge themselves if allowed to do so. The crop then becomes prominently distended and prone to tearing if traumatized.

In the process of hand-raising raptor chicks, careless overheating of formula in the microwave can lead to burns of the crop mucosa. Microwave ovens heat foods unevenly, creating occasional pockets of very hot formula. Surprisingly, chicks will swallow this hot food without signs of discomfort. To avoid crop burns, it is always better to warm the formula slowly in a hot-water bath. An even better alternative is to feed freshly killed, still warm animal parts.

The feeding of very cold foods can also lead to problems. Cold meat is retained in the crop for a longer period of time, and can therefore lead to digestive disorders.

Injuries, burns or capillaria abscesses in the distal esophagus frequently develop into crop fistulae. If only the crop wall is involved, food will escape into the subcutaneous tissues of the neck. This development is easily overlooked by a lay person and quickly leads to sepsis and death.

More commonly, the necrosis associated with penetrating crop injuries leads to complete fistulation including the skin. Crop fistulae of this kind present as broad crusty lesions located in the area between the head and the thoracic inlet (Fig. 13.43).

Crop fistulae require surgical debridement and closure to heal properly.

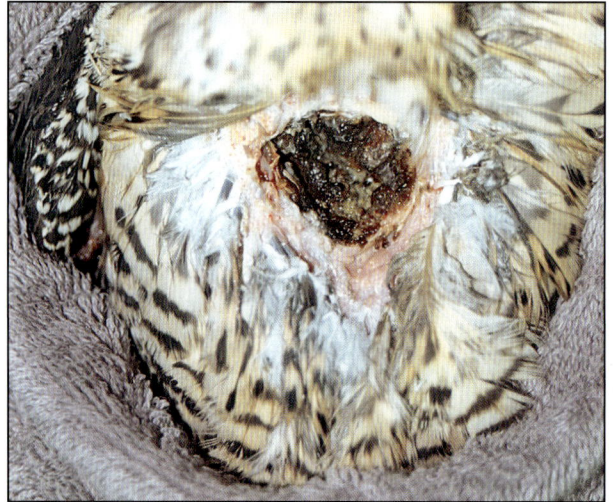
13.43

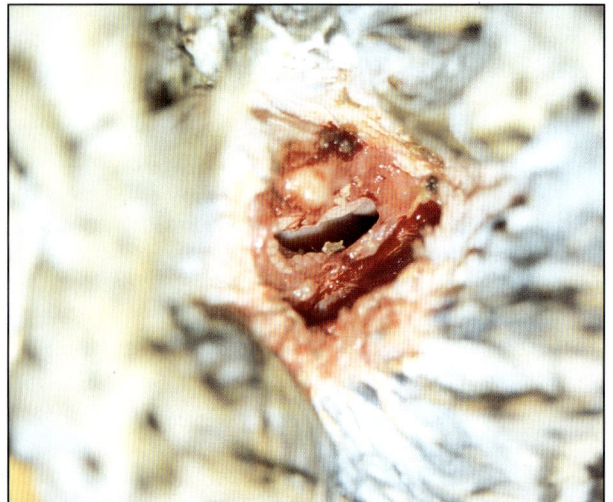
13.44

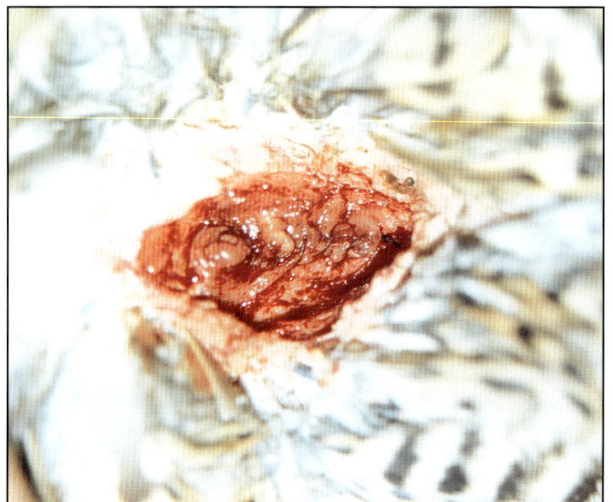
13.45

Figs. 13.43, 13.44 and 13.45: Esophageal or crop fistulae can have a variety of causes. They typically present as broad crusty lesions in the ventral neck region (13.43).
Surgical intervention is necessary to repair the defect and save the bird. The area is first cleaned and debrided (13.44). Sutures should be strong and tightly spaced (13.45) since the esophagus functions in the storage of food and must be able to withstand significant distention.
(Photos: Heidenreich)

Surgical repair of crop fistulae
The bird is placed in dorsal recumbency under general anesthesia. The feathers around the fistula can be moistened and pulled out of the way or plucked if necessary. Dry crusts and any necrotic tissue are gently removed until the edges of the defect are visible. Chronic crop fistulae frequently develop extensive adhesions between the esophageal wall and skin. The two layers should be carefully separated and grasped with forceps. The edges of the skin defect and the esophageal perforation are freshened by removing any necrotic tissue and approximately 1 mm of tissue all around (Fig. 13.24).

Closure of the esophagus is accomplished using absorbable suture material in an inverting layer oversewn with a simple continuous layer for additional strength. This double-layered closure is particularly important because it ensures a good seal and is better able to withstand tension during the healing period.

The skin is closed in a routine manner with simple interrupted absorbable sutures. The hawk should be kept off solid food for two or three days. Small, frequent meals of easily digested meat will minimize crop distention.

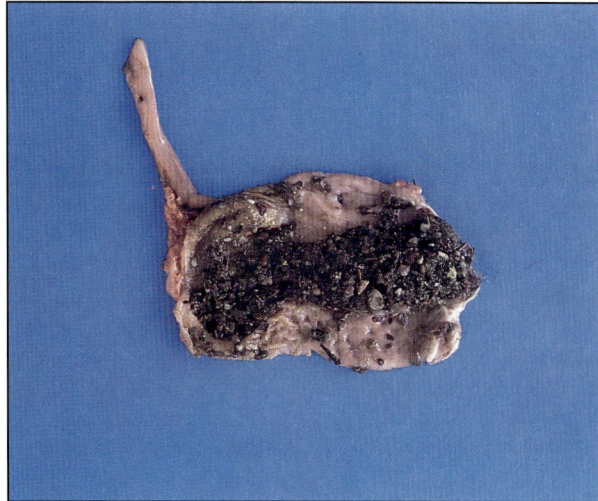

Fig. 13.46: Sand or fine gravel can adhere to cleaned meat and be ingested by a hawk. This type of grit cannot be formed into a pellet and presents a risk of gastric or intestinal obstruction and ileus.
(Photo: Heidenreich)

13.6.3   Proventriculus and ventriculus

The ventriculus (gizzard) of raptors does not have a thick muscular wall or distinct koilin layer like that of granivorous birds. Instead, it is thin-walled and elastic, similar to the proventriculus, or glandular stomach. As a result, the gastric wall is prone to perforation by sharp objects. Beyerbach (1990) reports that a peregrine falcon died after swallowing a pigeon's flight feather which penetrated the stomach wall.

13.6.3.1 Sand impaction

A direct consequence of improper feeding techniques is the ingestion and subsequent accumulation of sand or fine gravel in the proventriculus. Raw meat or skinned animals quickly get coated with gravel if they are placed on the ground for feeding. Larger gravel pieces are easily regurgitated by a hawk, but fine gravel or sand are not, nor are they incorporated into pellets. Thus, they either remain in the stomach to create impactions (Fig. 13.46), or pass through the intestinal tract where they may damage the mucosa or cause obstructions and ileus.

Clinical presentation
In the early stages, the bird may still be eating but no longer passing feces. The ingested food is vomited after several hours. Sometimes it remains in the upper digestive tract where it ferments and leads to further illness.

If the obstruction is at the intestinal level, the bird will refuse to eat and, if not properly treated, become sick and die within a few days.

Diagnosis
A presumptive diagnosis of sand impaction can be made from a good history and the absence of feces. Radiographs can confirm the diagnosis by revealing radioopaque mineral matter in the digestive tract (See Fig. 7.33).

Treatment
If sand or gravel are visible in the proventriculus or ventriculus but the bird is still eating relatively well, one can try giving fibrous casting material to promote expulsion of the stones. The neck skin of a pigeon works well. It is fed inside-out so that the feathers are on the inside. Some of the sand will get incorporated in the pellet formed from these feathers and be expelled. This treatment can be repeated several times if necessary.

If the impaction involves only the stomach and food is no longer passing through at all, gastric lavage will be necessary to remove the grit (see Ch. 4.4).

If intestinal ileus or obstruction are present, mineral oil can be administered to aid in lubricating the intestinal contents and promote passage of the foreign material. If the gravel has not passed within a few hours, surgical removal is indicated.

For an enterotomy, the anesthetized bird is placed in dorsal recumbency and an incision is made along the midline of the abdomen, starting just below the sternum. The duodenal loop, in which most impactions occur, is immediately visible. If the intestinal wall appears viable, a standard enterotomy will permit removal of the stones or sand easily. If the impaction has been present for more than three days, the intestinal wall is frequently necrotic and requires resection if the bird's life is to be saved.

With a healthy intestinal wall, gently clamping on either side of the impaction isolates the area to be cleaned out. The segment to be opened is exteriorized. Partial closure of the coelomic cavity will help minimize heat loss while preventing contamination and drying of tissues.

Since the avian intestine is very thin, the enterotomy incision should always be made transversely. Closure of the defect might otherwise lead to excessive narrowing of the lumen. The sand or gravel is gently removed using a small spoon or forceps. The area is then gently flushed with warm saline prior to closure with absorbable suture material (6–0) in a closely spaced, simple interrupted pattern.

Resection of devitalized bowel segments is always performed in areas of still healthy and well-perfused tissue. A simple interrupted suture pattern is used for the anastomosis as well. Irrigation with warm saline stimulates peristalsis and should be performed before replacing the intestine into the abdomen. The abdominal wall is closed in two layers, peritoneum and muscles first, then skin. Assuming its physical condition permits, the bird is kept off food for several days postoperatively.

Prevention

Impactions are easily avoided by providing hawks with suitable food animals that provide adequate casting material. At the very least, raptors should receive their food on feeding platforms. If a platform is not available, the meat, especially if cleaned, should be placed well away from gravel or sandy areas.

13.6.3.2 Feather and fur impactions

Ingestion of excessive amounts of fibrous material such as fur and feathers can result in impactions that have a similar clinical presentation as the sand impactions described above. Normally, the bird regurgitates feathers and fur after digestion is completed, taking its next meal only after having cast the pellet and thus emptied its proventriculus. Falconers are familiar with the problem of trying to fly a hawk that hasn't cast yet that day. The bird hunts well only after having expelled the indigestible portion of the previous day's

meal. The casting process can sometimes be accelerated by showing the bird food. Otherwise, the falconer is simply forced to wait.

Emaciated birds, or those that are ravenously hungry for other reasons such as thyroid hormone supplementation (see Ch. 13.1), frequently fail to wait until after casting the pellet before consuming more food. The ingestion of additional fur or feathers may result in significant gastric distention and the subsequent inability to regurgitate the accumulated fibrous material.

Radiographically, this type of impaction is difficult to identify. Fur and feathers are of similar density as other soft tissues. A contrast study using barium sulfate is usually required to confirm the diagnosis. The large pellet in the proventriculus rapidly becomes permeated with barium, but only a tiny thread of the contrast material is able to make its way into the small intestine (see Ch. 7, Fig. 7.33).

Their firm, tightly woven consistency makes mechanical removal of fibrous impactions via the esophagus rarely successful. A surgical gastrotomy is usually required to remove the mass.

The avian stomach is located near the left pelvis and its elasticity and firm structure make it easily accessible by an abdominal approach. The basic technique for a gastrotomy is similar to that for an enterotomy. Although it is desirable to keep the bird off food after the procedure, this is rarely possible. The degree of emaciation typically present in these birds necessitates immediate nutritional support. A liquid diet of bovine serum (Boviserin), egg yolk, blood or even canine and feline prepared liquid diets will help the bird recover while avoiding distention of the stomach for the first few days after surgery.

13.6.4   Cloacal prolapse

Prolapse of the cloaca is usually secondary to some other disease involving chronic diarrhea, tenesmus, or egg-binding. Treatment should therefore not be limited to replacing the prolapsed tissue. Any possible factors that may have precipitated the problem should be addressed as well. The clinical presentation and therapeutic options are similar to those described for prolapse of the oviduct (see Ch. 13.7.2.3).

13.7   The urinary tract and reproductive systems

Diseases primarily affecting the kidneys are rarely reported in birds of prey. Avian gout (see Ch. 9.2.2) and fatty liver syndrome of merlins (see Ch. 9.2.4) are the only exceptions to this rule. Nevertheless, the kidney is important in the excretion of wastes and is involved to some degree in many disease processes. The color and quality of the urates can be important indicators of diseases including toxicities or fungal and viral infections. The unmistakable pastel, almost neon green urates observed in seriously ill raptors (see Fig 7.11 in Ch. 7.4.1) are a strong indication of impending death. This unusual green color can be traced to total failure of the kidneys accompanied by renal hemorrhaging. The red hemoglobin pigment is converted into green verdiglobin and excreted with the urates. Birds showing this clinical sign usually die within 48 hours.

13.7.1   Male reproductive system

Although a variety of disease processes involving the phallus or gonads are described in other groups of birds, raptors rarely have problems of this kind. Part of the reason may be that such disorders are usually recognized in breeding birds, and raptor breeding programs, despite significant successes, are still in the early stages. The number of captive breeding birds is limited and many breeders, though careful and concerned, are not medically trained. Not every infertile tiercel is thoroughly examined to discover the source of the problem. Insufficient information may therefore be the reason for the paucity of reports on disorders of the male reproductive system in raptors.

13.7.2   Female reproductive system

Diseases involving the reproductive tract are definitely more common in female birds of prey. They usually occur in association with reproductive activity, especially during the egg-laying period.

13.7.2.1 Egg retention

Raptors lay their eggs at species-specific intervals. As a rule of thumb, the smaller the species, the shorter the interval between eggs. Small falcons and sparrowhawks produce eggs 1 or 2 days apart, while larger falcons have 2 or 3 day intervals, and eagles and vultures may have egg transit times of up to 4 days or more during the laying period.

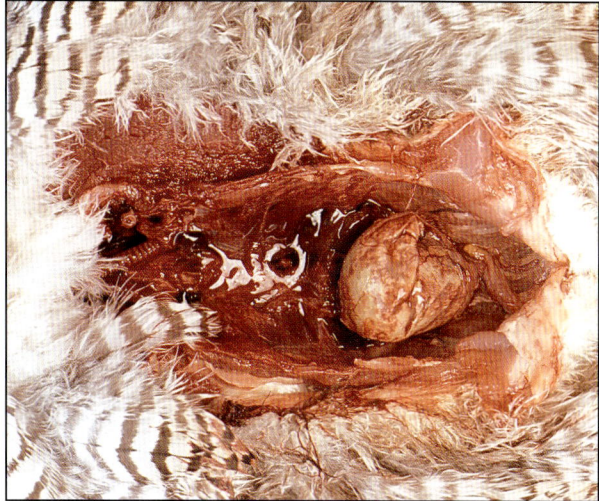

Fig. 13.47: An adult female hunting goshawk at necropsy. This bird died suddenly in January after capturing a rabbit. A fully developed egg was found in the caudal coelomic cavity. Presumably, the egg had been present since the breeding season in April of the previous year without causing clinical signs. During the struggle with the rabbit, the egg was broken and this resulted in the bird's death.
(Photo: Heidenreich)

If the interval between eggs is longer than expected, the possibility of egg retention should be considered. Unlike with egg-binding or dystocia, the causes off egg retention are usually difficult to determine. A delay of up to 24 hours can still be considered normal. If the breeder or veterinarian intervenes too early and subjects the bird to handling and examination, the stress to the bird may interfere with normal development of the un-laid egg. Waiting too long, on the other hand, can pose a risk to the bird, especially if it becomes egg-bound.

Stress of any kind or behavioral disturbances for the egg-laying female can produce delays in oviposition, even if the eggs have developed normally. As long as there are no abnormalities involving the egg shell or oviduct, such retained eggs are eventually always laid. Occasionally, they are not deposited in the nest, but are dropped from the perch or placed elsewhere in the breeding chamber instead. In some cases, complete eggs can remain within the reproductive tract for many months without causing obvious problems for the bird (Fig. 13.47).

13.7.2.2 Egg-binding (dystocia)

There are many possible reasons for a bird to become egg-bound and unable to expel a fully formed egg:

Atony of the uterus may keep the egg from moving forward and can be related to abnormalities in calcium metabolism or deficiencies in selenium.

Young females producing their first clutch are more prone to dystocia than older, more experienced birds. Strong temperature fluctuations can lead to problems in some of the smaller species. Infections involving the oviduct can impair function and result in adhesion between the egg shell and the mucosa. The most important factors, however, seem to be the shape of the egg and the structure of the shell.

The so-called "snake-eggs", which are eggs that fail to develop a mineralized shell, pose a particular problem. These soft, fluctuant structures provide no resistance to the peristaltic and uterine contractions and are therefore difficult to expel. Rough-shelled eggs, which can develop if there are problems during the last phase of shell development, also interfere with the ability of the uterus to push the egg out. Round eggs, or those that are propelled through the reproductive tract rounded end first, are more difficult to oviposit than eggs of normal shape and positioning.

Clinical signs
Only a few hours after the egg should have been laid, an egg-bound hawk will appear noticeably distressed and sick. The bird will be depressed and fluffed up, breathing heavily in or near the nest. Initial abdominal

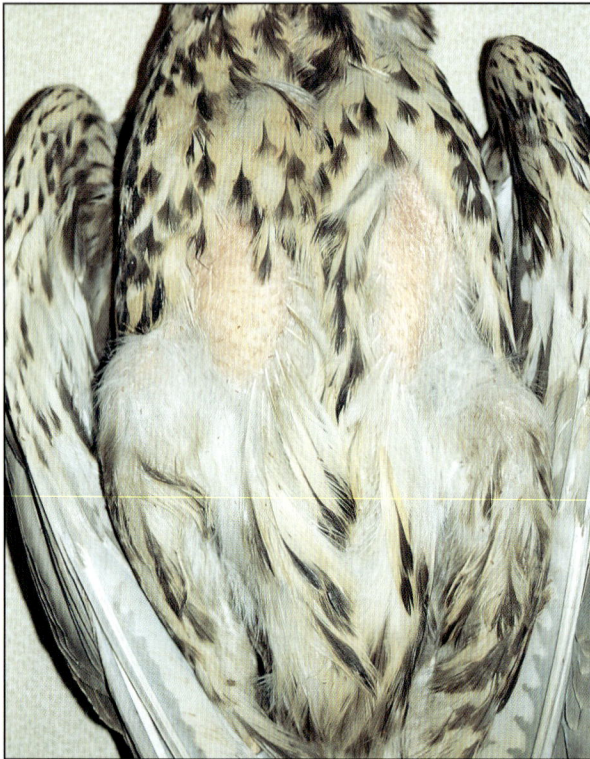

Fig. 13.48: During the incubation period, adult raptors develop an area of thickened, well-vascularized skin in the pectoral and abdominal regions. Large featherless patches called brood patches facilitate heat exchange between the bird's skin and its eggs.
(Photo: Heidenreich)

presses and bobbing movements of the tail become less frequent with time. If the condition is prolonged, the pressure created by the presence of the egg in the pelvis will affect the kidneys and impair blood flow through the large vessels in the caudal abdomen. Circulatory problems and even shock can result. Occasionally, prolapse of the oviduct or uterus (see below) occurs as a direct consequence of the continuous yet futile straining to expel the egg.

Diagnosis
An early diagnosis of dystocia is critical to a successful outcome. This usually depends on the watchfulness and experience of the breeder. Nevertheless, or maybe because of this, many birds are presented to the veterinarian only late in the process, when the condition has become very serious. If the egg has a normal mineralized shell and can easily be palpated in the abdomen, the diagnosis is simple. Eggs lacking a shell are more difficult to identify in this manner. In such cases, a differential diagnosis that includes tumors, ascites or hernias must be taken into account. Laying birds usually have a thickened and sometimes featherless brood patch on the chest and abdomen (Fig. 13.48). This can help make a diagnosis of egg-binding more likely.

Mineralized eggs can be easily seen radiographically as well. This additional procedure can sometimes waste precious time, however.

Treatment
It is always advisable to first try removing the egg by noninvasive means. Because the manipulations involved are very stressful for the hawk and elicit strong physical resistance, the bird should be anesthetized before attempting this.

Gentle massaging motions towards the cloaca are used to try to push the egg out. In simple cases, this will suffice, although some of the vaginal or uterine mucosa may be pushed out with the egg in this way. Careful separation of egg and mucosa followed by moistening of the tissues usually lets them return to their original position.

If gentle massage fails to produce the egg, further measures must be taken. Various techniques are mentioned in the literature (Joyner, 1994). Most of them are not recommended for birds of prey. The administration of oxytocin, vasotocin, or prostaglandins, all designed to stimulate uterine contractions, can easily lead to rupture of the uterus, especially in cases where the egg has adhered to the uterine mucosa. Ovocentesis is a procedure in which the contents of the egg are withdrawn with a needle and syringe, allowing the shell to be crushed and more easily delivered. It can lead to significant injury or hemorrhaging and should also be avoided.

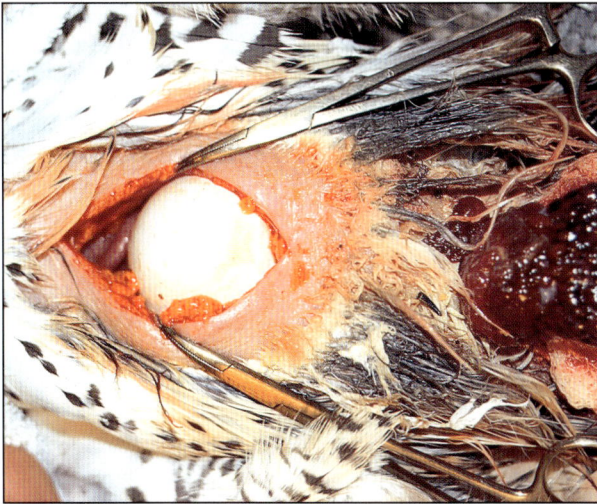

△ 13.49

13.50 ▽

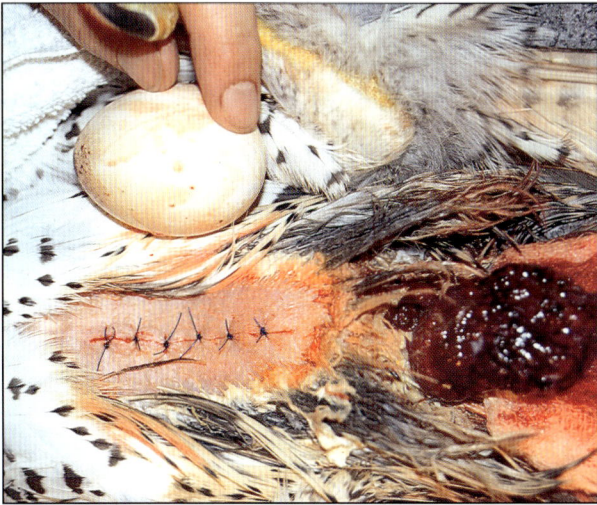

Figs. 13.49 and 13.50: A silver gyrfalcon (*Falco rusticolus*) suffered from egg-binding and strained so hard that she also prolapsed her oviduct. A ventral midline celiotomy permitted removal of the fully developed but unpigmented egg from the uterus (13.49). The uterus, abdominal muscles and skin were closed separately (13.50). (Photos: Heidenreich)

In the author's experience, the method of choice for treating dystocias in raptors is a hysterotomy. This technique permits removal of the egg with minimal risk of injury and the best chances of retaining normal reproductive abilities.

Surgical method: The bird is placed in dorsal recumbency under general anesthesia. The feathers over the abdomen are moistened and parted to expose the skin. The abdominal wall is opened directly over the palpable egg and then retracted to reveal the distended ivory-colored uterus immediately underneath. It is incised directly over the egg and the edges are immediately secured with clamps to prevent them from getting lost in the abdominal cavity (Fig. 13.49). The egg

is then quickly and easily lifted out of the abdomen. A thorough examination of the oviduct before closure will help identify any further eggs that may be present!

The uterus is closed using 5–0 absorbable suture material in a continuous inverting pattern. Peritoneum and abdominal muscles are apposed with 3–0 sutures in a closely spaced simple interrupted pattern. A continuous pattern is not safe as further eggs may be laid accompanied by abdominal pressing. Skin is closed using a simple interrupted pattern (Fig. 13.50). With some experience, the entire procedure should take no longer than 10 minutes.

All birds treated surgically in this way by the author continued to lay normal clutches the following season. In most cases, no further eggs were produced after surgery that same season. Presumably, the stress associated with egg-binding and the hysterotomy played a role in halting egg production. In one case, however, a golden eagle proceeded to lay another egg four days after surgery. The uterine sutures held and the egg was laid without complications.

13.7.2.3 Prolapse of the oviduct

Egg-binding is sometimes accompanied by prolapse of the oviduct or uterus (Fig. 13.50). If the oviductal mucosa is seen protruding from the vent, the hawk should be immediately captured and restrained. Covering the exposed tissues with moistened sterile gauze right away will help prevent further injury, desiccation or necrosis. The cloacal sphincter often closes tightly around the prolapsed tissues, interfering with venous drainage. The engorged oviduct can then become very difficult to replace. Cold compresses (ice water) can be applied to reduce the swelling.

Before attempting to reduce the prolapse, it must be determined whether an egg is still present in the oviduct. This would have to be removed first. The exposed tissue is then thoroughly cleaned with cold physiologic saline. In smaller raptors, lubricated cotton-tipped swabs can be used to push the oviduct gently back into place (Fig. 13.51). A gloved finger works well in the larger species.

Despite all efforts, it is common for the prolapse to recur only hours after a simple reduction. The uterus probably lacks the required muscle tone or has not contracted yet. It is therefore advisable to place a purse string suture or stay sutures in the cloacal opening to prevent the bird from pushing the oviduct out again. Care must be taken to leave enough of a gap that urates and feces can still be easily excreted. A purse string suture may be problematic in cases where another egg is expected. Close observation of the animal and a temporary release of the suture would be necessary to permit the egg to pass.

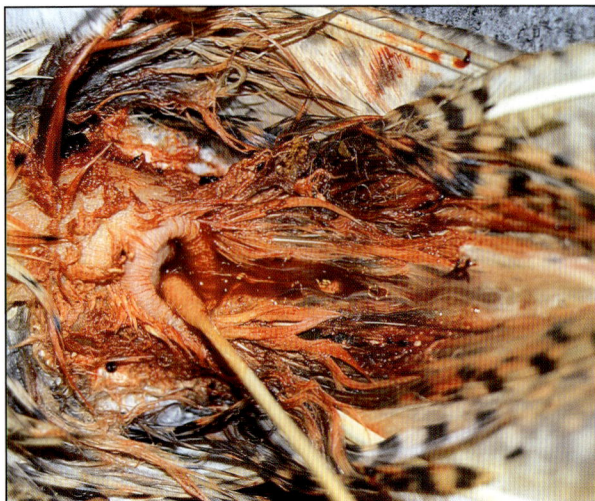

Fig. 13.51: The prolapsed oviduct in the bird depicted in Figs. 13.49 and 13.50 had been covered with moist gauze to protect it from drying during several hours of transport. It was easily replaced with a moist cotton-tipped swab. (Photo: Heidenreich)

13.7.2.4 Infections of the oviduct and ovary (salpingitis, metritis and oophoritis)

Both egg-binding and oviductal prolapse carry the risk of introducing pathogens to the reproductive tract. Prophylactic antibacterial therapy is therefore necessary after treating these disorders. Chlorhexidine or 1% tetracycline flushes have also proven helpful.

Artificial insemination requires eversion of the oviduct and can also result in salpingitis or metritis. The bacteria are generally introduced with dirty instruments or contaminated semen.

The clinical presentation will vary depending on the severity and location of the infection. Inflammation of the proximal oviduct affects early egg development. Yolks may fail to acquire a coat of albumin and remain in the oviduct, where they mummify to a rubbery consistency (Fig. 13.52). This can render the bird permanently sterile. Pathogens that ascend even farther, and reach the ovary, can result in life-threatening infections. Bacteria multiply very rapidly in the maturing follicles with their rich yolk and medical treatment usually arrives too late to save such birds.

13.7.3 Sterilization

As with other animals, birds of prey can, and sometimes should be rendered infertile. This may sound contradictory, since a great deal of effort and knowledge have gone into the breeding of such birds. Captive breeding has been reliably successful for barely two decades, and already there is discussion of surgically intervening to sterilize birds of prey.

Sometimes the breeders of very rare species approach veterinarians with an interest in having birds sterilized. They are probably hoping to maintain their monopoly on the market, preferring to sell infertile animals that cannot be used to found new breeding programs.

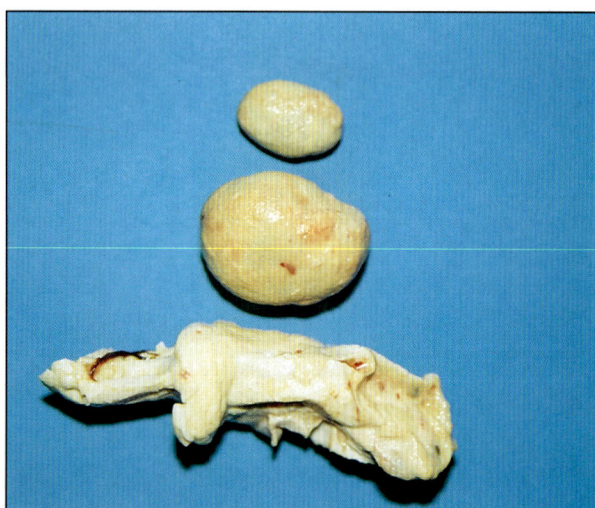

Fig. 13.52: Mummified ova from the oviduct of a saker falcon (*Falco cherrug*). They developed from yolks which entered the reproductive tract but failed for some reason to develop into normal eggs. (Photo: Heidenreich)

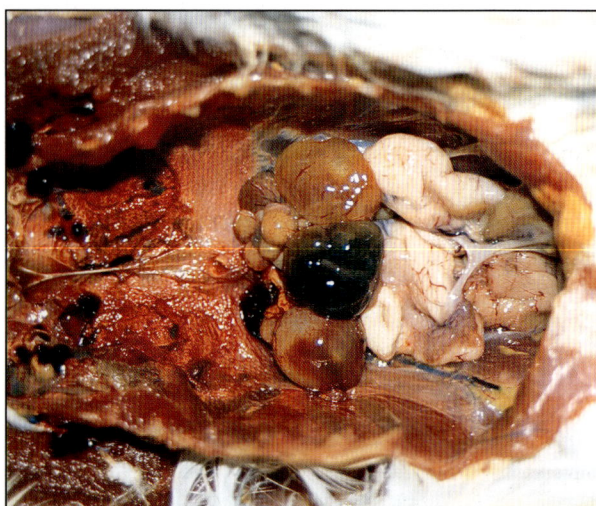

Fig. 13.53: Ascending bacterial infections can lead to metritis, salpingitis and infections of the ovary. Pathogens thrive in the rich, yolk-filled ova, as evident in the abnormal, darkly discolored follicles in this postmortem photograph. (Photo: Heidenreich)

A more valid reason for considering sterilization in raptors occurs with production of the many different hybrids possible among birds of prey (see Ch. 17.3.2). Conservation organizations and even local or federal authorities are concerned about possible crossbreeding between such hybrids that might escape to the wild, and natural populations. The introduction of genes from other species or subspecies would be undesirable in natural populations. Such concerns are certainly justified, especially with falcons. Unlike most others, hierofalcon subgroup hybrids can be propagated for an indefinite number of generations (Heidenreich et al., 1993).

Such concerns have already led to a ban on flying hybrid falcons in the Netherlands. In the United States, such birds must either be imprinted on man or sterilized to avoid possible interbreeding with native falcon populations (Saar, 1993).

There is always the risk that a bird will escape to the wild, especially if it is being used for falconry or otherwise flown free. Nevertheless, this happens only sporadically. The Arab practice of purposely releasing a hawk after the hunting season is completed has a much greater impact on this issue. Hundreds of falcon hybrids have been exported from the U.S., Canada and Europe to various Arab countries in the last few years. Presumably, these young hybrids have no difficulties joining native wild falcon populations after escaping or being released. Veterinarians with the Middle East Falcon Research Group in Abu Dhabi have recognized this problem and are evaluating the need to sterilize the predominantly female falcon hybrids popular in Middle Eastern countries (Samour, 1995).

Sterilization can be achieved in a number of ways.

Neutering

Neutering is a term that can be applied to either sex of an animal and usually pertains to the removal of the gonads, testes in the case of males, or ovaries in females.

This procedure used to be common in male chickens (caponizing) because it produced better weight gain in the birds. It was performed in one of two ways. The testes could be removed via a celiotomy approach between the last two ribs (Koenig, 1985), or the birds would be hormonally castrated by administering slow-release feminizing hormones under the cervical skin (SCHROEDER, 1965). Because the surgical technique was impractical on a large scale and hormones in food animals are now tightly controlled, castration in poultry is no longer common.

Neutering male birds of prey by the methods described above is certainly possible, but a number of health concerns make it inadvisable. Cason et al. (1988) and Fennell et al. (1990) were able to prove that removal of the male hormones has a strong nega-

tive effect on growth and overall development. Mase and Oishi (1991) found that castrating quail interfered with normal development of the bursa, an organ important in the immune system of birds.

Research of this kind has been performed only with domestic birds, and even there, has been relatively limited. The long term effects of neutering on moulting, for instance, have not been investigated. Castration in male birds of prey should therefore not be considered an option!

Sterilization

The term sterilization is generally used to indicate a method for making an animal infertile without necessarily removing the gonads. In females, this can be done by cutting or tying the oviduct, and in males the same can be done with the ductus deferens. Because these procedures do not interfere with the production of reproductive hormones, birds sterilized in this fashion continue to engage in normal pairing, mating and nesting behavior. They are infertile, however. Follicles no longer enter the oviduct and sperm are no longer able to travel along the ductus deferens.

These procedures can be performed with laparoscopic techniques in either sex. The bird must be sufficiently mature that its reproductive organs are well-developed and easily recognized and manipulated. Hawks should be full-grown, that is, fully feathered and dry (no pin feathers).

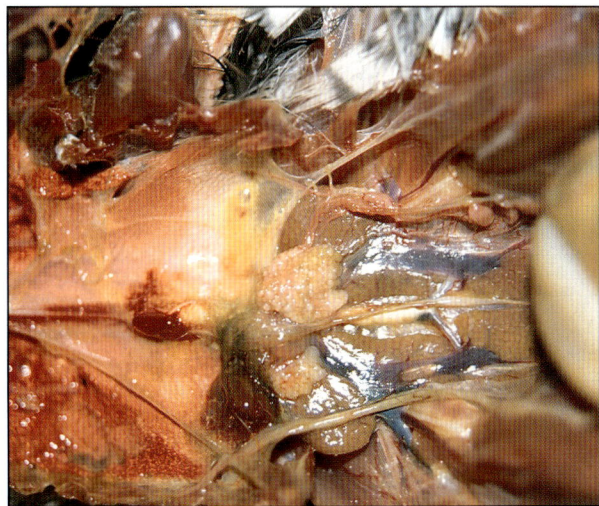

Fig. 13.54: An inactive ovary in an immature bird. The right ovary is still evident. It will atrophy completely by the time the bird reaches sexual maturity. The ligament that supports the infundibulum near the ovary is clearly visible (see also Fig. 13.55).
(Photo: Heidenreich)

Surgical technique for sterilizing the female hawk (from HEIDENREICH, 1994): The positioning and surgical approach are the same as that described for surgical sexing. The bird is placed in right lateral recumbency with the left hind limb extended backward. The celiotomy incision is made in the left flank area behind the last rib and in front of the left leg.

In juvenile birds, the ovary is a small, lumpy white structure located at the cranial pole of the left kidney (Fig. 13.54). The immature oviduct winds its way caudally from the ovary along the renal surface towards the cloaca. At this stage of development, the various anatomic divisions of the oviduct are not yet discernible. There is a ligament, however, that can be seen attached to the infundibulum and inserting on the second to last rib. It serves to support the infundibulum, which captures the ova at ovulation, in its position near the ovary. This ligament is grasped with a fine pair of hemostats (Fig. 13.55) and either transected or pulled from its attachment site on the rib. This releases the threadlike oviduct from its cranial attachment and allows it to retract caudally away from the ovary. The follicles no longer enter the oviduct at ovulation, falling instead into the coelomic cavity where they are presumably resorbed.

It is probably easier to grasp the oviduct somewhere along its course and transect it. However, this method carries the risk that the cranial part of the reproductive tract remains intact and capable of at least partially adding albumin and a shell to the ovum. The result would be an ectopic egg and iatrogenic dystocia.

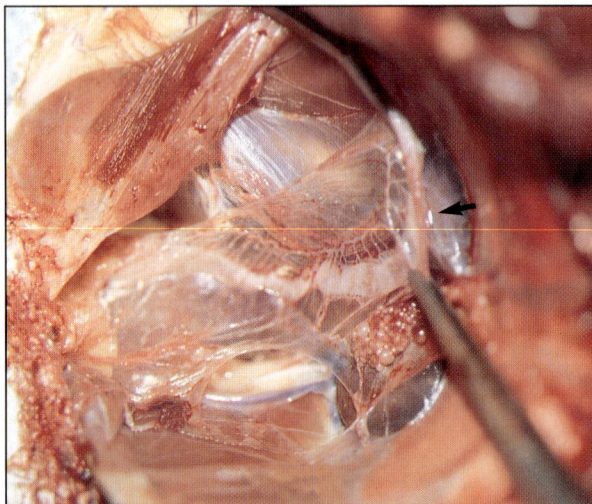

Fig. 13.55: An immature oviduct elevated to show the ventral ligament (arrow) which supports the infundibulum and must be transected during the sterilization procedure.
(Photo: Heidenreich)

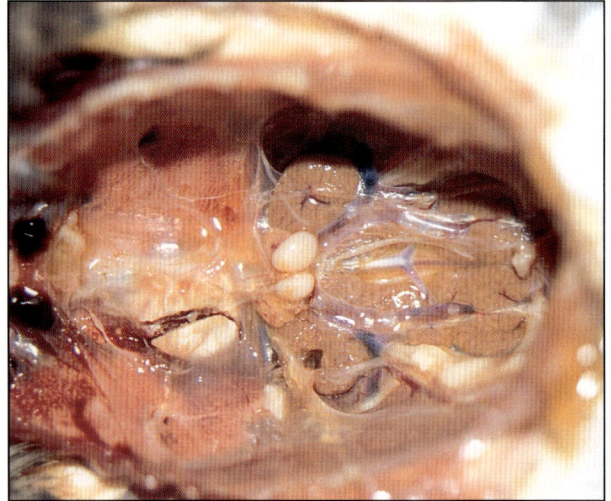

Fig. 13.56: The two enlarged testes of a three-year old peregrine falcon (*Falco peregrinus*) during breeding season.
(Photo: Heidenreich)

Surgical technique for sterilizing the male hawk (from Heidenreich, 1994): This procedure is considerably more difficult than the one described for females, especially in young tiercels. Their testes are still very small, lying tucked between the cranial pole of the kidney and the adrenal gland. The ductus deferens, a convoluted white tubule easily seen in mature birds, is so slight in juveniles that its traces can barely be recognized. Both structures are located retroperitoneally. The ductus, like the oviduct in females, runs along the kidney surface and can be dissected free and cut only with great delicacy and care. It is somewhat easier to transect the ductus deferens at its connection to the testis, near the epidydimis. The latter is a barely noticeable cone-shaped bump on the medial aspect of the testis. In any case, the peritoneum has to be lifted off the testis before the ductus can be transected. Because the immature reproductive organs in the young tiercel are not heavily vascularized, a ligature is not necessary. The ductus deferens is simply grasped with hemostats and separated from its attachment to the testis.

In contrast to the ovary, which is present only on the left side of the bird, this procedure in males must be repeated on the other side for the opposite gonad.

It is much easier to sterilize a tiercel during the breeding period. The testes and ductus deferens hypertrophy during this time and are better visualized and manipulated (Fig. 13.56). The approach then need not be repeated on the opposite side. Both the right and left ductus deferens are easily identified in the caudal kidney region and transected from one side.

References and literature of further interest

CASON, J.A., FLETCHER, D.L. and W.H. BURKE (1988):
Effects of caponization on broiler growth.
Poultry Science **67**, 979–981

FENNELL, M.J., JOHNSON A.L. and C.G. SCANES (1990):
Influence of androgens on plasma concentrations of growth
hormone in growing castrated and intact chickens.
General and Comparative Endocrinology **77**, 466–475

FRANKENHUIS, M.T. and H.J. KAPPERT (1980):
Infertility due to surgery on body cavity in female birds.
Causes and prevention.
Verh. Bericht XXII. Int. Symp. Erkr. Zootiere

HEIDENREICH, M. (1994):
Sterilisation von Falken - Eine Maßnahme zur Verhinderung
der Faunenverfälschung durch Hybridfalken.
(bislang unveröffentlicht)

HEIDENREICH, M., KÜSPERT, H., KÜSPERT, H.J. and R. HUSSONG
(1993):
Falkenhybriden. Deren Zucht, zum Verwandtschaftsgrad
verschiedener Falkenarten, sowie zum Thema der Faunenverfälschung durch Hybridfalken.
Beitr. Vogelkd. **39**, 205–226

JOYNER, K.L. (1994):
Theriogenology
in: Ritchie, B.W., G.J. Harrison u. L.R. Harrison (1994):
Avian medicine: principles and application
Wingers Publishing, Lake Worth, Florida

KÖNIG, H.E. (1985):
Die Kastration des Hähnchens.
Tierärztl. Praxis **13**, 307–311

MASE,Y. and T. OISHI (1991):
Effects of castration and testosterone treatment on the
development and involution of the bursa Fabricius in
Japanese quails.
General Comp. Endocr. **84**, 426–433

MILLER, L.E. and L.M. KRISTA (1985):
Effects of caponization on body weight, Atherosclerosis in
turkey lines.
Poultry Science **64**, 1002–1014

SAAR, C. (1993):
personal communication

SAMOUR, J. (1995):
The hybrid debate – Discussion on methods for sterilizing
falcon hybrids.
Falco **2**, 8

SCHRÖDER, K. (1965):
Zum Nachweis östrogenwirksamer Rückstände in chemisch
kapaunisierten Schlachthähnchen.
Vet. med. Diss., München

WILSON, S., GLADWELL, C. and R.T. CUNNINGHAM (1990):
Differential responses in castrated cockerels.
J. Endocrinology **125**, 139–146

13.8   The nervous system

Clinical signs indicative of central nervous system
(CNS) disease have often been described in birds of
prey. Greenwood (1973) divides CNS diseases in
raptors into five different categories based on their
cause: nutritional (e.g., calcium deficiency, see Ch.
11.2.1), infectious, (e.g., viral diseases, see Ch. 7), toxic
(see Ch. 12), injuries to the peripheral nervous system,
and injury involving the central nervous system. Goshawks and falcons are occasionally presented by falconers with clinical signs attributable to CNS disturbance. Definitive diagnostic tools, such as electro-
encephalography (EEG) and myelography, have not
yet been developed for use in raptors. The exact etiologies of the clinical syndromes described below therefore remain unclear.

13.8.1   Epilepsy in falcons

The term epilepsy is generally used to indicate a condition characterized by recurrent seizures caused by an
acquired or congenital intracranial cause. Hunting falcons have occasionally been reported to suffer from repeated convulsive episodes that can best be described
as epileptic. This disease has so far been described
only in male falcons.

In situations involving unusual excitement or stimulation, these birds suddenly become unable to fly. They
tumble to the ground and begin beating their wings
convulsively, seizuring for several minutes. Soon
thereafter, they spontaneously recover and return to
their normal behavior. In one particular falcon, these
episodes could be repeatedly induced by a loud call
from the falconer (CARTON, 1990). Presumably, the
call, which is generally used to alert a hunting hawk
to flushed quarry, produced such excitement in this
falcon that an epileptic seizure was triggered. Interestingly, PAULIK (1995) made similar observations in a
family of peregrine falcons. Only the tiercels in this
family developed clinical signs of epilepsy, making a
genetic, possibly sex-linked, etiology likely.

The author himself has seen a white gyrfalcon tiercel
which suffered from episodic seizures associated with
stimulation or excitement. During training, this bird
would fly at the lure in a normal fashion and with great

endurance. As soon as he actually struck the lure, the falcon would fall down convulsing, spread its tremoring tail and become completely unresponsive. Within seconds, he would regain consciousness and return to normal. Strangely enough, in a follow-up period of over two years, this falcon never showed these signs again.

13.8.2 "Goshawk paralysis"

Clinical signs

In every case, the goshawks developing this disease were still standing in the mews or had recently begun flying again after a period of inactivity. They demonstrated an acute onset lameness or stiffness in one leg, with balling of the toes in the affected foot (Fig. 13.57). Soon thereafter, often within 24 hours, the remaining leg became similarly affected. The birds sat or crouched on their hocks, but appeared otherwise unaffected. They continued accepting small morsels of food that were offered to them for several days before their condition deteriorated.

In many cases, the birds seemed unable to pass urates and feces. As a result, they became depressed and anorexic, losing weight and eventually dying after a period of fourteen days or so.

Diagnosis

The characteristic clinical presentation, together with the signalment and history, suffice for a diagnosis in most cases. Lead toxicity could potentially present with similar signs (see Ch. 12.1) and should be ruled out. Goshawks that have died of this paralytic disorder

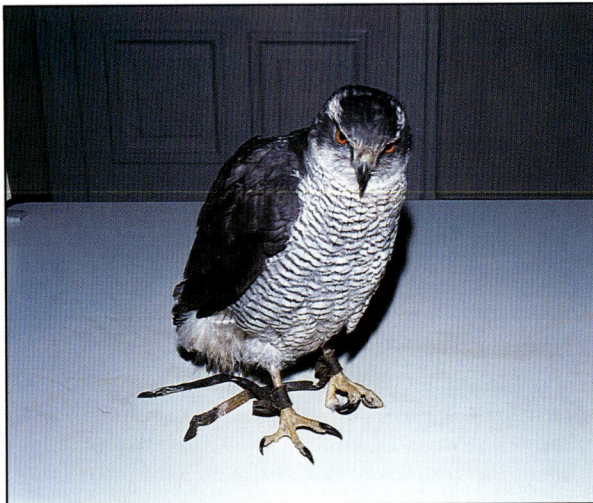

Fig. 13.57: Goshawk tiercel (*Accipiter gentilis*) in the early stages of goshawk paralysis showing paresis in one leg and "balling" of the affected foot.
(Photo: Heidenreich)

often show macroscopic petechial hemorrhages in the synsacral spinal cord. Damage to that part of the nervous system would certainly be compatible with the pelvic limb and perineal dysfunction observed in these birds. This problem is seen primarily in poorly conditioned goshawks, and it is tempting to speculate that the etiology may involve weakening or atrophy of the muscles that normally support the vulnerable junction between the fixed synsacrum and the more flexible thoracolumbar spine. When the hawk swoops low to land on the fist or an elevated branch, the lower back and legs are strongly extended, possibly stressing the spinal cord or damaging it by causing vertebral subluxation.

Treatment and prevention

The patient should be made as comfortable as possible on soft padded material or be outfitted with padded hock bandages to prevent pressure necrosis and injury to those joints. A dark, quiet box will help keep the hawk calm and minimize self-injury.

Good initial results have been obtained with the immediate administration of corticosteroids (prednisolone 2–5 mg/kg IM). This treatment can be repeated at two day intervals until recovery. B vitamins may also be administered. Although a vitamin deficiency is unlikely to be involved in this disease (see Ch. 11.1.2), B complex vitamins may aid in the regeneration of damaged nerves.

It is important to monitor hydration status and the passage of feces and urates. If necessary, the cloaca can be expressed manually. In anorectic birds, frequent force-feeding of small meals and fluid supplementation may become necessary.

In most cases, treatment is required for no more than 10 to 13 days. By then, the bird should be standing again. Any neurological deficits still present after this time bode ill for the overall prognosis, indicating possibly permanent spinal cord damage.

If the presumptive etiology of this disease is proven correct, hunting goshawks should be kept in larger flight cages even when not being flown, such as during the moulting period. This will prevent weakening of the musculature that supports the vertebral column. A wire and perch arrangement (see Ch. 3.3.3) may be preferable to the relatively small mews such birds are traditionally kept in.

References and literature of further interest

Böttcher, H. (1974):
Der Zehenkrampf beim Habicht.
Jb. Dtsch. Falkenorden, 50–51

Carton, F. (1990):
personal communication

Forbes, N.A. (1987):
Fits in the Harris hawk (*Parabuteo unicinctus*).
Vet. Rec. **120**, 264

Greenwood, A.G. (1973):
Veterinary medicine of birds of prey.
Proc. British Falc. Club Conf. 1973

Halliwell, W.H. (1969):
Epileptiform fits in falcons.
Hawk Chalk **8**, 42–43

Jessup, D.A. (1980):
Cranial nerve deficits in a rough-legged hawk.
Modern Vet. Pract. **61**, 240–241

Mikaelian, I. and J.J Thiebault (1990):
Pachymeningite ossifiante chez une buse variable
(*Buteo buteo*).
Point Vet. **21**, 909–910

Mundy, P.J. and C.M. Foggin (1981):
Epileptiform seizures in captive African vultures.
J. Wildl. Dis. **17**, 259–265

Paulik, J. (1995):
personal communication

Wallach, J.D. and G.M. Flieg (1970):
Cramps and fits in carnivorous birds.
Int. Zoo Yearbook **10**, 3–4

13.9 The endocrine system

The author has no personal experience with diseases involving endocrine dysfunction in birds of prey, and the pertinent literature provides very little information on this topic. A variety of studies have examined the influence of hormones on egg-laying and the moulting period in domestic poultry. Strict regulation of hormone supplementation in animals intended for human consumption, however, led to abandonment of this area of research.

Although the basic hormonal mechanisms probably function similarly in the many different groups of birds belonging to the class Aves, the use of hormones and the animal's reaction to them varies greatly between species. Lumeij (1994) therefore cautions against simply assuming that doses and responses valid in one avian species can be applied to another.

Diabetes mellitus has been separately addressed in Chapter 11.2.3.

13.9.1 Thyroid gland

The paired thyroid glands are located near the thoracic inlet on either side of the trachea. Among birds, problems most commonly arise in the form of hypothyroidism, or insufficient production of thyroid hormones. In raptors, this disease is most commonly caused by an iodine deficiency. The thyroid glands respond to the lack of necessary iodine by enlarging (hyperplasia), a condition which results in the characteristic goiter also recognized clinically in man and many other animals. Wisser and Ippen (1991) identified thyroid hyperplasia in 9 of 137 birds of prey whose thyroids were examined. Wadsworth and Jones (1979) also histologically diagnosed thyroid hyperplasia in a common buzzard (*Buteo buteo*).

Other avian species with goiters have been reported to develop dyspnea as a result of impingement by the enlarged thyroid glands on the trachea. Hypothyroidism also results in decreased activity, drowsiness, and a propensity for weight gain. In pet birds, this condition is generally treated with iodine supplementation in the food or water.

Hyperthyroidism, a condition of excess thyroid hormone production (see Ch. 13.1.1), presents the opposite clinical picture. The bird becomes hyperactive, ravenously hungry and loses weight rapidly if not supplied with adequate amounts of high quality food. Treatment for this condition in birds has not been reported.

13.9.2   Parathyroid glands

The two parathyroid glands lie very close to the thyroid glands and produce parathyroid hormone, which is involved in maintaining the calcium balance in the body. If serum calcium levels drop below normal (hypocalcemia), secretion of this hormone helps rectify the situation by stimulating calcium release from the bones and calcium retention by the kidneys. The only disorder involving this gland known in raptors is nutritional secondary hyperparathyroidism, described by Kumashiro and Amimoto (1987) and Long et al. (1983).

In one case, an osprey nestling was hand raised on a diet of cleaned raw meat. The bird developed weakness and drooping wings with spontaneous fractures of the wing bones. Reportedly, oral supplementation with calcium and vitamins resulted in recovery within eight weeks. This condition probably involved some degree of malformation in the growing bones (rickets, see Ch 11.2.1) and it is unlikely that fractures involving the long bones of the wings healed correctly on their own. Such reports must therefore be evaluated with some skepticism.

As described in other avian species, calcium deficiency in adults leads to demineralization of the bones (osteomalacia) and fibrous osteodystrophy.

13.9.3   Gonads

Pathologic changes involving the gonads (ovaries in the female, testes in the male) have been previously described in Chapter 13.7.

Breeders occasionally inquire about the possibility of hormonally influencing or even inducing egg-laying in females or improving fertility in males. All attempts at such manipulations in birds thus far have been unsuccessful. This may be attributable to our limited understanding of the avian endocrine system as well as to the fact that many of the commercially available mammalian hormones are ineffective in birds.

Tiercels demonstrating poor mating behavior can be stimulated to improve their performance by administering injectable testosterone. A dose of 8 mg/kg will result in stronger mating activity within two to three days. Testosterone does not affect the avian sperm count. Pair bonding, however, may be enhanced by the hormone's positive effect on male dominance.

Long-term administration of testosterone will result in a reduction or complete cessation of endogenous male hormone production. Impotence and infertility may result and such use of testosterone should therefore be avoided.

References and literature of further interest

Kumashiro, H. and A. Amimoto (1987):
Successful treatment of a few months old osprey (*Pandion*) suspected of nutritional secondary hyperparathyroidism.
J. Japan Vet. Med. Ass. **40**, 701–703

Long, P., Choi, G. and R. Rehmel (1983):
Oxyphil cells in a red-tailed hawk (*Buteo jamaicensis*) with nutritional secondary hyperparathyroidism.
Avian Dis. **27**, 839–843

Lumeij, J.T. (1994):
in: Ritchie, B.W., Harrison, G.J. and L.R. Harrison (1994):
Avian medicine: principles and application. 582–605
Wingers Publishing, Lake Worth, Florida

Wadsworth, P.F. and D.M. Jones (1979):
Some abnormalities of the thyroid gland in non-domesticated birds.
Avian Pathol **8**, 279–284

Wisser, J. and R. Ippen (1991):
Zum Vorkommen von Strumen bei Zoovögeln.
Wiener Tierärztl. Mschrift. **78**, 362–365

13.10   The musculoskeletal system

The musculoskeletal system of birds of prey, especially the wings and legs, has great demands placed upon it. Diseases involving this system occur most commonly in captive birds and are frequently the result of improper management and/or a poor diet.

13.10.1   Spraddle leg in chicks

Hand-raised raptor chicks (see Ch. 4.2) occasionally develop deformities of the pelvic limbs. In severe cases, the legs are no longer kept in their normal position tucked under the body, but are splayed out on one or both sides. This condition primarily affects chicks only a few days old, but if not corrected, it can lead to permanent changes in leg function and cripple the animal for life.

The development of spraddle leg has been linked to slippery nesting material or excessively large nests or boxes that allow the birds' legs to slide out from underneath them. It is easily avoided by placing very young chicks in an appropriately sized bowl padded with some kind of rough, easily cleaned or easily replaced material. Their legs thus remain firmly tucked underneath them until their muscles and bones have become strong enough to provide support.

Perosis (usually seen later and often unilateral) and rickets (also more common in older chicks, see Ch. 11.2.1.1) should be included in the differential diagnosis and ruled out by physical exam and radiographs.

Once spraddle leg has occurred, the chick should be kept in a close, nest-like container as described above. In addition, a hobble constructed so that the two legs are maintained a normal distance apart can be helpful. Such orthopedic devices should be applied for no more than five hours a day.

13.10.2   Alular malpositioning

Another problem sometimes encountered in young birds is malpositioning of the alula, or first wing digit. This small bone near the avian carpus turns so that it lies abnormally **under** the wing instead of extending **straight** along the anterior aspect of the metacarpals. This change in position can occur unilaterally or bilaterally and becomes obvious only after juvenile development has been completed and the bird is fully feathered (Fig. 13.58). Although the alula can be manually pushed back into its correct place, it soon returns to the abnormal position. Affected birds do not seem disabled in any way and appear to fly complete-

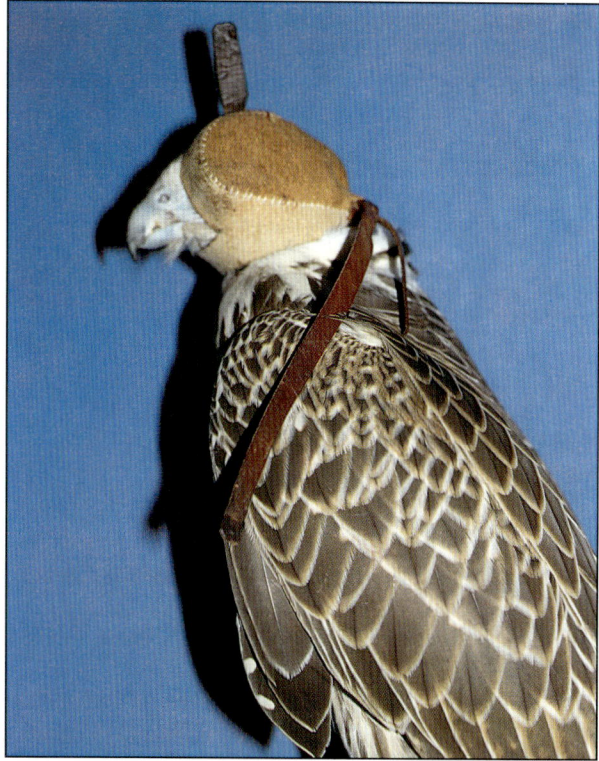

Fig. 13.58: The causes for malpositioning of the alula, as seen in this young hybrid falcon (saker falcon X gyrfalcon), have not been clearly determined. (Photo: Heidenreich)

ly normally. During flight, the alula, which is connected to four small feathers, is used for minor adjustments, primarily during steep descents. Close observation has revealed that the malpositioned digit is not noticeable during flight, presumably because the air pressure underneath the wing pushes it back into its intended position. Only at rest does the alula revert to its abnormal position.

The cause of this condition is unknown. It is noteworthy that alular malpositioning develops primarily in young birds raised in small aviaries that do not provide enough room for the growing birds to engage in adequate stretching and flapping of wings before they can fly. It seems likely that this is a preventable problem associated with inadequate housing for young birds raised in captivity.

Treatment is possible, but depends on the age of the hawk and the severity of the problem. The alula is pushed forward into its normal position and then stabilized with tape along the cranial edge of the wing. Most birds will soon notice this device and try to remove it. This should be prevented for at least the first few hours. A hood can be helpful in this situation, especially if it is fitted with a beak protector. Young birds, whose musculoskeletal system is still amenable to adjustment, require only a few days of fixation.

13.10.3   Perosis

Perosis, also known as "leg weakness", chondrodystrophy, or "slipped tendon" is seen occasionally in domestic and wild birds. It has been reported most commonly among young broiler chickens, male turkey poults and ostriches and involves changes in the hock joint that lead to medial luxation of the extensor tendon. Affected birds are unable to walk and their legs rotate laterally. Siegmann (1992) lists excessively rapid growth with insufficient exercise and certain nutritional deficiencies (manganese, choline, biotin) as possible causes of this condition.

In raptors, perosis has been described in a young lanner falcon (Kummerfeld, 1982) and in three gyrfalcons from the same clutch (Saar, 1990).

Clinical disease

Initial signs usually involve a unilateral lameness in nestlings several weeks or months old. The young birds will prefer to bear weight on the normal leg and rotate the affected leg outwards. As the condition progresses, they become unable to stand on the abnormal leg at all, frequently developing pododermatitis secondarily in the weight-bearing foot. Closer examination will reveal lateral bowing of the bones on either side of the affected hock joint. The joint itself is often warm, swollen and painful.

The birds appear otherwise unaffected, with normal appetites and good body condition.

Diagnosis

The clinical signs described above frequently allow a rapid presumptive diagnosis to be made. Abnormal lateral rotation of the distal leg and identification of the displaced tendon by palpation help confirm it. Radiographs can clarify the situation by ruling out rickets and revealing bony changes in the tibiotarsal-tarsometatarsal joint typical of perosis.

Treatment and prevention

Successful treatment of this disease is generally not possible. The bony and cartilagenous changes are not reversible by the time such birds are recognized and presented for treatment. Although not grossly visible, the leg abnormality often has a negative impact on the development of the bird's entire musculoskeletal system.

If nutritional deficiencies should play a role in this disease in raptors, as they do in poultry, close attention to the quality of the diet may help prevent further development of the disease and avoid its occurrence in other young birds. Manganese (3 mg/kg/day) can be added as a supplement to the food. Excess consumption of calcium and phosphorus has also been linked to perosis. Care should therefore be taken not to give growing birds excessive amounts of mineral supplements.

13.10.4   Pododermatitis (bumblefoot)

13.10.4.1 Pododermatitis in falcons

Pododermatitis in falcons, better known as bumblefoot, is a disease affecting the plantar metatarsal pad of the foot. It usually begins with swelling and inflammation of the area, complicated by secondary bacterial infections as ulcers form and the disease progresses. Eventually, infection and necrosis of the deep tendinous and bony components of the foot develop and can lead to permanent impairment of the bird's grasping ability, even after recovery. If not treated, advanced cases may even lead to systemic illness and death (Fig. 13.59).

Bumblefoot has been a problem in captive birds of prey since the earliest days of falconry. Ancient and medieval authors described this problem exactly (Al Gitrif, 744; Zapata, 1566; D'Arcussia, 1617), although they limited themselves to discussing its treatment and avoided examining the possible causes.

Modern science has brought with it a better understanding of physiological and pathological processes, and many publications examining the etiology of this often deadly disease have been produced. Some of the theories proposed have been unusual indeed.

Proposed causes for pododermatitis

RAETHEL (1962) proposed that small injuries to the skin allow bacteria to enter the foot and initiate a chronic infection.

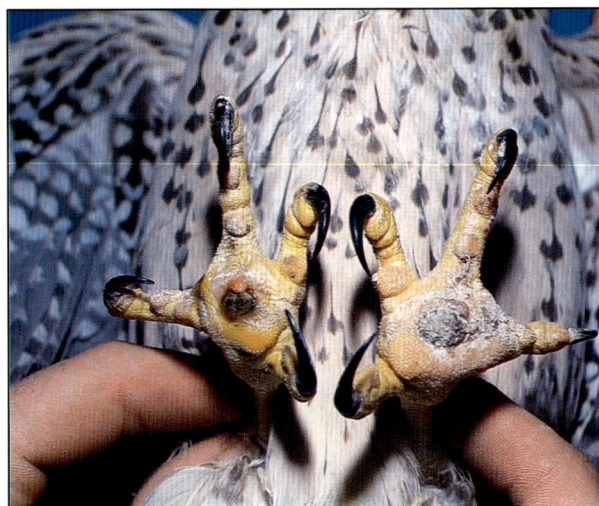

Fig. 13.59: End stage disease in a lanner falcon (*Falco biarmicus*) with pododermatitis or "bumblefoot". (Photo: Heidenreich)

Cooper (1978) suggested that these small injuries to the feet could be self-induced, caused when the hawk closed its foot and punctured it with the talon of the hallux. A bacterial infection would then follow. Experiments with starlings that he conducted resulted in bumblefoot-like lesions in the feet after local injection of *Staphylococcus aureus* bacteria. This theory was not changed in the more recent edition of his book (1985).

Although Woodford (1987) agreed with most of Cooper's ideas, he also mentioned gout as a possible cause for pododermatitis in falcons, postulating that uric acid deposits in the feet could result in the swelling and other changes seen in the early stages of this disease. Stehle (1965) had also discussed a possible connection with gout in this context.

These theories were supported by Williams (1986), who added an additional hypothesis regarding possible sources of injury. He suggested that trained falcons may puncture their metatarsal pads with the talon of their relatively short hallux when they grasp at a lure and just barely miss, too late to avoid clenching their feet. He recommended coping that talon to prevent this from occurring.

Two different possible causes were put forth by Trommer (1991). He suggested the possible involvement of parasites, especially air sac filariids, which would explain why bumblefoot seems to be more common in wild-caught birds. These parasites are ubiquitous among falcons in Arab countries. How these parasites would get into the feet was not explained. The second theory pertained to the use of block perches and suggested that the anatomical differences between the hierofalcon group and peregrine falcons might explain why the former are more commonly affected. He recommended distributing the pressure more evenly over the bottom of a falcon's foot by providing block perches with convex surfaces. The same suggestion had already been made by Bruell (1937) and was based on the idea that improper perching surfaces could play a role in the etiology of this disease. This theory had many supporters. Kiel (1982) also mentioned improperly designed block perches as possibly contributing to the development of pododermatitis. He also thought that puncture wounds to the foot pad could be caused by a falcon's sharp talons as they curl inward in the relaxed, raised foot.

All authors seem to agree that bumblefoot is not a significant problem in accipiters, and occurs primarily in falcons. Only Kummerfeld and Gruenhagen (1986) mention a case in which there were lesions of the toes (but no swelling of the metatarsal pad) in a wild European sparrowhawk. This was probably not a true case of bumblefoot.

Personal observations

The condition known as bumblefoot was common in earlier times, when wild-caught falcons were easily imported to Europe. Nowadays falconers fly almost exclusively captive-bred birds and veterinarians are only rarely presented with falcons suffering from pododermatitis. This shift has occurred although husbandry practices have really not changed much in this time. Unsuitable perch construction is therefore unlikely to be a factor in the disease. The same block perches are still used today.

Why, then, do captive bred falcons suffer much less frequently from bumblefoot than wild-caught birds do?

Wild-caught falcons, i.e., those captured in the autumn of their hatch year or even haggards, differ from captive-bred birds in one main respect. They are more accomplished fliers. They fly better because they have spent a part of every day for the past months or years in the air, regardless of weather, moult or other factors. Captive-bred birds, on the other hand, even if flown to the lure regularly, get no more than a few minutes of exercise daily. The average session involves a few minutes of initial free flight, then 50 passes to the lure, which may take no more than 10 minutes or so.

Until now, there have been no proven reports of pododermatitis among falcons in the wild. If, as suspected by Trommer, parasites were a possible cause, then wild birds should be particularly susceptible. This is not the case. On the contrary, it has been documented that affected falcons that were released to the wild recovered completely without human interference.

In areas where wild-caught falcons are still commonly used for hunting, primarily the Arab countries, bumblefoot is greatly feared. It typically occurs just after the hunting season when the falcons are rested for the moult, many months after their initial capture. This goes against the theories that propose self-injury as a factor, especially since birds are particularly well known for the rapidity and ease with which their injuries heal. Unlike mammals, birds almost never suffer from wound infections and heal well from surgeries, even if performed with minimal attention to sterile procedure.

Figures 13.60 and 13.61 show the feet of two gyrfalcons that had suffered extensor tendon injuries and subsequently pressed the sharp talon of their hallux into the foot pad for **two years**. The only sign of damage was callus formation (hyperkeratosis) at the site of irritation. Bumblefoot did not occur.

Everyone seems to agree that the treatment options for bumblefoot are limited and frequently unsuccessful. This, too, seems to indicate that the actual etiology of this disease is still not understood. Treatment tends

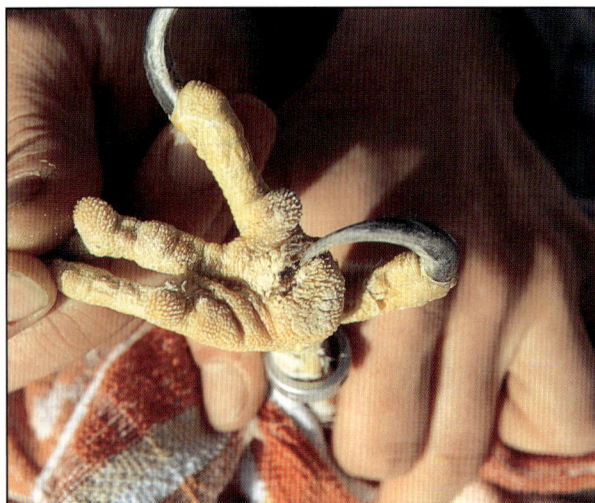

△ **13.60**

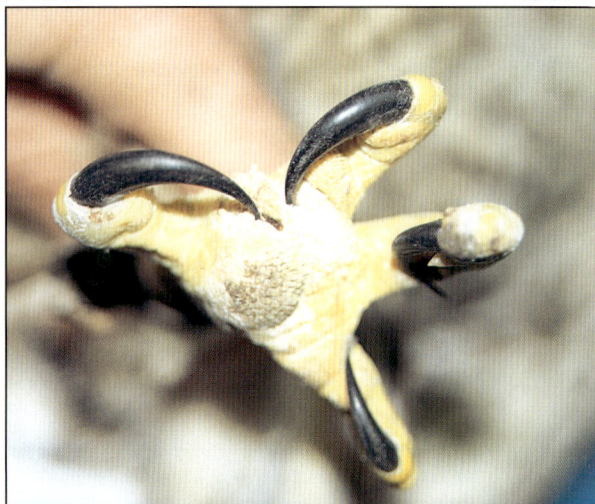

13.61 ▽

Figs. 13.60 and 13.61: In these two falcons, extensor tendon injuries to the hallux resulted in years of pressure by the affected talon on the sole of the foot. Despite this, the birds did **not** develop bumblefoot. (Photos: Heidenreich)

excess cardiac capacity, physical inactivity and changes in diet, are difficult to compensate for. Fluid escapes into the tissues from small blood vessels. The dependent edema that then develops collects in the lowest body parts, in this case, the feet. Similar fluid buildup is seen in well-trained horses suddenly forced to spend several days confined to a stall. Human performance athletes, too, know that they must come off a strenuous training program gradually to avoid major cardiovascular problems.

The cardiovascular development of a captive-bred falcon, on the other hand, corresponds exactly with its level of training. There is no excess capacity.

The reason that wild-caught falcons seem to develop bumblefoot after the hunting season is over might thus be explained. As long as the bird continues to be flown right after its capture and on into the hunting season, the circulatory system continues to function at levels approximating what it was accustomed to. The inevitable problems involving the feet and the bird as a whole occur only after the animal is forced to become inactive. The suddenly sedentary life style and plentiful food result in rapid weight gain. These abrupt changes in activity level and body weight would never occur under natural conditions.

The reason that accipiters seem to get pododermatitis less often than falcons may be related to the fact that they are short-distance hunters whose cardiovascular fitness level, even in the wild, is less well developed than that of falcons, who tend to be long-distance hunters. The discrepancy between the cardiovascular demands on accipiters in the wild and in captivity may not be so vastly different. Wild eagles and vultures, on the other hand, do spend a great deal of time flying. As expected, under captive conditions, they too occasionally suffer from bumblefoot (see below).

to be symptomatic rather than being aimed at eliminating the underlying causes of the problem.

Personal hypothesis regarding the etiology of pododermatitis

The more susceptible wild-caught falcons differ from the relatively resistant captive-bred ones primarily in their overall conditioning, including metabolic rate and cardiovascular fitness. A wild falcon brought into captivity has been flying daily over months or years to hunt for its food. Such a bird has a level of cardiovascular fitness comparable to that of a highly trained athlete. If the animal is then suddenly restricted to a life of inactivity, metabolic imbalances and massive circulatory disorders are likely to result. These circulatory problems, which result from a combination of

13.62

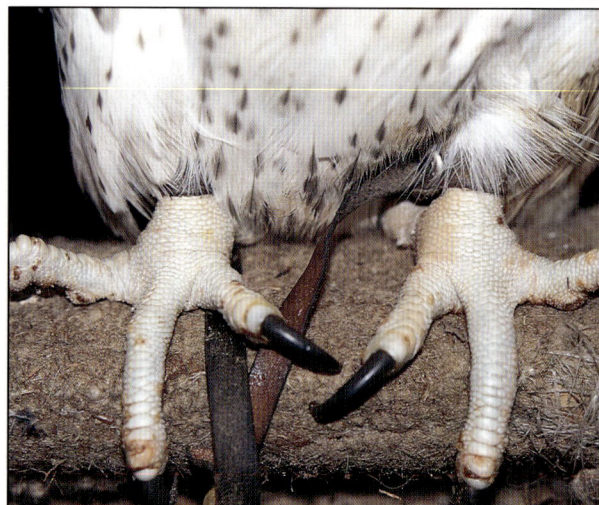

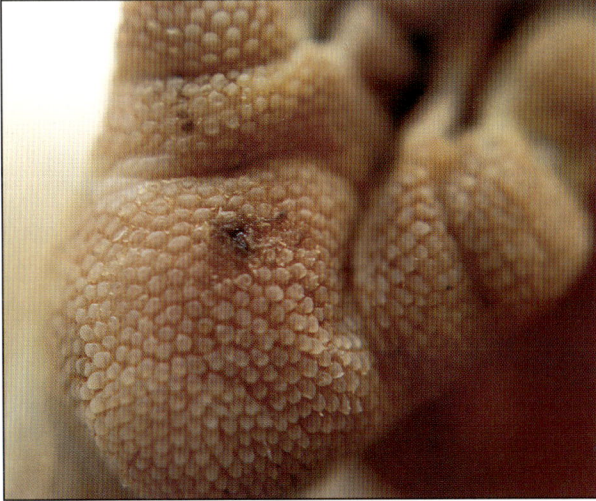
13.63

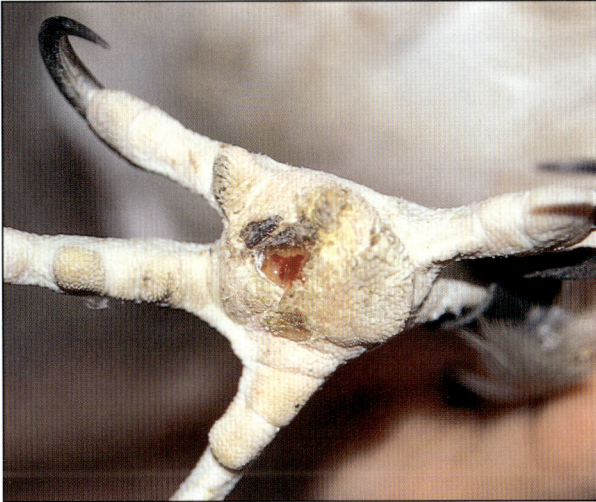
13.64

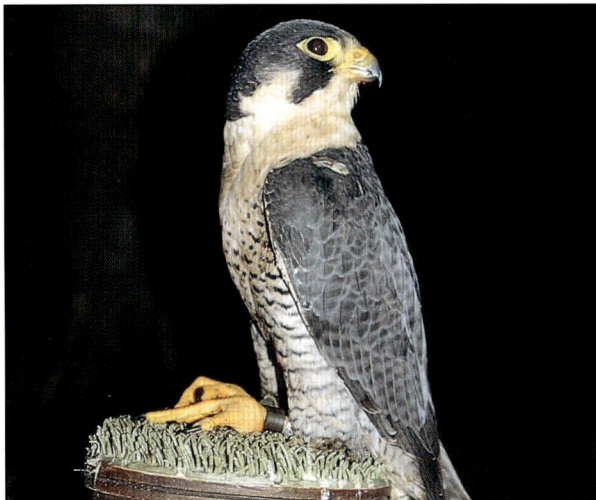
13.65

Clinical signs

Frequently, the patient is presented only after swelling or infection of the feet has become obvious. The subtle earlier signs typically pass unnoticed. The overall disease generally unfolds as follows:

0. Being flown hard yesterday, tied to the block perch and inactive today
1. Development of circulatory problems for which the body is unable to compensate, metabolic imbalances resulting from surplus protein availability and insufficient utilization of energy
2. Dependent edema involving the lower portions of the body, swelling of the metatarsal pads and toes
3. Pressure necrosis at weight bearing points **independent** of substrate
4. Bacterial invasion of crusty necrotic lesions
5. Purulent inflammation involving the entire foot, normal immune function not possible in the edematous areas due to inadequate blood flow, therefore response to antibiotic therapy and surgical intervention generally unsatisfactory
6. The bird crouches on hocks or becomes recumbent due to painful feet
7. Necrosis of the tendon sheaths and tendons resulting in inability to move toes
8. Generalized sepsis and death or euthanasia of the bird.

Figures 13.62–13.65 show the chronological development of pododermatitis in falcons. This condition can extend over many months and occasionally resolve spontaneously or at least stabilize, until some kind of stress reactivates the disease process.

Treatment

The success of therapy is directly dependent on the stage of the disease and the overall condition of the patient.

Figs. 13.62, 13.63, 13.64 and 13.65: The clinical progression of pododermatitis in falcons is depicted in this series of pictures. The initiating cause is **not** self-injury, but rather a generalized metabolic and cardiovascular imbalance that initially results in dependent edema (13.62). The edema is not always this obvious. Inadequate perfusion of the foot allows tiny foci of necrosis to develop (13.63) **independent** of the type of surface upon which the bird stands. Pathogens can now easily invade the necrotic tissue (13.64). The bacteria proliferate quickly because the lack of circulation to these areas limits immune system function. The tissues of the foot are rapidly destroyed, causing severe pain. Eventually, the falcon's overall health is affected and death may result. (Photos: Heidenreich)

Acute phase without bacterial involvement: The bird should immediately be brought down in weight and flown for exercise, or at least placed in a large aviary that permits ample activity to stimulate the metabolism. If this is not possible, daily rubbing in of ointments that stimulate blood flow (e.g., Capsolin®) will suffice in many cases. The actual massaging and rubbing of the area is as important as the ointment itself! REDIG (1993) recommends applying a mixture composed of 5 ml DMSO (dimethylsulfoxide), 4 mg dexamethasone and 1 g piperacillin dissolved in 3 ml of physiologic saline for birds that are in the early stages of bumblefoot. In the author's experience, daily soaking in warm soapy baths combined with local topical application of heparin-containing gels (Tensolvet®) is also effective in helping resolve mild cases of the disease.

Acute phase with bacterial involvement

In these cases, surgical debridement of the necrotic and infected tissues of the foot is usually indicated (Fig. 13.66). Careful removal of the damaged and discolored tissue should be performed while preserving the tendons inside their tendon sheaths as much as possible.

There is some disagreement regarding whether to close the surgical wound after such procedures. GERLACH (1982) recommends leaving it partially open to allow for drainage of secretions. Riddle and Hoolihan (1993) and Remple (1993) also recommend treating it as an open wound if indicated. For this situation, they developed a specific bandaging technique which leaves the actual wound open and prevents it from bearing any pressure during the healing process (Fig. 13.67).

In the author's experience, each case must be approached individually. As long as there is no joint involvement and joint fluid is not expected to be draining from the wound, primary closure is not a problem (Fig. 13.68). Further protection is then provided with appropriate bandaging. Since avian pus is caseous rather

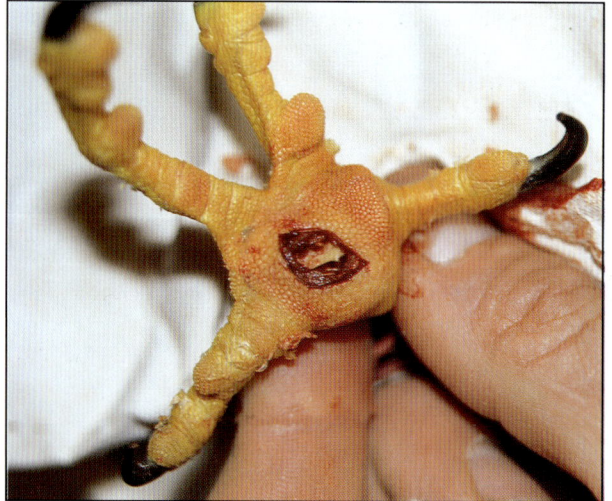

13.66

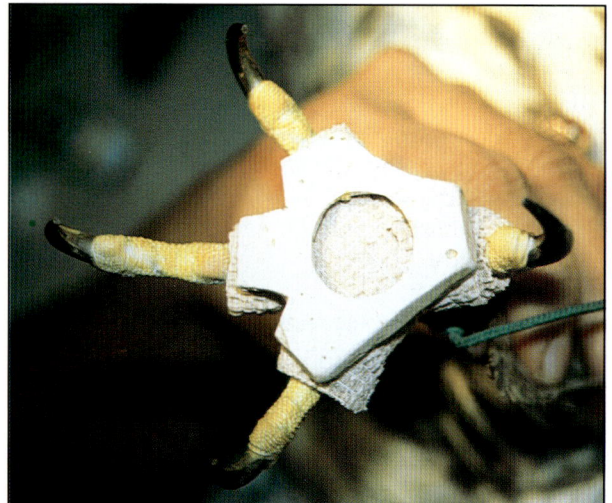

13.67

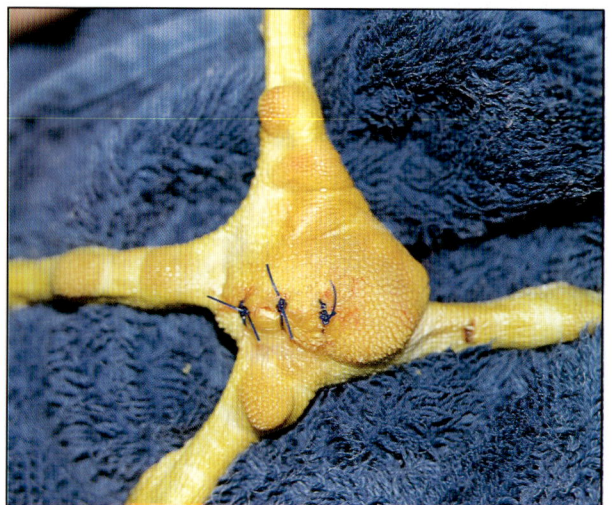

13.68

Figs. 13.66, 13.67 and 13.68: The prognosis for a successful outcome of treatment for bumblefoot depends directly on the severity of the condition. In the early stages of pododermatitis with bacterial infection, surgical debridement and closure can be very effective. A spindle-shaped incision is made around the area of necrosis (13.66) and necrotic debris and caseous exudate are removed carefully, making sure that tendons and tendon sheaths are preserved. A sample should be obtained for bacterial culture and sensitivity before instilling broad-spectrum antibacterial drugs into the surgical site. The wound is closed with fine suture material (13.68) and bandaged. Concurrent systemic therapy with appropriate antibiotics is absolutely necessary.

To reduce pressure on the surgery site and promote healing, specially constructed foot pads (from Remple) with a central opening can be included in the bandage (13.67). (Photos: Heidenreich, Lierz)

than liquid as in mammals, drainage of purulent material is not to be expected from wounds in any case.

A bacterial culture and sensitivity should be performed on the material removed from the foot, and antibiotic therapy should be based on the results. *Staphylococcus aureus* is one of the major pathogens typically found in bumblefoot lesions. It is often surprisingly resistant to many of the commonly used antibacterial agents, even in birds that have not been previously treated with such drugs. Antibiotic therapy should be kept up for longer periods of time, at least 14 days or more depending on the severity of the lesion and the rate of healing.

Prevention
In trying to prevent the occurrence of bumblefoot, one of the most important measures is the **gradual** buildup of body weight after the hunting season. Excessively rapid weight gain must be avoided. As a rule, the rate of gain should not exceed 5–10 grams per day. This means that the falcon must continue to be weighed regularly for approximately two more weeks after the end of the falconry season.

If clinical signs of pododermatitis are already present, the bird's weight should immediately be brought down to hunting season levels. Daily flight training should be resumed to stimulate the circulatory system and thus improve perfusion and immune system function in the feet. Every falconer has probably experienced that a falcon's feet are often cool to the touch prior to its flying, In contrast, the heat radiating from them after exercise can sometimes be felt right through the leather glove. Personal experience has convinced the author that housing bumblefoot patients in large circular aviaries greater than 30 meters in diameter and at least 6 meters in height promotes recovery so well that birds placed in such aviaries early enough often recover without requiring surgery at all (Fig. 13.69).

> In the author's opinion, chronic pododermatitis in falcons is the external manifestation of a generalized metabolic and cardiovascular disturbance whose origin lies in a failure to acknowledge the physiological and pathological processes occurring in the bird. By definition, it therefore involves a failure to meet the basic feeding, exercise and maintenance needs of the species!

13.10.4.2 Pododermatitis in vultures and eagles

Disease processes involving the feet similar to those described above in falcons are also seen in vultures and eagles. While the classic form of bumblefoot in falcons occurs primarily in the metatarsal pad of the foot, lesions involving the toes are a common component of this disorder in the larger species (Figs. 13.70–13.72). The causes of the problem are likely to be the same as those described for falcons. In these large birds the disease seems to occur during periods of inactivity and abundant food intake. Although the therapeutic approach is the same as that described for falcons, the rate of recovery in eagles and vultures is significantly higher.

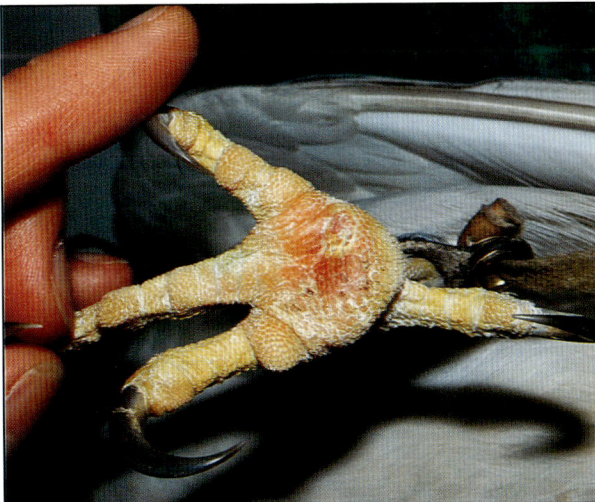

Fig. 13.69: Mild and moderate degrees of pododermatitis in falcons can resolve spontaneously if the bird is given plenty of flying time and exercise so that circulation to the feet improves. This can be accomplished in large flight cages or by falconry techniques for free flight. After a few weeks, the deep necrotic lesions will have healed and only some scars will be left.
(Photo: Heidenreich)

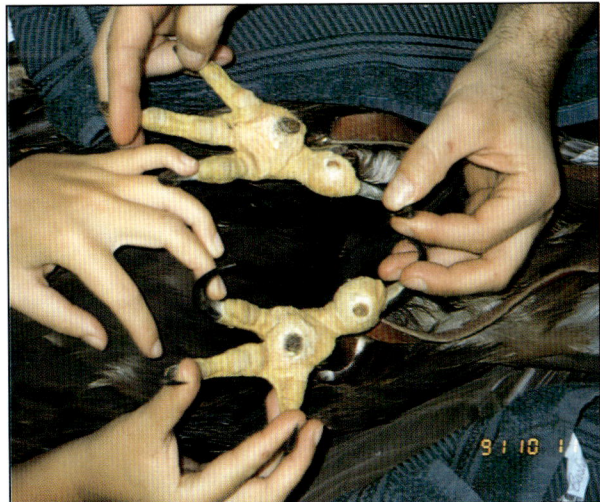

Fig. 13.70: Golden eagles (*Aquila chrysaetos*) trained for falconry also suffer from pododermatitis. As with falcons, the problem occurs most commonly when the hunting season ends. Eagles very easily put on weight and get fat, a tendency which may contribute to the development of this disease.
(Photo: Heidenreich)

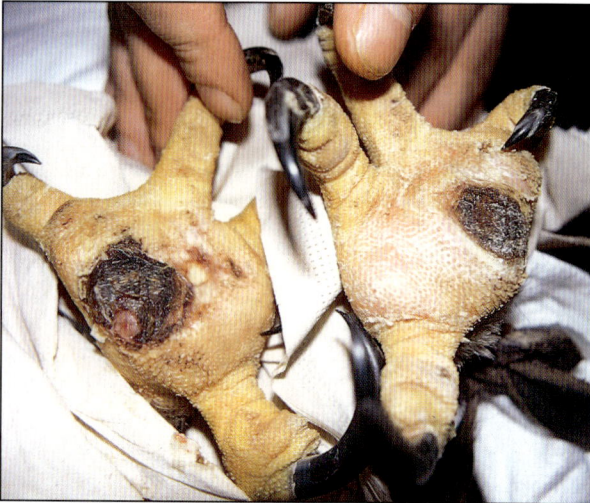

Fig. 13.71: This 22 year-old golden eagle (*Aquila chrysaetos*) was flown several times daily for years as part of a public show at a raptor center. After he attacked and injured a dog, the eagle was no longer permitted to fly and was placed in an aviary. After only six weeks, the first signs of pododermatitis were noticed on its feet. Regrettably, the bird was not presented for treatment until many months later, too late for effective therapy. (Photo: Heidenreich)

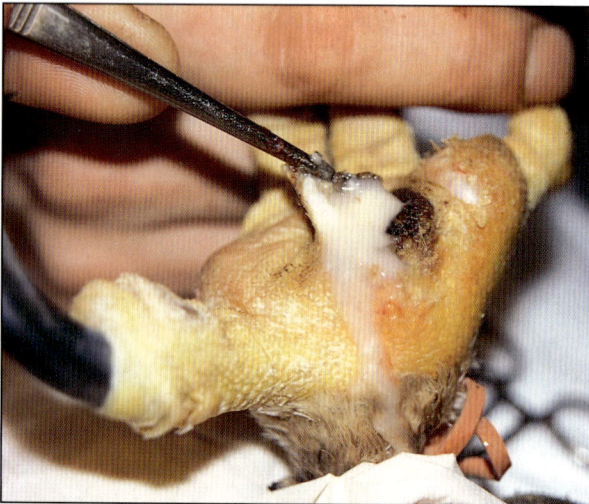

Fig. 13.72: In advanced cases of pododermatitis, joints and tendon sheaths are often involved in the disease process. On removing the superficial crust, purulent synovial fluid exudes from the wound. (Photo: Heidenreich)

13.10.4.3 Pelvic limb edema in accipiters

No disease comparable to bumblefoot as seen in falcons, vultures and eagles has been reported in accipiters. This is all the more surprising, as wild caught goshawks are commonly used in falconry, and the disease should appear in them as it does in falcons if they suffered from the same metabolic imbalances.

The condition described below has never been reported before. It occurs exclusively in wild-caught goshawks and its cause and significance have in the past been interpreted wrongly due to its localization in the legs of the bird.

Clinical disease
A few days after the goshawk is withdrawn from hunting activity, placed on a block perch and given access to excessive amounts of food, its legs become painfully swollen. They feel soft and doughy to the touch. Within days, the swelling resolves and localized bump-like lesions become visible (Fig. 13.73). Because of their location on the bird's legs, such lesions have in the past been ascribed to improperly fitted jesses.

Radiographic examination of the affected leg often reveals that the periosteum covering the bone underneath these bumps shows signs of being involved in the process. In advanced cases, even the keratin scales covering the leg in that area can flake off. Surprisingly, the hawk does not seem to favor the swollen leg in any way and continues to function normally.

Treatment
Topical therapy with ointments that encourage blood flow to the area (Capsolin®) works rapidly to reduce the swelling and usually leads to complete resolution of the lesion within a few weeks (Fig. 13.74). Presumably, the body's adjustment to a less active lifestyle also helps resolve the problem.

Prevention
As with falcons, eagles and vultures, goshawks, especially wild-caught ones, should be gradually brought down to an inactive phase. A slow gain of weight from hunting levels to molting condition is also important.

13.10.5 Muscular atrophy

A decrease in muscle tone and size always occurs after prolonged disuse of a particular body part. Depending on its location, an injury can often result in significant loss of mobility for a bird, producing a noticeable loss of muscle in the pectoral area or pelvic limbs within a short time. These changes can easily be reversed when the affected limb regains mobility.

A special form of muscle atrophy occurs in hunting hawks which are reduced in weight to prepare them for hunting.

Some falconers still believe that they can judge their bird's condition by palpating the pectoral (breast) muscles. A common rule is that the muscle belly should always be convex to the touch. If it becomes concave, then the bird has become too thin (Fuente, 1986). Such vague criteria for judgment have often resulted in

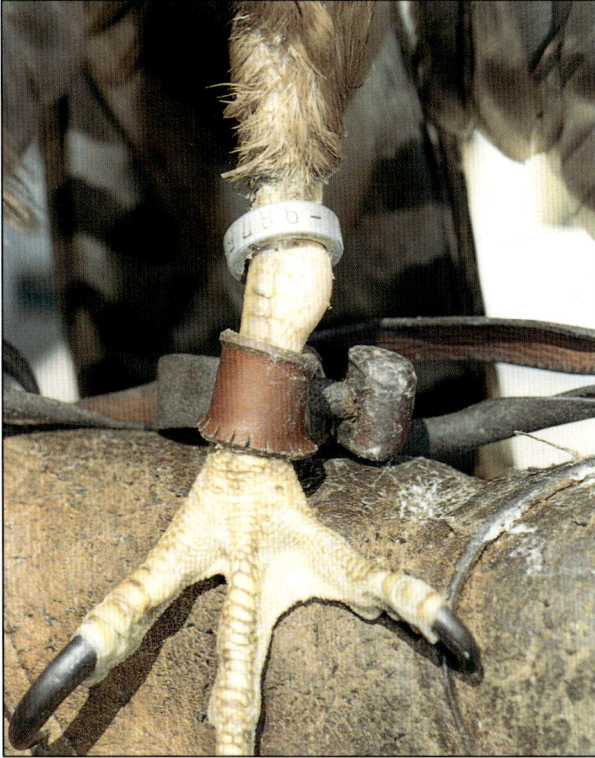

Figs. 13.73 △ **and 13.74** ▽: As with wild-caught falcons, sudden decreases in activity level also lead to disease in previously active wild-caught goshawks. Problems do not arise in the feet, however, but involve the legs instead. Edematous bumps (13.73) appear only days after regular exercise ceases and may take weeks to resolve (13.74). (Photos: Heidenreich)

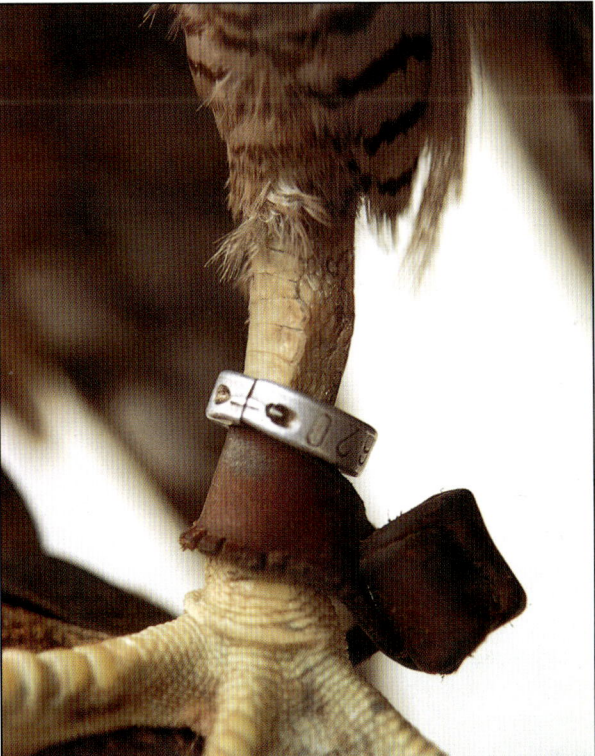

real damage to the hawk's health. Thankfully, most falconers now use scales to determine their bird's exact weight and no longer simply rely on palpation of muscles.

13.10.6   Frostbite

Various tropical raptor species have special temperature requirements (see Ch. 3.2.4) and do not tolerate cold weather. Body parts not covered with feathers and distal extremities, especially toes, are vulnerable to frostbite. Species such as the king vulture (*Sarcoramphus papa*), the Indian black vulture (*Sarcogyps calvus*) and the bateleur (*Terathopius ecaudatus*) are particularly vulnerable.

Initial signs primarily involve swelling of the affected digit. Later, blackening and necrosis of the tissue (dry gangrene) become apparent. The dead portions of the toe eventually fall or break off or require amputation (Fig. 13.75).

If frostbite is suspected or identified early enough, slow warming of the affected body parts can help minimize the damage to the tissues. Gentle massage in first cold, the gradually warmer water baths for 20–30 minutes will stimulate blood flow to the digits and help prevent their complete devitalization.

13.10.7   Power line injuries

Our modern landscapes are crisscrossed with wires and wild birds of prey as well as free-flying hunting hawks are always at risk of colliding with unseen high tension power lines or electric railroad cables. Such contact puts them at risk of burns or even death by electrocution. Haas (1993) estimated that 17% of the raptors killed in Germany fall victim to this type of death. Hammer (1991) examined the various types of poles and towers designed to suspend power lines and discussed their relative risks.

Raptors, in particular, favor very tall perching sites and therefore like to fly to the tall metal towers that carry high tension power lines. During landing or take-off, the bird's wings are spread and can easily come in contact with electrified parts. In rain or fog, a spark can jump even more easily onto the hawk. Severe burns involving the appendages (Fig. 13.76) or even death can result.

13.10.8   Congenital anomalies

There have been a few reports of congenital anomalies of the musculoskeletal system in birds of prey. Tegtmeier (1995), for instance, produced a red kite (*Milvus*

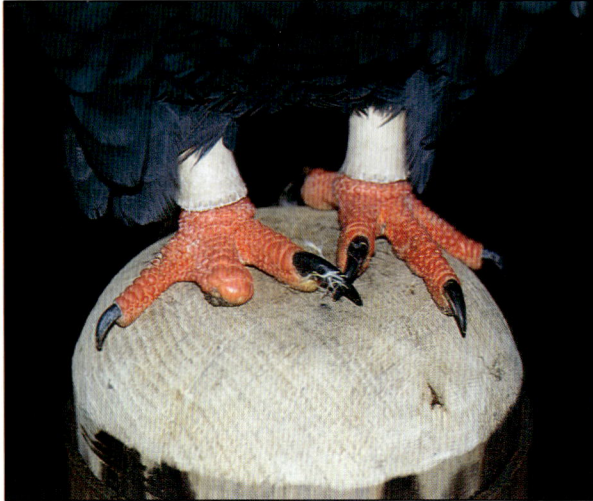

Fig. 13.75: Cold sensitive, tropical raptor species (in this case a bateleur, *Terathopius ecaudatus*) can easily lose toes to frostbite in European or North American winters. (Photo: Heidenreich)

milvus) with five toes (polydactyly). It was not a heritable trait, as the offspring of this bird all had normal feet. Bednarek (1974) reported an anomaly involving the bones of the wing in a wild goshawk (*Accipiter gentilis*). On one side only, this bird had an extra alula and shortened carpometacarpals. It did not survive into adulthood, being completely dependent for food on its parents, and starved to death once they ceased feeding it. The primary feathers arising from this goshawk's abnormally short carpometacarpus were so densely packed that the bird was unable to fly.

Saar (1974) and Bednarek (1974a) noted some presumably genetically based abnormalities in the tail feathers of a peregrine falcon (*Falco peregrinus*) and a common kestrel (*Falco tinnunculus*). While normal

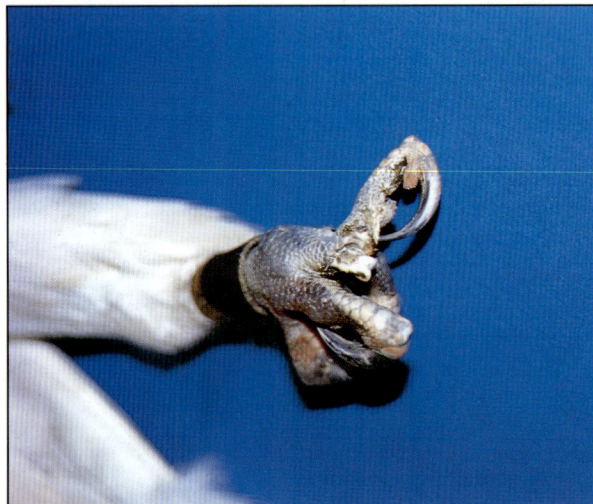

Fig. 13.76: This young white gyrfalcon (*Falco rusticolus*) was literally electrocuted after contacting a high-tension wire. Note the burned foot.   (Foto: Heidenreich)

peregrine falcons have 12 tail feathers, this particular bird had 14. The kestrel had the normal number of feathers, but they displayed a distinctly abnormal banding pattern.

13.10.9   Luxations and fractures

Dislocations (luxations) of limb joints in raptors occur with perosis (see Ch. 13.10.3) and due to trauma. Most common are luxations of the elbow or of the shoulder, where the humerus comes together with the scapula, coracoid and clavicle in a complex joint. This type of injury can occur when a hawk strikes an object such as a wire with outspread wings.

The avian shoulder joint relies primarily on muscles, tendons and ligaments to connect the humerus to the trunk. Luxations at this site always involve tearing of this connective apparatus and are difficult if not impossible to repair. Fixing the affected wing in a normal position to the body with a bandage may occasionally allow some recovery of the bird's ability to fly. Rarely is it enough to allow the bird to return to hunting or be released.

Elbow luxations usually involve the ulna. They are more easily reduced and stabilized and have a better prognosis for return to normal function if treated early.

Fractures, or interruptions in the normal continuity of bone structure, are seen in raptors from the wild and in captivity. They are usually caused by trauma (raptors with metabolic bone disease being the exception, see Ch. 11.2.1.1), and most commonly involve the long bones of the wing or leg.

Fractures in very young birds, whose bones are still relatively soft, tend to be "greenstick", or bending fractures, where the periosteum covering the bone remains intact. The prognosis for such fractures is quite good if they are corrected promptly.

The older a bird gets, the harder its bones become. In addition, avian bones have particularly thin cortices, an adaptation that helps minimize body weight for these flying animals. As a result, fractures in adult birds are usually compounded by extensive splintering of the bone.

The pneumatic, or air-filled, humerus and femur are connected with the air sac system of the bird and present additional complications in case of fracture. Open fractures, i.e., those in which the sharp ends of broken bone or some other injury have resulted in penetration of the skin, usually have an even poorer prognosis for return to normal function. The exposed bone suffers from drying of the periosteum and pathogens gain access to the injured bone and surrounding tissues, making repair of the fracture much more difficult. Healthy periosteal tissue is vital to external callus formation, a particularly important fact in pneumatic bones, which are less able to form endosteal callus because they are filled with air.

Closed fractures (no penetration of skin) involving marrow-filled bones are significantly easier to repair, if the surrounding nerves, blood vessels and ligaments have not been too severely damaged. Because the integrity of these soft tissues is so important to the outcome of the case, all birds that have suffered a fracture should immediately be placed in a dark, quiet location to prevent further damage. The injured limb should be gently immobilized in a normal position using light, breathable bandage materials. Smaller species with suspected wing fractures can be temporarily restrained inside a close-fitting elastic nylon stocking. Nonadherent elastic bandage material (Tesakrepp, Vetwrap) has also proven very useful for temporarily immobilizing injured limbs.

Diagnosis

Detailed evaluation of a fracture requires radiography. At least two views and detailed radiographic technique are required to get a good picture of the fracture, including fragments and fissures in the bone.

Fractures involving the sternum, or keel, are especially challenging to identify. They require exact ventrodorsal positioning as well as a lateral view to be identified. Injuries of this kind are particularly common in emaciated birds whose keel juts out sharply due to atrophy of the breast musculature. As the pectoral muscles that attach to the sternum are the biggest flight muscles in the avian body, hawks suffering from this type of fracture will present unable to fly although no injuries to either wing are apparent.

Treatment options

There is a great variety of treatment options for fractures. The choice depends on the type and location of the break in the bone, as well as the size and temperament of the bird. The goal in any case is to reestablish the original anatomic structure of the bone and surrounding soft tissues as closely as possible and restore the injured body part to normal function. There are various ways to achieve this.

Conservative methods: Modern medicine offers us many surgical options for fracture repair, including pinning, plating and external fixation. These are elegant, complicated methods that may not always be necessary. The decision whether such surgical methods are really indicated should be made on a case-by-case basis. Sometimes simpler, less invasive techniques can achieve the same purpose.

Immobilization: In some cases it may suffice to keep the bird quiet until healing is completed. Fractures in-

volving the sternum and the clavicle or coracoid can often be treated this way. The hawk should be prevented from using its wings for two to three weeks. A darkened box that permits the entry of only enough light that the bird can find and eat its food can serve such a purpose. In addition body wrapping one or both wings can help immobilize the injured bone and prevent unwanted motion during cleaning of the box or handling and examination of the bird.

Bandages and splints: In many cases, simple fractures of the extremities can be easily reduced and aligned without having to resort to surgical approaches and implants. Nevertheless, even closed reductions must be performed under full anesthesia so that there is complete muscle relaxation. In cases with compound fractures or if the injury is not recent, and muscles and tendons have significantly contracted, other options will have to be considered. It is easiest to evaluate and perform closed reductions on bones that have minimal surrounding muscle tissues, such as those of the lower leg and foot.

After realigning the fracture ends, the limb must be kept firmly bandaged for at least two or three weeks,

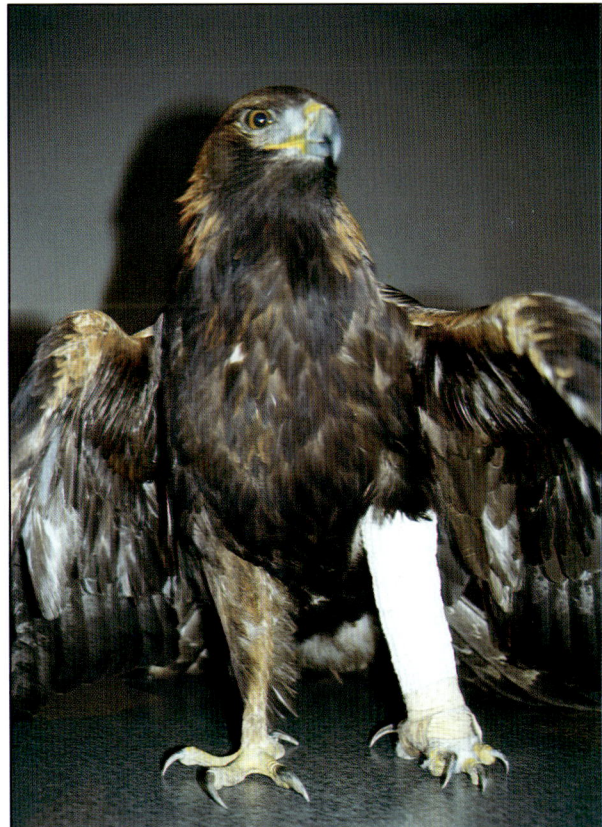

Fig. 13.77: Modern bandage materials made of synthetic polymers are light, strong and easy to apply. This makes them ideal for casting and splinting in birds of prey such as this golden eagle (*Aquila chrysaetos*).
(Photo: Heidenreich)

depending on the age of the bird and the rate of healing. Adequate padding of splinted limbs is important to prevent pressure necrosis of the thin avian skin. The splints themselves should be made of very light but strong materials. Plaster casts such as were used in the past are unsuitable for use in birds, both because of their weight and their required thickness. Modern materials such as Hexcelite®, Baycast®, Lightcast® or Deltacast® have proven useful in raptors. These casting materials are made of lightweight synthetic materials that harden upon exposure to air or ultraviolet light or after softening in hot water. They can be molded to the desired shape and provide good stability (Fig. 13.77).

Splints can also be made from plastic cylinders that are cut in half lengthwise and placed on the limb over some type of padding material. Although such devices provide adequate stability, they have the drawback that they do not conform to the anatomy of the bird's leg and generally fail to immobilize the joints above and below the fracture. They are most useful for fractures of the tarsometatarsus.

Adequate stability at the fracture site is the most important factor in permitting rapid healing of the bone to take place. Bandages and splints should be applied such that the bone ends cannot slide out of alignment while at the same time avoiding excessive pressure on the surrounding tissues. Pressure leads to inadequate perfusion of the area and pressure necrosis. Checking the limb daily for swelling, especially in the toes, is also very important.

Since the synthetic casting materials recommended above are all relatively radiolucent, radiographic reexamination of the fractured bones is easily performed without having to remove the bandages and potentially disrupting the healing process.

Fractures involving the radius, ulna or carpometacarpus are also often successfully treated using external coaptation. If only one of the two parallel running bones, radius or ulna, is fractured, the other one helps act as a natural splint. The wing should be placed in a figure eight bandage and then wrapped to the body in a normal position using Vetwrap or some similar nonadherent bandage material. The other wing need not be incorporated in the bandage and will help the bird maintain its balance. Body wraps should run only over the breast muscles and avoid the thoracic inlet and the abdomen. If necessary, the bandage can be cut out in those areas to permit normal expansion of the esophagus and crop with food and maintain freedom of movement for the legs.

Surgical methods: If the type or location of the fracture indicates that splinting and bandaging would not suffice to keep the bone ends aligned and immobile during the healing process, a surgical approach and placement of fixators may be indicated. The thin corti-

ces of avian bones make plating impractical in most raptor species. The screws are unable to obtain sufficient hold in the bone and adequate stability is therefore difficult to achieve. Intramedullary pinning offers a better alternative.

Various sizes of stainless steel Kirschner wires and Steinmann pins are available for intramedullary use in birds. The technique is relatively simple. The first step involves identification and gentle freeing of the two fractured ends of bone from the surrounding tissues. The pin can be placed in medullary cavity of the proximal fragment by retrograde or normograde insertion. Great care must be taken that the pin does not enter the articular (joint) space while being seated in the end of the bone!

Placement of a single pin that fills a large portion of the medullary canal does not prevent rotational instability. It is therefore preferable to use stack-pinning or Rush-pinning techniques, where several pins of smaller diameter are placed in the bone such that rotational instability is better controlled.

Placement of the pins into the distal fragment occurs one at a time by pushing them from proximal to distal while holding the broken bone in apposition. Either positive profile threaded or unthreaded pins can be used. In either case, they must be firmly anchored in the distal cortex, again without compromising any joint spaces. Radiographs should be taken during or after surgery to assure correct pin placement.

The long pin ends exposed proximally are cut off close to the bone, leaving enough length to permit grasping and removal when indicated in the future. If adequate stability has been achieved, additional bandaging is not required. This also facilitates frequent examination of the surgery site and avoids the undesirable muscle atrophy and joint ankylosis that usually occur with prolonged immobilization of limbs.

Besides stack-pinning, various authors have described the use of bone cement in the repair of avian fractures (Lind, 1988; Kuzma and Hunter, 1989; Degernes et al., 1993). The polymethylmethacrylate cement is used in combination with polypropylene intramedullary rods to provide lightweight, rotationally stable fixation of fractured long bones without the need of later fixator removal. This technique has several drawbacks. Care must be taken that no cement is left between the apposed ends of the fractured bone, as this would interfere with callus formation and bone healing. This technique cannot be used in open or infected wounds. Also, the semi-flexible polymer rods are sometimes not rigid or long enough to provide the stability required for avian long bones.

Some types of fractures, such as those occurring close to a joint, those involving infection, or those that are

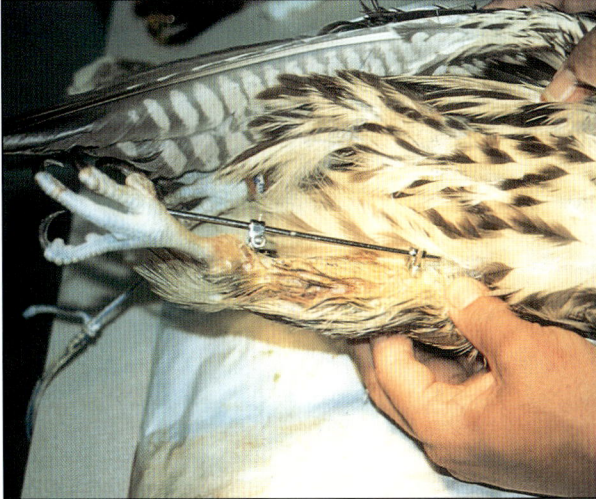

Fig. 13.78: If intramedullary pinning is not an option, external fixation of a fracture, as in this saker falcon (*Falco cherrug*), may provide a good alternative. (Photo: Lierz)

severely comminuted, may not be amenable to fixation using intramedullary pins alone. For these, external fixators provide an excellent alternative or additional form of stabilization.

External fixation involves driving at least two and preferably three or more pins through the soft tissues and both cortices of the bone on either side of the fracture. The pins should never be placed through an existing wound or surgical site, as that would increase the risk of infection.

After placement, the exposed pins can be used to aid in closed reduction of the fracture segments. Open reduction is often required in older or contaminated fractures even if they are being repaired with external fixation techniques.

The fixator pins are then stabilized with an external bar made of metal (Kirschner-Ehmer apparatus, Fig. 13.78) or, more easily, using polymethylmethacrylate inside plastic tubing, synthetic casting materials or dental acrylic. The bars should be placed such that they do not interfere with normal function and carriage of the limb.

The advantages of this technique include being able to avoid opening the fracture site, thus minimizing further soft tissue damage to the area, reduced need for additional external bandaging, helping retain mobility and strength in the affected limb, less risk of articular damage, and easy removal once bone healing is complete.

The lightweight construction of avian bones makes them relatively prone to complex fracturing and fissuring, especially in older birds. Compound, oblique and spiral fractures are common. Small bony sequestra that

cannot be incorporated into the fixation should be removed. Callus formation will fill in for these small defects. Larger fragments and fissures can be stabilized using cerclage wiring techniques.

Inadequately stabilized fractures result in delayed healing and excess callus formation at best and in malunions or nonunions (pseudoarthroses, Fig. 13.79) at worst. The result is frequently a nonfunctional limb for the bird. Surgical repair of malunions and nonunions is difficult and carries a guarded to poor prognosis for return to normal function.

13.10.10 Tendon injuries

Partial or complete disruption and tearing of tendons occurs occasionally in raptors, especially in the hallux. Occasionally, unilateral or bilateral tendon tears can be traced back to improperly fitted jesses in which the metal grommet proves to be a source of chronic irritation to the extensor tendon. Frequently the cause is unknown.

Rupture of the extensor tendon of the hallux results in an inability to pull the toe back and out from under the foot. The unopposed action of the flexor tendon keeps the hallux pulled forward (Fig. 13.80). Surgical attempts to repair the disrupted tendon are generally not successful. The stresses placed on this tendon are simply too great and the torn ends do not heal well.

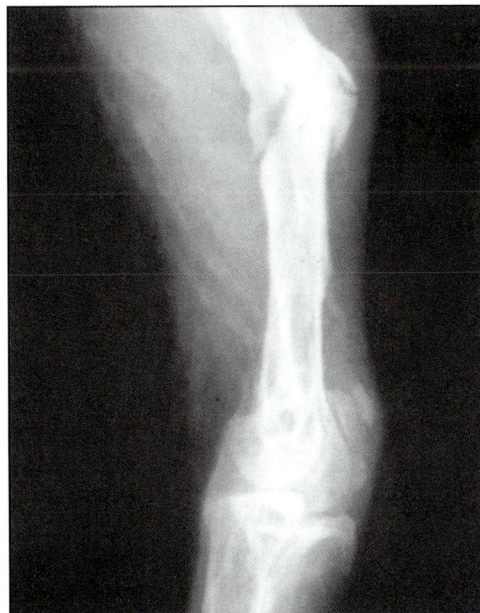

Fig. 13.79: Improperly treated fractures can easily develop into permanently unstable nonunions. This radiograph shows a nonunion in the tibiotarsus of a golden eagle (near the top of the picture). (Photo: Heidenreich)

13.10.11 Injuries caused by bands

The bands or rings used for purposes of identification in raptors (see Ch. 4.1) are inherently associated with some risk. Some of the larger species such as vultures and eagles can seriously injure themselves in attempting to remove these devices from their legs. Even bands that are tolerated by the bird can result in injury under some circumstances. Mild swelling of the legs, as seen with minor injuries for example, can result in constriction and vascular compromise to the distal leg and toes. The natural shedding of leg scales can result in an accumulation of keratin under the ring that may also lead to constriction. In advanced cases, the band can almost grow into the leg as granulation tissue proliferates up and around the metal.

The removal of problematic bands such as these always involves some risk to the leg and foot of the bird. With open bands, the two ends must be carefully grasped with strong pliers and gently pulled apart. Closed rings are cut open first, then pulled apart in a similar manner. Clipping or cutting the metal rings is often very difficult, requiring careful use of a variable speed hobby tool with a fine tip cutting bit. Because most birds will tend to struggle during the procedure and risk fracturing a leg, general anesthesia is recommended during band removal.

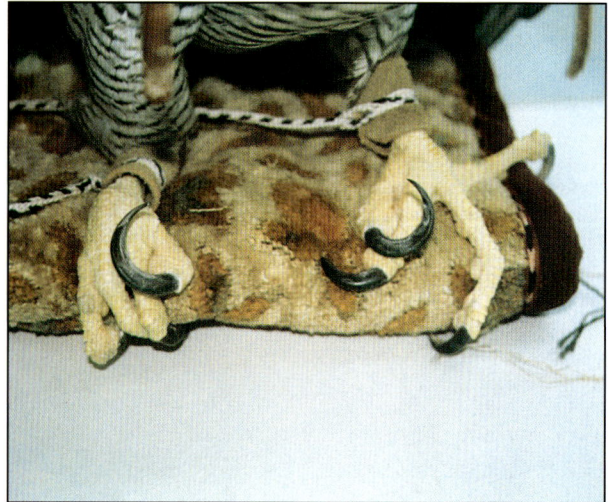

Fig. 13.80: Strains or tears of the extensor tendon of the hallux result in the "folding under" of these toes. The talons quickly become overgrown from lack of normal wear. (Photo: Lierz)

Leg bands on birds are fundamentally problematic and can result in injury to the bird in many different ways. Perry (1994) goes so far as to decline using them at all and recommends their removal as a preventive measure before problems arise.

References and literature of further interest

AL GITRIF (744):
Die Beizvögel.
Reprint: G. Olms Verlag, Hildesheim,1988

BEDNAREK, W. (1974):
Anomalie des Handskeletts bei einem männlichen Habicht
(*Accipiter gentilis*).
Jb. Dtsch. Falkenorden 48–49

BEDNAREK, W. (1974a):
Abweichende Großgefiederzeichnung bei einem jungen
Turmfalken *(Falco tinnunculus).*
Jb. Dtsch. Falkenorden 49–50

BRÜLL, H. (1937):
Krankheiten der Beizvögel
In: Waller, R.
Der wilde Falk ist mein Gesell.
Verlag Neumann-Neudamm

COLES, B. (1988):
Innere Medizin und Chirurgie bei Vögeln.
Gustav Fischer Verlag, Jena

COOPER, J.E. and J.R. NEEDHAM (1976):
An investigation into the prevalence of *S. aureus* on avian feet.
Vet. Rec. **98**, 172–174

COOPER, J.E. (1980):
Pathologie und Therapie von Ballenentzündungen bei
Greifvögeln.
Prakt. Tierarzt **61**, 966

COOPER, J.E. (1980):
Surgery of the foot in falcons: an historic operation.
Ann. Royal Colleg. Surg. England **62**, 445–448

COOPER, J.E. (1987):
Pathological studies on avian pododermatitis (bumblefoot).
Int. Symp. Erkrank. Zootiere **29**,107–113

DEGERNES, L.A., LIND, P.J. and P.T. REDIG (1993):
Raptor orthopedics using methyl methacrylate and polypropylene rods.
in: Redig, P.T. et al. (1993): Raptor biomedicine 122–127
Chiron Pub., Keighley West Yorkshire, England

FUENTE, F.R. DE LA (1986):
El arte de cetrería.
2. Aufl. Librería Noriega, Mexiko

GARNER, M.M. (1989):
Bumblefoot associated with poxvirus in a wild golden eagle
(*Aquila chrysaetos*).
Compan. Anim. Pract. 19, 17–20

GERLACH, C. (1982):
Erfahrungen und neue Versuche bei der Heilung der Vogelhaut und der dicken Hände bei Greifvögeln.
Prakt. Tierarzt **63**, 440, 442–444

GRIMM, F. and W. SIEBELS (1986):
Perkutane Osteosynthese beim Vogel mit optimiertem »Fixateur externe«.
DVG, V. Tagung Vogelkrankh. 213–216

HAAS, D. and M. TRAH (1988):
Knochenzement in der Vogelorthopädie – ein Beitrag zur operativen Frakturversorgung bei größeren Vögeln (Fallberichte).
Kleintierpraxis **33**, 179–182

HAAS, D. (1993):
Clinical signs and treatment of large birds injured by electrocution.
in: REDIG, P.T. et al. (1993):
Raptor biomedicine 180-183
Chiron Pub. Ltd., Keighley, West Yorksire, England

HALLIWELL, H.W. (1975):
Bumblefoot Infections in Birds of Prey.
J. Zoo Animal Medicine **6**, 8–10

HAMMER, W. (1991):
Greifvogel-Unfälle an elektrischen Freileitungen.
Greifvögel und Falknerei 42–50
Verlag Neumann-Neudamm, Morschen-Heina

HEIDENREICH, M. (1993):
Hypothese zur Ätiologie der »Dicken Hände« bei Falken.
Greifvögel und Falknerei 56–60
Verlag Neumann-Neudamm, Morschen-Heina

HOWARD, P.E. (1990):
The use of bone plates in the repair of avian fractures.
J. Amer. Animal Hospital Ass. **26**, 613–622

KIEL, H. (1982):
Greifvogelkrankheiten
In: Waller, R.
Der Wilde Falk ist mein Gesell
Verlag Neumann-Neudamm

KIEL, H. (1985):
Die Ballengeschwulst (»Dicke Hände«) bei Greifvögeln.
Tierärztl. Praxis **13**, 171–176

KOC, B., ALKAN, Z. and N. GUZEL (1989):
Surgical repair of fractures of wild birds (peregrines, eagles, hawks).
Vet. Hekimler Dernegi Dergisi. **59**, 90–98

KOCK, M.D. (1983):
The use of a modified Kirschner-Ehmer apparatus in avian fracture repair.
J. Small Animal Practice, **24**, 383–390

KÖSTERS, J. (1974):
Haltungsbedingte Krankheiten bei Greifvögeln.
Prakt. Tierarzt **55**, 31–33

KUMMERFELD, N. (1982):
Perosis bei einem Lannerfalken *(Falco biarmicus)*.
Prakt. Tierarzt **63**, 449–452

KUMMERFELD, N. and H. GRÜNHAGEN (1986):
Ballenentzündung »Bumble foot« bei einem Wild-Sperber *(Accipiter nisus)*
Jahrb. Dtsch. Falkenorden, 54–55

KUZMA, A. and B. HUNTER (1989):
Avian fracture repair using intramedullary bone cement and plate fixation.
Proc. Ass. Avian Vet. Seattle, Wash. 177–181

LAIR, S. (1990):
Le traitement chirurgical de la pododermatite chez les oiseaux de proie.
Med. Vet. Quebec **20**, 57

LIND, P.J., GUSHAWA, D.A. and J.A. VANEK (1988):
Fracture repair in two owls using polypropylene rods and acrylic bone cement.
Ass. Avian Vet. Today **2**, 128–132

NIE, G.J.-VAN (1981):
Tuberculose bij een buizerd met bumblefoot.
Tijdschr. Diergeneeskde **106**, 1033–1036

OAKS, J.L. (1989):
Treatment of a falcon for localized tetanus secondary to bumblefoot.
J. Ass. Avian Vet. **3**, 140–141

PERRY, R.A. (1994):
The avian patient.
in: Ritchie, B.W. et al. (1994):
Avian medicine: principles and application 26–44
Wingers Pub., Lake Worth, Florida

RAETHEL, H.S. (1962):
Krankheiten der Beizvögel und deren Behandlung
In: Brüll, H. Die Beizjagd
Verlag Paul Parey Hamburg und Berlin

REDIG, P.T. (1987):
Treatment of bumblefoot and the management of aspergillosis and various other problems commonly seen in raptors.
Proc. Am. Ass. Zoo Vet. 309–316

REDIG, P.T. (1993):
Bumblefoot treatment in raptors.
in: Fowler, M.E. (1993):
Zoo and wild animal medicine.
W.B. Saunders Company, Philadelphia, USA

REMPLE, J.D. and C.J. REMPLE (1987):
Foot casting as adjunctive therapy to surgical management of bumblefoot in raptorial species.
J. Am. Anim. Hosp. Ass. **23**, 633–639

REMPLE, J.D. (1993):
Raptor bumlefoot: a new treatment technique
in: Raptor biomedicine 154–160
Chiron Pub. Ltd. Keighley, West Yorkshire, England

RIDDLE, K.E.(1981):
Surgical Treatment of Bumble Foot in Raptors.
In: Recent Advances in the Study of Raptor Diseases.
Proc. I. Int. Symp. Diseases Birds of Prey, 67–78
Chiron Pub. Ltd. Keighley, West Yorkshire, England

RIDDLE, K.E. and J. HOOLIHAN (1993):
A form-fitting, composite-casting method for avian
appendages.
in: Raptor biomedicine 161–164
Chiron Pud. Ltd., Keighley, West Yorkshire, England

RITCHIE, B.W., LATIMER, K.S., OTTO, C.M. and D.T CROWE
(1990):
A technique of entraosseous cannulation for intravenous
therapy in birds.
Comp. Continuing Educ. Pract. Vet. **12**, 55–58

ROWLEY, J, BROWN, R.D. and S.E. WHITE (1985):
Bumblefoot in raptors.
Avian/Exotic Pract. **2**, 5–7

SAAR, C. (1974):
Wanderfalke mit 14 Staart-Pennen.
Jb. Dtsch. Falkenorden, 50

SAAR, C. (1990):
personal communication

SATTERFIELD, W.C. and K.I. O'ROURKE (1981):
Staphylococcal bumblefoot [claw disease of birds]:
vaccination and immunomodulation in the early treatment
and management.
J. Zoo Anim. Med. **12**, 95–98

SATTERFIELD, W.C. and K.I. O'ROURKE (1981):
Immunological considerations in the management of
bumblefoot [Staphylococcus aureus infection].
in: Recent advances in the study of raptor diseases. 123–129
Chiron Pub. Ltd., Keighley, West Yorkshire, England

SATTERFIELD, W.C. and K.J. O'ROURKE (1980):
Immunological considerations in the management of
bumblefoot.
in: Cooper, J. E. and A. G. Greenwood
Recent advances in the study of raptor diseases.
Chiron Pub. Ltd. , Keighley, West Yorkshire, England 123–129

SIEGMANN, O. (1992):
Kompendium der Geflügelkrankheiten.
5. Aufl. Verlag Paul Parey, Berlin u. Hamburg

STEHLE, S. (1965):
Krankheiten bei Greifvögeln und Eulen, mit Ausnahme
der parasitären Erkrankungen.
Vet. med. Diss, Hannover

TEGTMEIER, A. (1995):
personal communication

TROMMER, G. (1991):
Zur Entstehungsgeschichte der »Dicken Hände« bei Falken.
Jb. Dtsch. Falkenorden, 6–9

WILLIAMS, M.H. (1991):
Health and Disease.
In: Glasier, Ph. Falconry and Hawking. 278–280
Batsford, London, England

WOODFORD, M.H. (1987):
A Manual of Falconry, 156–158
A+C Black, London, England

ZAPATA, L. (1566):
Libro de cetrería.
Biblioteca Nacional de Madrid

14 Neoplasms

While tumors are common in some avian species, especially budgerigars and chickens, they are reported only occasionally in birds of prey. This chapter lists some examples derived from the author's own repertoire of cases. Several of these neoplasms have not previously been described in birds of prey.

Lipoma in a saker falcon (*Falco cherrug*)
Over a period of several months, this 16-year-old falcon developed a slowly enlarging mass on the dorsal aspect of the left wing. The bird's overall attitude was unaffected. The tumor was soft and had the approximate size of a pigeon's egg (Fig. 14.1). It did not seem painful on examination. During excision, the lipomatous neoplasm was found to be well-circumscribed and limited to the subcutaneous tissues.

Fibroma in a common kestrel (*Falco tinnunculus*)
An adult kestrel suffered repeated trauma to the cere over many months due to inappropriate housing in a wire-mesh enclosure. On initial presentation, the cere had developed a firm enlargement that was presumed to be an abscess. On palpation, however, the mass was very firm rather than doughy or fluctuant like an abscess.

This fibroma probably originated in the exuberant granulation tissue that developed at the site of repeated injury.

Nasolacrimal duct adenoma in a hybrid falcon (*Falco rusticolus X Falco cherrug*)
This 7-year-old successful breeding falcon slowly developed a mild swelling in the area between the eye and nostril. The mass slowly enlarged until it became big enough to interfere with normal functioning (Fig. 14.2). At this point it was surgically removed. Underneath a tight covering of skin, the soft grayish mass was easily identified in the area of the nasolacrimal duct. The nasolacrimal duct normally drains tears and other ocular secretions from the eye into the nose.

Complete removal of the neoplasm was not possible, leaving the concern that it would recur. However, since it took several years to reach this size, this was considered an acceptable risk.

Osteosarcoma in a hybrid falcon (*Falco rusticolus X Falco cherrug*)
This 20-week-old bird was being flown to the lure and initially appeared normal. Then he suddenly began favoring the right wing during flight. There was no

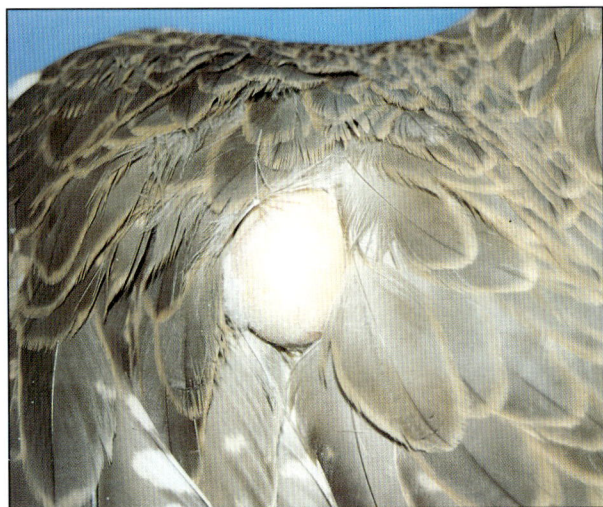

Fig. 14.1: A lipoma on the wing of a saker falcon (*F. cherrug*).   (Photo: Heidenreich)

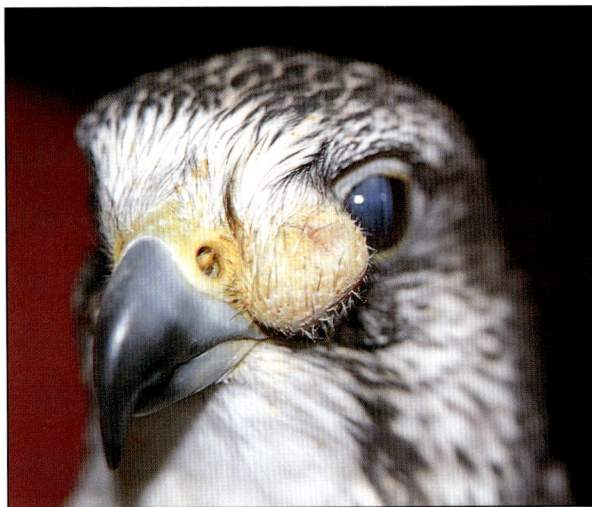

Fig. 14.2: A hybrid falcon with a nasolacrimal duct adenoma.   (Photo: Heidenreich)

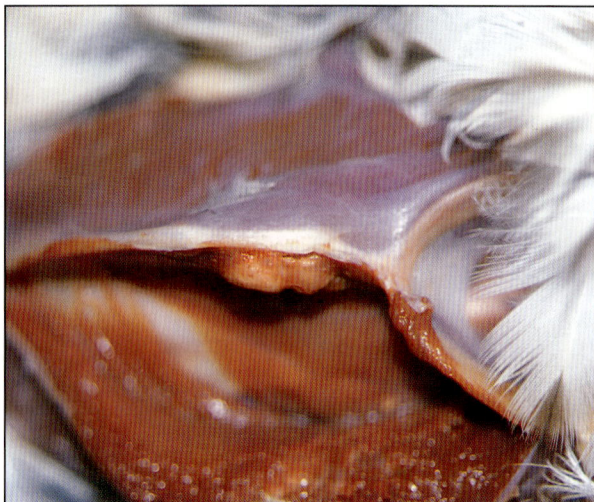

Fig. 14.3: A sternal osteosarcoma in a hybrid falcon. The pectoral muscles on the affected side have been removed prior to this postmortem photograph. (Photo: Heidenreich)

Adenocarcinoma in a peregrine falcon
(Falco peregrinus)

An 8-year-old female peregrine developed a flaccid paralysis of the left leg over a period of several days. At that time it was noticed that the bird was markedly underweight. A walnut-sized tumor was found near the cranial pole of the left kidney during postmortem examination. This renal neoplasm was impinging on the left sciatic nerve, thereby causing the lameness observed in this bird.

Similar renal tumors are common in budgerigars between 4 and 6 years of age. They are rare in raptors.

history of trauma and the wing was kept in a normal position at rest. Radiographs revealed bony changes involving the keel. Shortly thereafter the falcon died of a herpesvirus infection and was necropsied. A pea-sized bony mass was present on the right side of the keel (Fig. 14.3). A diagnosis of osteosarcoma was confirmed histologically. The cleaned sternum clearly shows the proliferative bony character of the neoplasm (Fig. 14.4). No metastases were found elsewhere in the body.

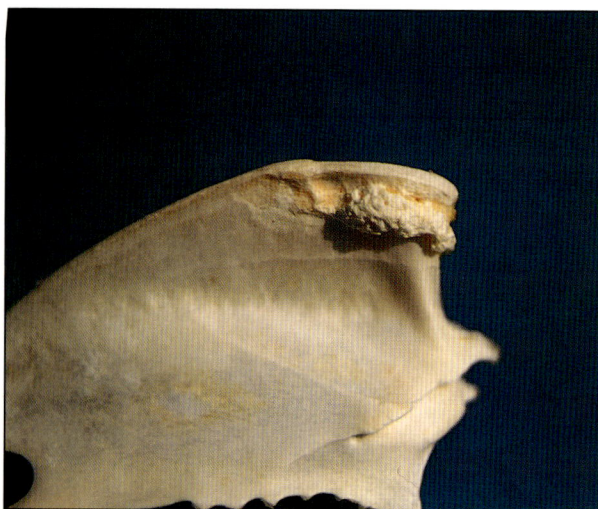

Fig 14.4: The cleaned bony keel of the young falcon depicted in Figure 14.3. (Photo: Heidenreich)

References and literature of further interest

COOPER, J.E., WATSON, J. and L.N. PAYNE (1978):
A mixed cell tumour in a Seychelles kestrel (*Falco araea*).
Avian Pathology **7**, 651–658

COOPER, J.E. (1978):
An adenocarcinoma in a buzzard (*Buteo buteo*).
Avian Pathology **7**, 29–34

COOPER, J.E. (1979):
An oviduct adenocarcinoma in a Mauritius kestrel (*Falco punctatus*).
Avian Pathology **8**, 187–191

COOPER, J.E. and S.L. PUGSLEY (1984):
A mesothelioma in a ferruginous hawk (*Buteo regalis*).
Avian Pathology **13**, 797–801

COOPER, J.E., WILKENS, W. and K. LAWRENCE (1993):
Four cases of neoplasia in birds of prey.
in: REDIG, P.T. et al. (1993): Raptor biomedicine 32–33
Chiron Pub. Ltd., Keighley, West Yorkshire, England

HIGGINS, R.J. and D.A.R. HANNAM (1985):
Lymphoid leukosis in a captive merlin (*Falco columbarius*).
Avian Pathology **14**, 445–447

KUFUOR-MENSAH, E. and G.L. WATSON (1992):
Malignant melanomas in a penguin (*Eudyptes chrysolphus*) and a red-tailed hawk (*Buteo jamaicensis*).
Vet. Path. **29**, 354–356

ROSSKOPF, W.J., WOERPEL, R.W., BONDE, J., WATER, D.-VAN-DE, MARTIN, S., LA-BONDE, J. and D. VAN-DE-WATER (1987):
Malignant lymphoma in a peregrine falcon-a case report.
Proc. Int. Conf. Zool. Avian Med. 325–331

WADSWORTH, P.F. and D.M. JONES (1980):
A renal carcinoma in an Augur buzzard (*Buteo rufofuscus augur*).
Avian Pathology **9**, 219–223

15 Anesthesia

In raptors the use of sedative or anesthetic drugs to eliminate stress and pain is important not only during surgery. It can make diagnostic procedures or other manipulations such as bandage changes easier and safer as well. Birds of prey, whether wild or captive, are not accustomed to veterinary procedures and react very defensively. There are various methods of reducing the stress and risk involved in examination for both animal and handler, while at the same time permitting a more accurate diagnosis to be reached.

15.1 Sedation

Sedative drugs that have an overall calming effect without necessarily providing analgesia, have proven useful in the treatment of poisoned birds. Strong convulsions or seizures that could result in injury to the animal can be controlled with various medications. Diazepam (Valium®) at a dose of 0.5–1.5 mg/kg PO SID will reduce the likelihood of epileptic episodes. It can be used at the same doses intravenously or intramuscularly, particularly in efforts to control an ongoing seizure. At doses of 0.5 mg/kg IM or 2.5 mg/kg PO SID, diazepam can be used as a behavior modifier to reduce aggressive behavior between hawks in a group.

Ketamine is a rapid-acting anesthetic that should never be used as a sedative. Although low doses of 3 to 10 mg/kg appear to calm an animal down briefly, the recovery period is often associated with excitement, ataxia and salivation.

15.2 Local anesthesia

There is generally no advantage to local anesthesia in treating birds of prey. In addition, most birds seem to tolerate local anesthetics very poorly. The administration of lidocaine or procaine can result in death.

15.3 General anesthesia

General anesthesia is of critical importance not only in permitting veterinarians to perform safe and painless surgical procedures, but also in allowing them to take appropriately positioned radiographs, to treat wounds or to change bandages. Ideally, this type of anesthesia is easily controlled while providing complete analgesia and muscle relaxation. The goal is to choose the safest anesthetic drugs possible, specifically those with a wide therapeutic index and minimal undesirable physiologic side effects. Fitzgerald and Blais (1993) were probably correct in stating that there is no ideal anesthetic for all situations and that the selection of drugs and routes of administration depends on the individual case and on the experience of the person administering them.

Prior to anesthetizing a bird, it should be thoroughly examined, including basic bloodwork if necessary. The patient should have an empty stomach. In smaller raptors that means 12 hours off food, in larger ones, a 24 hour fast is recommended. The hawk should also have cast since its last meal. These measures will minimize the chance that food or casting material are regurgitated during anesthesia or afterward, possibly obstructing the airway or leading to aspiration. An empty stomach also facilitates visualization and manipulations involved in abdominal surgery. In emergencies where an empty stomach cannot be guaranteed, the esophagus can be packed off with gauze (remember to remove it afterwards!) and the airway should be intubated.

Emaciated and/or dehydrated birds are at greater risk during anesthesia and every effort should be made to stabilize them first. The intravenous administration of fluids and electrolytes half an hour before surgery can be lifesaving. Fluids can also be given during and after the procedure in cases where a delay is contraindicated or anesthesia is prolonged. Sinn (1994) assumes that all sick or injured raptors are at least 10% dehydrated and uses this to calculate their immediate fluid needs as follows:

Body weight (grams) X 0.1 = Fluid volume (ml)

A rough guideline for more prolonged fluid therapy in birds of prey is 50 ml/kg/day. These fluids should not be given orally and even subcutaneous administration, as advocated by GYLSTORFF and GRIMM (1987), is discouraged by Sinn on the grounds that fluids given this way are unlikely to enter the circulation to raise blood volume quickly enough.

Sinn also recommends giving lactated Ringer's solution rather than 5 % glucose because the glucose is rapidly metabolized, leaving behind only water. All fluids should be warmed to body temperature before being given. The maximum that can be administered at one time in healthy birds is 90 ml/kg/hr, which amounts to a drip rate of 1.5 ml/kg/min. Rates greater than this are poorly tolerated (see Chapter 6.3).

With endangered species or those that are known to be sensitive to the drug, the initial anesthetic dose should be at the low end of the recommended range. Additional amounts can then be given until the desired effect is achieved. The patient should be as calm as possible during induction. Loud noises and frightening visual stimuli should be avoided. If possible, keeping the hawk hooded will help. With injectable drugs, the patient can be returned to the transport box or darkened cage after the injections have been given. Once the initial effects of the anesthetic are noticeable, the patient can be taken back out.

Patient monitoring during anesthesia involves observing respiration and heart rates and checking reflexes to assess anesthetic depth. Respiratory rates will vary depending on the species and among individuals, so that normal values can not be given. Some birds may become apneic under normal levels of gas anesthesia, requiring intermittent positive pressure ventilation. In general, the quality of an anesthetized patient's respiration is more important than the frequency. These observations apply to the heart as well. In very small raptors, heart rates can exceed 200 beats per minute, while they tend to range between 70 and 100 beats/min in larger birds of prey.

The regular monitoring of reflexes is the best way to assess anesthetic depth:

In a **lightly** anesthetized patient, stimulation of various body parts will result in a reflex response, although the animal is immobile and not consciously aware of the event. Palpebral and corneal reflexes or cloacal sphincter muscle contraction are seen in response to gentle stimulation. Pinching between the toes causes the foot to contract and a pupillary light response is present.

The **ideal** anesthetic depth has been reached when the eyelids are closed, the pupils have dilated and the nictitans responds slowly to corneal stimulation. All muscles are relaxed and pain reflexes are absent. The bird is breathing slowly and deeply.

Normal thermoregulatory mechanisms are usually impaired during anesthesia, resulting in a drop in body temperature. The animal should therefore be kept warm both during and after the anesthetic episode. Hypothermia is a particular risk with small birds and heat lamps or heating pads are important with these patients.

During the recovery period, which may take only a few minutes with inhalant anesthetics but is generally longer with injectable drugs, the patient should be carefully monitored and protected from self-injury during potentially violent phases. Wrapping the bird gently in a towel and placing it in sternal recumbency is helpful. The head should be easily visible so that one can rapidly assist the animal if hypersalivation or vomiting threaten the airway (Fig. 15.1). When the patient is alert enough to emerge from the rolled towel on its own, it can safely be returned to an appropriate cage or box.

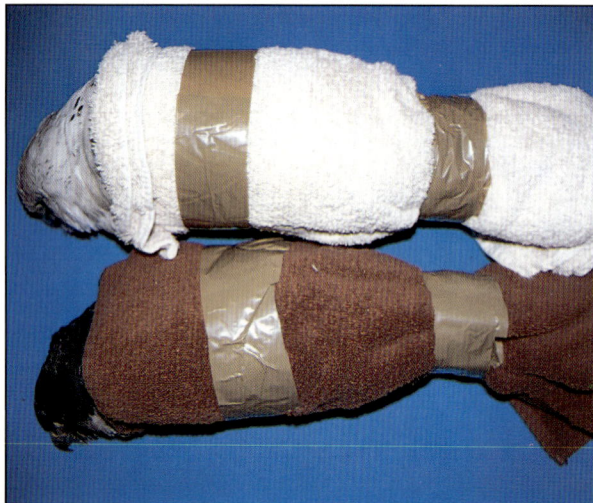

Fig. 15.1: Recovery from injectable anesthetics can occasionally be accompanied by excitement and uncontrolled activity. To prevent self-injury, the bird can be wrapped in a soft towel which is gently fastened without interfering with respiration. Once the bird is alert and coordinated enough to free itself from the towel, it can be placed in an appropriate container or transport box.
This method of wrapping a bird is not to be used for the transport of unanesthetized birds. The animals would overheat and most certainly die!
(Photo: Heidenreich)

15.3.1   Injectable anesthesia

In the early days of avian anesthesia, anesthetic agents used in mammals were indiscriminately administered to birds as well. Soon thereafter, both HEIDENREICH (1978) and KOLLIAS and MCLEISH (1978) reported on the use of ketamine in raptors. Other drugs such as chloral hydrate, chloralose, pentobarbital, methomidate and others were found to be unsuitable for use in birds and relegated to the realm of history.

The use of ketamine alone has a variety of disadvantages. Among them are sometimes violent recoveries, hypersalivation and poor muscle relaxation. Ketamine is therefore combined with other drugs such as xylazine or diazepam to produce a gentler, more readily controlled form of anesthesia. Reversal agents for some of these anesthetic agents have become available in the last few years, making it even easier to control or end an anesthetic episode as required. This has been particularly useful in shortening the recovery phase and reducing the excitement sometimes seen during this period. In fact, injectable anesthesia has become so safe and effective in birds of prey that it compares well with gas anesthesia.

In the author's experience, intravenous administration of a combination of ketamine (7 mg/kg) and xylazine (0.6 mg/kg) is very effective in falcons, goshawks, vultures and eagles. It produces rapid anesthesia and good muscle relaxation without excitement or other difficulties during induction. The period during which a surgical plane of anesthesia is maintained lasts about 30 minutes and can be extended as needed by additional doses of the drug combination. Once the procedure has been completed, 0.1 mg yohimbine given IV permits recovery within a few minutes. The bird will be standing in 5 minutes and ready for transport in half an hour. Yohimbine is a reversal agent for xylazine only. Its use may result in some excitatory behavior during recovery as the unopposed effects of the ketamine are seen.

Table 15.1 gives an overview of injectable anesthetic protocols used in birds of prey.

Redig (1993) no longer uses different ratios of ketamine and xylazine in raptors. Instead, he advocates the use of a stock solution at a ratio of 5 parts ketamine to one part xylazine which can be made by combining equal volumes of ketamine (100 mg/ml) and xylazine (20 mg/ml). For anesthesia, this stock solution is then administered intravenously on the basis of species and body weight (see Table 15.2).

Table 15.1: Reports of injectable anesthetics used in birds of prey

Combination of anesthetic agents [per kg body weight]	Species	Authors
15–30 mg ketamine + 2–8 mg climazolam IM	various raptors	GUTZWILLER et al. (1984)
8–15 mg ketamine + 0.5–1 mg diazepam IM	falcons	GÖLTHENBOTH (1995)
30–40 mg ketamine + 1–1.5 mg diazepam IM	various raptors	REDIG and DUKE (1983)
3–8 mg ketamine + 0.5–1 mg diazepam IM	eagles and vultures	GÖLTHENBOTH (1995)
10 mg ketamine + 1 mg xylazine IM Reversal: tolazoline	turkey vultures	ALLEN and OOSTERHUIS (1986)
4.4 mg ketamine + 2.2 mg xylazine IV Reversal: yohimbine 0.10 mg i.v.	red-tailed hawk	DEGERNES ET AL. (1988)
50 mg ketamine + 4 mg xylazine IM	lethal to goshawks!	LUMEIJ (1986)
4.83 mg ketamine + 0.38 mg xylazine IV 18.43 mg ketamine + 1.52 mg xylazine IV	vultures small raptors	PETRUZZI (1988)
3–5 mg ketamine + 0.05–1 mg medetomidine IM or 2–4 mg ketamine + 0.025–0.07 mg medetomidine IV Reversal: atipamezole	various avian species	JALANKA (1991) BERTHIER (1993)
Sedation: xylazine 1.0–20 mg IV or 2.5–20 mg IM Reversal: yohimbine 0.2 mg IV	vultures, small falcons and buteos	FREED and BAKER (1989)

15.3.2 Inhalant anesthesia

Unlike injectable anesthesia, where a variety of different drug combinations have proven effective, only one gas can be recommended for inhalant anesthesia – **isoflurane**.

The other two gases, methoxyflurane and halothane, have been found unsuitable for use in birds. Methoxyflurane is associated with prolonged induction and recovery periods and can cause liver and kidney damage, not only in the patient, but also in humans exposed to the gas during the procedure. A scavenger system is therefore essential when using this gas.

Halothane has a shorter induction period, but recovery can still take up to 20 minutes, depending on the length of the procedure. In addition, this gas can depress cardiac and respiratory function. This makes it unsuitable for use in patients with cardiac or circulatory system abnormalities or those with diseases of the respiratory system.

Isoflurane is minimally metabolized in the body (only 3%, compared to 15% for halothane and 50% for methoxyflurane!) and is therefore not associated with liver or kidney pathology. It is also less soluble in blood, resulting in very rapid induction and recovery times.

The equipment needed for isoflurane anesthesia is relatively modest. An isoflurane vaporizer (a cleaned and re-calibrated halothane vaporizer can also be used), an oxygen source with a control valve, a flow meter and various sizes of endotracheal tubes and masks. Face masks can be made from plastic cups fitted with an attachment for the gas tubing at the narrow end and covered with an elastic membrane over the wide open end. An X-shaped cut in the membrane allows the bird's head to be placed inside the mask while minimizing the escape of gas around its neck.

Calm, hooded falcons or eagles often allow the mask to be placed over their head as they stand on the fist. Other birds will require some form of restraint. These animals should be induced as quickly as possible using vaporizer settings as high as 4 or 5%. As soon as the bird is anesthetized, the level is reduced to maintenance values between 1 and 2% (Pascoe, 1985). Sinn (1994) recommends that any patient to be kept anesthetized longer than 10 minutes be intubated. In raptors, this is relatively simple because the glottis is easily visualized by gently pulling the tongue forward (Figs. 15.2–15.3).

During surgical procedures involving the neck or upper airway (foreign body removal, for example), it may not be possible to intubate the trachea. In such cases, a tube can be inserted into the caudal abdominal air sac. The approach is the same as that used for endoscopic sexing (see Chapter 7.6).

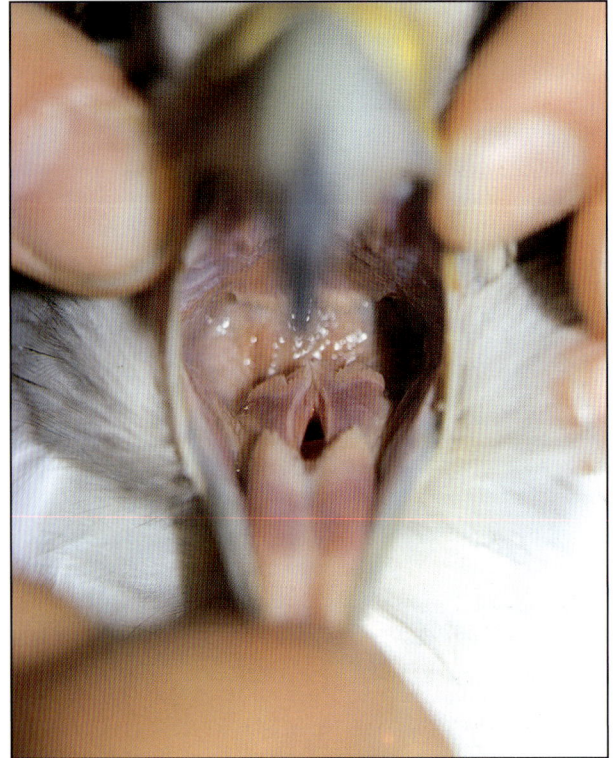
△ **15.2**

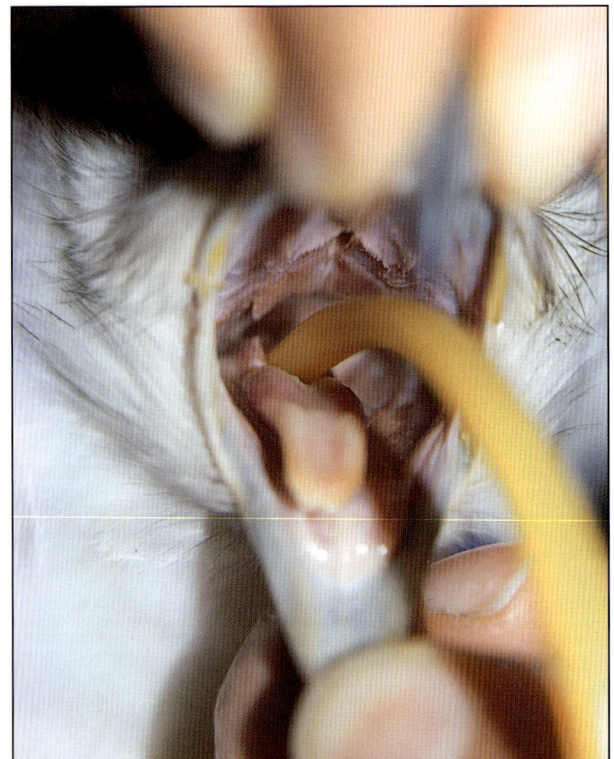
15.3 ▽

Figs. 15.2 and 15.3: Gently pulling the tongue forward allows visualization of the avian glottis (15.2) and permits easy tracheal intubation (15.3). The endotracheal tube can be fastened to the lower beak with adhesive tape during anesthesia.
(Photos: Heidenreich)

15.3.3 Anesthetic emergencies

Despite all precautions, life-threatening incidents can occur at any time during anesthesia. In case of respiratory arrest more than 10 seconds in duration, ventilatory assistance is immediately necessary. In birds that are intubated, this is usually done manually using the reservoir bag on the anesthetic machine. Levels of isoflurane should be reduced or turned off.

Hawks under injectable anesthesia can be ventilated by gentle intermittent manual compression of the sternum. If spontaneous respiration does not return promptly, the bird should be intubated and ventilated as described above. Ventilation can also occur through a tube placed in the caudal abdominal air sac, if necessary. Immediate administration of the appropriate reversal agent should be considered. Sinn (1994) recommends applying a few drops of doxapram to the tongue to stimulate respiration. With cardiac arrest, all attempts at resuscitation are futile.

Table 15.2: General anesthesia (1 hour) with ketamine/xylazine (5:1) in various birds of prey (from REDIG, 1993)

Species	Body weight [g]	Dose [ml]	Comments
Buteos (*Buteo* spp.)			
Broad-winged hawk (*B. platypterus*)	350–400	0.08	
Red-shouldered hawk (*B. lineatus*)	800–1000	0.08–0.10	
Rough-legged hawk (*B. lagopus*)	800–1100	0.08–0.10	
Red-tailed hawk (*B. jamaicensis*)	650–1500	0.06–0.10	
Ferruginous hawk (*B. regalis*)	900–1700	0.10–0.12	
Accipiters (*Accipiter* spp.)			caution!
Sharp-shinned hawk (*A. striatus*)	100–150 (m) 175–250 (f)	0.04–0.06	
Cooper's hawk (*A. cooperi*)	250–350 (m) 350–500 (f)	0.08–0.10	difficult to maintain
Northern goshawk (*A. gentilis*)	600–800 (m) 800–1200 (f)	0.05 0.07	the most sensitive species – long recovery period
Eagles (*Haliaeetus* spp., *Aquila* spp.)			
Bald eagle (*H. leucocephalus*)	3000–4500	0.25–0.50	cardiac arrhythmias, respiratory depression, safe nevertheless
Golden eagle (*A. chrysaetos*)	3000–4500	0.40–0.70	rapidly metabolized, may need additional doses
Falcons (*Falco* spp.)			tolerate this combination well
American kestrel (*F. sparverius*)	90–125	0.05	rapidly metabolized
Merlin (*F. columbarius*)	150–250	0.06	rapidly metabolized
Prairie falcon (*F. mexicanus*)	500–700 (m) 800–950 (f)	0.10 0.20	
Peregrine falcon (*F. peregrinus*)	500–700 (m) 800–1050 (f)	0.10 0.20	prolonged effects in older birds
Gyrfalcon (*F. rusticolus*)	950–1500	0.25	
Gyrfalcon hybrids			same as purebred gyrfalcons
Others			
Osprey (*Pandion haliaetus*)	1200–1500	0.12–0.20	
Turkey vulture (*Cathartes aura*)	1200	0.15	

References and literature of further interest

ADDIS, F., MORTELLARO, C.M. and G. VANOSI (1990):
Anestesia negli animali »insoliti«. Anestesia generale nei rapaci.
Summa., **7**, 79–84, 86

ALLEN, J.L. and J.E. OOSTERHUIS (1986):
Effect of tolazoline on xylazine-ketamine-induced anesthesia
in turkey vultures.
J. Amer. Vet. Med. Ass. **189**, 1011–1012

BEDNARSKI, R.M., LUDDERS, J.W., LEBLANC, P.H., PICKETT, P.
and C.J. SEDGWICK (1985):
Isoflurane-nitrous oxide-oxygen anesthesia in an Andean
condor (*Vultur gryphus*).
J. Amer. Vet. Med. Ass. **187**, 1209–1210

BERTHIER, J.L., DEMONTOY-BOMSEL, M.C. and R. PERRIN (1993):
L'association medétomidine-ketamine et l'atipamézole dans
l'anesthsie des oiseaux.
VISZ **35**, 281–285

CLUTTON, R.E. (1986):
Prolonged isoflurane anesthesia in the golden eagle.
J. Zoo Anim. Med. **17**, 103–105

DEGERNES, L.A., KREEGER, T.J., MANDSAGER, R. and
P.T. REDIG (1988):
Ketamine-xylazine anesthesia in red-tailed hawks with
antagonism by yohimbine.
J. Wildl. Dis. **24**, 322–326

FITZGERALD, G. and D. BLAIS (1993):
Inhalation anaesthesia in birds of prey.
in: Redig, P.T. et al. (1993): Raptor biomedicine 128–135
Chiron Pub., Keighley, West Yorkshire, England

FORBES, N.A. (1984):
Avian anaesthesia. (Correspondence concerning ketamine and
diazepam for Falconiformes).
Vet. Rec. **115**, 134

FREED, D.F. and B. BAKER (1989):
Antagonism of xylazine hydrochloride sedation in raptors by
yohimbine hydrochloride.
J. Wildl. Dis. **25**, 136–138

GÖLTHENBOTH, R. (1995):
in: Gölthenboth, R. u. H.G. Klös (1995):
Krankheiten der Zoo- und Wildtiere
Blackwell Wissenschafts-Verlag, Berlin

GRIMM, F. (1987):
Anästhesie beim Vogel.
Tierärztl. Praxis **15**, 381–384

GUTZWILLER, A., VÖLLM, J. and B. HAMZA (1984):
Einsatz des Benzodiazepins Climazolam bei Zoo- und Wildtieren.
Kleintierpraxis **29**, 381–340

GYLSTORFF, I. and F. GRIMM (1987):
Vogelkrankheiten.
Eugen Ulmer Verlag, Stuttgart

HEERDEN, J., KOMEN, J.VAN-, MYER, E. and J.VAN-HEERDEN (1987):
The use of ketamine hydrochloride in the immobilisation of the
cape vulture (*Gyps coprotheres*).
J. South Afric. Vet. Ass. **58**, 143–144

HEIDENREICH, M. (1978):
Narkose bei Greifvögeln und Eulen mit Ketaminhydrochlorid.
Prakt. Tierarzt. **59**, 672–680

JALANKA, H.H. (1991):
Medetomidine-ketamine und atipamezole – a reversible method
for chemical restraint in birds.
Proc. Europ. Ass. Avian Vet. 102–105

JAYADEVAPPA, S.M., SRINIVAS, V. and P.H.T. REDDY (1983):
Amputation of the wing of a falcon under halothane
anaesthesia – a case report.
Indian J. Vet. Surgery **4**, 74–75

KOLLIAS, G.V. and I. MCLEISH (1978):
Effects of ketamine hydrochloride in red-tailed hawks (*Buteo
jamaicensis*). I. Arterial blood gas and acid base. II. Biochemical and hematologic.
Comp. Biochem. Physiol. **60 C**, 57–59

LUMEIJ, J.T. (1986):
Anesthetic fatalities in goshawks.
Tagung über Vogelkrankheiten, Giessen **5**, 201–207

MIKAELIAN, J. (1991):
Intravenously administered propofol for anesthesia of the
common buzzard (*Buteo buteo*), the tawny owl (*Strix aluco*),
and the barn owl (*Tyto alba*).
Proc. Conf. Europ. Com. Ass. Avian Vet. **1**, 97–101

PASCOE, P.J., DYSON, D., WAELCHLI-SUTER, C. and T. DOHERTY
(1985):
Avian anaesthesia.
Vet. Rec. **116**, 58

PETRUZZI, V., CODA, S., XIMENES, L.A. and P. NAITANA (1988):
Ketamine-xylazine combination in general anaesthesia of
raptors. Evaluation of certain vital parameters.
Obiettivi Doc. Vet. **9**, 59–62

REDIG, P.T. and G.E. DUKE (1983):
Intravenously administered ketamine HCl and diazepam for
anesthesia of raptors.
J. Amer. Vet. Med. Ass. **169**, 886–888

REDIG, P.T. (1993):
Medical management of birds of prey.
Raptor Center, Minnesota 27–32

SAMOUR, J.H. (1984):
Comparative studies of the use of some injectable anaesthetic
agents in birds.
Vet. Rec. **7**, 6–11

SINN, L.C. (1994):
Anesthesiology.
in: Ritchie, B.W., Harrison, G.J. u. L. R. Harrison (1994):
Avian medicine: principles and application.
Wingers Publishing, Lake Worth, Florida

16 Rehabilitation of wild birds of prey

Orphaned, sick or injured wild raptors are often found by well-meaning people and taken into captivity to be raised, cared for or medically treated. The ultimate goal of any such efforts at rehabilitation should be to return the animals to the wild as soon as possible. This goal is predicated on the bird's ability to survive on its own. To release an unprepared or crippled animal is both inappropriate and inhumane.

Wild birds of prey must be in excellent physical condition to hunt successfully, defend themselves from potential enemies and undertake sometimes very long migrations. Prior to release, strong consideration must therefore be given not only to the resolution of the animal's original problem, but also to its overall strength, endurance and skill in flying and hunting.

Even periods of inactivity as short as one week can result in a significant loss of physical condition, threatening a raptor's chances of survival in nature. Other things such as feather condition and environmental factors can also play a role. A great deal of knowledge and effort is therefore required to prepare a bird of prey successfully for release into the wild.

16.1 Rehabilitation and release of adult raptors

Once a bird is considered healthy, it can begin an appropriate training program designed to prepare it for release into the wild. The first step is always a thorough physical exam to assess the animal's attitude, body condition, plumage, senses, nervous system (especially reflexes) and to check on the resolution of specific illnesses or injuries. Bloodwork, including a hematocrit and white blood cell count at the very least, will add valuable information to an evaluation of the bird's releasability.

Of critical importance is an assessment of the hawk's ability to fly. The first requirement is intact plumage. Many types of feather damage can be repaired using traditional falconer's techniques such as feather imping. The actual flight tests are initially done in an enclosed space such as an aviary or flight cage and start over small distances of a few meters. The bird flies back and forth between two perches (modified saw-horses work well and are easily moved around) and various aspects of flight are evaluated:
1. Symmetry and strength of the wing beats.
2. Balance during flight.
3. Position of the legs during flight (they are normally extended beneath the tail).
4. Height and speed of flight (strong birds will tend to fly upward at first and then descend to land on the other perch).
5. Style of landing (should be soft and coordinated, using both feet).
6. Respiratory effort on landing, both initially and after several flights. Strength and endurance over multiple consecutive flights. Both are an indication of physical fitness.

Most wild birds will need a little time to become accustomed to flying between two such perches, especially in the presence of humans.

Larger raptors like eagles and vultures may be difficult or impossible to assess over such short distances. They usually need to be evaluated outdoors. This involves fitting them with jesses and a swivel and then attaching a creance approximately 30 to 50 meters long. A light but strong nylon cord is ideal. The free end of the creance is held by an assistant or tied to an object that the bird can drag for a short distance, but that is heavy enough to stop its flight eventually. The line should never be attached to an immovable object. Some rehabilitators have successfully used some type of spool or other mechanism that allows the creance to unwind as the bird flies and that can be controlled or stopped and rewound afterward.

The bird to be evaluated is released into the wind and observed for flight ability and endurance as described above. Near the end of the creance, or before the bird reaches the limit of the open space available, the assistant should gradually increase the tension on the line, forcing the flying bird to slow down and land. Most hawks will head towards the nearest trees, but should never be permitted to actually reach them. Rapid fliers like falcons, goshawks and sparrowhawks are not well-suited to creance flying. They can achieve very rapid flight speeds over short distances and are thus prone to injury if suddenly forced to land.

For falcons and other birds of prey, manning and falconry training techniques have proven to be the best method for pre-release conditioning. The birds are flown to the lure just like hunting hawks in training. This permits a thorough evaluation of their physical ability and conditioning, and provides an ideal technique for preparing them for release. Exercise of this kind also helps the bird develop or recover its hunting skills. A raptor's ability to survive in nature is directly dependent on its ability to hunt successfully, and it should not be released until it has demonstrated its skill in doing so. This may involve the capture of wild game, the killing of live mice offered inside an aviary or flight cage (for buteos) or the pursuit and capture of live pigeons (for falcons).

It is often argued that birds trained in this manner become too tame and lose their natural fear of humans. This concern is completely unfounded. Previously wild birds of prey return to their natural behavior very quickly and will keep a safe distance away from humans only a few days after being released.

Conditioning programs that assess physical fitness, based in part on blood lactic acid levels, have been used in training human athletes, race horses or racing greyhounds. Redig (1993) applied similar techniques to birds of prey and developed the following training program for pre-release conditioning:

Training program

Phase I:
Initially the bird is flown over a distance of 30 meters for 3 to 5 consecutive flights **one minute apart**. This procedure is repeated three times a week. Once the bird can complete this exercise on its own without tiring, it can move on to Phase II.

Phase II:
The flight distance is now extended to 60 meters. For birds weighing over 1 kg, this distance is flown 6 or 7 times with one-minute intervals. Smaller species less than 1 kg in weight should fly the distance 10 times. This exercise regimen is repeated every other day.

Phase III:
The distance is again increased, this time to 90 meters. When the bird is able to fly this length ten times in a row without tiring for several days in a row, it should be released **immediately**.

In recent years it has become feasible to obtain small radio transmitters weighing only a few grams, that can be fastened to the tail feathers or leg of a bird. They are used to track flight and migration patterns or, among falconers, to locate lost hunting hawks (Klüh, 1993). The receiver's range will vary depending on local topography, but typically covers a distance of at least 10 or 20 kilometers.

These types of transmitters can be useful in raptor rehabilitation as well, permitting observation and recapture of a released raptor that is not functioning adequately in the wild. If the bird does well, the transmitter is lost. Much can be learned about rehabilitation this way. However, since these devices cost around $200, they are not often used in this way.

A rehabilitated bird that is able to fly well may suffer from other limitations that preclude its return to the wild. Most common among these are eye injuries, seen frequently in birds of prey that have suffered head trauma. Eye injuries such as detached retinas are difficult to detect unless a fundic exam is performed. They are probably much more common than most rehabilitators know.

Fully functional binocular vision is a fundamental requirement for successful hunting, permitting a hawk to judge distances to objects such as perches or prey animals accurately. Fast-flying aerial hunters such as falcons and accipiters are unable to survive with only one functional eye and should never be released in that condition.

Crippled or missing feet and toes also usually impair hunting and perching ability enough to prevent release of the affected bird. Frequently they also result in uneven weight-bearing and lead to pododermatitis. Many of these birds must be euthanatized.

Anything that impairs normal flight ability, including improperly healed fractures, reductions in joint mobility or permanently damaged feather follicles affecting primary or secondary feather function, is cause not to release a bird.

Redig (1993) suggested that a raptor be evaluated for the following release parameters before being set free:

A. Physical condition
    1. Feather condition
    2. Feet and talons
    3. Wings

B. Hematology
    1. Hematocrit 40–45%
    2. Total protein 3.4–4.5 g/l
    3. Total white blood cells under 12×10^9 /l

C. Radiographic evaluation

D. Antiparasitic treatment

E. Training
    1. Endurance
    2. Respiratory activity and recovery rate
    3. Lactic acid measurements

16.2   Rehabilitation and release of nestlings

Falconers involved in reintroduction projects with endangered birds of prey have developed several techniques that permit the successful training and release of young raptors into the wild (Saar, 1993).

Adoption by adult birds

The simplest method is the placement of captive nestlings with wild adult pairs of the same species. It is important that the adoptive parents have nestlings of their own of approximately the same age, and that the total number of young in the nest not exceed the parents' ability to supply them with food.

Hacking

If no wild eyries are available, the young birds may have to be hand-raised. It is very important that the nestlings not become too accustomed to humans or even imprinted. For this reason it is best to keep several young birds together and to minimize their visual exposure to humans. Dummies of adult birds can help provide the appropriate imprinting. Sometimes captive adults will tolerate or even feed unrelated chicks and thus help make this stage of captive rearing easier.

Once the young birds can stand and eat whole food on their own, they are placed in an artificial nest or box at a suitable hacking site. Typically, the box is raised on some type of platform or tower and permits an open view of the surrounding area from at least one side. Initially, a mesh is used to prevent the chicks from leaving their new home. After a period of acclimatization, this barrier is removed carefully. Feeding takes place through a trap door or pipe that prevents the birds from seeing humans or associating them with food.

As the birds mature they will leave the hack box and begin spending time on the surrounding platform. Even after fledging, they will keep returning to the hack site for food (Figs. 16.1–16.2).

Although it varies somewhat with species and sex, the young birds generally take only a few weeks to develop their own hunting skills to the point where they no longer need to return to the hacking tower at all.

Unlike those adopted into wild nests, these young raptors will lack the warnings and protection from predators normally provided by the parent birds. This results in higher rates of mortality for nestlings released from hacking towers. A more detailed description of hacking methods is provided by Sherrod et al. (1987).

Clearly, the conscientious rehabilitation of injured or orphaned wild birds of prey is difficult and requires a large amount of patience and empathy, a thorough understanding of the animal's natural history and behavior, a working knowledge of falconry and access to knowledgeable veterinary care. Many of the animals treated belong to endangered or threatened species or populations. The individuals brought into captivity for treatment can teach us much about the natural or man-made problems facing these birds of prey in their natural habitats. Rehabilitation efforts will only succeed with the cooperation of specialists including veterinarians, falconers, biologists, and government wildlife officials.

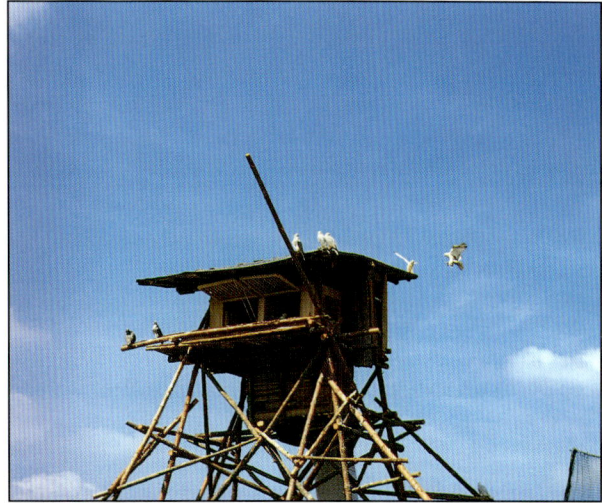

△ 16.1   16.2 ▽

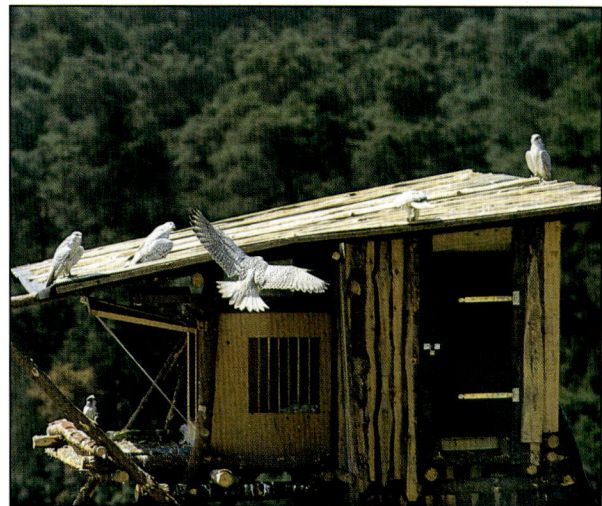

Figs. 16.1 and 16.2: The release of young raptors by the hacking method can be done from buildings, tree nests or specially-constructed hacking towers (16.1). These pictures show a group of young gyrfalcons (*F. rusticolus*) that were not actually intended for release. They were permitted to fly free for approximately four weeks and then recaptured before they began hunting on their own and left.
(Photos: Heidenreich)

Too many raptors treated at state or private wildlife rehabilitation centers, or by individual rehabilitators, are released after being apparently "healed". Although this may make their success rate look good, the actual outcome of these cases is rarely known and hardly ever looked into. Rehabilitators, veterinarians, falconers and government wildlife officials should work together to achieve their common goal of truly helping wild raptors. This must involve learning more about their needs, their problems and the possible solutions, both for individual animals and on a population level.

References and literature of further interest

CHAPLIN, S.B. (1990):
Guidelines for exercise in rehabilitated raptors.
Wildl. J. **12**, 17–20

CHAPLIN, S.B., MUELLER, L. and L. DEGERNES (1990):
Physiological assessment of rehabilitated raptors prior to release.
Wildl. J. **12**, 7–18

COOPER, J.E. and L. GIBSON (1980):
The assessment of health in casualty birds of prey intended for release.
Vet. Rec. **106**, 340–341

FREY, H. and W. WALTER (1989):
The reintroduction of the bearded vulture *Gypaetus barbarus* into the Alps.
Raptors in The Modern World, 341–344
WWGBP, Berlin

KLÜH, P.N. (1993):
Zum Einsatz der Telemetrie in der Falknerei.
Greifvögel und Falknerei, 43–56
Verlag Neumann-Neudamm, Morschen-Heina

LUDWIG, D.R. (1982):
Selection of release sites and post-release studies for rehabilitated wildlife.
Wildlife rehabilitation.
Proc. Nat. Wildl. Rehab. Symp., 25–36

REDIG, P.T. (1993):
Methods of evaluating the readiness of rehabilitated raptors for release.
Brochure, Minnesota Raptor Center, 157–160

SAAR, C. (1993):
Wanderfalken-Auswilderungsbericht 1993.
Greifvögel und Falknerei, 32–43
Verlag Neumann-Neudamm, Morschen-Heina

SHERROD, S.K., HEINRICH, W.R., BURNHAM, W.A., BARCLAY, J.H. and T.J. CADE (1987):
Hacking: A method for releasing Peregrine falcons and other birds of prey.
The Peregrine Fund, Boise, Idaho

17 Forensics

All birds of prey are protected by national and international agreements (see Ch. 18) and ownership of such birds is subject to many legal restrictions. Nevertheless, they are frequently maintained in captivity for display, breeding, sport and other purposes. Increasingly, unscrupulous collectors or animal traders in search of large profits ignore the regulations that legally protect these birds, forcing the authorities responsible to increase their vigilance, and leading to more inspections, confiscations, and court cases.

In the process of investigating such cases, the wildlife authorities and the courts often employ experts to assist in definitively identifying the raptors, especially as to age and species.

In general, anyone deemed knowledgeable in the field and appointed as such by the court can be an expert witness. In some countries, such experts are appointed by the government based on their knowledge of national laws and international treaties pertaining to the animals involved. These people are available to assist the courts, the local authorities and even private persons with questions or concerns regarding birds of prey.

A variety of questions or concerns may arise as part of the inspections or investigations performed by the authorities responsible for enforcing the laws pertaining to birds of prey. Experts in the field are often called upon to help resolve them. This chapter discusses some of the subjects that are important in such cases, especially those involving forensics.

17.1 Age determination

The life span of wild raptors is difficult to determine since few of them are continuously observed and weak, old or sick individuals quickly fall prey to other predators. The maximum life span that might be expected under optimal captive conditions is therefore almost never reached in the wild. Records obtained from zoos or private individuals are better indicators of possible life spans for various species and report some surprisingly long-lived individuals, as indicated in Table 17.1. It appears that there is a direct correlation between body size and life span among raptors. The bigger the species, the longer it tends to live.

More important than knowing the possible life span, however, is determining the age of an individual bird as accurately as possible.

Table 17.1: Maximum recorded life spans of selected raptor species

Raptor species	Life span (years)
White-tailed sea eagle (*Haliaeetus albicilla*)	95, egg-laying until 42 years of age
Bateleur (*Terathopius ecaudatus*)	>55
Andean condor (*Vultur gryphus*)	>52
Golden eagle (*Aquila chrysaetos*)	>48
Red kite (*Milvus milvus*)	38
Saker falcon (*Falco cherrug*)	29, egg-laying until 24 years of age
Northern goshawk (*Accipiter gentilis*)	>28
Common buzzard (*Buteo buteo*)	24
Peregrine falcon (*Falco peregrinus*)	24, egg-laying until 18 years of age
Common kestrel (*Falco tinnunculus*)	14
Merlin (*Falco columbarius*)	12, egg-laying until 10 years of age

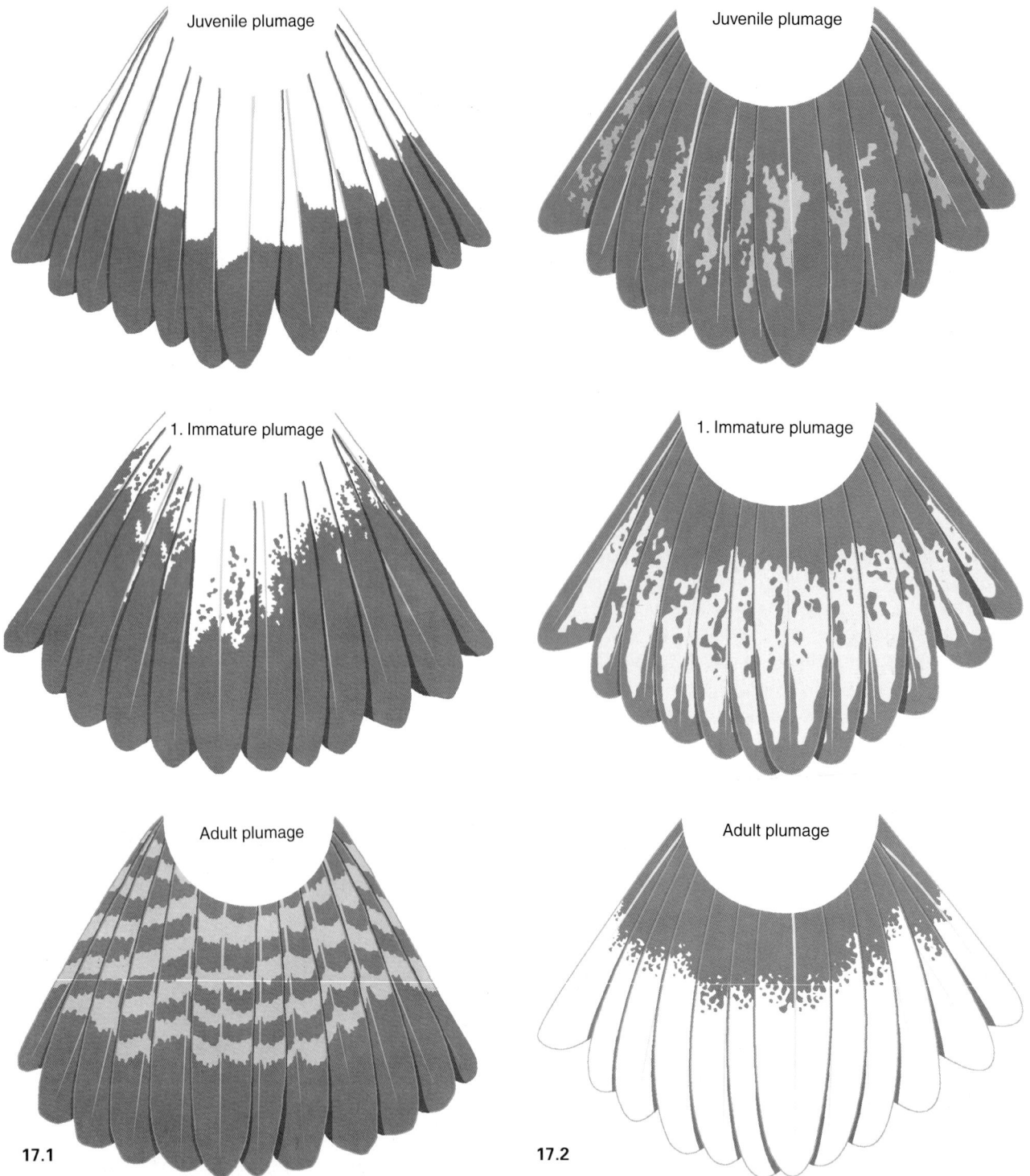

Figs. 17.1 and 17.2: While golden eagles (*Aquila chryseatos*) (left) have a light-colored tail when young and acquire dark feathers only after 5 or 6 years, the white-tailed sea eagle (*Haliaeetus albicilla*) (right) starts out dark and acquires a white tail with maturity.
(Illustration: R. Gattung-Petith and A. Gattung)

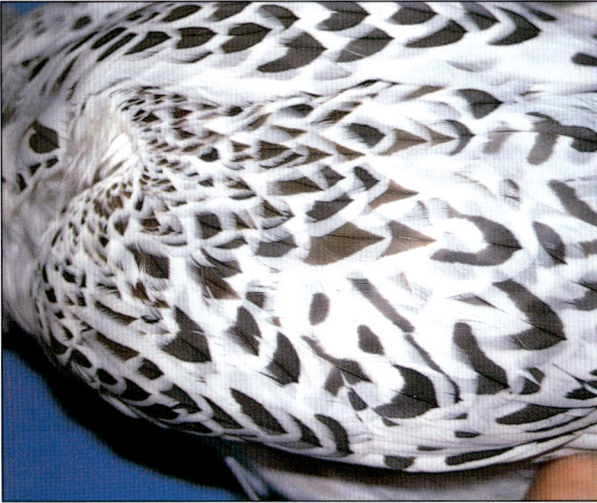

Fig. 17.3: A white gyrfalcon (*F. rusticolus*) near the completion of its molt showing a few remnants of the brown juvenile plumage among the scapular covert feathers. (Photo: Heidenreich)

17.1.1   Plumage characteristics

Many raptor species have differing feather patterns and colors that make up their juvenile, subadult and adult plumage. This has been adequately described and depicted in the relevant reference books (see Ch. 19), and will therefore not be discussed here in detail.

Much of the literature pertaining to this subject does not indicate at which ages these feather changes take place. It may take several years for some species to reach their adult plumage. Golden eagles (Fig. 17.1)

and white-tailed sea eagles (Fig. 17.2) are a good example of this. In general, raptors tend to achieve their final adult feather patterns at about the same time as they reach sexual maturity.

Smaller birds of prey lose their immature plumage more rapidly, usually completely molting into the adult pattern by the autumn of their second year. This first adult plumage frequently retains a few scattered juvenile feathers, making an exact age determination in these birds still possible.

Example:
The birds depicted in Figures 17.3 and 17.4, a white gyrfalcon (*Falco rusticolus*) and a northern goshawk (*Accipiter gentilis*), are both in adult plumage, but both also retain a few feathers from their immature set.

The birds hatched in year X and wore their juvenile plumage until their first molt. The molt begins in the spring of the following year (X + 1) and is completed by autumn of that same year. The year after that (X + 2), molt begins again in spring, and this time, even the last few juvenile feathers are lost. This means that an exact determination of a bird's age is possible until it is about $2^1/_2$ years old. After that, age can only be estimated.

In goshawks, the black and white banding pattern of the breast feathers also changes with time, becoming narrower or finer with age. Although this can be helpful, it is not an exact indicator of age.

Young European black vultures have much down on their heads (Fig. 17.5), but gradually lose it as they get older, until they are left only with a small downy cap.

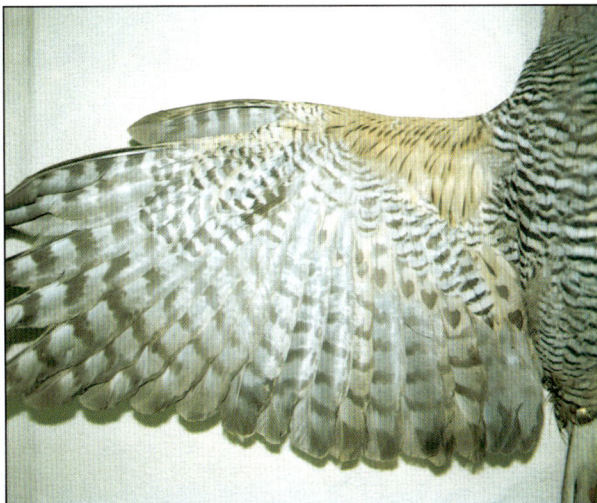

Fig. 17.4: Only the undersides of the wings still carry some remaining feathers from this northern goshawk's (*Accipiter gentilis*) immature plumage. (Photo: Heidenreich)

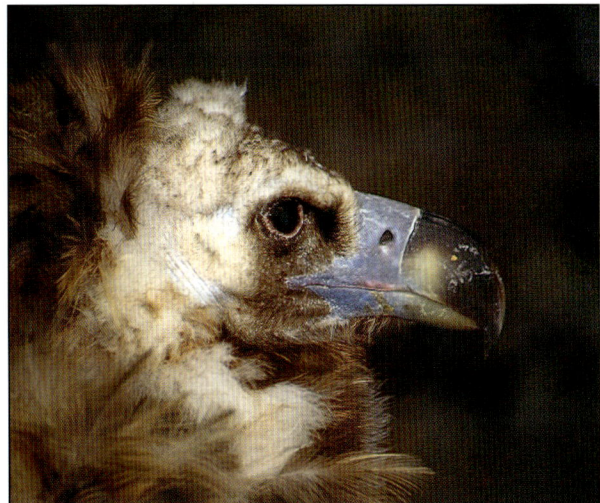

Fig. 17.5: Juvenile European black vultures (*Aegypius monachus*) differ from adults in that their head is covered with a dense layer of downy feathers. (Photo: Heidenreich)

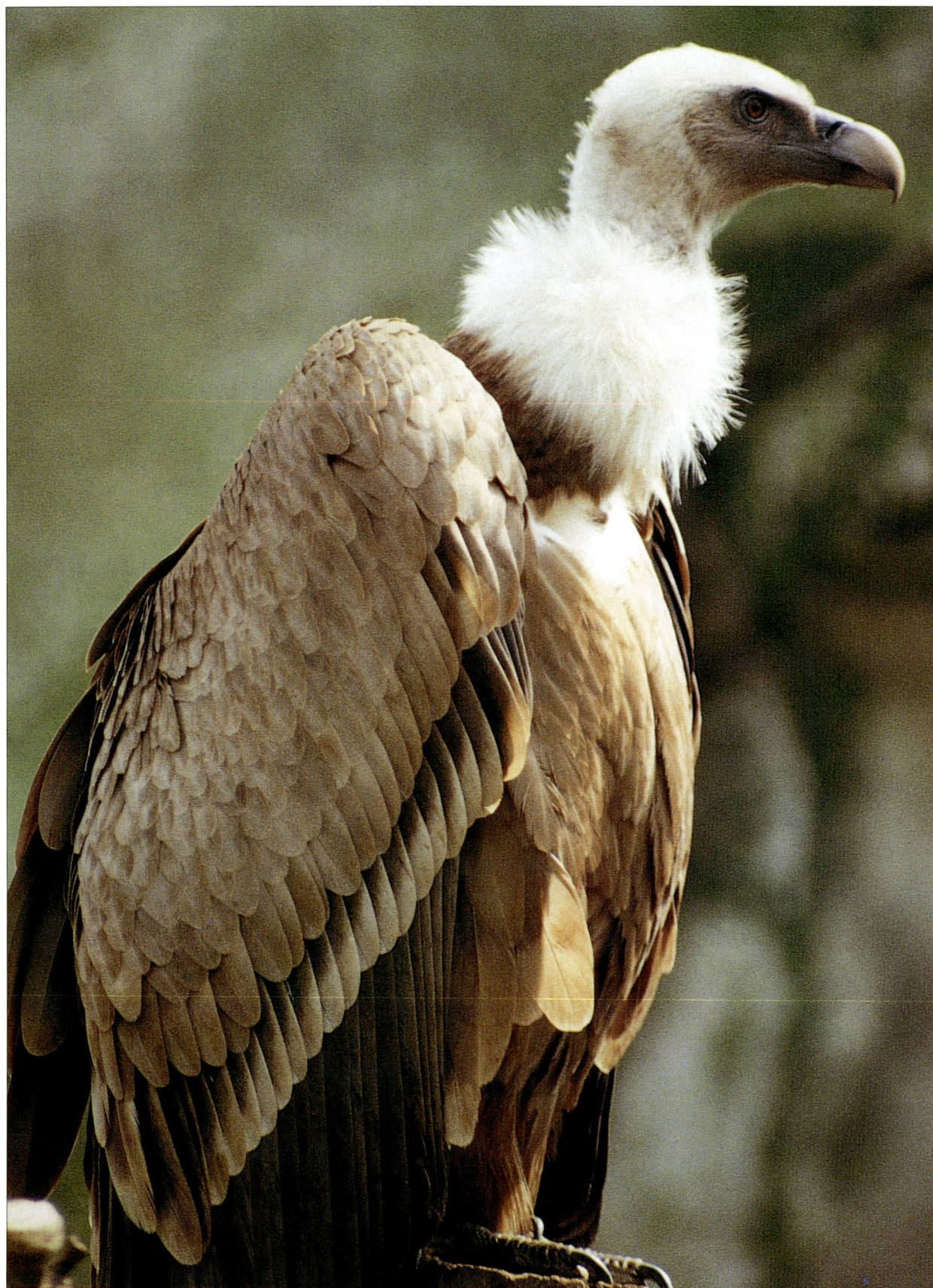

Fig. 17.6: The typical white neck ruff seen in adult griffon vultures (*Gyps fulvus*).

(Photo: Heidenreich)

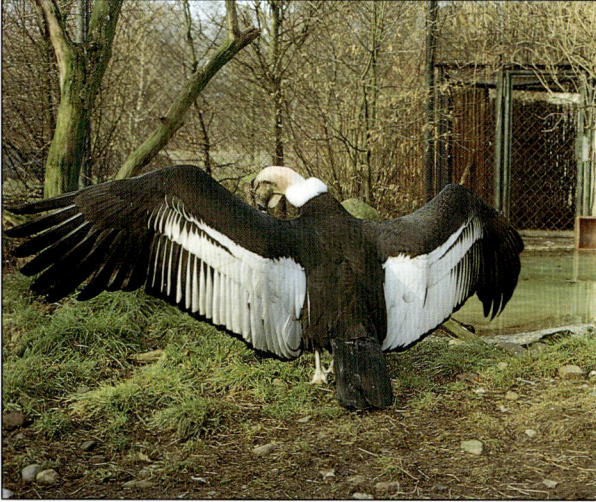

Fig. 17.7: Andean Condors (*Vultur gryphus*) are 8 to 10 years old before they attain their adult plumage with its characteristic white wings.
(Photo: Heidenreich)

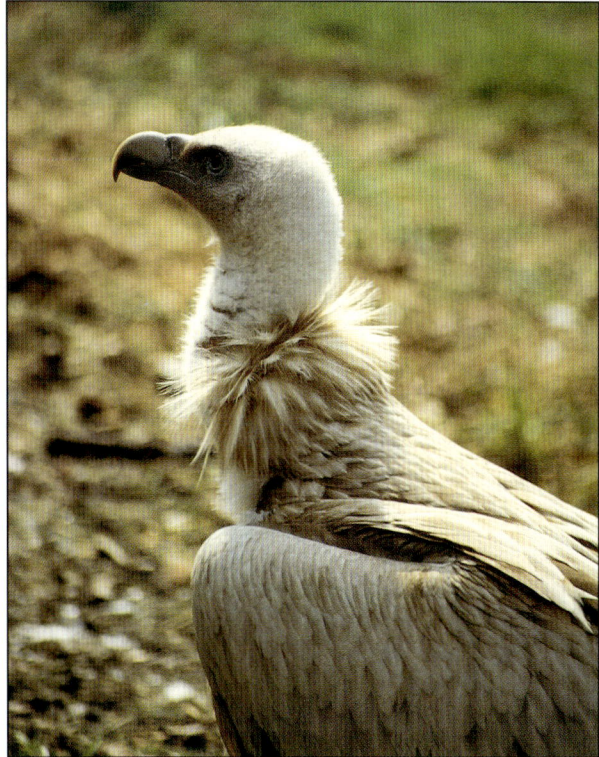

Fig. 17.8: Older griffon vultures (*Gyps fulvus*) have a fuzzy white neck ruff (see Fig. 17.6), while young birds have a scruffy brownish one.
(Photo: Heidenreich)

Juvenile Andean condors also have a downy head which eventually becomes completely bald as they mature. The typical pattern of white secondary feathers and coverts on the wings (Fig. 17.7) appears at approximately 8 to 10 years of age when they become sexually mature.

Almost all vultures of the genus *Gyps* have a feathery brown neck band when young (Fig. 17.8). With maturity, this band of feathers becomes white and fuzzy (Fig. 17.6).

Immature harpy eagles have a closely banded tail. The bands become fewer with each molt, until adults are left with only three widely spaced bands on their tails.

17.1.2 Cere and leg color

Many birds of prey are born with a yellowish coloration of the cere and unfeathered portions of the legs and feet. The hierofalcons are an exception to this rule, having distinctly bluish legs and ceres when young (Fig. 17.9). With adulthood, they too turn yellow (Fig. 17.10). The rate at which this change occurs is not the same in all birds, but it always begins with their first molt the year after hatching. The yellow coloration depends on various factors besides age. The presence of carotene in the diet appears to be important. Birds on varied diets, especially those that eat day-old chicks rich in yolk, will develop the yellow coloration earlier than those that primarily eat rats, for example.

The color of the cere and legs is therefore only a general indicator of age, and cannot be used for the exact determinations often required by a court of law.

17.1.3 Eye color

The color of the iris changes with age in many accipiters and buteos. Juvenile red-tailed hawks have a pale yellowish iris that takes several years to change to a dark brown color. Goshawk nestlings have gray eyes that become pale yellow by the time they fledge (Fig. 17.11). Over time, the iris becomes deeper yellow, eventually turning orange or even deep red in older goshawks (Fig. 17.12).

These changes in iris pigmentation have been ascribed purely to age. They may, in fact, be related more closely to cumulative light exposure. The more intense the exposure to light, the more rapid is the color change. This theory is based on evidence obtained from a case in which a 7-year old goshawk suffered from fusion of the eyelids of one eye since birth. The open eye developed the characteristic orange color seen in older accipiters, but when its lids were surgically separated, the closed eye still had the pale yellow juvenile coloration (Fig. 17.13).

Eye color is therefore not a reliable indicator of age in birds of prey.

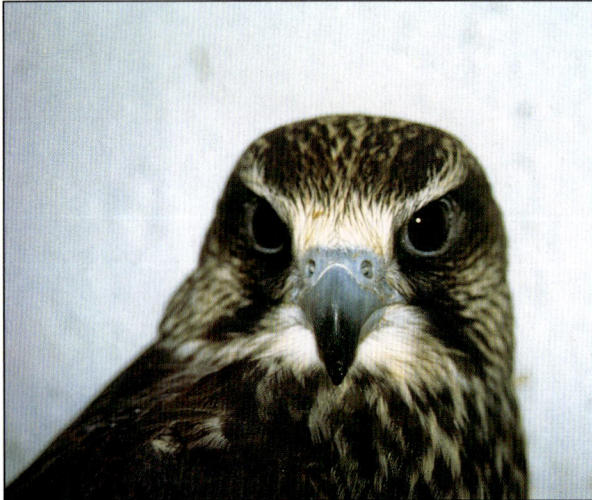

△ 17.9   17.10 ▽

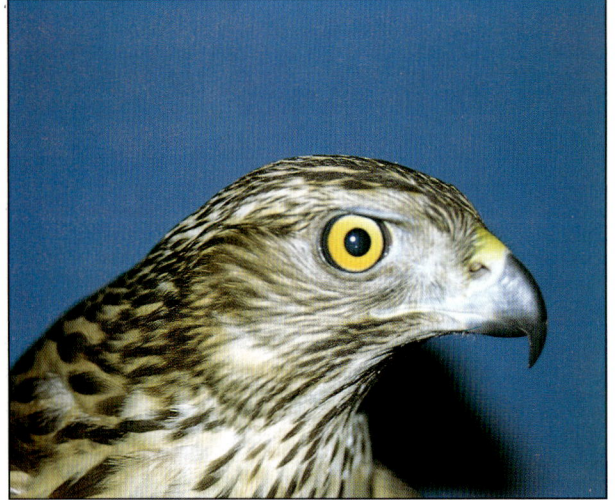

17.11

Figs. 17.11 and 17.12: The iris of northern goshawks (*Accipiter gentilis*) is light yellow in juveniles (17.11) and gradually turns red in adults (17.12). (Photos: Heidenreich)

17.12

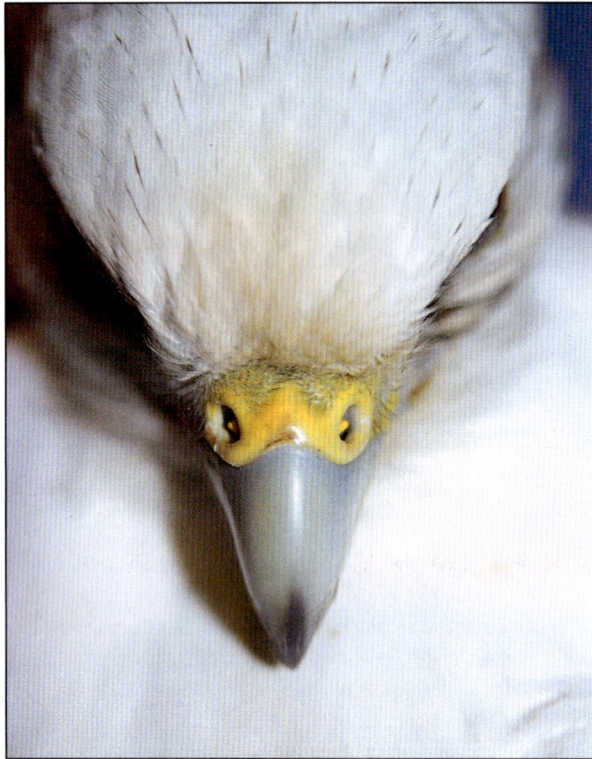

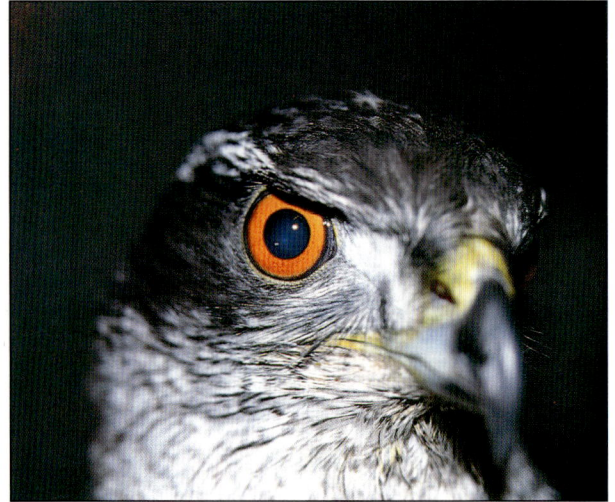

Figs. 17.9 and 17.10: Young hierofalcons (17.9, *F. cherrug*) have a distinctly bluish-gray cere in the first year of life. After that, it becomes yellow (17.10, *F. rusticolus*). (Photo: Heidenreich)

17.2   Sex determination

Some raptor species are sexually dimorphic. In others, the sexes cannot be told apart by external appearance.

As a rule, male birds of prey are smaller than females. There can be significant overlap in the weight ranges for the two sexes, however, so that weight alone does not always permit an exact determination of sex.

The New World vultures have an unusual pattern, males being distinctly larger than females in this group of birds (see also Ch. 2).

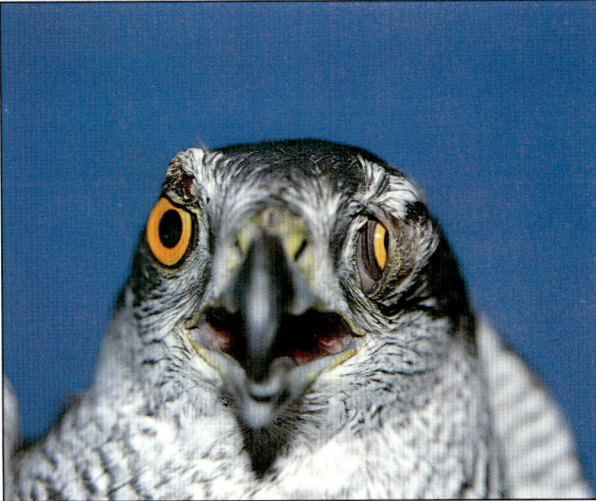

Fig. 17.13: The degree of change in iris pigmentation seems to depend on exposure to light. The normal right eye of this bird is already deep orange, while the left one, which was covered by the eyelids since birth, still appears yellow.
(Photo: Heidenreich)

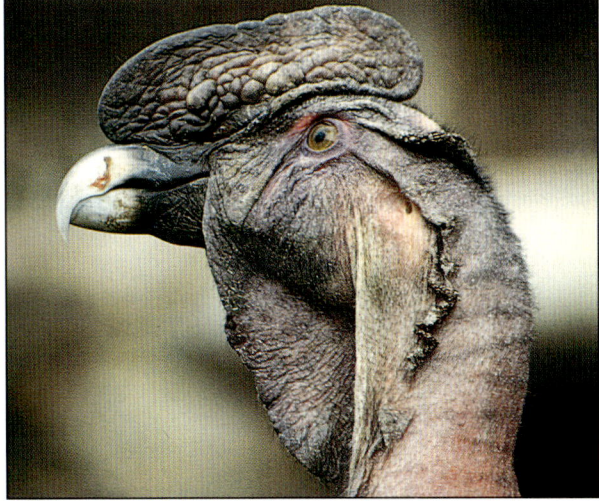

Fig. 17.15: Only a few raptor species show distinct sexual dimorphism. Adult male Andean condors are easily identified by the fleshy comb on their head.
(Photo: Heidenreich)

Species in which both sexes are of similar size can sometimes be told apart by beak size and shape. In eagles, for instance, the female's beak is bulkier and forms a straight extension of the top line of the head.

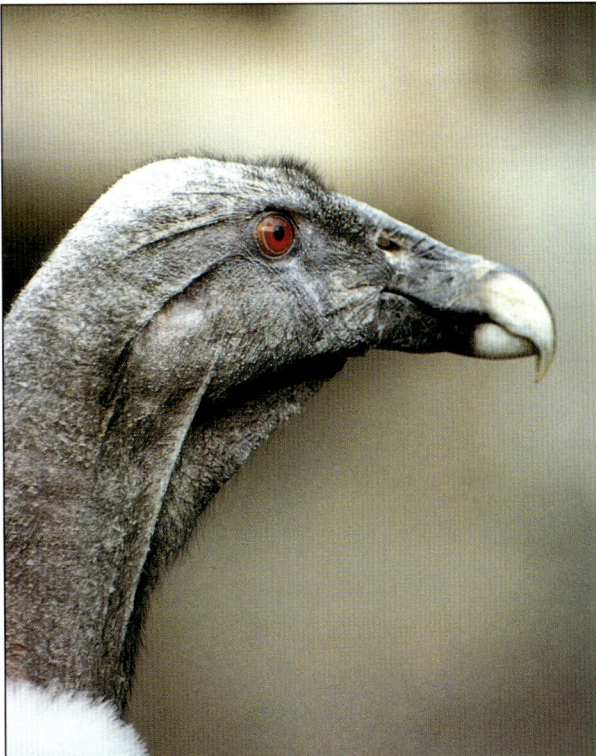

Fig. 17.14: Andean condor female.
(Photo: Heidenreich)

Males have a more slender beak that comes off the head somewhat lower.

Some raptor species show phenotypic distinctions between the sexes when they reach maturity (Figs. 17.14 and 17.15). Some of the more common ones and their determining characteristics are presented in Table 17.2.

Those raptors in which there is no sexual dimorphism must be surgically sexed.

17.3   Species identification

The identification of purebred raptor species is generally straightforward and there are many well-illustrated guide books to help with this task. Problems can arise in trying to identify captive falcons, however. Hybrids that closely resemble pure species are now very common (see below). On the other hand, small deviations from the species description do not always mean that one is dealing with a hybrid falcon. The reference books often distinguish between the various subspecies of a particular falcon species. In the process of captive breeding, however, these distinctions have become blurred, so that pure subspecies are hardly ever found in captivity. Even purebred individuals belonging to a single species are thus a mixture of various subspecies groups.

The peregrine, saker and gyrfalcons are presented here as examples of common falconry birds that are extensively bred in captivity and whose variations are sometimes confusing and difficult to identify.

17.3.1   Purebred species

17.3.1.1   Peregrine falcons (*Falco peregrinus*)

There are 18 peregrine falcon subspecies distributed all over the world. The phenotypic distinctions between them are sometimes very small. For legal purposes, these distinctions are usually of no importance. The law pertains only to the species *Falco peregrinus*, in which the not yet definitively classified desert falcons *Falco pelegrinoides pelegrinoides* (Barbary falcon) and *Falco pelegrinoides babylonicus* (red-naped shaheen) are included. It is therefore sufficient to be able to identify a peregrine falcon as such.

Figures 17.16 through 17.25 give an overview of the various types of adult purebred peregrines and present one bird in immature plumage.

17.3.1.2   Gyrfalcons (*Falco rusticolus*)

Gyrfalcons occur in a wide range of color phases ranging from dark to almost completely white. These variants are generally considered to be "types" rather than subspecies. The white gyrfalcon from Greenland, for example, is called the "candicans type" while the grayish one from Iceland is known as the "islandus type".

Figures 17.26 through 17.31 show the various color phases of adult gyrfalcons and one bird in immature plumage.

White gyrfalcons are very popular for hybrid breeding as well. They are usually crossed with saker falcons to produce bigger, lighter offspring that still retain most of the saker qualities.

Too often, experts asked to identify gyrfalcons classify birds that differ slightly from the illustrations presented in the reference books as hybrids. The set of figures 17.32-17.37 shows the variability in tail feather patterns seen even in purebred white gyrfalcons.

Table 17.2: Sexually dimorphic characteristics in selected raptor species

Raptor species	Male	Female
Andean Condor (*Vultur gryphus*)	distinct comb-like caruncle	no comb (caruncle)
Osprey (*P. haliaetus*)	narrower, lighter breast band	darker, wider breast band
Secretary bird (*S. serpentarius*)	red-rimmed eye, longer crest and tail than female	yellow-rimmed eye
Snail kite (*R.sociabilis*)	bluish-black plumage	reddish-brown plumage
Bateleur (*T. ecaudatus*)	black primaries	brown primaries
Marsh harrier (*C. aeruginosus*)	secondaries bluish-gray	secondaries brown
Hen harrier (*C. cyaneus*)	plumage light blue	plumage brown
Pallid harrier (*C. macrourus*)	plumage light gray	plumage light brown
Montagu's harrier (*C. pygargus*)	plumage light blue	plumage brown
European sparrowhawk (*A. nisus*) and other small accipiters	smaller body size, rusty underbelly, bluish-gray back	larger body size, gray back
Bonelli's eagle (*H. fasciatus spilogaster*)	dark primaries, more contrasting plumage	gray primaries, lighter overall
Lesser kestrel (*F. naumanni*)	blue head, red back, tail blue with black band	uniformly brown
American kestrel (*F. sparverius*)	wings blue, tail red with single black band	brown, multiple bands on tail
Common kestrel (*F. tinnunculus*)	blue head and tail, single black band on tail	brown, multiple bands on tail
Red-footed falcon (*F. vespertinus*)	sooty black head and back, red belly and legs	brown head, distinctly banded tail
Merlin (*F. columbarius*)	blue head and back, rusty breast	uniformly brown
European Hobby (*F. subbuteo*)	plain reddish-brown legs	streaked legs

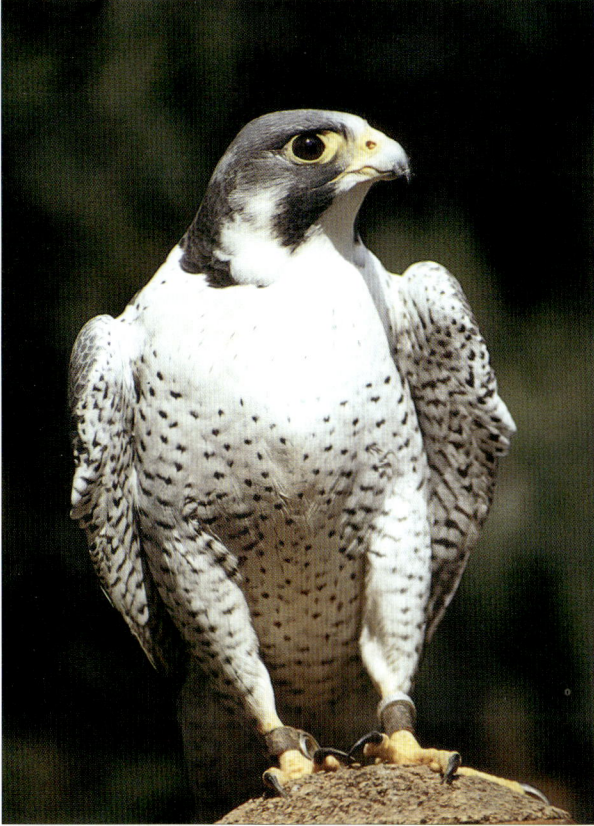

17.16

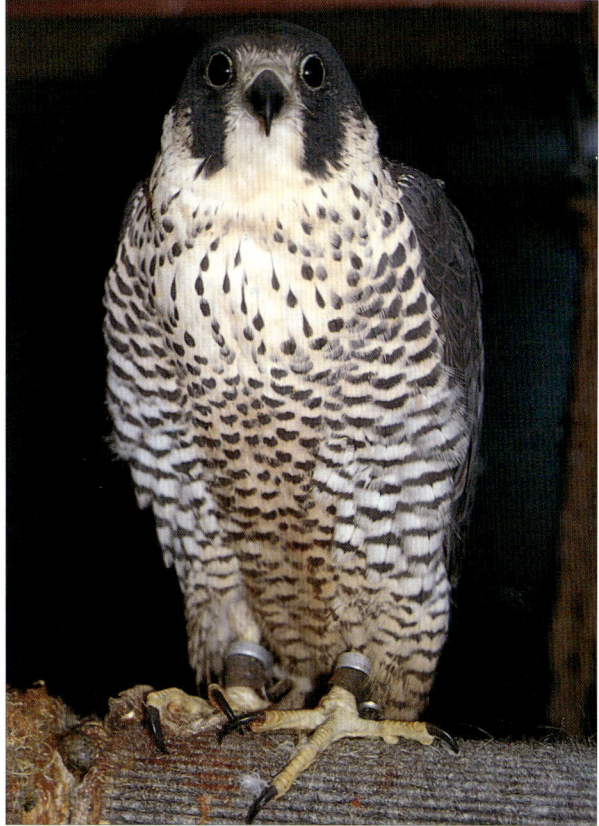

17.17

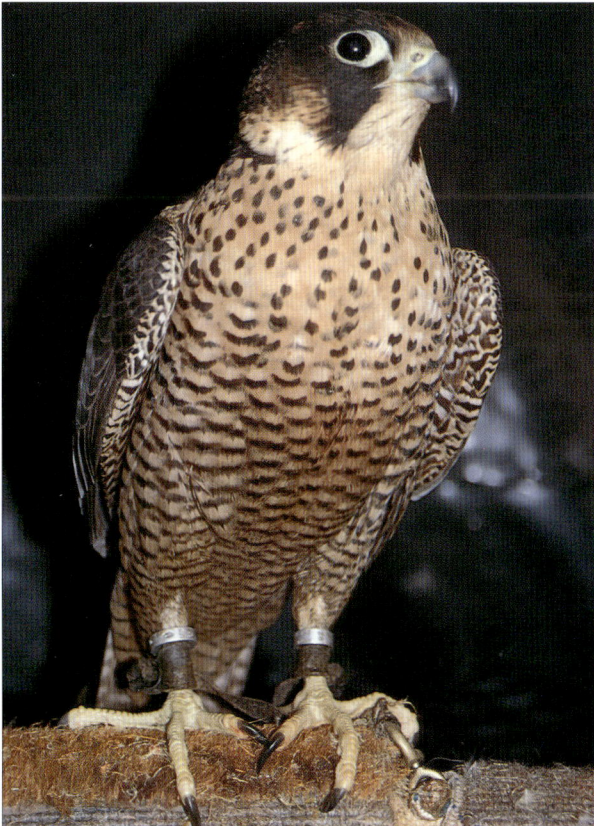

17.21

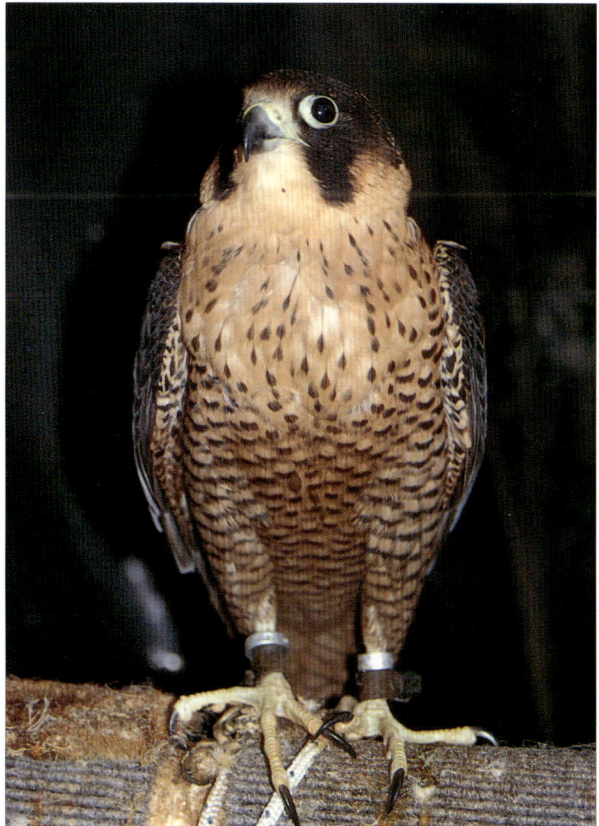

17.22

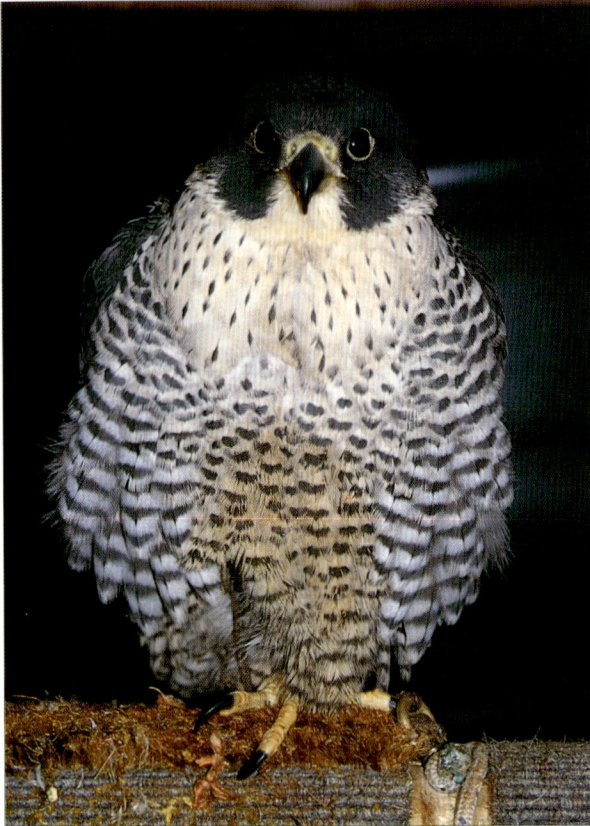

17.18

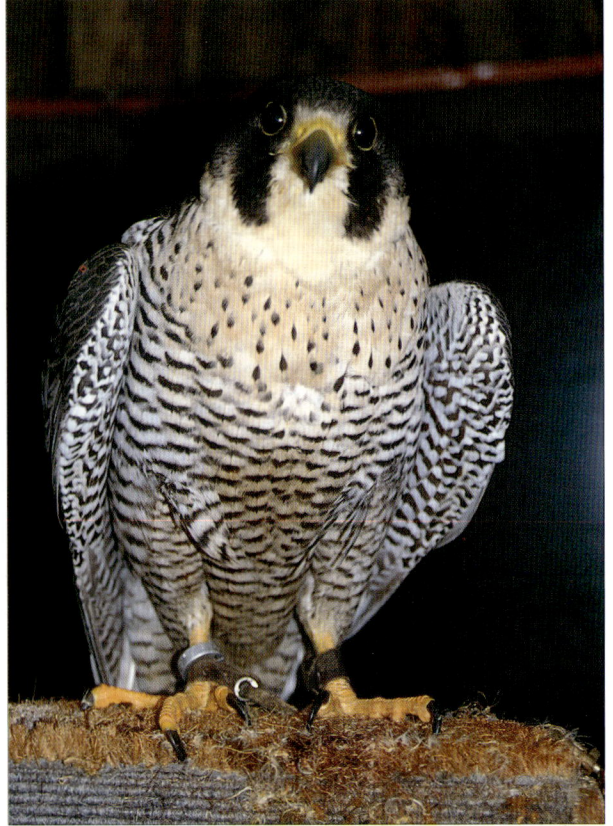

17.19

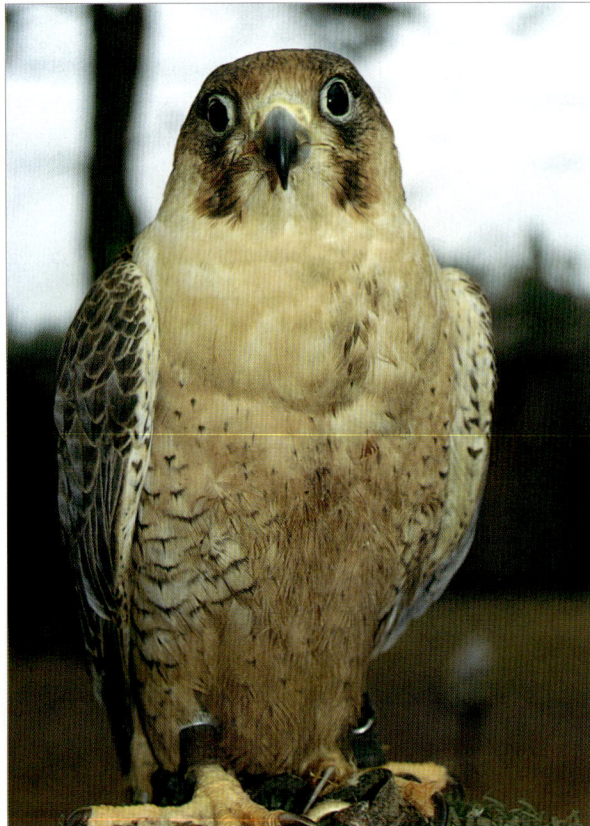

17.23

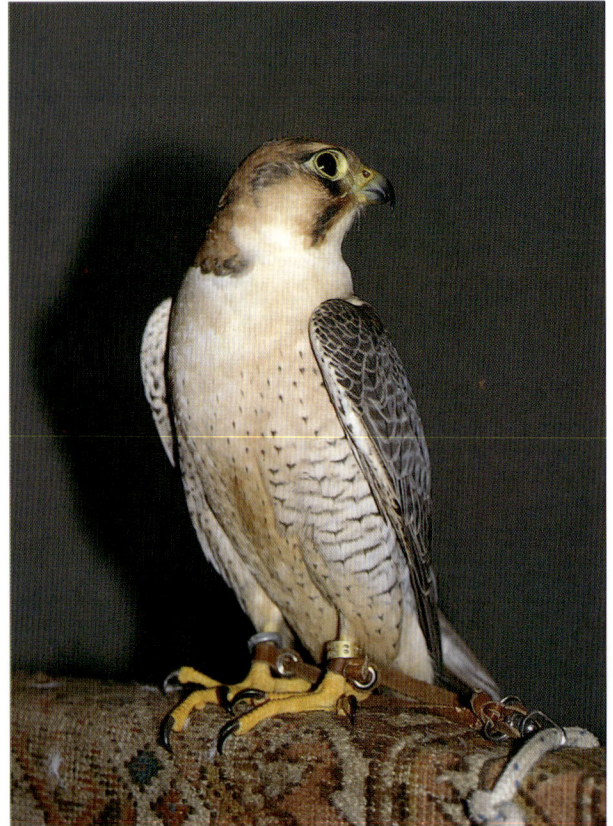

17.24

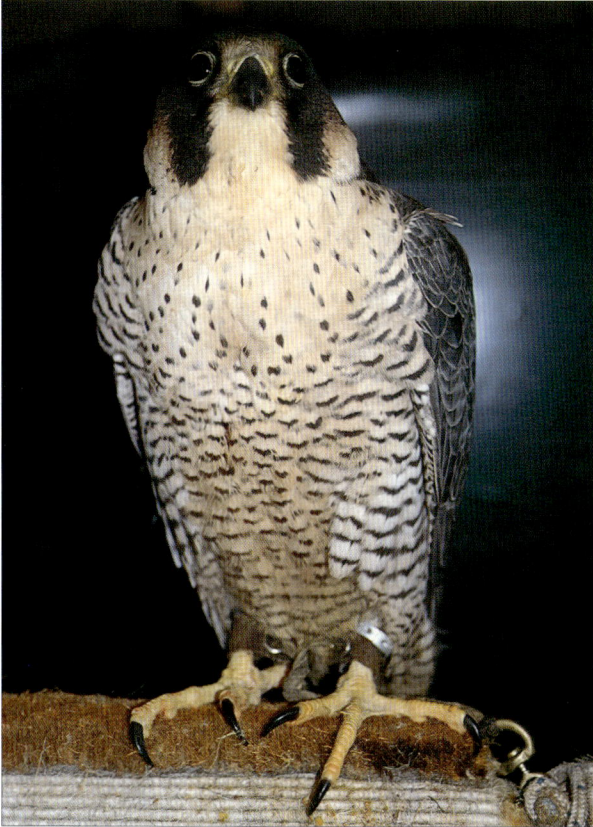

17.20

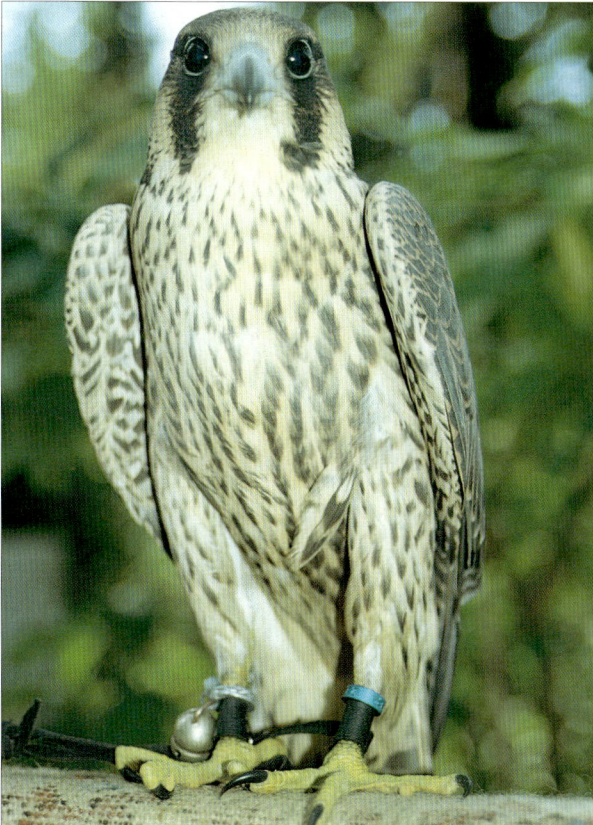

17.25

Figs. 17.16, 17.17, 17.18, 17.19, 17.20, 17.21, 17.22, 17.23, 17.24, and 17.25: Captive-bred peregrine falcons usually no longer conform to distinct subspecies standards and only roughly resemble the various classified groups presented in reference books.
A light "calidus" type (17.16), a normal "peregrinus" type (17.17), a "peregrinus" type with a shortened moustachial stripe (17.18), crosses between "peregrinus" and "brookei" types with varying degrees of red coloration (17.19 and 17.20), typical "brookei" type (17.21), very red "brookei" type (17.22), pure red-naped shaheen (*F. pelegrinoides babylonicus*) (17.23), Barbary falcon phenotype (*F. pelegrinoides pelegrinoides*) (17.24), peregrine falcon in juvenile plumage (17.25).
(Photos: Heidenreich)

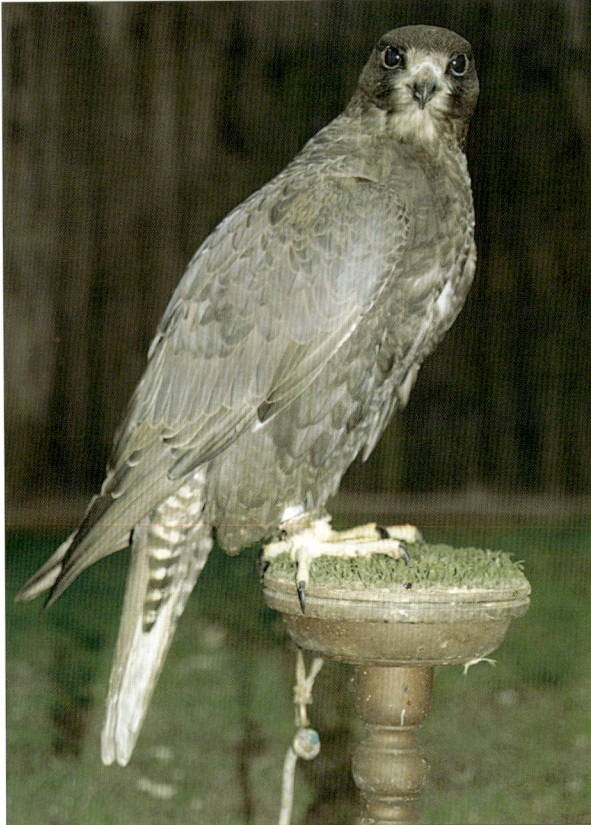

17.26

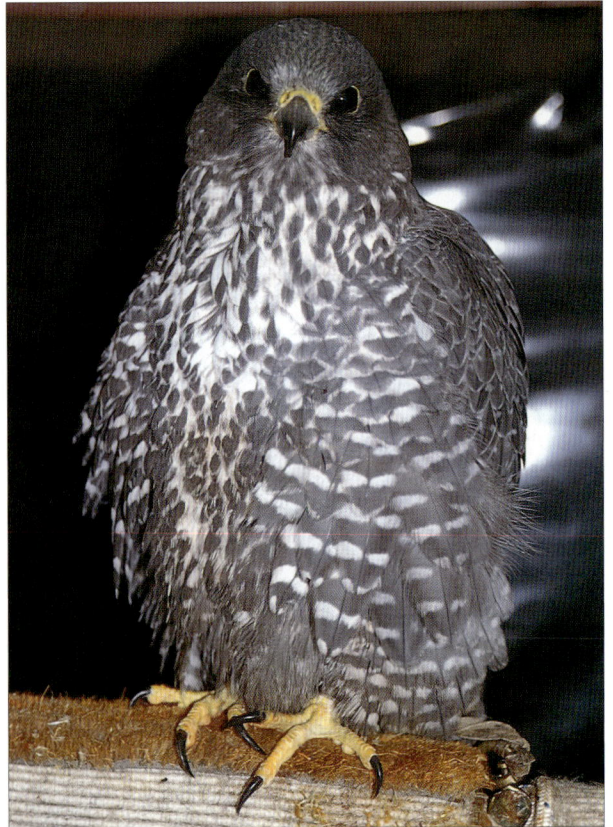

17.27

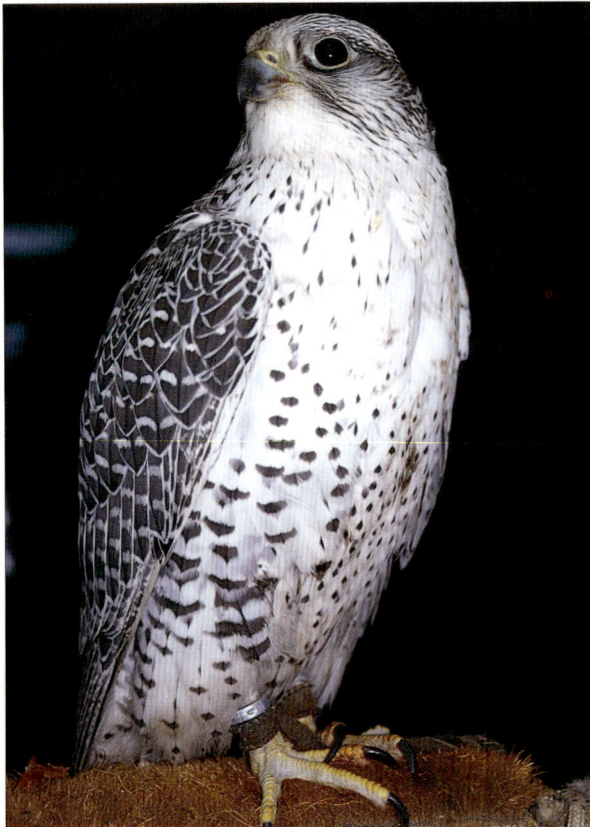

17.29

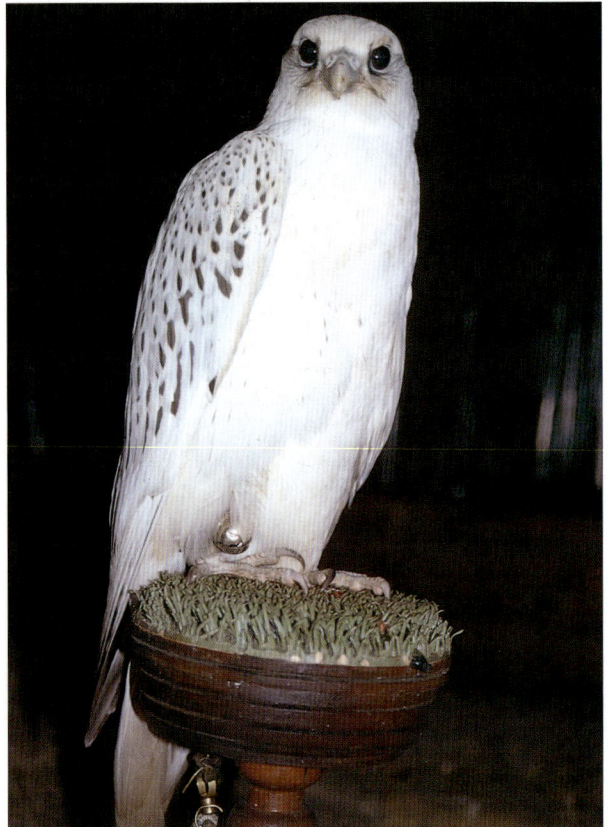

17.30

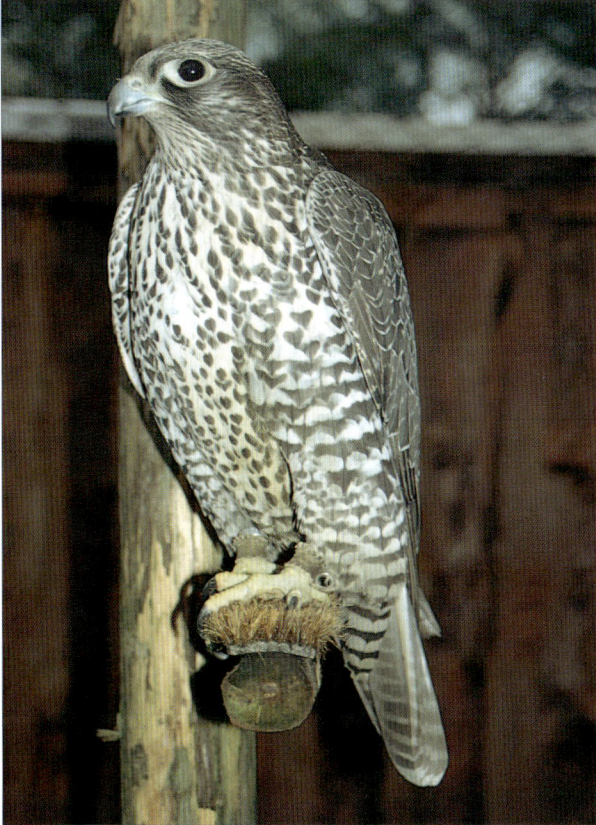

17.28

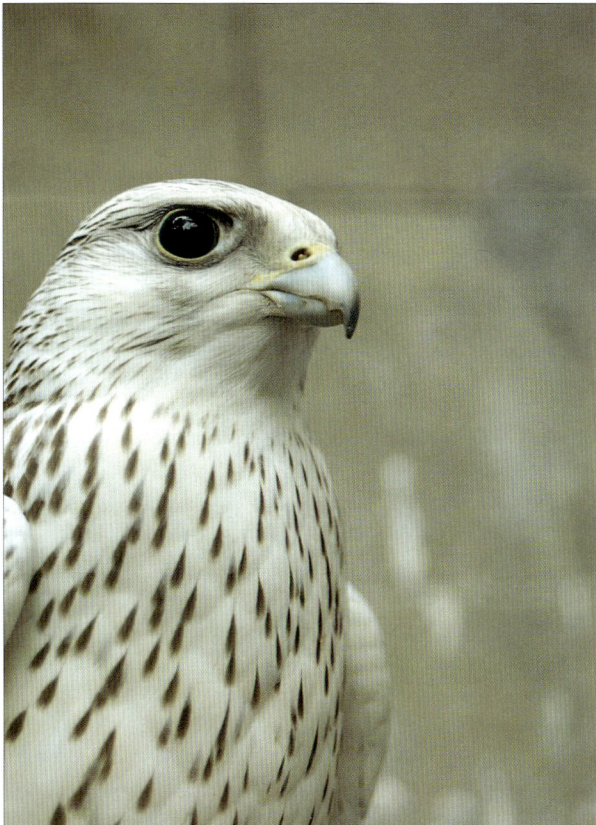

17.31

Figs. 17.26, 17.27, 17.28, 17.29, 17.30 and 17.31:
Captive-bred gyrfalcons are also usually mixtures of
various geographical races or types. They are often
cross bred this way to obtain birds of specific colors.
Dark gyrfalcon types (17.26-17.28), white gyrfalcon types
(17.29 and 17.30), and an immature white gyrfalcon in
its second year of life already showing a change in cere
color (17.31).
(Photos: Heidenreich)

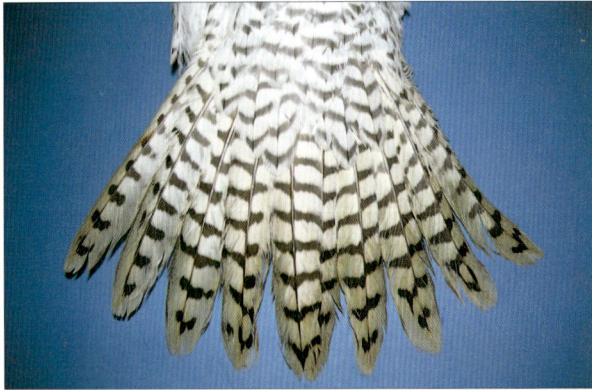

17.32

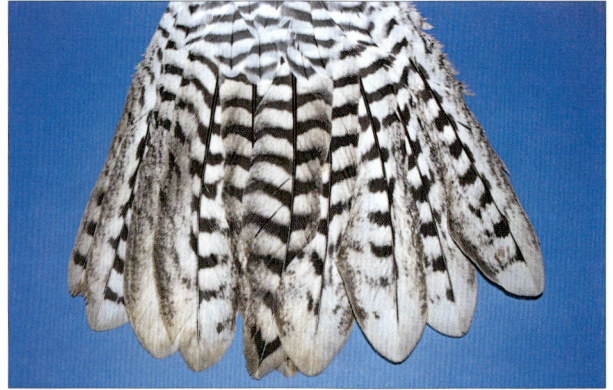

17.33

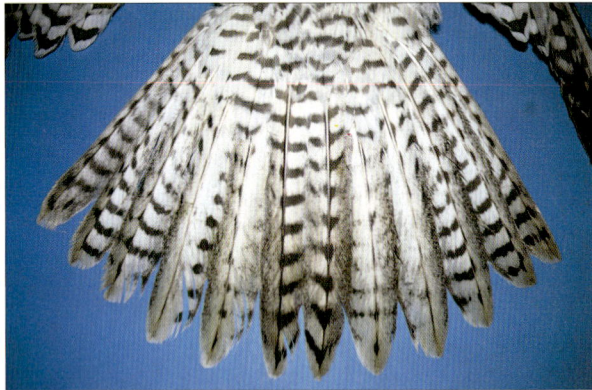

17.34

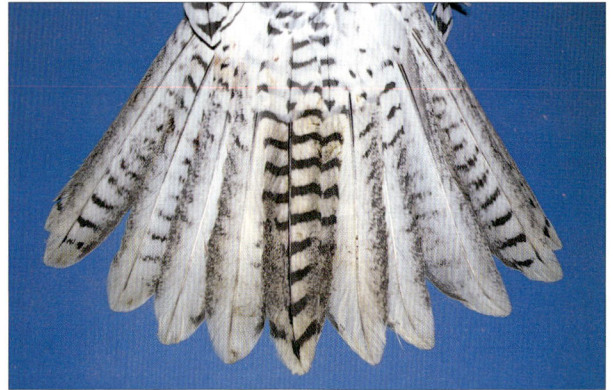

17.35

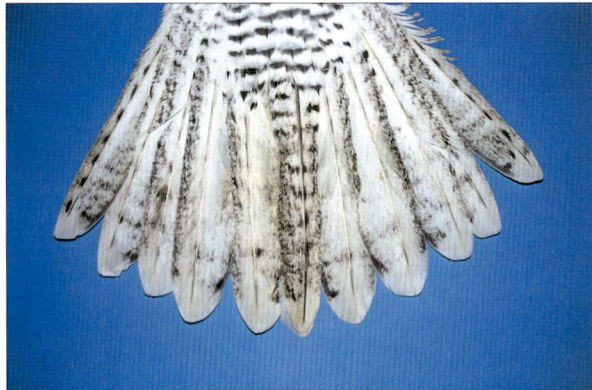

17.36

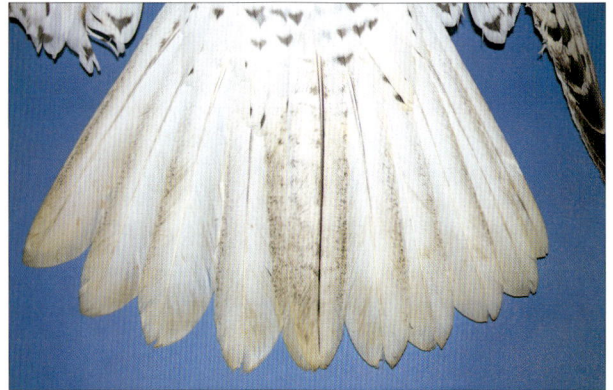

17.37

Figs. 17.32, 17.33, 17.34, 17.35, 17.36 and 17.37: The various color patterns found in the tail feathers of white gyrfalcons do not indicate hybridization. They merely reflect the wide range of natural variation in this species. (Photos: Heidenreich)

17.3.1.3   Saker falcons (*Falco cherrug*)

Like gyrfalcons, saker falcons exist in a variety of color variations and types. They can range from almost white to very dark in plumage. The Altai saker falcon (*Falco cherrug altaicus*) is especially difficult to classify. This type looks more like a gyrfalcon, but has meanwhile been accepted as a saker falcon subspecies.

Various color variations seen in adult sakers are depicted in Figs. 17.38 to 17.43. One bird in immature plumage is also shown. Figs. 17.44 through 17.49 show several different tail feather patterns encountered among saker falcons.

Table 17.3: Hybridizations between raptor species (from ROSENKRANZ, 1981; BUNELL, 1986; CADE, 1988; HEIDENREICH et al.,1993, PÖPPELMANN, 1994; v. PÖLNITZ, 1995 and BRÜNING, 1995)

Peregrine falcon (*Falco peregrinus*)	X	Lanner falcon (*Falco biarmicus*)
	X	Saker falcon (*Falco cherrug*)
	X	Prairie falcon (*Falco mexicanus*)
	X	Red-naped shaheen (*Falco pelegrinoides*)
	X	Bat falcon (*Falco rufigularis*)
	X	Gyrfalcon (*Falco rusticolus*)
	X	Laggar falcon (*Falco jugger*)
	X	Merlin (*Falco columbarius*)
	X	American kestrel (*Falco sparverius*)
Gyrfalcon (*Falco rusticolus*)	X	Red-naped shaheen (*Falco pelegrinoides*)
	X	Saker falcon (*Falco cherrug*)
	X	Merlin (*Falco columbarius*)
Prairie falcon (*Falco mexicanus*)	X	Gyrfalcon (*Falco rusticolus*)
	X	Red-naped shaheen (*Falco pelegrinoides*)
Common kestrel (*Falco tinnunculus*)	X	Lesser kestrel (*Falco naumanni*)
	X	Gyrfalcon (*Falco rusticolus*)
Golden eagle (*Aquila chrysaetos*)	X	Imperial eagle (*Aquila heliaca*)
	X	Tawny eagle (*Aquila rapax*)
Imperial eagle (*Aquila heliaca*)	X	Tawny eagle (*Aquila rapax*)
Northern goshawk (*Accipiter gentilis*)	X	European sparrowhawk (*Accipiter nisus*)
	X	Common buzzard (*Buteo buteo*)
Red kite (*Milvus milvus*)	X	Black kite (*Milvus migrans*)
	X	Common buzzard (*Buteo buteo*)
Harris' hawk (*Parabuteo unicinctus*)	X	Ferruginous hawk (*Buteo regalis*)
	X	Cooper's hawk (*Accipiter cooperii*)
	X	Red-tailed hawk (*Buteo jamaicensis*)

17.3.1.4   Photo documentation

Experts on birds of prey are occasionally asked to identify a raptor species based on a photographic image. Many of these pictures are of poor quality or otherwise insufficient for a definitive identification.

Some examples of proper photographic techniques and documentation are presented in Figs. 17.50 through 17.55 (pages 250–251) This type of documentation makes species identification somewhat easier for a person who can not examine the bird itself.

17.3.2   Hybrids

The crossing of raptor species to produce hybrid offspring has long been practiced among breeders. This involves both the mixing of subspecies and the hybridization of birds classified as separate species.

Morris and Stevens (1971) were the first to report on the successful mating between a female saker falcon and peregrine falcon tiercel who had pair-bonded in captivity. In 1975, Boyd and Boyd succeeded in producing a prairie falcon X peregrine falcon hybrid with artificial insemination techniques. Cade and Weaver obtained two hybrid offspring from a gyrfalcon X peregrine falcon breeding in 1976. Table 17.3 lists some of the raptor hybrids that have been produced so far.

Because many of the falcon hybrids are fully viable and fertile birds, various second-generation hybrid combinations have been produced as well. Table 17.4 lists the F_2 generation hybrids that have been reported so far. Other types of raptors have rarely been known to have viable second-generation offspring from hybrid parents.

Table 17.4: Multiple hybridizations reported among falcons (females listed first)

(red-naped shaheen X prairie falcon) X prairie falcon	BUNELL (1986)
(peregrine falcon X gyrfalcon) X gyrfalcon	BUNELL (1986)
(peregrine falcon X prairie falcon) X merlin	HAAK (1980)
saker falcon X (red-naped shaheen X gyrfalcon)	MÜLLER (1984)
(red-naped shaheen X merlin) X prairie falcon	MÜLLER (1987)
saker falcon X [saker falcon X (red-naped shaheen X gyrfalcon)]	KÜSPERT (1990)
[(red-naped shaheen X prairie falcon) X prairie falcon] X gyrfalcon	BUNELL (1986)

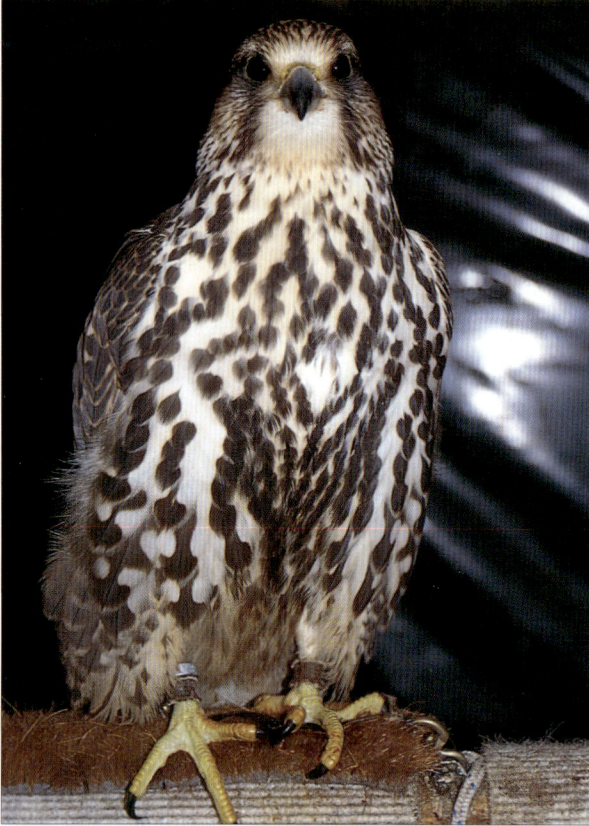

17.38

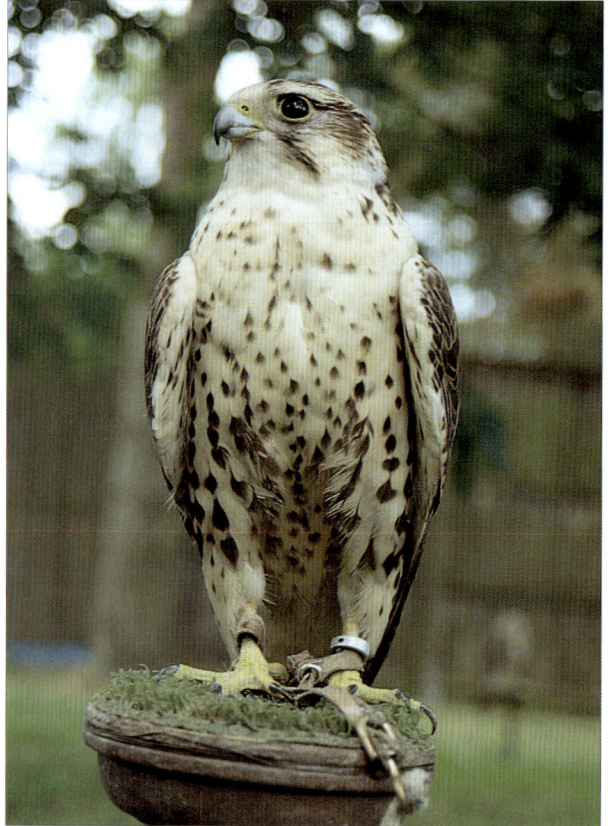

17.39

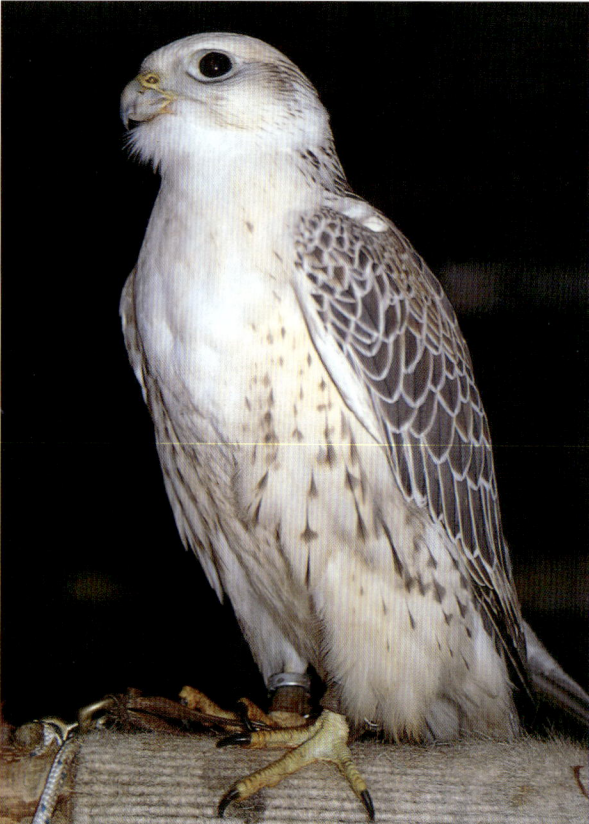

17.41

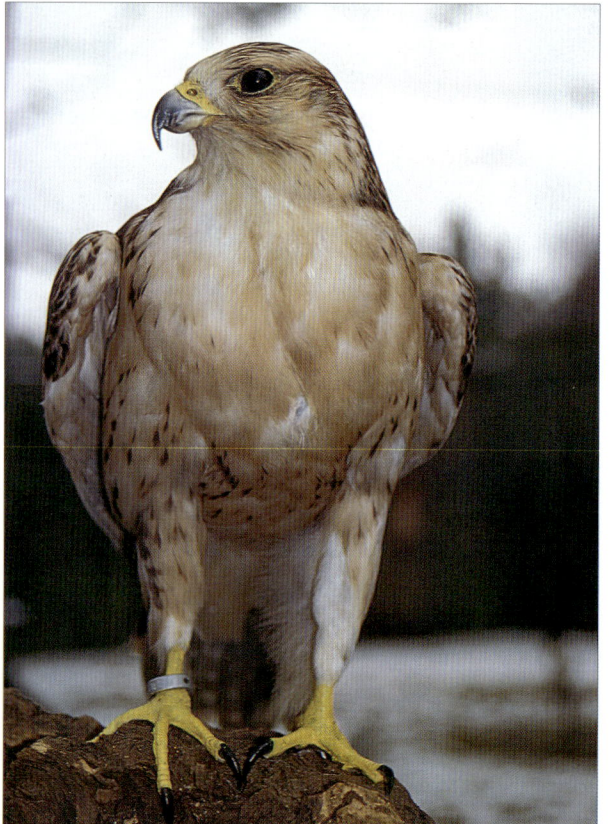

17.42

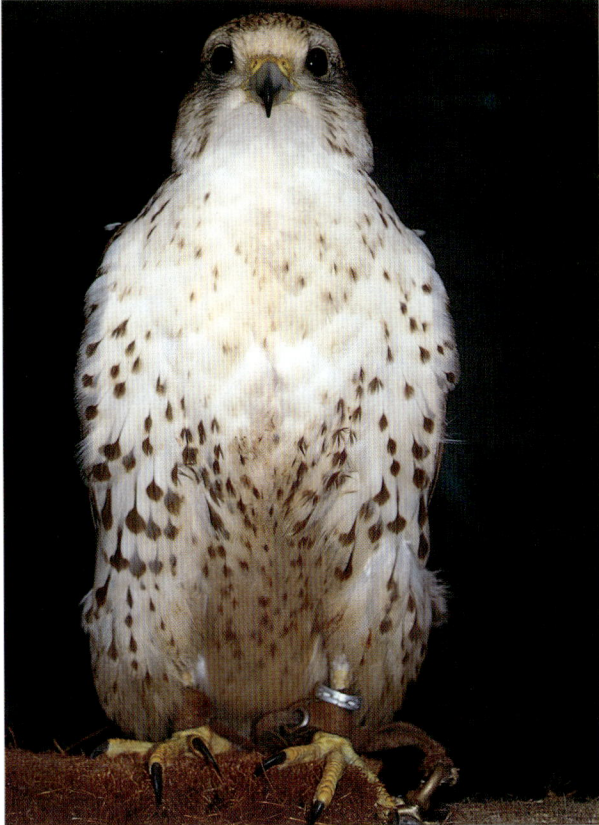

17.40

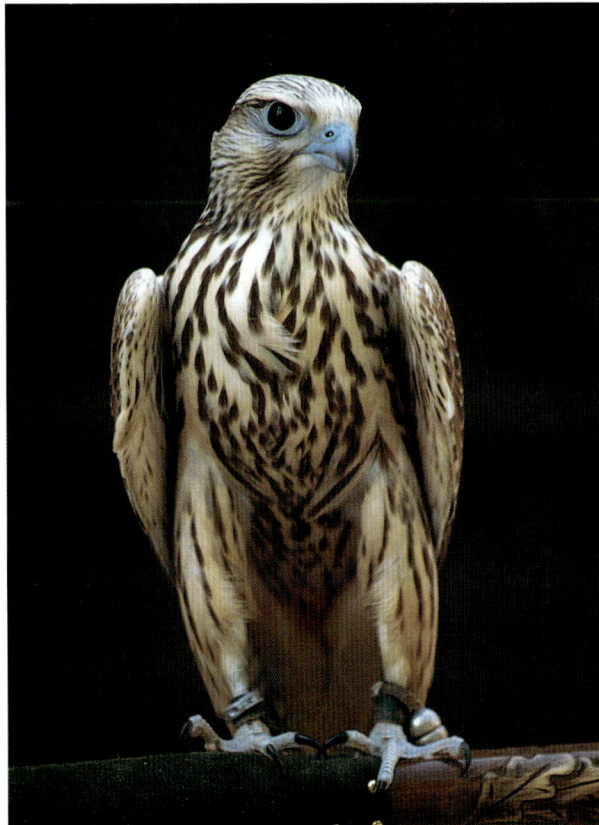

17.43

Figs. 17.38, 17.39, 17.40, 17.41, 17.42 and 17.43:
Pure saker falcons can vary in color from very light
to dark. Fig. 17.42 shows a stuffed specimen known
to come from Mongolia. A juvenile saker falcon
is shown in Fig. 17.43 (Photo: von Pölnitz).
(Photos: Heidenreich)

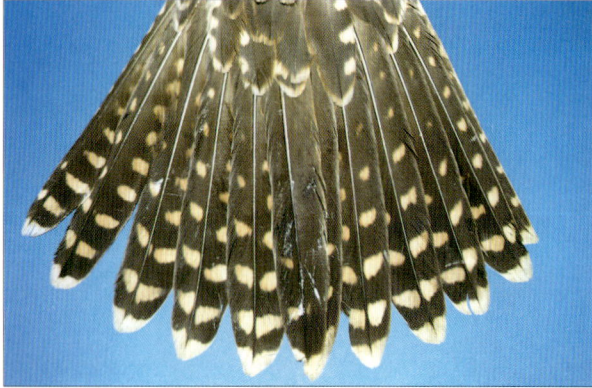

17.44

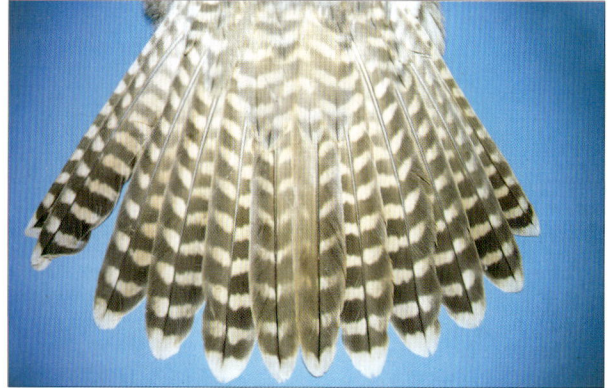

17.45

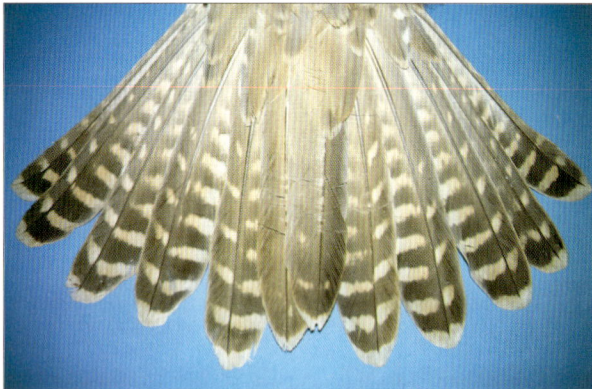

17.46

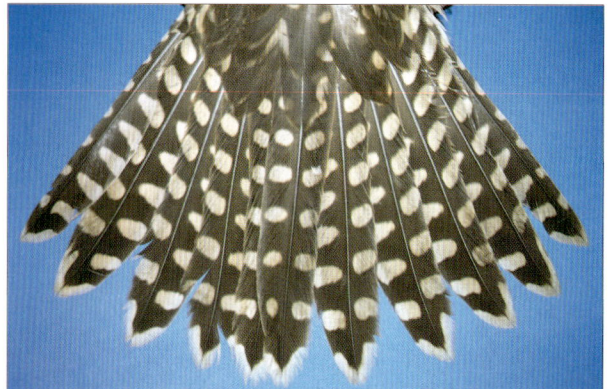

17.47

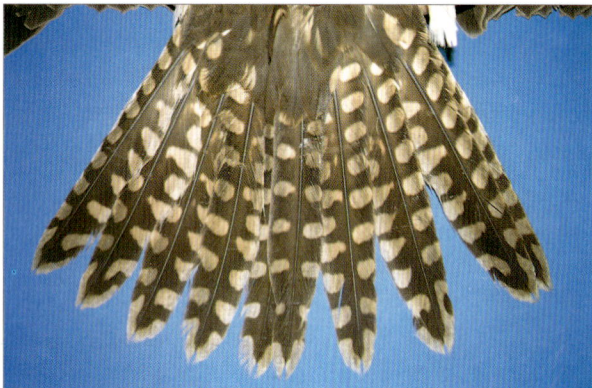

17.48

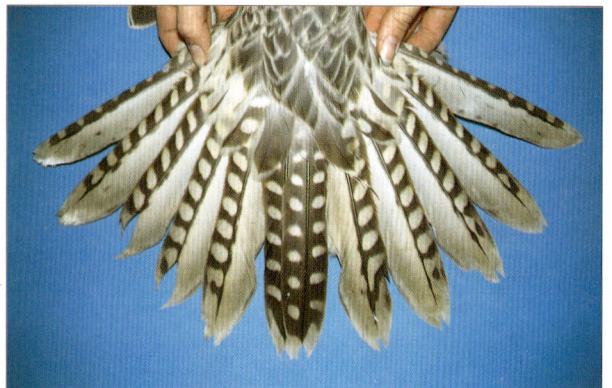

17.49

Figs. 17.44, 17.45, 17.46, 17.47, 17.48 and 17.49: The literature describes saker tail feathers as typically being marked with a pattern of "eyes". As with gyrfalcons, however, the tail patterns among sakers can vary substantially (see especially 17.49).
(Photos: Heidenreich)

Back in 1988, Cade and others expressed concern that raptor hybridization was being attempted and reported without providing comments or information regarding the methods employed or the success rates of the various combinations. This is particularly regrettable, since hybrid breeding studies could potentially provide interesting information regarding the phylogenetic relationships among the various species (Bednarek, 1991). Hardaswick and Smith (1981) did publish a paper discussing the breeding of F₁ hybrids between prairie and peregrine falcons.

Soon after people became aware of the success of falcon hybrids, concerns arose regarding the potential for such "artificial" breeds to escape and mate with wild falcons, thereby potentially altering the gene pool of these wild populations. It was therefore significant that Rafuse (1986) observed the natural pairing of a wild peregrine tiercel and prairie falcon female in Saskatchewan, Canada. This pair produced two young in 1985 and five in 1986.

Fischer (1967) and Baumgart (1971) reported on interspecific pairing of various falcon species in Mongolia and Bulgaria, although there appeared to be no successful offspring.

Seibold et al. (1993) used gene sequencing of mitochondrial DNA to analyze the possible phylogenetic relationships between various falcon species. Their results suggest that saker falcons may have hybridized with other species in the distant past.

Heidenreich and Kuespert (1992) determined in breeding experiments that hybrids resulting from the crossing of peregrine falcons with birds of the hierofalcon group are fertile, but that breeding them is rarely successful. Although these F₂ eggs are fertile, the embryos usually don't survive the incubation period. The few chicks that do hatch die in the first few days of life. Rosenkranz (1995) confirmed these observations. His pair of gyrfalcon-peregrine hybrids produced eight fertilized eggs, but all the embryos died before hatching.

Within the hierofalcon group, however, hybrids are completely fertile and can be hybridized for an indefinite number of generations, even without the use of artificial insemination. For instance, a gyrfalcon X saker falcon hybrid was successfully crossed with a lanner falcon X laggar falcon hybrid to produce viable offspring. Fig. 17.56 outlines our current understanding of falcon hybridization.

In the early days of captive raptor breeding, people were producing primarily hybrid falcons. One reason for this was the relatively limited number of breeding animals available, which may have forced some breeders to try interspecific matings. Another reason may have related to the strict laws protecting birds of prey. These laws pertained to purebred species, but did not apply to hybrids. Such animals were therefore exempt from the rules and regulations governing the ownership and sale of raptors. Since then, the laws have been changed and all hawks are now protected.

Today, the law states that a hybrid bird is protected by the same laws pertaining to the more highly protected of its two parents. A gyrfalcon X saker falcon hybrid, for example, is protected under Appendix I of CITES (see Ch. 18), as is its gyrfalcon parent, even though saker falcons are listed under Appendix II.

These regulations are difficult to enforce. It is not easy for a lay person to distinguish a hybrid like the one mentioned above from a pure saker falcon. Such a bird can thus be reported to the authorities as belonging to a group that is subject to lower levels of protection, permitting the owner to obtain otherwise illegal export permits, for example.

One last reason for producing hybrid birds of prey is to satisfy a demand for such birds from the falconry community. Experience has shown that certain hybrid combinations, gyrfalcon/peregrine crosses for example, make excellent hunting hawks. They are therefore in high demand. Arab falconers, who have traditionally caught wild saker falcons for training as hunting birds, have come to appreciate the hybrids' outstanding qualities and have been purchasing increasing numbers of them. By crossbreeding with gyrfalcons, breeders can produce phenotypic saker falcons that show the light coloration and higher body weights that the Arabs prefer.

In this context, however, there is great concern regarding the Arab practice of releasing unwanted hunting hawks at the end of the hunting season. Captive-bred hybrids set free after one season in this way are skilled hunters and have no problem surviving and

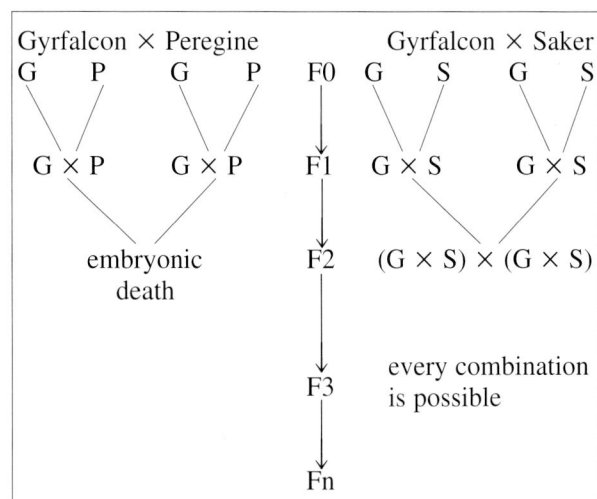

Fig. 17.56: Variations on hybrids

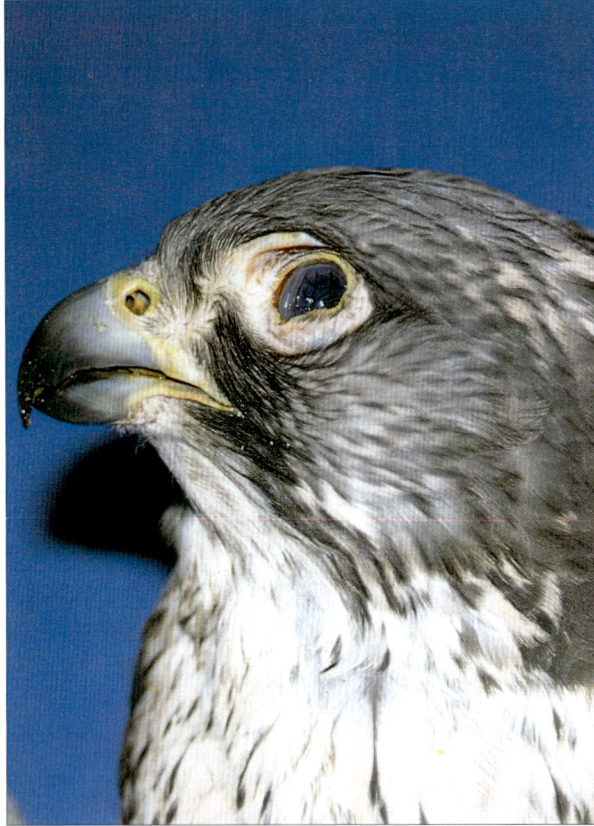

17.50

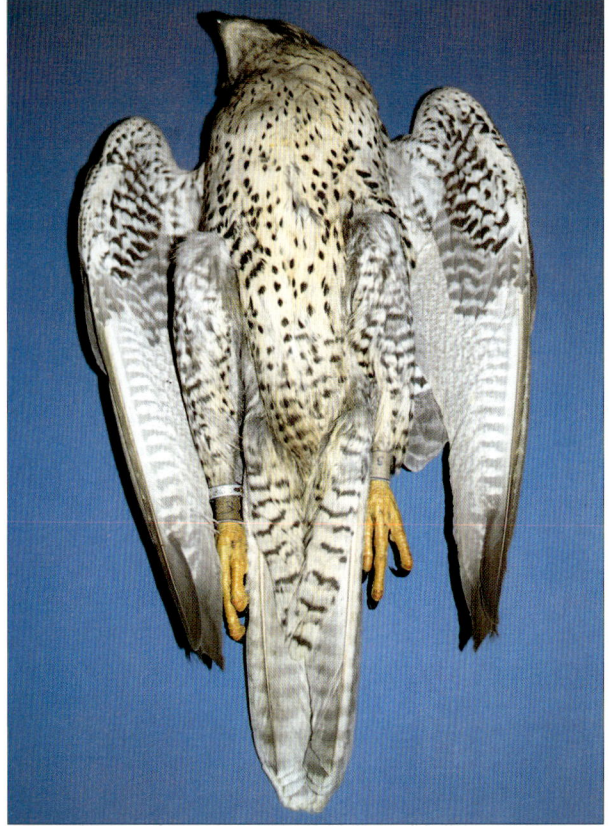

17.51

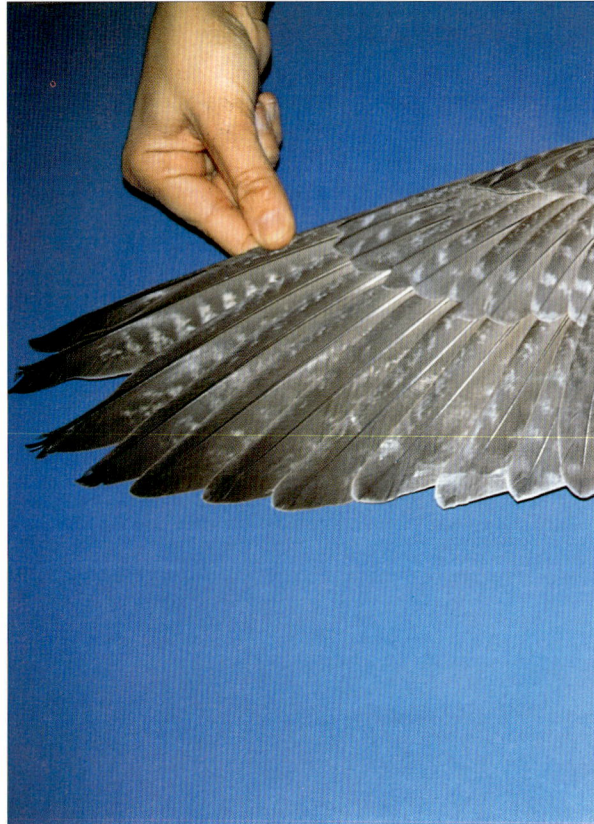

17.53

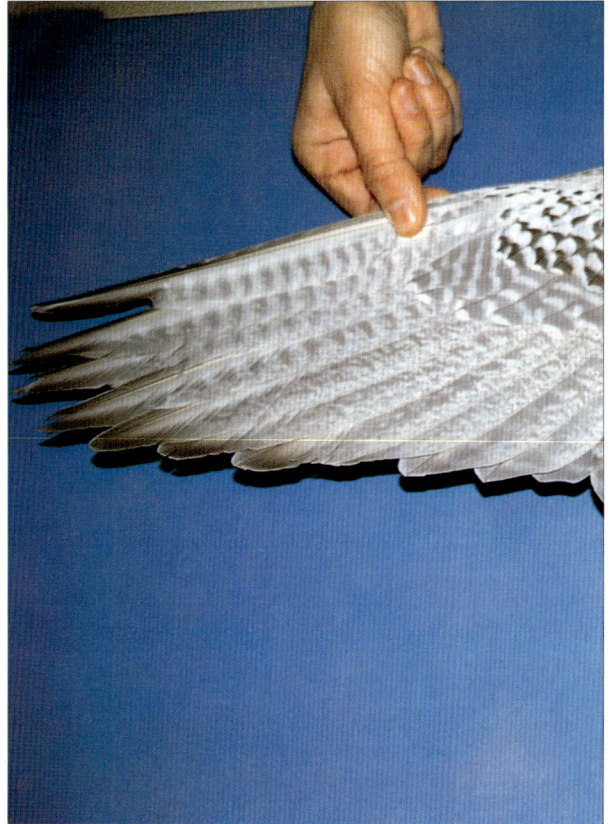

17.54

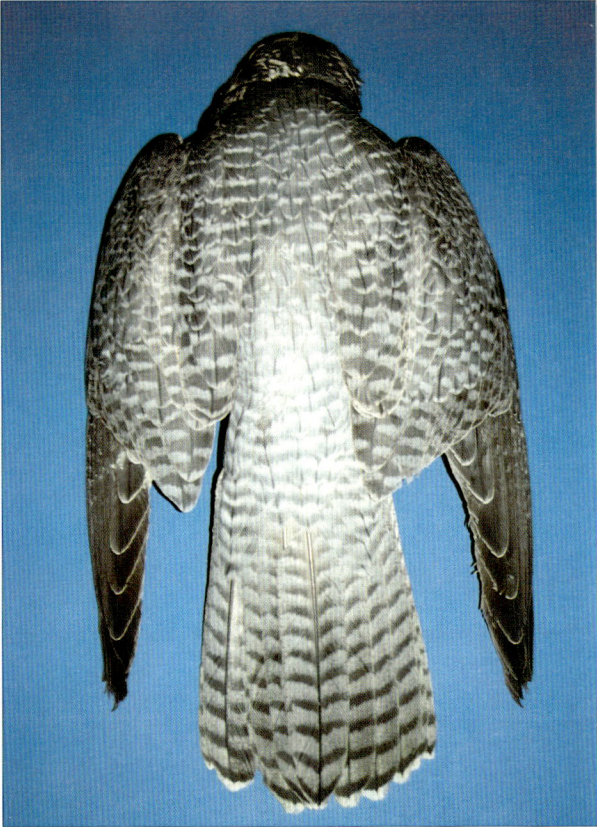

17.52

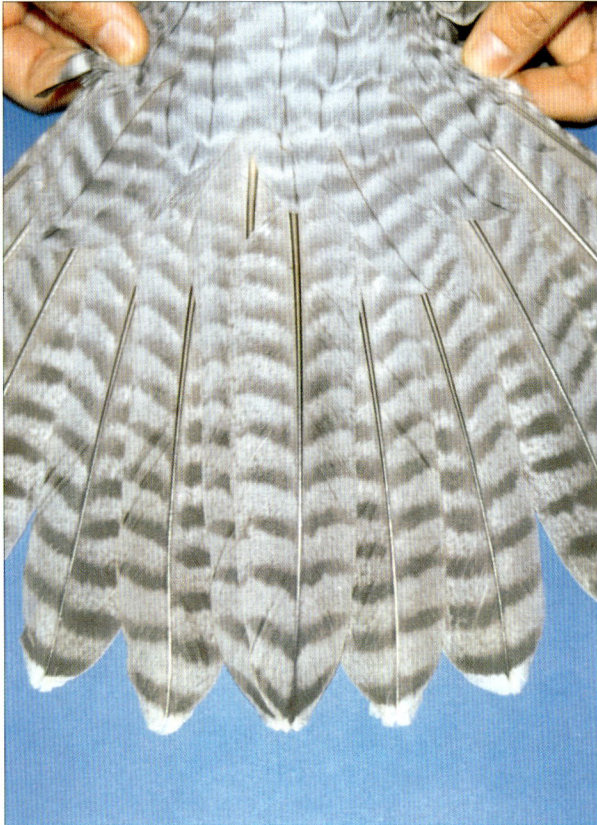

17.55

Figs. 17.50, 17.51, 17.52, 17.53, 17.54 and 17.55:
Great care must be used in photographically document-
ing a bird for identification in a court of law. Besides
depicting the various body parts and plumage as shown,
the bird's weight and length measurements should be
recorded. This series of photos depicts a pure gray
gyrfalcon tiercel (*F. rusticolus*).
(Photos: Heidenreich)

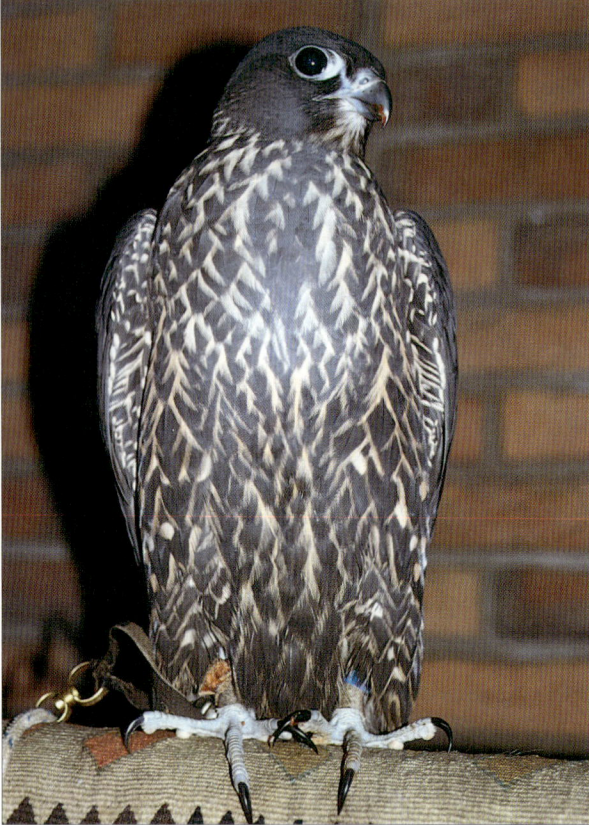

17.57

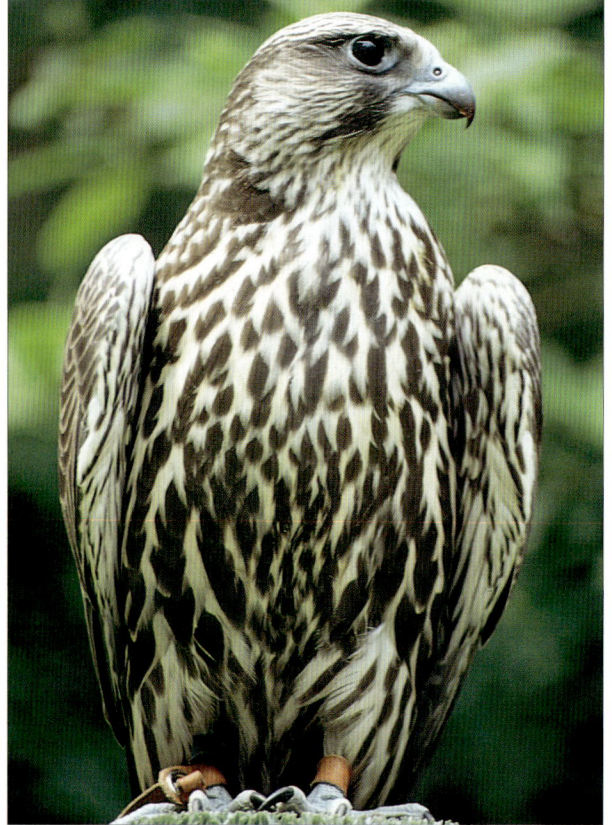

17.58

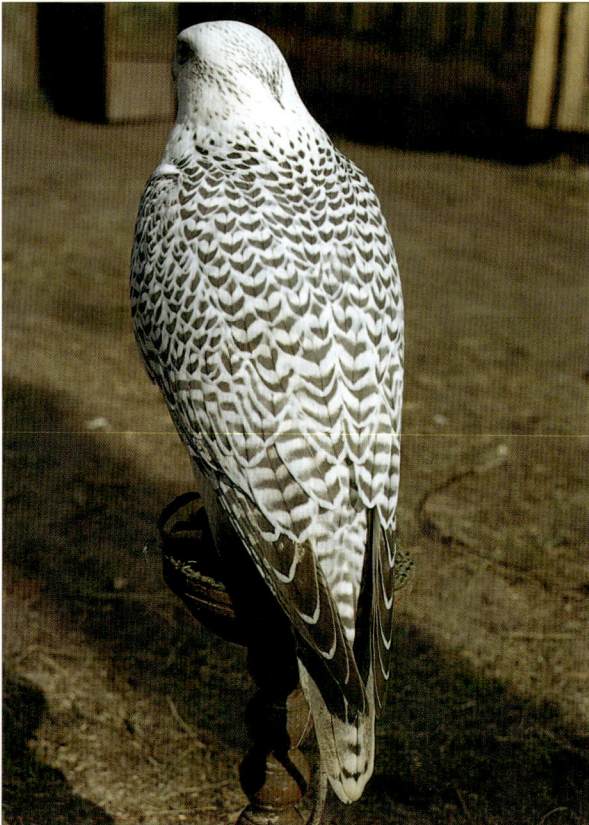

17.60

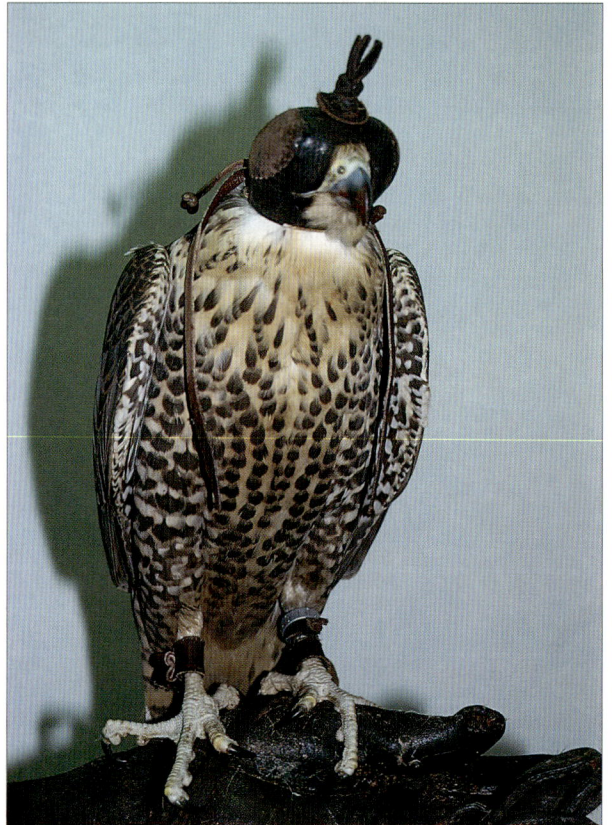

17.61

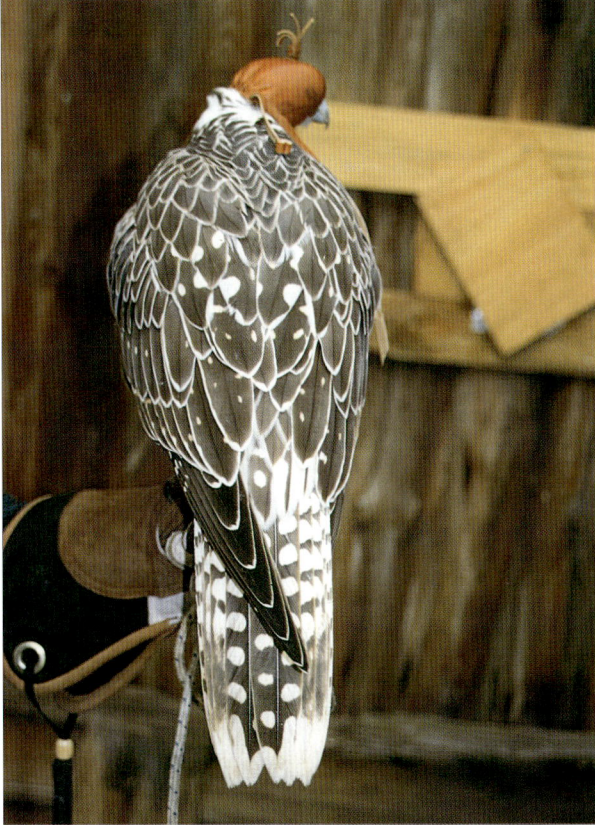

17.59

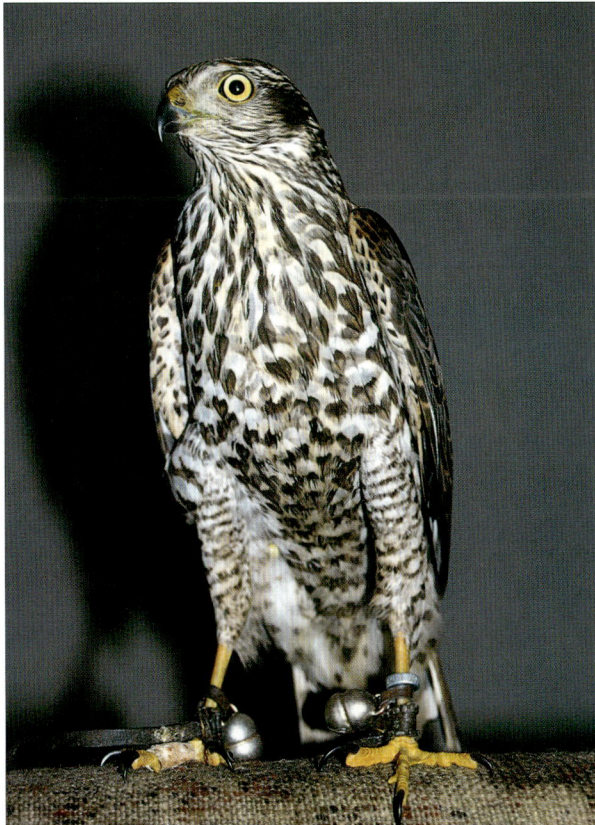

17.62

Figs. 17.57, 17.58, 17.59, 17.60, 17.61 and 17.62: A juvenile dark peregrine X gyrfalcon hybrid (17.57), juvenile saker X gyrfalcon (17.58), light juvenile $^3/_4$ saker X gyrfalcon [saker falcon X (saker X gyrfalcon)] (17.59), an adult white $^3/_4$ gyrfalcon X saker [(saker X gyrfalcon) X gyrfalcon] (17.60) which can not be visually distinguished from a pure gyrfalcon, an adult peregrine X laggar falcon (17.61), juvenile European sparrowhawk X northern goshawk (17.62).
(Photos: Heidenreich)

joining wild saker populations. This could indeed interfere with the purity of the wild population.

One possible approach to dealing with this problem would involve sterilizing such birds before selling them (see sterilization of female falcons and tiercels, Ch. 13.7.3).

The exact identification of raptor hybrids based only on phenotypic characteristics is difficult, and occasionally impossible, even for experts. The appearance of these birds varies so much that the best one can usually do is indicate a presumptive species origin. The hybrid types shown in Figs. 17.57–17.62 (pages 252–253) should therefore not be taken as rigid guides to hybrid raptor identification. They merely give an overall impression of the variety of phenotypes encountered among these birds.

Hybrid identification (saker falcon X gyrfalcon or lanner falcon)
The tail banding pattern can be useful in identifying the offspring of saker falcons and gyrfalcons or lanner falcons. Many saker falcons have a characteristic, so-called "eye" pattern on the feathers of the tail (see Fig. 17.47, page 248). In any case, they never show the definite straight bands seen in other species.

Hybrid saker offspring tend to inherit the straight banding pattern of the other parent, and rarely retain the saker "eye" pattern (Figs. 17.63–17.65, page 255).

Nevertheless, hybrids inside this hierofalcon group are very difficult or impossible to identify definitively, especially if they are multiple generation hybrids.

Hybrid identification (hierofalcon X peregrine falcon)
As discussed in Chapter 13, peregrine falcons differ from the hierofalcon group in the relative lengths of their primary flight feathers. Hierofalcons have the pattern **9 > 8 > 10 > 7**. In peregrines, the relationship is **9 > 10 > 8 > 7** (Dementiew, 1960).

Some hybrids of these two falcon types will have feathers that conform to the peregrine pattern, making the wings appear more pointed, even though the bird may otherwise look more like a hierofalcon. Others may have the hierofalcon pattern of primary feathers, but look more like peregrines (Figs. 17.66–17.68).

Juvenile hybrids in this group always have the same bluish-gray feet and legs seen in young hierofalcons as well. Presumably this is inherited as a dominant trait. Purebred peregrines have yellowish legs, even as youngsters. The only exception is *Falco peregrinus pealei,* whose legs are also blue as juveniles.

17.3.3   Egg shell identification

During inspections of raptor breeding facilities in one case, the authorities were presented with egg shells from which certain young birds in question were supposed to have hatched. This ruse was intended to fool the inspectors into believing that the birds had been captive-bred at that facility.

In another case, eggs that had supposedly been laid by a captive lanner falcon were sold to an egg collector. The eggs, however, appeared to be gyrfalcon eggs.

Since the eggs of large falcons are all very similar in size, color and appearance, such claims have been difficult to refute. In the hope of finding a method of distinguishing such eggs to the level of species, it was theorized that falcon eggs should differ in structure at the microscopic level. This theory was based on the fact that fertile eggs from northern falcons differ from Central European and Mediterranean species in the humidity levels required for incubation. Gyrfalcon eggs need lower humidity levels and therefore probably have a dense shell with few pores. Lanner and saker falcons, on the other hand, need a more porous shell to achieve the evaporation rates of at least 15% required for hatching.

Hussong (1995) examined this problem as part of his dissertation. By examining the shells of the various types of eggs under an electron microscope, he was able to identify clear structural differences between the species. At that level of magnification, the egg shells of saker, lanner, peregrine and gyrfalcons can easily be differentiated from each other and from those of other species (Figs. 17.69–17.72, page 256).

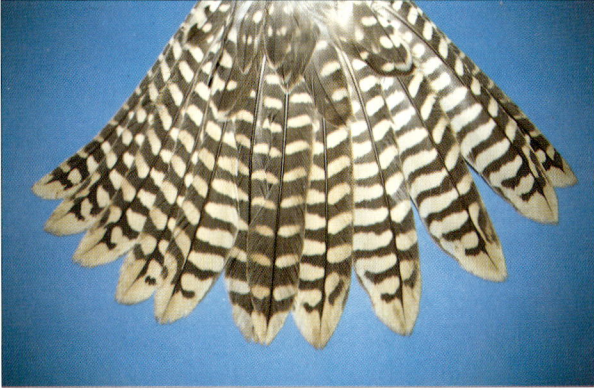

17.63

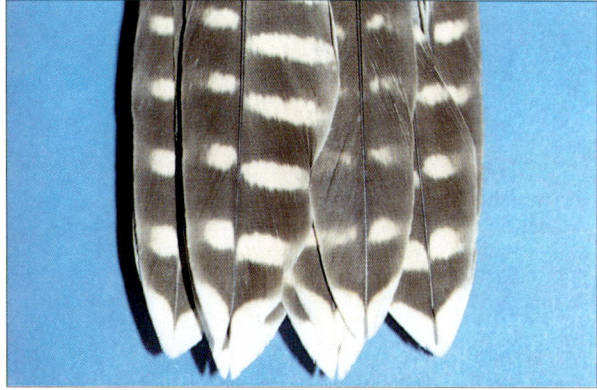

17.64

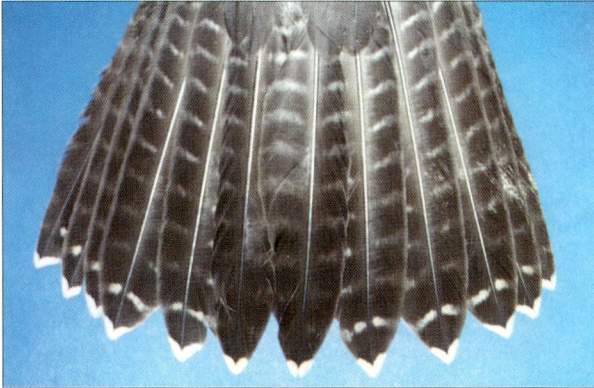

17.65

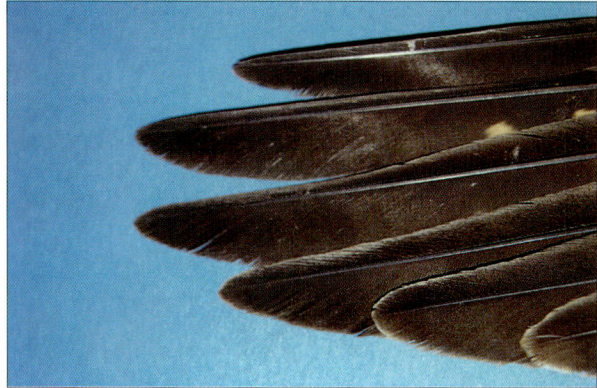

17.66

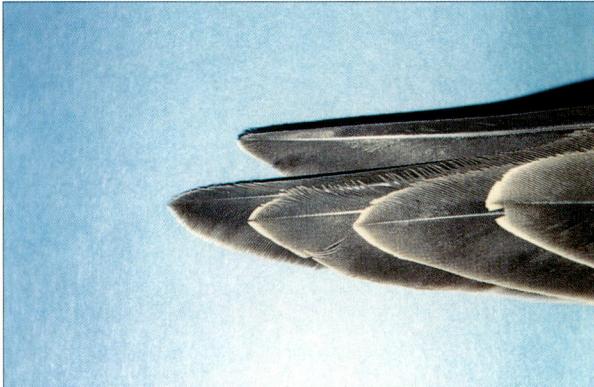

17.67

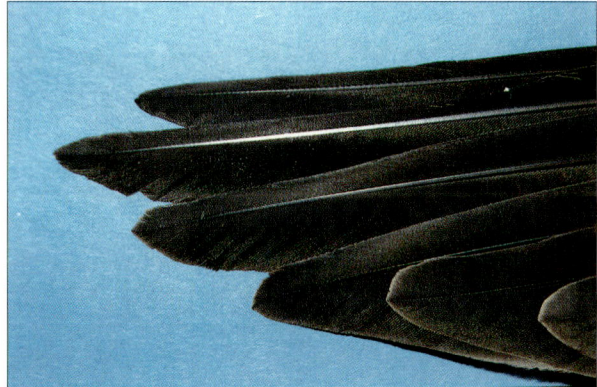

17.68

Figs. 17.63, 17.64, and 17.65: Tail feathers of a juvenile saker X gyrfalcon hybrid (17.63), a saker X lanner falcon hybrid (17.64) and a saker X peregrine falcon hybrid (17.65). The pattern seen in Fig. 17.65 is very similar to that seen in some gray gyrfalcon crosses.
(Photos: Heidenreich)

Figs. 17.66, 17.67 and 17.68: The relative lengths of primary feathers in a saker falcon (17.66) are representative of the hierofalcon group in general. The primaries from a peregrine falcon (17.67) and a peregrine X gyrfalcon hybrid (17.68). The latter has the peregrine configuration.
(Photos: Heidenreich)

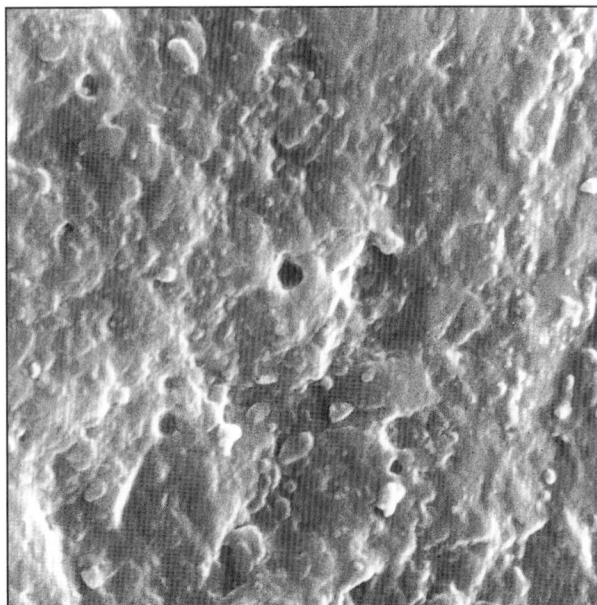

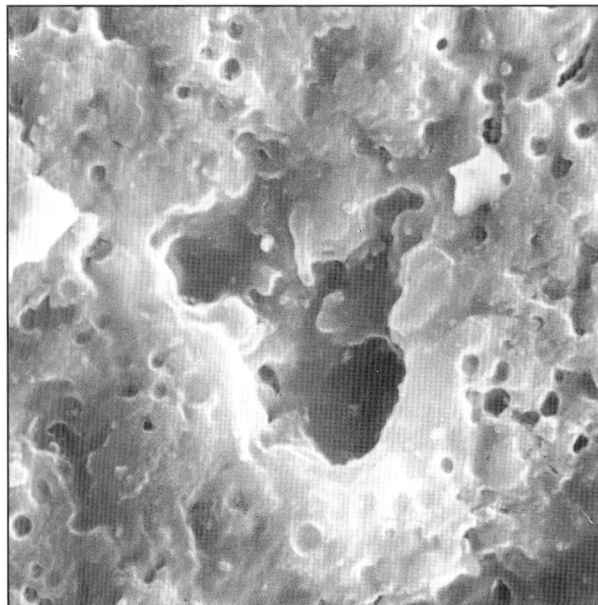

△ 17.69   17.70 ▽   △ 17.71   17.72 ▽

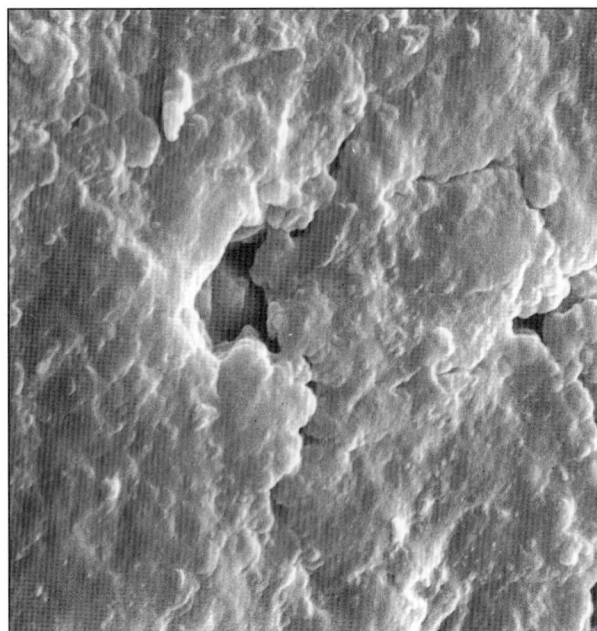

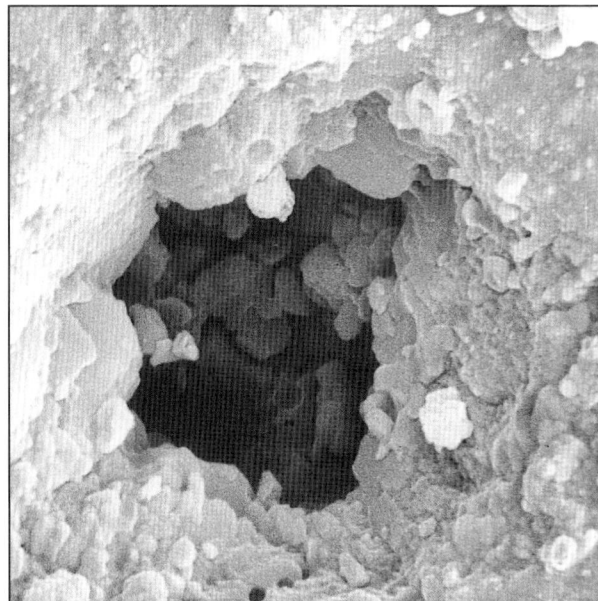

Figs. 17.69, 17.70, 17.71 and 17.72: Peregrine falcon eggs have a relatively dense, compact shell with many small pores (17.69, enlarged 6000X).
Gyrfalcon egg shells are also dense, but tend to be coarser and have larger pores than peregrine shells (17.70, enlarged 5000X).
The shells of lanner falcon eggs are even coarser and more porous (17.71, enlarged 5000X).
Saker falcon eggs have the largest pores and most loosely constructed shell of all (17.72, enlarged 5000X).
(Photos: Hussong)

References and literature of further interest

BAUMGART, W. (1971):
Beitrag zur Kenntnis der Greifvögel Bulgariens.
Beitr. Vogelkd. **17**, 33–70

BAUMGART, W. (1975):
Die Bedeutung funktioneller Kriterien für die Beurteilung der taxonomischen Stellung paläarktischer Großfalken.
Jb. Dtsch. Falkenorden, 68–77

BEDNAREK, W. (1991):
Zuchtbericht 1991
Jb. Dtsch. Falkenorden, 18–21

BOYD, L.L. and N. BOYD (1975):
Hybrid Falcons.
Hawk Chalk **14**, 53–54

BRÜNING, H. (1995):
personal communication

BUNNELL, S. (1986):
Hybrid Falcon Overview - 1985.
Hawk Chalk **25**, 43–47

CADE, T. (1974):
Plans for Managing the Survival of the Peregrine Falcon.
Raptor Res. Report **2**, 89–104

CADE, T. (1987):
Wiederansiedelung als eine Methode des Naturschutzes.
Jb. Dtsch. Falkenorden, 35–45

CADE, T. (1988):
Vermehrung von Taggreifvögeln In Gefangenschaft.
Jb. Dtsch. Falkenorden, 17–31

CADE, T. and J.D. WEAVER (1976):
Gyrfalcon X Peregrine Hybrids Produced by Artificial Insemination
J. North Amer. Falc. Assoc. **15**, 42–47

DEMENTIEW, G.P. (1960):
Der Gerfalke.
A. Ziemsen Verlag, Wittenberg Lutherstadt

DEMENTIEW, G.P. and A. SCHAGDASUREN (1965):
Über die mongolischen Würgfalken und die taxonomische Stellung des Altaigerfalken.
Samml. Arbeit Zoolog. Mus. Universität Moskau, **9**, 3–37

FISCHER, W. (1967):
Beobachtungen am Sakerfalken (*Falco cherrug*) in der Mongolei.
Beitr. Vogelkd. **12**, 420–428

HAAK, W. (1980):
Hybrid Falcons.
J. North Am. Falc. Assoc. **19**, 74–83

HARDASWICK, V.J. and D.S. SMITH (1981):
Peregrine X Prairie Hybrids.
North. Amer. Falc. Ass. 4–11

HEIDENREICH, M. and H. KÜSPERT (1992):
Métodos de la reproducción en cautividad de las diferentes especies de halcones. El problema de los híbridos y la cooperación entre criadores y autoridades.
Proc. Congr. Nac. Cria. Aves Cetrería **1**, 15–17

HEIDENREICH, M., KÜSPERT, H., KÜSPERT, H.J. and R. HUSSONG (1993):
Falkenhybriden. Deren Zucht, zum Verwandtschaftsgrad verschiedener Falkenarten, sowie zum Thema der Faunenverfälschung durch Hybridfalken.
Beitr. Vogelkd. **39**, 205–226

HUSSONG, R. (1995):
Speziesspezifische Eischalenmerkmale verschiedener Falken
Vet. Med. Diss., München (in Vorbereitung)

KALTENPOTH, H. and W. SCHULENBURG (1988):
Muli oder Maulesel?
Beitrag zur Morphologie der Spermatozoen der sog. Hybridfalken.
Jb. Dtsch. Falkenorden 36-37

KLEINSCHMIDT, O. (1901):
Der Formenkreis *Falco Hierofalco* und die Stellung des ungarischen Würgfalken in demselben.
Aquila **8**, 1–49

KNÖFERL, J. (1976):
Kreuzung zwischen Rotschwanz- und Mäusebussard.
Der Falkner **25/26**, 35

KÜSPERT, H. (1990):
personal communication

MORRIS, J. and R. STEVENS (1971):
Successful cross-breeding of a Peregrine Tiercel and a Saker Falcon.
Cap. Breed. Diurn. Birds of Prey **1** 5–7

MÜLLER, E. (1984 U. 1987):
personal communication

PÖLNITZ, V., N. (1995):
personal communication

PÖPPELMANN; B. (1994):
Hybridzucht: Sperber mal Habicht.
Tinnunculus **2**, 13

RAFUSE, B. (1986):
Directors Reports.
Hawk Chalk **24**, 26

RAFUSE, B. (1986a):
Directors Reports.
Hawk Chalk **25**, 9

ROSENKRANZ, D. (1981):
personal communication

SEIBOLD, I., HELBIG, A.J. and M. WINK (1993):
Molecular Systematics of Falcons (Family *Falconidae*)
Naturwissenschaften **80**, 87–90

SEIBOLD, I. (1994):
Untersuchungen zur molekularen Phylogenie der Greifvögel anhand von DNA-Sequenzen des mitochondriellen Cytochrom b-Gens.
Diss., Heidelberg, Hartung-Gorre Verlag, Konstanz

18 Legal issues regarding birds of prey

Legislation protecting birds of prey has been established in international agreements, the regulations of the European Union and in many western countries, as well as at federal and state levels.

The laws regarding birds of prey are intended to protect them and impose severe penalties on those who are caught in violation of the mandates. Anyone working with or owning such birds must therefore carefully observe the applicable regulations. The many articles and paragraphs that comprise this legislation are so diverse, far-reaching and open to interpretation in various ways, that it becomes almost impossible for a lay person to make sense of them. This chapter is intended to help clarify the situation, especially regarding the regulations in place on an international level.

The author is particularly grateful to State Councilor Anette Schmidt-Räntsch and Dr. habil. Rainer Blanke for reviewing this important chapter with regard to legal accuracy.

18.1 International agreements (CITES)

The international trade in endangered species is a profitable enterprise that threatens the survival of many species all over the world. The regulation of such trade, particularly as it pertains to species whose populations are at risk, is the goal of the **Convention on International Trade in Endangered Species of Wild Fauna and Flora** (**CITES**), dated March 3, 1973.

Regular conferences held by the member states of this agreement continue to improve, extend and modify the set of regulations codified by the treaty. Further recommendations are issued at such meetings in the form of resolutions. While the treaty's text is binding for all member-states, the legal basis of the subsequent resolutions is not absolutely clear. Nevertheless, according to Emonds (1986), in practice they must be observed.

The CITES agreement depends on trade prohibitions, the requirement of special permits for those who trade in endangered species and the development of common permit requirements to carry out its regulations. For this purpose, all species of wild animals

have been listed in three appendices according to the degree of their endangerment in the wild. The following criteria for ranking were agreed upon at the 9th meeting of the Conference of Member States held November 7 to 18, 1994 in Fort Lauderdale, Florida, USA. (Conf. 9.24):

Appendix I contains all species threatened with extinction whose survival is, or could be, impaired by trade.

A. The survival of a species could or would be impaired by trade if:

1. it is known to be traded commercially, or
2. it is probably being traded commercially, although no clear evidence therefore is available, or
3. a potential international demand exists for specimens of this species, or
4. it would likely be traded in the absence of controls established by the framework described in Appendix I.

B. Additionally, there are certain biological criteria that apply to all species listed in Appendix I, or those that could be added to it. A species can be regarded as threatened by extinction if it meets, or is likely to meet, at least one of the following criteria:

1. The wild population is small and exhibits at least one of the following traits:
   a) an already observed, foreseeable or expected decline in the number of individuals, or the size and quality of their habitat; or
   b) every existing subpopulation consists of a very small number of individuals; or
   c) during one or more of their life stages, the majority of individuals are concentrated in a specific subpopulation, or
   d) the number of individuals is prone to strong short-term fluctuations, or
   e) high vulnerability as a consequence of the biology or behavior of the species (including migration)
2. The wild population has a limited area of distribution and exhibits at least one of the following traits:

a) fragmentation or incidence at very few sites; or

b) large fluctuations in the area of distribution or the number of subpopulations; or

c) high vulnerability as a consequence of the biology or the behavior of the species; or

d) an already existing, beginning or expected decline in one of the following factors: area of distribution, number of subpopulations, number of individuals, area, extent or quality of the habitat, or reproductive potential.

3. There is a decline in the number of individuals living in the wild, that is either

a) in progress or has occurred in the past (and could potentially occur again); or

b) has shown initial signs of occurring or is to be expected based on the following conditions:
   – a decrease in the size or quality of the natural habitat; or
   – the manner and intensity of utilization; or
   – external threats, e.g. the introduction of potential pathogens, competing organisms, parasites, predators, hybridization, introduced species or the effects of harmful substances and toxins; or
   – a reduced reproductive potential.

4. The status of the respective species is such that, unless it is added to Appendix I, one or more of the above criteria are likely to apply within the next five years.

Appendix II includes less threatened species for which careful management is required to ensure sustainable trade. A species would be listed in this Appendix when it meets one of the following criteria:

A. It is known, becoming apparent or to be expected that, without stricter regulations, trade in this species will soon cause it to meet at least one the criteria listed in Appendix I.

B. It is known, becoming apparent, or to be expected that the removal of wild specimens belonging to that species for purposes of international trade has, or could have, a negative impact on that particular species, in so far as either

1. a sustainable rate of removal will be exceeded over an extended period of time; or

2. the population is thereby reduced to the extent that its survival could be endangered by other factors.

Also included in Appendix II are species which resemble another species from Appendix II or Appendix I so closely that they can not be easily distinguished by a lay person.

Appendix III includes species regulated by independent legislation within one of the convention states, but for which international trade is not sufficiently controlled in this manner, making additional CITES regulation necessary.

The CITES treaty requires special permits for trade with specimens of protected animal species. The exact identification and scientific classification of the animals involved is therefore very important. While birds of prey are usually relatively easily identified, there are some cases where the scientific designation is uncertain. CITES member states therefore agreed to standardize the classification. The publication listed below has been designated the standard for use in classifying birds (class Aves) for this purpose:

Sibley, C. G. and B. L. Monroe (1990): *Distribution and Taxonomy of Birds of the World.* New Haven & London.

The classification of hybrids can become difficult if the parent animals are not listed in the same appendix, e.g., Peregrine Falcon (Appendix I) X Saker Falcon (Appendix II). Resolution 2.13 was created to resolve this problem: hybrids of this kind are classified according to the parent possessing the higher protective status. All gyr- or peregrine falcon hybrids, for example, are listed automatically in Appendix I.

The concept of a "specimen" covers not only living and dead birds of prey, but also any readily identifiable parts or artifacts made from them, including pelts, feathers and eggs!

Table 18.1 lists the raptor species protected by CITES according to their classification in the appendices.

The regulation of commerce
The following regulations are established by **Article III** of the CITES agreement for international commerce in the wild birds of prey listed in Appendix I:

*(2) The **export** of a specimen of a species listed in Appendix I requires the advance issue and presentation of an export permit. An export permit is granted only if the following conditions are met:*

a) a scientific authority from the exporting country has certified that this export will not endanger the survival of the species.

b) the responsible authorities from the exporting country have verified that the specimen was not acquired in violation of the regulations established by that country to protect its animal and plant life.

c) the responsible authorities from the exporting country have assured themselves that each living specimen has been prepared for transport and shipped in such a way that the risks of injury, illness or cruelty are eliminated to the greatest extent possible.

d) the responsible authorities from the exporting country have verified that an import permit has been issued for this specimen by the country of destination.

*(3) The **import** of a specimen from a species listed in Appendix I requires the advance issue and presentation of an import permit and either an export permit or a re-exportation certificate. An import permit is granted only if the following conditions are met:*
(a) a scientific authority from the importing country has certified that the intended purpose of the import will not endanger the survival of the species.
b) a scientific authority of the importing country has verified that, in the case of a living specimen, the recipient has available appropriate facilities for its housing and care, and
c) the responsible authorities of the importing country have verified that the specimen will not be used primarily for commercial purposes.

These strict regulations have led to the almost complete disappearance of legal commerce with the wild raptor species listed in Appendix I.

Birds of prey listed in Appendix II, which make up the majority, can in principle be traded without defining the objective of the importation. Free trade is permitted, the only condition being the presentation of an export permit from the country of origin.

All statements made so far concern only birds of prey obtained from the wild. Significantly fewer restrictions are imposed on birds bred in captivity. Article VII, Paragraph 4 of CITES states that:
Specimens of an animal species listed in Appendix I that have been captive bred for purposes of trade ... are considered as specimens of Appendix II species.

Consequently, they can be commercially traded using the same documentation required for wild specimens listed in Appendix II of CITES. Only an export permit from the country of origin is required (Res. 2.12).

No export and import permits are required for trade in captive bred animals from Appendix II. According to Article VII, Paragraph 5, a breeding certificate is sufficient (CITES-Certificate).

According to Schmidt-Räntsch and Schmidt-Räntsch (1990), this relaxation of trading restrictions for animals bred in captivity presents some incentive for misuse. It is therefore important in writing these permits to establish a functional definition of captive breeding.

The text of the CITES treaty itself does not define the concept of captive breeding, but resolutions 2.12. (Costa Rica) and 4.15. (Gabarone) later addressed this issue. They establish that captive bred specimens are only those which come from a breeding facility that is reliably able to produce second generation offspring (F_2 generation). This does not necessarily mean that

Table 18.1: Birds-of-prey listed in the CITES appendices

Appendix I	Appendix II	Appendix III
Cathartidae California condor (*Gymnogyps californianus*) Andean condor (*Vultur gryphus*) ***Accipitridae*** Western imperial eagle (*Aquila (heliaca adalberti)*) Eastern imperial eagle (*Aquila heliaca*) Wilson's hook-billed kite (*Chondrohierax uncinatus wilsonii*) White-tailed sea eagle (*Haliaeetus albicilla*) Bald eagle (*Haliaeetus leucocephalus*) Harpy eagle (*Harpia harpyja*) Philippine monkey-eating eagle (*Pithecophaga jefferyi*) ***Falconidae*** Seychelles kestrel (*Falco araea*) Laggar falcon (*Falco jugger*) Aldabra kestrel (*Falco newtoni aldabranus*) Barbary falcon (*Falco p. pelegrinoides* and *babylonicus*) Peregrine falcon (*Falco peregrinus*) Mauritius kestrel (*Falco punctatus*) Gyrfalcon (*Falco rusticolus*)	all *Falconiformes* except the New World vultures (*Cathartidae*)	King vulture (*Sarcoramphus papa*) Honduras

the specimen itself must be from the F_2 or later generations (Emonds, 1986).

In the case of birds listed in Appendix I, these so-called "commercial breeding facilities" in member states must be reported to and certified by the CITES Secretariat.

The rules discussed above do not apply to species listed in Appendix II. They need only have been bred in captivity.

Permits and certificates
Permits and certificates for trade must conform to the requirements established in **Article VI**:

2) An export permit must contain all the information specified in the example given in Appendix IV. It must be used for export within six months of the date of issue.

3) Every permit or certificate must include the title of this treaty (CITES, author's note)*, the name and stamp of the issuing authority, and an assigned control number.*

4) Copies of permits or certificates issued by the responsible authorities must be clearly identified as such and cannot be used in place of the originals – except to the extent specified in the document itself.

5) A separate permit or certificate is required for each shipment of specimens.

6) The responsible authority of the receiving country must invalidate and retain the export permit or re-importation certificate as well as the import permit presented upon arrival of a specimen.

7) To the extent practicable and possible, the responsible authority may mark a specimen for identification. A "marking" in this context means an indelible imprint, a band or some other form of identification not easily amenable to unauthorized duplication.

The text of the CITES treaty is binding for all member states and must be integrated into their respective legislation. According to **Article XIV**, each country is free to issue more stringent regulations to govern the trade, receivership, ownership or transport of specimens of the species listed in the Appendices. Many countries in the European Union have exercised this option.

18.2   European law

EWG Decree Nr. 3626/82 of December 3, 1982, which went into effect on January 1, 1984, embodies the CITES regulations within the European Union. In addition, **EWG Decree Nr. 3418/83**, the so-called form decree, is also in effect for all EU states. Both were created with the intention of uniformly establishing the CITES regulations for all EU member states, including those which have not yet joined the CITES agreement (Ireland).

<u>Applications</u>
According to **Article 2**, this decree applies to the following specimens:

(a) any living or dead animal ... belonging to a species listed in Appendix I of the CITES agreement, or parts or products derived from such animals, listed in Appendix B of this decree, as well as any other product for which there is evidence in the packaging, the brand name, the labeling or some other circumstance, that it may contain parts or products made of animals ... belonging to these species;

(b) any living or dead animal ... belonging to a species listed in Appendices II or III of the CITES agreement, or parts and products derived from such animals, listed in Appendix B of this decree, as well as any other product for which there is evidence in the packaging, the brand name, the labeling or some other circumstance, that it may contain parts or products made from animals ... belonging to these species, with the exception of those parts or products which the regulations of the agreement exempt based on specific references laid out in Appendices II and III of CITES.

<u>Category of protection for birds of prey</u>
EWG Decree Nr. 3626/82 lists all birds of prey from Appendices I and II of CITES in its own Appendix C, Part I. **Article 3** of this decree establishes the following regulations:

(1) Specimens listed in Appendix C, Part I are to be treated like specimens of species listed in Appendix I of CITES.

This means that all raptors except the five New World vulture species not listed in CITES are considered equal and subject to the legal requirements imposed on species in Appendix I of CITES.

Trade within the European Community
Commerce among members of the European Community requires documents as prescribed by Article 29 of EWG Decree Nr. 3418/83 (Nr. 262, color blue), even for captive-bred specimens. This must include CITES documentation which attests to the specimen's breeding.

Trade with countries outside the European Community
Commerce with countries outside the European Community is regulated by **Article 5** and establishes the following:

(1) During the import of specimens into the European Community as described in Articles 2 and 3, an import permit or an import certificate as required by Article 10 (order Nr. 261, color gray) must be presented to the customs office.

(2) During the export or re-export of specimens from the European Community as described in Article 2, a document as required by Article 10, paragraph 3 (order Nr. 261, color gray) must be presented to the customs office.

(3) The customs officials receiving the permits must send them on to the responsible authorities of the member state under whose authority they operate.

Restrictions and exceptions
Article 6 regulates commercial uses. It expressly forbids the display of raptors for commercial purposes in amusement parks, falconry centers, etc., as well as their sale, housing prior to sale, offering for sale or promotion of sale. Exceptions are possible in EU member states only under the following conditions:

(a) The specimens were obtained under treaty regulations and brought into the territories which are subject to this decree before it went into effect (prior ownership).

(b) the specimens of a species were bred in captivity ... or the specimens are parts of such animals ... or were made from such animals;

(c) the specimens are intended for purposes of <u>research, teaching, or breeding</u>;

(d) the specimens originated in a member state and have been taken from the wild in accordance with the laws or by permission of the authorities of that member state (legal removal from the wild);

(e) the specimens were obtained under treaty regulations and brought into the territories subject to this decree after it went into effect and are <u>not</u> intended for mainly <u>commercial purposes</u>.

Certification
Article 11 empowers the relevant authorities to hand out the required certifications upon request:

(a) certification that a certain specimen was brought into the territories for which the decree is valid prior to its taking effect, but in accordance with treaty regulations, or that it was obtained before the treaty applied to this species (prior ownership);

(b) certification that a certain specimen of a species was born <u>and</u> bred in captivity or ... that a specimen is part of such an animal ... or was made from such an animal.

EWG Decree Nr. 3626/82 extensively regulates trade in protected species. **Article 15** gives member states of the European Union the right to establish further controls. Some countries, including Germany, have taken advantage of this opportunity. The details of the legislation protecting birds of prey in each individual country are not covered here. Nevertheless, they are important and should be familiar to anyone dealing with or owning raptors in these states.

References and literature of further interest

BLANKE, R. (1989):
Grenzüberschreitender Greifvogelhandel in der Bundesrepublik Deutschland.
Greifvögel und Falknerei, 25–29
Verlag Neumann-Neudamm, Morschen-Heina

EMONDS, G. (1986):
CITES-Bescheinigungen und Greifvogelhandel.
NuR **4**, 141–144

HAMMER, W. (1988):
Nochmals: Internationales und nationales Artenschutzrecht.
Mzschr. Dtsch. Recht **42**, 907–908

HAMMER, W., HEIDENREICH, M., KÖSTERS, J. and G. TROMMER (1988):
Empfehlungen zur tierschutzgerechten Haltung von Greifvögeln und Eulen.
Tierärztliche Praxis **17**, 59–70

SCHMIDT-RÄNTSCH, A. and J. SCHMIDT-RÄNTSCH (1990):
Leitfaden zum Artenschutzrecht.
Bundesanzeiger-Verlag, Köln

19 Additional references

AL GITRIF (1988):
Die Beizvögel.
Georg Olms Verlag, Hildesheim, Zürich, New York

ALLEN, M. (1980):
Falconry in Arabia.
Orbis Publishing, London

AL-NAHAYAN, ZAID BIN SULTAN (1976):
Falconry as a sport. Our arab heritage. Abu Dhabi 1976–1396
Westerham Press Ltd., Westerham, Kent, England

AL-TIMIMI, F.A. (1987):
Falcons and falconry in Qatar.
Ali Bin Ali Printing Press, Qatar

BAUMGART, W. (1991):
Der Sakerfalke.
A. Ziemsen Verlag, Wittenberg Lutherstadt

BEEBE, F.L. (1992):
The compleat falconer.
Hancock House Publishers, Blaine, WA, USA

BEEBE, F.L. (1992):
A falconry manual.
Hancock House Publishers, Blaine, WA, USA

BROWN, A.F. (1988):
Kunstbrut. Handbuch für Züchter.
Verlag M.+H. Schaper

BROWN, L. and D. AMADON (1968):
Eagles, hawks and falcons of the world.
Country Life Books, Hamlyn House, Feltham, Middlesex, England

BRÜLL, H. (1962):
Die Beizjagd.
Verlag Paul Parey, Hamburg

CHAMBERLAT, DE, C.A. (1987):
Falconry and art.
Philip Wilson Publishers, London

CHANCELLOR, R.D. and B.-U. MEYBURG (1986, 1991):
Birds of prey. Bulletins Nrr.: 3 und 4
World Working Group on Birds of Prey, Berlin, London, Paris

COOPER, J.E. (1978):
Veterinary aspects of captive birds of prey.
Standfast Press, Saul, Gloucestershire

COX, J. (1985):
Observations on falconry in Pakistan.
Pilot Publishing, Karachi, Pakistan

D'ARCUSSIA, CH. (1980):
Falconaria
Fourier Verlag, Wiesbaden

DEMENTIEW, G.P. (1960):
Der Gerfalke.
A. Ziemsen Verlag, Wittenberg Lutherstadt

ECKERT, J., KUTZER, E., ROMMEL, M., BÜRGER, H-J. and W. KÖRTING (1992):
Veterinärmedizinische Parasitologie
4. Auflage, Verlag Paul Parey, Berlin und Hamburg

FISCHER, W. (1976):
Stein-, Kaffern- und Keilschwanzadler.
A. Ziemsen Verlag, Wittenberg Lutherstadt

FISCHER, W. (1977):
Der Wanderfalke.
A. Ziemsen Verlag, Wittenberg Lutherstadt

FISCHER, W. (1980):
Die Habichte.
A. Ziemsen Verlag, Wittenberg Lutherstadt

FIUCYNSKI, D. (1987):
Der Baumfalke.
A. Ziemsen Verlag, Wittenberg Lutherstadt

FUENTE, F. R. DE LA (1986):
El arte de cetrería.
Librería Noriega, México

GABRISCH, K. and P. ZWART (1987):
Krankheiten der Wildtiere.
Schlütersche Verlagsanstalt und Druckerei, Hannover

GLASIER, P. (1991):
Falconry and hawking.
Batsford Ltd., London

GÖLTHENBOTH, R. and H.G. KLÖS (1995):
Krankheiten der Zoo- und Wildtiere.
Blackwell Wissenschafts-Verlag, Berlin

GRANDE, J.L.G. and F. HIRALDO (1987):
Las rapaces ibéricas.
Centro de Fotografía de la Naturaleza, Madrid

GYLSTORFF, I. and F. GRIMM (1987):
Vogelkrankheiten
Verlag Eugen Ulmer, Suttgart

HAAK, B.A. (1992):
The hunting falcon.
Hancock House Publishers, Blaine, WA, USA

HARTING, J.E. (1989):
Hints on the management of hawks and practical falconry.
Nimrod Press, Alton, Hampshire, England

HEIDENREICH, M. (1982):
Diseases of parrots.
T.F.H. Publications, Neptune, USA

HENTSCHEL, P. (1980):
Beizvogelkrankheiten, Vorbeuge und
Behandlung.
Jagdinformationen 1–2
Institut für Forstwissenschaften, Eberswalde

HOHENSTAUFEN, F. II. V. (1240):
De arte venandi cum avibus.
Nachdruck 1964: Insel Verlag, Frankfurt/M.

HOLLINSHEAD, M. (1993):
Hawking ground quarry.
Hancock House Publishers, Blaine, WA, USA

KRONBERGER, H. (1978):
Haltung von Vögeln, Krankheiten der Vögel.
Gustav Fischer Verlag, Jena

LASCELLES, G. (1892):
Falconry
in: Coursing and Falconry.
Ashford Press Publishing, Shedfield, Hampshire

LINK, H. (1986):
Untersuchungen am Habicht (*Accipiter gentilis*).
Verlag Dtsch. Falkenorden

MAVROGORDATO, J. (1982):
Behind the scenes.
Element Books Ltd., Salisbury, Wiltshire, England

MAVROGORDATO, J. (1985):
A hawk for the bush.
C.W. Daniel Ltd., Saffron Walden, Essex, England

MICHELL, E.B. (1988):
Introducing falconry.
Nimrod Press Ltd., Alton, Hants, England

ORTLIEB, R. (1979):
Die Sperber.
A. Ziemsen Verlag, Wittenberg Lutherstadt

ORTLIEB, R. (1989):
Der Rotmilan.
A. Ziemsen Verlag, Wittenberg Lutherstadt

PARRY-JONES, J. (1993):
Falconry, care, captive breeding and conservation.
David and Charles, Devon

PETRAK, M.L. (1988):
Diagnostik und Chirurgie beim Ziervogel.
Ferdinand Enke Verlag, Stuttgart

PIECHOCKI, R. (1991):
Der Turmfalke.
A. Ziemsen Verlag, Wittenberg Lutherstadt

REDIG, P.T., COOPER, J.E., REMPLE, J.D. and D.B. HUNTER
(1993):
Raptor Biomedicine
Chiron Publications Ltd:, Keighley, West Yorkshire, England

REMPLE, D. and C. GROSS (1993):
Falconry and birds of prey in the gulf.
Motivate Publishing, Dubai

RICHTIE, B.W., HARRISON, G.J. and L.R. HARRISON (1994):
Avian medicine: principles and application.
Wingers Publishing, Lake Worth, Florida

SALVIN, F.H. and W. BRODRICK (1855):
Falconry in the British Isles.
John van Voorst, London, England

SAVAGE, C. (1993):
Falken.
Gerstenberg Verlag, Hildesheim

SCHMIDT-RÄNTSCH, A. and J. SCHMIDT-RÄNTSCH (1990):
Leitfaden zum Artenschutzrecht.
Bundesanzeiger Verlags-Gesellschaft, Köln

SCHÖNEBERG, H. (1994):
Falknerei. Der Leitfaden für die Falknerprüfung.
Eigenverlag, Ampermoching

SHERROD, S.K., HEINRICH, W.R., BURNHAM, W.A.,
BARCLAY, J.H. and T.J. CADE (1987):
Hacking: A method for releasing Peregrine Falcons and other
birds of prey.
The Peregrine Fund, USA

SIEGMANN, O. (1993):
Kompendium der Geflügelkrankheiten.
5. Auflage, Verlag Paul Parey Berlin und Hamburg

STEVENS, R. (1987):
Observations on modern falconry.
Pilot Publishing, England

TENNESEN, M. (1992):
Falken
Westermann Verlag, Braunschweig

UPTON, R. (1980):
A bird in the hand.
Debrett's Peerage Ltd., London, England

UPTON, R. (1987):
O for a falconer´s voice.
Crowood Press, Ramsbury, Marlborough, England

UPTON, R. (1990):
Falconry. Principles and practice.
A & C Black, London

VÖGELE, H.H. (1931):
Die Falknerei.
Verlag Neumann-Neudamm, Melsungen

WALLER, R. (1937):
Der wilde Falk ist mein Gesell.
Verlag Neumann-Neudamm

WEBSTER, H.M. and J.H. ENDERSON (1988):
Game hawking ... at its very best.
Windsong Press, Denver, CO, USA

WEICK, F. (1980):
Die Greifvögel der Welt
Verlag Paul Parey, Berlin und Hamburg

WOODFORD, M.H. (1987):
A manual of falconry.
A & C Black Ltd. London, England

ZAPATA, L. (1566):
Libro de cetrería.
Biblioteca Nacional de Madrid

20   Glossary of falconry terms

aylmeri
: leather anklets closed with grommets through which straps can be pulled to create jesses.

bating
: jumping or flying off the fist in response to some perceived threat.

bell
: a bell attached to the hawk's leg.

bewits
: short thin strips of leather used to fasten the bells to the hawk's legs.

block
: a cylindrical or cone-shaped piece of wood with a ring on it and a metal spike at the bottom. The hawk is often set on this type of perch outdoors to "weather" or while out in the field during hunting or training.

blood feathers
: developing feathers that still have a shaft filled with blood or pulp.

bow perch
: a perch generally used outdoors for accipiters and buteos and constructed in a ring or semi-circular shape.

cadge
: a rectangular wooden frame on which hawks are transported hooded.

call off
: to call or whistle to lure a bird off a perch or someone else's fist.

casting
: used as a noun, synonymous with pellet. Used as a verb, it denotes the act of regurgitating a pellet.

cast off
: to let the bird fly from the fist.

cere
: the waxy, featherless skin above the beak surrounding the nostrils.

coping
: cutting or filing the sharp or excessively long points off beak and talons

contour feathers
: the small feathers covering most of a bird's body.

covert feathers
: the small contour feathers found in rows on the wings and tail.

creance
: a long line attached to the hawk via the swivel and jesses. Typically used in training hawks which can not yet be trusted loose.

crop
: the dilatation of the esophagus that initially holds the food ingested by a bird.

eyas
: see under nestling.

eyrie
: the nesting place of a bird of prey.

falconry
: the art of hunting with birds of prey.

falconer
: one who practices the art of falconry. Often requires a period of training and a license in Western countries.

fledgling
: a young bird that has left the nest recently.

flight feathers
: the large, stiff feathers of the wings and tail that are required for flight.

footing
: to clutch or grasp with the talons and hold.

fret marks
: also called stress marks, these transparent lines that cross the vane of a feather are evidence of stress to the bird during feather growth.

full-summed	the state a bird is in when all new feathers are full length and no longer filled with pulp.
glove	also called a gauntlet. A leather covering for the falconer's fist on which the hawk sits.
hack	a state of liberty in which young hawks are allowed to live free and supplied with food for a few weeks in order to acquire flying skills before being trained. Also used as a method for reintroducing captive-bred eyasses back into the wild.
haggard	a hawk that has been captured from the wild after molting into its adult plumage
hallux	the first digit in a hawk's foot, it opposes the other three toes and permits grasping and perching.
hatchling	a recently hatched young bird.
hierofalcons	a grouping of phylogenetically similar falcons that includes gyrfalcons, saker falcons, lanner falcons and laggar falcons.
hood	used as a noun it refers to the leather cap used to cover hawks' eyes to tame them and calm them. used as a verb, hooding refers to the placement of the hood over the bird's head.
imping	a method of repairing broken flight or tail feathers in which a new feather is attached to the base of the bird's own by means of a small pin and some glue.
jesses	the short narrow leather straps that are fastened to the legs of a hawk.

leash	a narrow cord attached to the jesses and used for tying a bird to the perch or block.
lure	also called a drawer. A weighted quarry-like object tied to the end of a line and garnished with a piece of meat. It is swung aloft in training or to lure the hawk back to the falconer.
manning	also called training or reclaiming. Taming a hawk so that it is accustomed to man's presence.
mail	a hawk's breast feathers.
mantle	to spread the wings over the food to hide it while eating, seen mostly in young birds.
mews	a place where hawks are kept.
nestling	also called an eyas. A young hawk that is still or would normally still be in the nest, i.e. it has not fledged yet.
moult	used as a noun or verb, it refers to the annual process whereby the bird loses its old feathers and replaces them with new ones.
mutes	the droppings or excrement of a hawk.
nares	nostrils.
passage-hawk	a wild hawk caught during migration, usually still in immature plumage.
pellet	also called a casting. The regurgitated remains of indigestible fur, feathers and bone produced by a hawk after digesting a meal.
pluming	to pluck the quarry
perch	a structure upon which the bird stands when not on the fist. Sometimes applied only to those found in the aviary or mews.

preen	to straighten and rearrange the feathers using the beak.
primary feathers	also called primaries, beam feathers or phalangeal feathers. The remiges or flight feathers that attach to the metacarpal bone of the wing.
quarry	the game or prey flown at by the hawk.
rectrices	the large tail feathers.
screen perch	a perch generally used indoors or under cover. It has a cloth or screen suspended underneath that prevents the leash from getting twisted around the perch and helps the bird remount if it has jumped off.
secondary feathers	also called secondaries or flags. The remiges or flight feathers that attach to the ulna of the wing.
stoop	also called swoop. The swift descent of a falcon upon its quarry.
swivel	a metal device that attaches to jesses and leash and prevents them from getting twisted.
talons	the long sharp claws of a hawk.
tiercel	the male bird of prey. Used on its own it denotes a male peregrine falcon.
train	the tail of a hawk.
weather	to place a bird upon its perch outdoors.

21 Index

Numbers in *italics* refer to captions of illustrations and numbers in *italics* plus *t* refer to tables